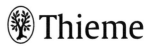

An Evidence-based Approach to Phytochemicals and Other Dietary Factors

Jane Higdon, PhD †
Linus Pauling Institute
Oregon State University
Corvallis, Oregon, USA

Victoria J. Drake, PhD
Manager
Micronutrient Information Center
Linus Pauling Institute
Oregon State University
Corvallis, Oregon, USA

2nd edition

33 illustrations

Thieme
Stuttgart · New York

Library of Congress Cataloging-in-Publication Data is available from the publisher.

Important note: Medicine is an ever-changing science undergoing continual development. Research and clinical experience are continually expanding our knowledge, in particular our knowledge of proper treatment and drug therapy. Insofar as this book mentions any dosage or application, readers may rest assured that the authors, editors, and publishers have made every effort to ensure that such references are in accordance with **the state of knowledge at the time of production of the book.**

Nevertheless, this does not involve, imply, or express any guarantee or responsibility on the part of the publishers in respect to any dosage instructions and forms of applications stated in the book.

Every user is requested to examine carefully the manufacturers' leaflets accompanying each drug and to check, if necessary in consultation with a physician or specialist, whether the dosage schedules mentioned therein or the contraindications stated by the manufacturers differ from the statements made in the present book. Such examination is particularly important with drugs that are either rarely used or have been newly released on the market. Every dosage schedule or every form of application used is entirely at the user's own risk and responsibility. The authors and publishers request every user to report to the publishers any discrepancies or inaccuracies noticed. If errors in this work are found after publication, errata will be posted at www.thieme.com on the product description page.

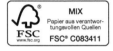

1st English Edition 2007

© 2013 Georg Thieme Verlag KG,
Rüdigerstrasse 14,
70469 Stuttgart, Germany
http://www.thieme.de
Thieme Medical Publishers, Inc.,
333 Seventh Avenue,
New York, NY 10001, USA
http://www.thieme.com

Some of the product names, patents, and registered designs referred to in this book are in fact registered trademarks or proprietary names even though specific reference to this fact is not always made in the text. Therefore, the appearance of a name without designation as proprietary is not to be construed as a representation by the publisher that it is in the public domain.

Cover design: Thieme Publishing Group
Typesetting by primustype Robert Hurler GmbH, Notzingen, Germany
Printed in Germany by CPI books

ISBN 978-3-13-141842-5
eISBN 978-3-13-169712-7

Foreword

Accuse not Nature!
She has done her part;
Do thou but thine!
John Milton, *Paradise Lost*, 1667

Archeology reveals that ancient peoples recognized that certain foods could promote health and treat disease. The use of decoctions, distillates, extracts, and infusions of plant foods, spices and related botanicals in apothecary, Ayurvedic, Chinese, Native American, and other traditional medicines reflects the early application of this knowledge regarding their bioactive constituents. Today, exciting advances in nutrition and medicine, as well as numerous reports in popular books and the media, have stimulated a general interest in phytochemicals and other dietary factors. New recipes emphasizing phytochemical-rich dishes, common foods fortified with these "functional" ingredients, and dietary supplements formulated with a variety of these compounds seem to be appearing every month. However, this profusion of choices is often accompanied by confusion about their efficacy and safety. Thus, the need for ready access to sound, evidence-based science by consumers and healthcare professionals is more critical than ever before.

We now appreciate that our evolution in a world of edible plants allowed our bodies not only to forego the energy necessary for synthesizing many critical compounds (that we now call "essential nutrients") but also to take advantage of other natural constituents in these foods beyond their provision of basic nutritive value. For example, it is interesting to note how our retina employs the carotenoid lutein to filter phototoxic blue light and near-ultraviolet radiation in the same way that lutein protects the plants from which we obtain it. Nutrition scientists are now working to understand the enormous complexity and health implications of thousands of phytochemicals and other dietary factors, including their bioavailability, distribution, metabolism, excretion, mechanisms of ac-

tion, and interactions with one another within individual foods and whole diets. It is worth noting that research indicates that many of these compounds have the potential to influence the expression of mammalian genes, suggesting phytochemicals can influence fundamental aspects of our cellular function, despite their not being "essential" to us. It can appear an overwhelming challenge to document the myriad of fruits, grains, legumes, nuts, seeds, and vegetables and the ways in which they serve to support our physical well being and our mental state. However, the first publication of this book by Dr. Jane Higdon, now updated by Dr. Victoria Drake in this second edition, makes this task much easier by providing a concise synthesis of the basic, observational, and clinical data now available and organizing the material in a practical fashion both by foods and by bioactive constituents and their applications to health promotion and therapy.

The worldwide, demographic imperative of the aging population is readily reflected in the shift during the last century from a situation where most mortality resulted from communicable diseases to one where mortality is more often a result of chronic disease. The promise of the power of nutrition lies in our being able to understand the benefits offered not only by essential macronutrients and micronutrients but by other dietary factors, especially phytochemicals like carotenoids, chlorophylls, glucosinolates, organosulfurs, phytosterols, and polyphenols, as well compounds like α-lipoic acid, L-carnitine, choline, and ubiquinone (coenzyme Q_{10}). All of these compounds, and the foods that contain them, are described in this book. In addition to their own expertise, Drs. Higdon and Drake have ensured the accuracy of this material by having each chapter reviewed by an authority in that field.

The application of this knowledge about phytochemicals and other dietary factors will provide a sound foundation for new dietary guidelines and also the requisite scientific substantiation for the development of new food products, sometimes called designer foods, functional foods, pharmafoods, or nutraceuticals, as well as for dietary supplements. However, a great deal more research must still be done to demonstrate not only the efficacy but also the safety of these ingredients and how they are formulated into new products that offer to enhance our biological defense mechanisms, promote optimal physiological responses, reduce the risk of specific diseases, and even slow the processes associated with aging. While regulations concerning labeling and claims of benefit made for food products seem often to be controversial, there is no doubt that evaluating the emerging scientific information with sound judgment, as is done in this book, will help health-care providers, especially dietitians, nurses, and physicians, apply it today and allow policymakers and researchers to plan for the future in a rational manner.

Whether counseling patients about their diets or developing more healthful food products, a two-pronged approach is required: reducing ingredients with negative attributes, such as refined sugars, saturated and *trans*-fatty acids, and sodium, and increasing ingredients with positive attributes, including phytochemicals and other dietary factors. However, this is difficult, not only because issues of convenience, cost, and taste must be considered but also because our knowledge of exactly which healthful ingredients to incorporate is still quite limited, including their effective doses, forms, combinations, and safety. Nonetheless, many elements are now converging to ensure these challenges will be met: the requirement of both the private and public sector to reduce health-care costs, the demands of consumers for "natural" solutions to live longer and better lives, and the drive of food companies and the stores that sell their products to respond to their customers' needs. Drs. Higdon and Drake have given us a book that is authoritative but easy to read and provides a solid background for those wanting to understand how phytochemicals and other dietary factors may offer some solutions to this problem.

Jeffrey Blumberg, PhD, FASN, FACN, CNS
Friedman School of Nutrition Science and Policy
Jean Mayer USDA Human Nutrition Research
Center on Aging
Tufts University
Boston, Massachusetts
USA

Preface to the Second Edition

I am honored to revise and update Dr. Jane Higdon's book, *An Evidence-based Approach to Dietary Phytochemicals*. Since the first edition was published in 2007, the literature on the role of plant foods and phytochemicals (literally, plant chemicals) in health and disease has greatly expanded. In this second edition, all 20 chapters of the first edition have incorporated new information from the relevant, more recently published peer-reviewed studies, especially studies with human subjects. Moreover, this edition has been expanded to include new chapters on other dietary factors, including choline, coenzyme Q_{10}, L-carnitine, and lipoic acid. The first part of this book discusses the evidence for the health effects of various plant foods and beverages: fruits and vegetables, cruciferous vegetables, legumes, nuts, whole grains, coffee, and tea. The second section focuses on individual phytochemicals and classes of phytochemicals, and the third section covers key nutrients (essential fatty acids and choline), as well as other dietary factors (coenzyme Q_{10}, L-carnitine, and lipoic acid) that the body synthesizes but that are also found in dietary and supplementary sources.

The importance of a plant-based diet in maintaining optimum health and preventing chronic disease is now well recognized. Plant foods not only provide essential vitamins and minerals but also contain countless phytochemicals, as well as dietary fiber, that benefit health. It is critical that people—health professionals and the general public alike—have access to scientifically accurate and peer-reviewed information regarding how plant foods and their constituents affect health. Additionally, as the availability and popularity of functional foods and dietary supplements increases, it is necessary to consider their safety profiles, including potential drug and nutrient interactions. This extensively referenced book concisely synthesizes a large amount of experimental, epidemiological, and clinical research on the health effects of plant foods, phytochemicals, and other dietary factors, and also provides the reader with practical information on sources (dietary and supplemental), nutrient and drug interactions, and possible adverse effects.

Acknowledgments

I wish to thank the faculty, staff, and students of the Linus Pauling Institute for their editorial advice and support in the revision of this book, especially Balz Frei, PhD, director and endowed chair; Stephen Lawson, administrative officer; and Barbara McVicar, assistant to the director. I am very appreciative to all of the distinguished scientists listed as the Editorial Advisory Board, who reviewed the contents of each chapter and provided helpful comments. I would also like to thank James W. Anderson, MD, and Martijn B. Katan, PhD, for reviewing the information presented on legumes and coffee, respectively. Finally, I am extremely grateful for the careful and comprehensive work by Dr. Higdon in writing the first edition of this book. I hope that readers find this new edition adds successfully to her legacy.

Victoria J. Drake, PhD
Manager, Micronutrient Information Center
Linus Pauling Institute
Oregon State University
Corvallis, Oregon
USA

Preface to the First Edition

Plant foods, including fruits, vegetables, legumes, whole grains, and nuts, are prominent features of healthy dietary patterns. In addition to providing energy and essential micronutrients (vitamins and minerals), plant foods contribute thousands of phytochemicals to the human diet. Although the term "phytochemicals" literally means plant chemicals, it is often used to describe plant-derived compounds that may affect health but are not essential nutrients. Although there is ample evidence to support the health benefits of diets rich in plant foods, evidence that these benefits are due to specific phytochemicals is more limited. Because plant foods are complex packages of biologically active compounds, the health benefits of individual phytochemicals cannot always be separated from those of the foods that contain them. Consequently, the first section of the book discusses the evidence for the health benefits of plant foods and beverages, including fruits and vegetables, legumes, nuts, whole grains, coffee, and tea.

Scientific research on the potential for specific dietary phytochemicals or classes of dietary phytochemicals to prevent and treat chronic diseases has expanded rapidly over the past decade. In some cases, the results of preclinical research have been promising enough to warrant clinical trials designed to examine the bioavailability, safety, and efficacy of high doses of isolated phytochemicals in humans. In the United States and other countries, supplements and extracts containing concentrated doses of isolated phytochemicals are available to the public as dietary supplements without a prescription. The market for functional foods, such as phytosterol-enriched margarines, is also rapidly expanding. As the popularity of these products increases, health and nutrition professionals need accurate information about potential health benefits, risks, and interactions associated with these phytochemicals. The second section of this book reviews the scientific and clinical evidence for the health benefits of individual dietary phytochemicals and classes of phytochemicals. Because high doses of isolated phytochemicals may have unexpected effects, the available evidence regarding the safety of these Compounds is also reviewed.

My goal in writing this book was to synthesize and organize the results of thousands of experimental, clinical, and epidemiological studies to provide an overview of current scientific and clinical knowledge regarding the role of plant foods and phytochemicals in human health and disease. An expert in the field covered in each chapter has reviewed the text to ensure its accuracy. The names and affiliations of these scientists are listed in the Editorial Advisory Board. Throughout this book, human research published in peerreviewed journals is emphasized. Where relevant, the results of experimental studies in cell culture or animal models are included. Although randomized controlled trials provide the strongest support for the efficacy of phytochemicals, it is not always ethical or practical to perform a randomized, double-blind, placebo-controlled trial. Observational studies also provide important information about relationships between plant food and phytochemical intakes and human health and disease. In reviewing the epidemiological research, more weight is given to the results of large prospective cohort studies, such as the Nurses' Health Study and Health Professionals Follow-up Study, than retrospective case-control or cross-sectional studies. When available, the results of systematic reviews and meta-analyses, which summarize information on the findings of many similar studies, are also included.

This book could not have been written without the collaboration and support of the scientists and staff of the Linus Pauling Institute at Oregon State University. The Institute was founded in 1973 by Linus Pauling, Ph.D., the only individual ever to win two, unshared Nobel Prizes (Chemistry, 1954; Peace, 1962). In 1996, the Linus Pauling Institute moved to the campus of Oregon State University (Dr. Pauling's undergraduate alma mater) and now operates as one of the University's Research Centers and Institutes. More than 35 years ago, Dr. Pauling proposed that dietary factors, such as vitamin C, could play a significant role in enhancing human health and preventing chronic disease. The basic premise that an optimum diet is the key to optimum health continues today as the foundation of the Linus Pauling Institute at Oregon State University. Scientists at the Linus Pauling Institute investigate the roles that micronutrients and phytochemicals play in human aging and chronic diseases, particularly cancer, cardiovascular disease, and neurodegenerative disease. The goals of the research at the Linus Pauling Institute are to understand the molecular mechanisms behind the effects of nutrition on health and to determine how micronutrients and phytochemicals can be used in the prevention and treatment of diseases. In particular, scientists at the Linus Pauling Insti-

tute's Cancer Chemoprotection Program are working to understand the mechanisms by which dietary phytochemicals may prevent or treat cancer and to identify novel dietary phytochemicals that may protect against cancer. The Linus Pauling Institute is also dedicated to training and supporting new researchers in the interdisciplinary science of nutrition and optimum health, as well as to educating the public about the science of optimum nutrition.

Jane Higdon, PhD
The Linus Pauling Institute
Oregon State University
Corvallis, Oregon
USA

Editorial Advisory Board

Contents

How To Use This Book

Chapter Organization

Information on the health benefits of various classes of plant foods can be found in Chapters 1 to 5. Chapters 6 and 7 provide information on the phytochemical-rich beverages coffee and tea. Information on individual dietary phytochemicals or classes of dietary phytochemicals can be found in Chapters 8 to 19. Chapters 20 to 24 provide information on specific nutrients or other dietary factors.

Plant Foods
(Chapters 1 to 5)

Each chapter on plant foods contains the following sections:
- Introduction
- Disease Prevention—a review of the evidence that diets rich in certain plant foods play a role in chronic disease prevention
- Intake Recommendations—a review of intake recommendations from government or health-oriented agencies, for example, the 2010 Dietary Guidelines for Americans or recommendations by the National Cancer Institute
- Summary
- References

Coffee and Tea
(Chapters 6 and 7)

Chapters on coffee and tea contain the following sections:
- Introduction
- Bioactive Compounds—a discussion of some of the phytochemicals thought to contribute to the health effects of these beverages

- Disease Prevention—a review of the evidence that these beverages play a role in disease prevention
- Safety—a discussion of potential adverse effects of high intakes of these beverages, including drug and nutrient interactions
- Summary
- References

Phytochemicals
(Chapters 8 to 19)

Each chapter on phytochemicals contains the following sections:
- Introduction
- Bioavailability and Metabolism[1]—a review of the available information on absorption, metabolism, and elimination as it relates to bioavailability in humans
- Biological Activities—a discussion of the biological activities, often identified in cell culture or animal experiments, that may contribute to the health effects of a phytochemical
- Disease Prevention—a review of the evidence that specific phytochemicals play a role in disease prevention
- Disease Treatment[2]—a review of the evidence that specific phytochemicals may be useful in disease treatment
- Sources—information about foods and supplements that contain the phytochemical of interest; when available, information about supplement doses is included
- Safety—information about adverse effects and drug and nutrient interactions
- Summary
- References

---

[1] Chapter 16 (Fiber) does not contain a section on Bioavailability and Metabolism.
[2] Chapters 11 (Flavonoids), 13 (Isothiocyanates), 15 (Lignans), 17 (Garlic), and 19 (Resveratrol) do not contain a section on Disease Treatment.

Nutrients and Other Dietary Factors (Chapters 20 to 24)

Each chapter contains the following sections:
- Introduction
- Function[1] or Biological Activities[2]—current scientific understanding of the function or biological activity of the nutrient or dietary factor, with respect to maintaining health and preventing disease
- Deficiency—signs, symptoms, and physiological effects of frank deficiency of the nutrient; for the chapters on dietary factors that can also be endogenously synthesized, genetic and acquired conditions of deficiency are discussed
- Disease Prevention[3]—a review of the evidence that specific nutrients or dietary factors play a role in disease prevention
- Disease Treatment—a review of the evidence that specific phytochemicals may be useful in disease treatment
- Sources—information on endogenous biosynthesis, dietary, and supplemental sources of the nutrient or dietary factor; when available, this section includes a table of dietary sources
- Safety—information about adverse effects and drug and nutrient interactions
- Summary
- References

Appendices

Several appendices have been included to facilitate the use of this book:
- Glycemic Index and Glycemic Load—a review of the evidence that the blood glucose-raising potential of carbohydrate in different foods plays a role in their health effects
- Quick Reference to Diseases—a chart that allows the reader to locate information on plant foods, phytochemicals, or dietary factors by disease or health condition
- Drug Interactions—a table summarizing known drug interactions with the phytochemicals or dietary factors discussed in this book
- Nutrient Interactions—a table summarizing known nutrient interactions with the phytochemicals or dietary factors discussed in this book
- Quick Reference to Foods Rich in Phytochemicals or Other Dietary Factors—a chart that allows the reader to identify foods that are rich in a variety of phytochemicals and dietary factors
- Glossary

---

[1] Chapters 21 (Choline) and 22 (Coenzyme Q_{10}) contain a section on Function.

[2] Chapters 20 (Essential Fatty Acids), 23 (L-Carnitine), and 24 (Lipoic Acid) contain a section on Biological Activities.

[3] Chapter 24 (Lipoic Acid) does not contain a section on Disease Prevention.

Table of Measures

In the metric system, a microgram (μg, mcg, or sometimes ug) is a unit of mass equal to one millionth (1/1 000 000) of a gram or one thousandth (1/1000) of a milligram. It is one of the smallest units of mass (or weight) commonly used. The abbreviation "μg" conforms to the International System of Units.

Weight	
Metric	**English (US)**
1 mg (1000 μg)	0.002 grain (0.000035 oz)
1 g (1000 mg)	0.04 oz
1 kg (1000 g)	35.27 oz (2.2 lb)
English (US)	**Metric**
1 grain	64.8 mg
1 oz	28.4 g
1 lb	453.6 g (0.45 kg)
Volume	
Metric	**English (US)**
1 mL	0.03 oz
1 L (1000 mL)	2.12 pt
1 L	1.06 qt
1 L	0.27 gal
English (US)	**Metric**
1 fl oz	30 mL
1 pt	470 mL
1 qt	950 mL
1 gal	3.79 L
Liquids	
Metric	**English (US)**
1 mL	⅕ tsp
5 mL	1 tsp
15 mL	1 tbsp
30 mL	⅛ cup
60 mL	¼ cup
100 mL (1 dL)	About ⅖ cup
120 mL	½ cup
240 mL	1 cup
480 mL	1 pt

Abbreviations:

dL	deciliter	μg	microgram
fl oz	fluid ounce	mL	milliliter
g	gram	oz	ounce
gal	gallon	pt	pint
kg	kilogram	qt	quart
L	liter	tbsp	tablespoon
lb	pound	tsp	teaspoon
mg	milligram		

Abbreviations

AA	arachidonic acid	CYP	cytochrome P450
AARP	American Association of Retired Persons	DADS	diallyl disulfide
		DAS	diallyl sulfide
ABC	ATP-binding cassette	DASH	Dietary Approaches to Stop Hypertension (study)
AFB_1	aflatoxin-B_1		
AhR	aryl hydrocarbon receptor	DATS	diallyl trisulfide
AI	adequate intake	DBP	diastolic blood pressure
AIDS	acquired immunodeficiency syndrome	DGLA	dihomo-γ-linolenic acid
		DHA	docosahexaenoic acid
AITC	allyl isothiocyanate	DHHS	(US) Department of Health and Human Services
ALA	α-linolenic acid		
ALCAR	acetyl-L-carnitine	DHLA	dihydrolipoic acid
ALT	alanine aminotransferase	DIM	3,3'-diindolylmethane
AMD	age-related macular degeneration	DM	diabetes mellitus
AMP	adenosine monophosphate	DRI	dietary reference intake
AP-1	activator protein 1	EC	epicatechin
APC	adenomatous polyposis coli	ECG	epicatechin gallate
ARE	antioxidant response element	EFA	essential fatty acid
AREDS	Age-Related Eye Disease Study	EGC	epigallocatechin
Arnt	AhR nuclear translocator protein	EGCG	epigallocatechin gallate
ATBC	Alpha-Tocopherol Beta-Carotene (trial)	eNOS	endothelial nitric oxide synthase
		EPA	eicosapentaenoic acid — (US) Environment Protection Agency
ATP	adenosine triphosphate		
BHMT	betaine-homocysteine methyltransferase	EPIC	European Prospective Investigation into Cancer and Nutrition (study)
BITC	benzyl isothiocyanate	EPO	erythropoietin
BMD	bone mineral density	ER	estrogen receptor
BMI	body mass index	ER+	estrogen receptor positive
BPH	benign prostatic hyperplasia	ERE	estrogen response element
CABG	coronary artery bypass graft	ESR	erythrocyte sedimentation rate
CACT	carnitine:acylcarnitine translocase	FDA	(US) Food and Drug Administration
CAN	cardiovascular autonomic neuropathy	FEV_1	forced expiratory volume (in 1 second)
CARET	β-Carotene and Retinol Efficacy Trial	FNB	Food and Nutrition Board
CAT	carnitine acetyltransferase	FRDA	Friedrich ataxia
CFTR	cystic fibrosis transmembrane conductance regulator	GCL	γ-glutamyl cysteine ligase
		GLA	γ-linolenic acid
CHD	coronary heart disease	GLUT4	glucose transporter-4
CIN	cervical intraepithelial neoplasia	GRAS	generally recognized as safe
CoA	coenzyme A	GST	glutathione S-transferase
COMT	catechol-O-methyltransferase	GTP	guanosine triphosphate
COPD	chronic obstructive pulmonary disease	HbA_{1c}	glycosylated hemoglobin
		HDL	high-density lipoprotein
COX	cyclooxygenase	HFCS	high-fructose corn syrup
CPT	carnitine palmitoyltransferase	HIV	human immunodeficiency virus
CT	cyclic trimer		

HMG-CoA	3-hydroxy-3-methyl-glutaryl-coen-zyme A		**PAD**	peripheral arterial disease
HPFS	Health Professionals' Follow-up Study		**PAH**	polycyclic aromatic hydrocarbon
			PCB	polychlorinated biphenyl
HPV	human papilloma virus		**PDH**	pyruvate dehydrogenase
HRV	heart-rate variability		**PEITC**	phenethyl isothiocyanate
IBS	irritable bowel syndrome		**PEMT**	phosphatidylethanolamine N-meth-yltransferase
IC	intermittent claudication		**PKB**	protein kinase B
I3C	indole-3-carbinol		**PLA$_2$**	phospholipase A$_2$
ICZ	indolo[3,2-b]carbazole		**PPAR**	peroxisome proliferator-activated receptor
IgA	immunoglobulin A			
iNOS	inducible nitric oxide synthase		**PSA**	prostate-specific antigen
INR	international normalized ratio		**PUFA**	polyunsaturated fatty acid
IR	insulin receptor		**RDA**	recommended dietary allowance
IU	international unit		**RNS**	reactive nitrogen species
LA	linoleic acid/α-lipoic acid		**ROS**	reactive oxygen species
LDL	low-density lipoprotein		**RRP**	recurrent respiratory papillomatosis
LOX	lipoxygenase		**SAM**	S-adenosyl methionine
LVEF	left ventricular ejection fraction		**SAMC**	S-allylmercaptocysteine
LXR	liver X receptor		**SBP**	systolic blood pressure
MI	myocardial infarction		**SCD**	sudden cardiac death
MMP	matrix metalloproteinase		**SFA**	saturated fatty acid
MS	multiple sclerosis		**SFN**	sulforaphane
NAD	nicotinamide adenine dinucleotide		**SLE**	systemic lupus erythematosus
NCEP	(US) National Cholesterol Education Program		**SREBP**	sterol regulatory element-binding protein
NF-κB	nuclear factor kappa B		**TCA**	tricarboxylic acid
NHANES	(US) National Health and Nutrition Examination Survey		**tHcy**	total homocysteine
			THF	tetrahydrofolate
NHS	Nurses' Health Study		**α-TOH**	α-tocopherol
NIH	(US) National Institutes of Health		**UDP**	uridine diphosphate
NKF	(US) National Kidney Foundation		**UGT**	UDP-glucuronosyl transferase
NO	nitric oxide		**UL**	tolerable upper intake level
NSAID	nonsteroidal anti-inflammatory drug		**USP**	United States Pharmacopeia Convention
NTD	neural tube defect		**VIN**	vulvar intraepithelial neoplasia
16αOHE1	16α-hydroxyestrone		**VLDL**	very low-density lipoprotein
2OHE1	2-hydroxyestrone		**XRE**	xenobiotic response element
OSL	observed safe level			

1 Fruits and Vegetables

Despite all of the controversy surrounding the optimal components of a healthy diet, there is little disagreement among scientists regarding the importance of fruits and vegetables. The results of numerous epidemiological studies and recent clinical trials provide consistent evidence that diets rich in fruits and vegetables can reduce the risk of chronic disease.[1] On the other hand, evidence that very high doses of individual micronutrients or phytochemicals found in fruits and vegetables can do the same is inconsistent and relatively weak. Fruits and vegetables contain thousands of biologically active phytochemicals that are likely to interact in several ways to prevent disease and promote health.[2] Fruits and vegetables are rich in antioxidants, which help protect the body from oxidative damage induced by pro-oxidants. The best way to take advantage of these complex interactions is to eat a variety of fruits and vegetables.

Disease Prevention

Cardiovascular Disease

Dietary patterns characterized by relatively high intakes of fruits and vegetables are consistently associated with significant reductions in the risk of coronary heart disease (CHD) and stroke. A meta-analysis that combined the results of 11 prospective cohort studies found that people in the 90th percentile of fruit and vegetable intake (approx. five servings per day or more) had a risk of myocardial infarction (MI) that was around 15% lower than for those in the 10th percentile of intake.[3] Among more than 126 000 men and women participating in the Health Professionals' Follow-up Study and the Nurses' Health Study, those who consumed eight or more servings of fruits and vegetables daily had a risk of developing CHD over the next 8–14 years that was 20% lower than those who consumed less than three servings daily.[4] In the same cohort, the risk of ischemic stroke (stroke caused by a reduction in blood flow to part of the brain) was 30% lower in those who consumed at least five servings of

fruits and vegetables daily than in those who consumed less than three servings daily.[5] Based on the results of the Health Professionals' Follow-up Study and the Nurses' Health Study (NHS), eating one extra serving of fruits or vegetables daily would decrease one's risk of CHD by approximately 4% and decrease the risk of ischemic stroke by 6%. In a meta-analysis designed to estimate the global burden of disease attributable to low fruit and vegetable consumption, epidemiologists concluded that increasing individual fruit and vegetable consumption (excluding potatoes) up to 600 g/day (approx. seven servings per day) could decrease the risk of CHD by 31% and the risk of ischemic stroke by 19%.[1] Three recent meta-analyses have examined fruit and vegetable consumption and risk of CHD or stroke. In a meta-analysis that included nine cohort studies, an additional daily serving of fruit and vegetables was associated with a 4% decreased risk for CHD.[6] Another meta-analysis, which examined 12 separate studies, found that individuals who consumed more than five daily servings of fruit and vegetables experienced a 17% reduction in risk of CHD compared with those who consumed less than three servings daily.[7] In a meta-analysis of eight studies examining fruit and vegetable intake, individuals who consumed three to five daily servings or more than five daily servings had an 11% or 26% reduction in risk of stroke, respectively, when compared with those who consumed fewer than three servings daily.[8]

High blood pressure (hypertension) increases the risk of heart disease and stroke.[9] Adding more fruits and vegetables to a sensible diet is one potential way to lower blood pressure. In the Dietary Approaches to Stop Hypertension (DASH) study, 459 people with and without high blood pressure were randomly assigned to one of three diets: (1) a typical American diet that provided approximately three servings per day of fruits and vegetables and one serving per day of a low-fat dairy product, (2) a fruit and vegetable diet that provided eight servings per day of fruits and vegetables and one serving per day of a low-fat dairy product, or (3) a combination diet (now called the DASH diet) that provided nine servings per day of fruits and vegetables and three servings per day of low-fat dairy products.[10] After 8 weeks, the blood pressure of those on the fruit and vegetable diet (eight servings per day) was significantly lower than those on the typical American diet, while the blood pressure of those on the combination (DASH) diet (nine servings per day of fruits and vegetables) was lower still.

Several compounds may contribute to the cardioprotective effects of fruits and vegetables, including vitamin C, folate, potassium, fiber, and various phytochemicals.[11] However, supplementation of individual micronutrients or phytochemicals has not generally resulted in significantly decreased incidence of cardiovascular events in randomized controlled trials. Thus, in the case of fruits and vegetables, the "benefit of the whole may be greater than the sum of its parts."

Type 2 Diabetes Mellitus

In addition to other complications, type 2 diabetes mellitus (DM) is associated with increased risk of cardiovascular disease—the leading cause of death in type 2 diabetes.[12] Although the evidence for a beneficial effect of a diet rich in fruits and vegetables on diabetes is not as consistent as it is for heart disease, the results of a small number of studies suggest that higher intakes of fruits and vegetables are associated with improved blood glucose control and lower risk of developing type 2 DM. In a cohort of almost 10000 adults in the United States, the risk of developing type 2 DM over the next 20 years was around 20% lower in those who reported consuming at least five daily servings of fruits and vegetables compared with those who reported consuming none.[13] In another prospective cohort study that followed more than 40000 US women for an average of 9 years, fruit and vegetable intake was not associated with the risk of developing type 2 DM in the entire cohort, but higher intakes of green leafy and yellow vegetables were associated with significant reductions in the risk of type 2 DM in overweight women.[14] Higher fruit and vegetable intakes were weakly associated with a reduced risk of diabetes in a cohort of more than 20000 individuals followed for 12 years.[15] In a cohort of 71346 women participating in the NHS, total fruit and vegetable intake was not associated

with risk for diabetes, although further analysis revealed that intake of fruit or green leafy vegetables was individually associated with a modest reduction in risk of diabetes.[16] A systematic review and meta-analysis of five cohort studies found that fruit and vegetable intake was not associated with type 2 diabetes.[17] However, in a cross-sectional study of more than 6000 adults in the United Kingdom who did not have diabetes, those with higher fruit and vegetable intakes had significantly lower levels of glycosylated hemoglobin (HbA$_{1c}$), a measure of long-term blood glucose control.[18] Possible compounds in fruits and vegetables that may enhance glucose control include fiber and magnesium.

Cancer

The results of numerous case–control studies indicate that eating a diet rich in fruits and vegetables decreases the risk of developing several different types of cancer, particularly cancers of the digestive tract (oropharynx, esophagus, stomach, colon, and rectum) and lung.[19–21] The results of some of these studies were the foundation for the National Cancer Institute's "5 A Day" program, which was aimed at increasing the fruit and vegetable consumption of the American public to a minimum of five servings daily. The current US government campaign "Fruits & Veggies More Matters" has replaced the "5 A Day" program. In contrast to the results of case–control studies, many recent prospective cohort studies have found little or no association between total fruit and vegetable intake and the risk of various cancers.[22–44] There are several possible explanations for this discrepancy. Case–control studies, in which the past diets of people diagnosed with a particular type of cancer are compared with the diets of people without cancer, are more susceptible to bias in the selection of participants and dietary recall than prospective cohort studies, which collect information on the diets of large cohorts of healthy people and follow the development of disease in the cohort over time.[45] Although prospective cohort studies provide weak support for an association between total fruit and vegetable consumption and cancer risk, they provide some evidence that high intakes of certain classes of fruits or vegetables are associated with reduced risk of individual cancers. Higher intakes of fruits have been associated with modest but significant reductions in lung cancer risk in a pooled analysis of eight prospective cohort studies,[28] and with reductions in risk of bladder cancer in some studies.[46] In men, higher intakes of cruciferous vegetables have been associated with significant reductions in the risk of bladder cancer,[47] as well as prostate cancer,[48] and higher intakes of tomato products have been linked with significant reductions in the risk of prostate cancer.[49]

Osteoporosis

Several cross-sectional studies have reported that higher intakes of fruits and vegetables are associated with significantly higher bone mineral density (BMD) and lower levels of bone resorption (loss) in men and women.[50–53] In a study that followed BMD over 4 years, higher fruit and vegetable intakes were associated with significantly less decline in BMD at the hip in elderly men but not elderly women.[50] Fruits and vegetables are rich in precursors to bicarbonate ions, which serve to buffer acids in the body. When the quantity of bicarbonate ions is insufficient to maintain normal pH, the body is capable of mobilizing alkaline calcium salts from bone to neutralize acids consumed in the diet and generated by metabolism.[54] Increased consumption of fruits and vegetables reduces the net acid content of the diet and may preserve calcium in bones, which might otherwise be mobilized to maintain normal pH. However, the results of a recent placebo-controlled trial in 276 postmenopausal women suggest that supplementing the diet with alkali, either through supplemental potassium citrate or an additional 300 g/day of fruits and vegetables, did not increase BMD or blunt the age-associated bone loss over a 2-year period.[55] Results from the DASH study support a beneficial link between fruit and vegetable intake and bone health. In addition to decreasing blood pressure, increasing fruit and vegetable intake from approximately three to nine servings daily decreased urinary calcium loss by almost 50 mg/day[10] and lowered biochemical markers of bone turnover, particularly bone resorption, including serum levels of C-terminal telopeptide of type 1 collagen.[56] Taken together, the results of epidemiological studies and controlled clinical trials suggest that a diet rich in fruits and vegetables can help prevent bone loss, although the specific mechanisms are not known with certainty.

Age-Related Eye Diseases

Cataracts

Cataracts are thought to be caused by oxidative damage to proteins in the eye's lens, induced by long-term exposure to ultraviolet light. The resulting cloudiness and discoloration of the lens leads to vision loss that becomes more severe with age. The results of several large prospective cohort studies suggest that diets rich in fruits and vegetables, especially fruits and vegetables rich in carotenoid and vitamin C, are associated with decreased incidence and severity of cataracts.[57–60] In a study of male US health professionals, high intakes of both broccoli and spinach were associated with fewer cataract extractions.[57]

Macular Degeneration

Degeneration of the macula, the center of the retina, is the leading cause of blindness in people over the age of 65 years in the United States.[61] Lutein and zeaxanthin are carotenoids that are found in relatively high concentrations in the retina; these carotenoids may play a role in preventing damage to the retina caused by light or oxidants.[62] In two case–control studies, high intakes of carotenoid-rich vegetables, especially those rich in lutein and zeaxanthin, such as dark green, leafy vegetables, were associated with a significantly lower risk of developing age-related macular degeneration (AMD).[63,64] In a prospective cohort study of more than 118 000 men and women, those who consumed three or more servings of fruits daily had a 36% lower risk of developing AMD over the next 12–18 years than those who consumed fewer than 1.5 servings.[65] Interestingly, vegetable intake was not associated with the risk of macular degeneration in this cohort. In a more recent study, combined lutein and zeaxanthin intake was not associated with prevalence of intermediate AMD in a cohort of women aged 50–79 years.[66] However, further analysis of the data revealed that women younger than 75 years with stable intakes of lutein and zeaxanthin had a 43% lower risk of developing intermediate AMD.[66]

Table 1.1 Examples of one serving of fruits or vegetables

Fruit or Vegetable	Amount in One Serving
Fruit or vegetable juice	¾ cup (6 fl oz)
Apple	1 medium
Orange	1 medium
Banana	1 small
Salad greens, raw	1 cup
Chopped fruit or vegetables	½ cup
Cooked vegetables	½ cup
Cooked beans, peas, or lentils	½ cup
Dried fruit	¼ cup

Chronic Obstructive Pulmonary Disease

Chronic obstructive pulmonary disease (COPD) is a term that includes emphysema and chronic bronchitis, two chronic lung diseases that are characterized by airway obstruction. Although smoking is by far the most important risk factor for COPD, the results of several epidemiological studies suggest beneficial associations between vegetable and, more strongly, fruit intakes and COPD risk.[67] The results of several epidemiological studies in Europe indicate that higher fruit intakes, especially apple intakes, are associated with higher forced expiratory volume (FEV$_1$) values, indicative of better lung function.[68-70] In a study of 2500 middle-aged Welsh men, those who ate at least five apples weekly had a significantly slower decline in lung function than those who did not eat apples over a 5-year period.[69] In a study of 2917 European men followed over 20 years, each 100 g (3.5 oz) increase in daily fruit consumption was associated with a 24% decrease in the risk of death from COPD.[71] The reasons for the beneficial association between fruit intake and lung health are not yet known. Because oxidative stress is thought to play a role in the etiology of chronic obstructive lung disease, scientists are currently investigating the possibility that antioxidants and phytochemicals found in fruits, such as vitamin C or flavonoids, could play a protective role. Higher fruit and vegetable intake was inversely associated with risk of COPD in a small case–control study of male cigarette smokers,[72] providing support for the antioxidant hypothesis. Interestingly, when compared with a Western dietary pattern (refined grains, cured and red meats, French fries, and desserts), a prudent dietary pattern that emphasized fruits, vegetables, fish, and whole grains was associated with a 25%–50% reduction in COPD risk in large cohorts of men[73] and women.[74]

Neurodegenerative Disease

Although it is not yet clear whether a diet rich in fruits and vegetables will decrease the risk of neurodegenerative diseases like Alzheimer disease and Parkinson disease in humans, studies in animal models of these diseases suggest that diets rich in fruits like blueberries[75] or tomatoes may be protective.[76] Interestingly, a prospective study that followed 1836 older Japanese Americans for an average of 6.3 years found that regular consumption of fruit and vegetable juices was associated with a decreased risk of developing Alzheimer disease.[77] More studies are needed to determine whether fruit and vegetable consumption is protective against neurodegenerative diseases.

Intake Recommendations

Many agencies within the US government, including the Centers for Disease Control and Prevention, recommend eating a variety of fruits and vegetables daily; the recommended serving number depends on age, sex, and activity level.[78] **Table 1.1** provides some examples of a single serving of fruits or vegetables. Consumption of a variety of different fruits and vegetables is recommended, including dark green, red, orange, yellow, blue, and purple fruits and vegetables, as well as legumes (peas and beans), onions, and garlic. Moreover, certain groups of fruits and vegetables, such as cruciferous vegetables, may provide specific health benefits (see Chapter 2). Additionally, fiber-rich, whole fruits are recommended over high-sugar fruit juices.

Summary

- Dietary patterns characterized by high intakes of fruits and vegetables are consistently associated with significant reductions in cardiovascular disease risk.

- Although prospective cohort studies provide weak support for an association between total fruit and vegetable consumption and cancer risk, they provide some evidence that high intakes of certain classes of fruits or vegetables are associated with reduced risk of individual cancers.
- The results of epidemiological and controlled clinical trials suggest that diets rich in fruits and vegetables can help prevent bone loss.
- The results of prospective cohort studies suggest that high intakes of fruits and vegetables rich in vitamin C and carotenoids may be associated with decreased risk of age-related eye diseases, such as macular degeneration or cataracts.
- Many organizations, including the Centers for Disease Control and Prevention, recommend eating a variety of fruits and vegetables daily; the recommended serving number depends on total caloric intake, which is governed by age, sex, body composition, and physical activity level.

References

1. Lock K, Pomerleau J, Causer L, Altmann DR, McKee M. The global burden of disease attributable to low consumption of fruit and vegetables: implications for the global strategy on diet. Bull World Health Organ 2005;83(2):100–108
2. Liu RH. Potential synergy of phytochemicals in cancer prevention: mechanism of action. J Nutr 2004; 134(12, Suppl): 3479S–3485S
3. Law MR, Morris JK. By how much does fruit and vegetable consumption reduce the risk of ischaemic heart disease? Eur J Clin Nutr 1998;52(8):549–556
4. Joshipura KJ, Hu FB, Manson JE, et al. The effect of fruit and vegetable intake on risk for coronary heart disease. Ann Intern Med 2001;134(12):1106–1114
5. Joshipura KJ, Ascherio A, Manson JE, et al. Fruit and vegetable intake in relation to risk of ischemic stroke. JAMA 1999;282(13):1233–1239
6. Dauchet L, Amouyel P, Hercberg S, Dallongeville J. Fruit and vegetable consumption and risk of coronary heart disease: a meta-analysis of cohort studies. J Nutr 2006;136(10):2588–2593
7. He FJ, Nowson CA, Lucas M, MacGregor GA. Increased consumption of fruit and vegetables is related to a reduced risk of coronary heart disease: meta-analysis of cohort studies. J Hum Hypertens 2007;21(9):717–728
8. He FJ, Nowson CA, MacGregor GA. Fruit and vegetable consumption and stroke: meta-analysis of cohort studies. Lancet 2006;367(9507):320–326
9. Chobanian AV, Bakris GL, Black HR, et al; National Heart, Lung, and Blood Institute Joint National Committee on Prevention, Detection, Evaluation, and Treatment of High Blood Pressure; National High Blood Pressure Education Program Coordinating Committee. The Seventh Report of the Joint National Committee on Prevention, Detection, Evaluation, and Treatment of High Blood Pressure: the JNC 7 report. JAMA 2003;289(19):2560–2572
10. Appel LJ, Moore TJ, Obarzanek E, et al; DASH Collaborative Research Group. A clinical trial of the effects of dietary patterns on blood pressure. N Engl J Med 1997;336(16):1117–1124
11. Bazzano LA, Serdula MK, Liu S. Dietary intake of fruits and vegetables and risk of cardiovascular disease. Curr Atheroscler Rep 2003;5(6):492–499
12. Winer N, Sowers JR. Epidemiology of diabetes. J Clin Pharmacol 2004;44(4):397–405
13. Ford ES, Mokdad AH. Fruit and vegetable consumption and diabetes mellitus incidence among U.S. adults. Prev Med 2001;32(1):33–39
14. Liu S, Serdula M, Janket SJ, et al. A prospective study of fruit and vegetable intake and the risk of type 2 diabetes in women. Diabetes Care 2004;27(12):2993–2996
15. Harding AH, Wareham NJ, Bingham SA, et al. Plasma vitamin C level, fruit and vegetable consumption, and the risk of new-onset type 2 diabetes mellitus: the European prospective investigation of cancer–Norfolk prospective study. Arch Intern Med 2008; 168(14):1493–1499
16. Bazzano LA, Li TY, Joshipura KJ, Hu FB. Intake of fruit, vegetables, and fruit juices and risk of diabetes in women. Diabetes Care 2008;31(7):1311–1317
17. Hamer M, Chida Y. Intake of fruit, vegetables, and antioxidants and risk of type 2 diabetes: systematic review and meta-analysis. J Hypertens 2007; 25(12):2361–2369
18. Sargeant LA, Khaw KT, Bingham S, et al. Fruit and vegetable intake and population glycosylated haemoglobin levels: the EPIC-Norfolk Study. Eur J Clin Nutr 2001;55(5):342–348
19. Block G, Patterson B, Subar A. Fruit, vegetables, and cancer prevention: a review of the epidemiological evidence. Nutr Cancer 1992;18(1):1–29
20. World Cancer Research Fund. Food, Nutrition, and the Prevention of Cancer: a Global Perspective. Washington, DC: American Institute for Cancer Research; 1997
21. Liu C, Russell RM. Nutrition and gastric cancer risk: an update. Nutr Rev 2008;66(5):237–249
22. van Gils CH, Peeters PH, Bueno-de-Mesquita HB, et al. Consumption of vegetables and fruits and risk of breast cancer. JAMA 2005;293(2):183–193
23. Tsubono Y, Otani T, Kobayashi M, Yamamoto S, Sobue T, Tsugane S; JPHC Study Group. No association between fruit or vegetable consumption and the risk of colorectal cancer in Japan. Br J Cancer 2005; 92(9):1782–1784
24. Sato Y, Tsubono Y, Nakaya N, et al. Fruit and vegetable consumption and risk of colorectal cancer in Japan: The Miyagi Cohort Study. Public Health Nutr 2005;8(3):309–314
25. Lin J, Zhang SM, Cook NR, et al. Dietary intakes of fruit, vegetables, and fiber, and risk of colorectal cancer in a prospective cohort of women (United States). Cancer Causes Control 2005;16(3):225–233
26. Key TJ, Allen N, Appleby P, et al; European Prospective Investigation into Cancer and Nutrition (EPIC). Fruits and vegetables and prostate cancer: no association among 1104 cases in a prospective study of 130 544 men in the European Prospective Investigation into

Cancer and Nutrition (EPIC). Int J Cancer 2004; 109(1):119–124

27. Hung HC, Joshipura KJ, Jiang R, et al. Fruit and vegetable intake and risk of major chronic disease. J Natl Cancer Inst 2004;96(21):1577–1584

28. Smith-Warner SA, Spiegelman D, Yaun SS, et al. Fruits, vegetables and lung cancer: a pooled analysis of cohort studies. Int J Cancer 2003;107(6):1001–1011

29. McCullough ML, Robertson AS, Chao A, et al. A prospective study of whole grains, fruits, vegetables and colon cancer risk. Cancer Causes Control 2003; 14(10):959–970

30. Michaud DS, Pietinen P, Taylor PR, Virtanen M, Virtamo J, Albanes D. Intakes of fruits and vegetables, carotenoids and vitamins A, E, C in relation to the risk of bladder cancer in the ATBC cohort study. Br J Cancer 2002;87(9):960–965

31. Flood A, Velie EM, Chaterjee N, et al. Fruit and vegetable intakes and the risk of colorectal cancer in the Breast Cancer Detection Demonstration Project follow-up cohort. Am J Clin Nutr 2002;75(5):936–943

32. Smith-Warner SA, Spiegelman D, Yaun SS, et al. Intake of fruits and vegetables and risk of breast cancer: a pooled analysis of cohort studies. JAMA 2001; 285(6):769–776

33. Michels KB, Edward Giovannucci, Joshipura KJ, et al. Prospective study of fruit and vegetable consumption and incidence of colon and rectal cancers. J Natl Cancer Inst 2000;92(21):1740–1752

34. Larsson SC, Andersson SO, Johansson JE, Wolk A. Fruit and vegetable consumption and risk of bladder cancer: a prospective cohort study. Cancer Epidemiol Biomarkers Prev 2008;17(9):2519–2522

35. Michels KB, Mohllajee AP, Roset-Bahmanyar E, Beehler GP, Moysich KB. Diet and breast cancer: a review of the prospective observational studies. Cancer 2007; 109(12, Suppl):2712–2749

36. Freedman ND, Subar AF, Hollenbeck AR, Leitzmann MF, Schatzkin A, Abnet CC. Fruit and vegetable intake and gastric cancer risk in a large United States prospective cohort study. Cancer Causes Control 2008;19(5):459–467

37. George SM, Park Y, Leitzmann MF, et al. Fruit and vegetable intake and risk of cancer: a prospective cohort study. Am J Clin Nutr 2009;89(1):347–353

38. Holick CN, De Vivo I, Feskanich D, Giovannucci E, Stampfer M, Michaud DS. Intake of fruits and vegetables, carotenoids, folate, and vitamins A, C, E and risk of bladder cancer among women (United States). Cancer Causes Control 2005;16(10):1135–1145

39. Koushik A, Hunter DJ, Spiegelman D, et al. Fruits, vegetables, and colon cancer risk in a pooled analysis of 14 cohort studies. J Natl Cancer Inst 2007; 99(19):1471–1483

40. Larsson SC, Håkansson N, Näslund I, Bergkvist L, Wolk A. Fruit and vegetable consumption in relation to pancreatic cancer risk: a prospective study. Cancer Epidemiol Biomarkers Prev 2006;15(2):301–305

41. McCullough ML, Bandera EV, Patel R, et al. A prospective study of fruits, vegetables, and risk of endometrial cancer. Am J Epidemiol 2007;166(8):902–911

42. Rohrmann S, Becker N, Linseisen J, et al. Fruit and vegetable consumption and lymphoma risk in the European Prospective Investigation into Cancer and Nutrition (EPIC). Cancer Causes Control 2007;18(5):537–549

43. Weikert S, Boeing H, Pischon T, et al. Fruits and vegetables and renal cell carcinoma: findings from the European prospective investigation into cancer and nutrition (EPIC). Int J Cancer 2006;118(12):3133–3139

44. Boffetta P, Couto E, Wichmann J, et al. Fruit and vegetable intake and overall cancer risk in the European Prospective Investigation into Cancer and Nutrition (EPIC). J Natl Cancer Inst 2010;102(8):529–537

45. Willett W. Nutritional Epidemiology. 2nd ed. New York: Oxford University Press; 1998

46. Riboli E, Norat T. Epidemiologic evidence of the protective effect of fruit and vegetables on cancer risk. Am J Clin Nutr 2003; 78(3, Suppl):559S–569S

47. Michaud DS, Spiegelman D, Clinton SK, Rimm EB, Willett WC, Giovannucci EL. Fruit and vegetable intake and incidence of bladder cancer in a male prospective cohort. J Natl Cancer Inst 1999;91(7):605–613

48. Kirsh VA, Peters U, Mayne ST, et al; Prostate, Lung, Colorectal and Ovarian Cancer Screening Trial. Prospective study of fruit and vegetable intake and risk of prostate cancer. J Natl Cancer Inst 2007; 99(15):1200–1209

49. Giovannucci E, Rimm EB, Liu Y, Stampfer MJ, Willett WC. A prospective study of tomato products, lycopene, and prostate cancer risk. J Natl Cancer Inst 2002;94(5):391–398

50. Tucker KL, Hannan MT, Chen H, Cupples LA, Wilson PW, Kiel DP. Potassium, magnesium, and fruit and vegetable intakes are associated with greater bone mineral density in elderly men and women. Am J Clin Nutr 1999;69(4):727–736

51. New SA, Bolton-Smith C, Grubb DA, Reid DM. Nutritional influences on bone mineral density: a cross-sectional study in premenopausal women. Am J Clin Nutr 1997;65(6):1831–1839

52. New SA, Robins SP, Campbell MK, et al. Dietary influences on bone mass and bone metabolism: further evidence of a positive link between fruit and vegetable consumption and bone health? Am J Clin Nutr 2000;71(1):142–151

53. Prynne CJ, Mishra GD, O'Connell MA, et al. Fruit and vegetable intakes and bone mineral status: a cross sectional study in 5 age and sex cohorts. Am J Clin Nutr 2006;83(6):1420–1428

54. New SA. Nutrition Society Medal lecture. The role of the skeleton in acid-base homeostasis. Proc Nutr Soc 2002;61(2):151–164

55. Macdonald HM, Black AJ, Aucott L, et al. Effect of potassium citrate supplementation or increased fruit and vegetable intake on bone metabolism in healthy postmenopausal women: a randomized controlled trial. Am J Clin Nutr 2008;88(2):465–474

56. Lin PH, Ginty F, Appel LJ, et al. The DASH diet and sodium reduction improve markers of bone turnover and calcium metabolism in adults. J Nutr 2003; 133(10):3130–3136

57. Brown L, Rimm EB, Seddon JM, et al. A prospective study of carotenoid intake and risk of cataract extraction in US men. Am J Clin Nutr 1999;70(4):517–524

58. Christen WG, Liu S, Schaumberg DA, Buring JE. Fruit and vegetable intake and the risk of cataract in women. Am J Clin Nutr 2005;81(6):1417–1422

59. Jacques PF, Chylack LT Jr, Hankinson SE, et al. Long-term nutrient intake and early age-related nuclear lens opacities. Arch Ophthalmol 2001;119(7):1009–1019

60. Lyle BJ, Mares-Perlman JA, Klein BE, Klein R, Greger JL. Antioxidant intake and risk of incident age-related nuclear cataracts in the Beaver Dam Eye Study. Am J Epidemiol 1999;149(9):801–809

61. Cooper DA, Eldridge AL, Peters JC. Dietary carotenoids and certain cancers, heart disease, and age-related macular degeneration: a review of recent research. Nutr Rev 1999;57(7):201–214

62. Mares-Perlman JA, Millen AE, Ficek TL, Hankinson SE. The body of evidence to support a protective role for lutein and zeaxanthin in delaying chronic disease. Overview. J Nutr 2002;132(3):518S–524S

63. Seddon JM, Ajani UA, Sperduto RD, et al; Eye Disease Case-Control Study Group. Dietary carotenoids, vitamins A, C, and E, and advanced age-related macular degeneration. JAMA 1994;272(18):1413–1420

64. Snellen EL, Verbeek AL, Van Den Hoogen GW, Cruysberg JR, Hoyng CB. Neovascular age-related macular degeneration and its relationship to antioxidant intake. Acta Ophthalmol Scand 2002;80(4):368–371

65. Cho E, Seddon JM, Rosner B, Willett WC, Hankinson SE. Prospective study of intake of fruits, vegetables, vitamins, and carotenoids and risk of age-related maculopathy. Arch Ophthalmol 2004;122(6):883–892

66. Moeller SM, Parekh N, Tinker L, et al; CAREDS Research Study Group. Associations between intermediate age-related macular degeneration and lutein and zeaxanthin in the Carotenoids in Age-related Eye Disease Study (CAREDS): ancillary study of the Women's Health Initiative. Arch Ophthalmol 2006; 124(8):1151–1162

67. Romieu I, Trenga C. Diet and obstructive lung diseases. Epidemiol Rev 2001;23(2):268–287

68. Tabak C, Smit HA, Räsänen L, et al. Dietary factors and pulmonary function: a cross sectional study in middle aged men from three European countries. Thorax 1999;54(11):1021–1026

69. Butland BK, Fehily AM, Elwood PC. Diet, lung function, and lung function decline in a cohort of 2512 middle aged men. Thorax 2000;55(2):102–108

70. Tabak C, Arts IC, Smit HA, Heederik D, Kromhout D. Chronic obstructive pulmonary disease and intake of catechins, flavonols, and flavones: the MORGEN Study. Am J Respir Crit Care Med 2001;164(1):61–64

71. Walda IC, Tabak C, Smit HA, et al. Diet and 20-year chronic obstructive pulmonary disease mortality in middle-aged men from three European countries. Eur J Clin Nutr 2002;56(7):638–643

72. Celik F, Topcu F. Nutritional risk factors for the development of chronic obstructive pulmonary disease (COPD) in male smokers. Clin Nutr 2006;25(6):955–961

73. Varraso R, Fung TT, Hu FB, Willett W, Camargo CA. Prospective study of dietary patterns and chronic obstructive pulmonary disease among US men. Thorax 2007;62(9):786–791

74. Varraso R, Fung TT, Barr RG, Hu FB, Willett W, Camargo CA Jr. Prospective study of dietary patterns and chronic obstructive pulmonary disease among US women. Am J Clin Nutr 2007;86(2):488–495

75. Joseph JA, Denisova NA, Arendash G, et al. Blueberry supplementation enhances signaling and prevents behavioral deficits in an Alzheimer disease model. Nutr Neurosci 2003;6(3):153–162

76. Suganuma H, Hirano T, Arimoto Y, Inakuma T. Effect of tomato intake on striatal monoamine level in a mouse model of experimental Parkinson's disease. J Nutr Sci Vitaminol (Tokyo) 2002;48(3):251–254

77. Dai Q, Borenstein AR, Wu Y, Jackson JC, Larson EB. Fruit and vegetable juices and Alzheimer's disease: the Kame Project. Am J Med 2006;119(9):751–759

78. Centers for Disease Control and Prevention. Eat a Variety of Fruits & Vegetables Every Day. [Web page]. Available at: http://www.fruitsandveggiesmatter. gov/. Accessed April 30, 2012

2 Cruciferous Vegetables

Cruciferous or *Brassica* vegetables are so named because they come from plants in the family known to botanists as Cruciferae (Brassicaceae). Many commonly consumed cruciferous vegetables come from the *Brassica* genus, including broccoli, Brussels sprouts, cabbage, cauliflower, collard greens, kale, kohlrabi, mustard, rutabaga, turnips, bok choy, and Chinese cabbage.[1] Arugula, horseradish, radish, wasabi, and watercress are also cruciferous vegetables.

Cruciferous vegetables are unique in that they are rich sources of glucosinolates, sulfur-containing compounds that impart a pungent aroma and a spicy (or bitter) taste.[2] The hydrolysis (breakdown) of glucosinolates by a class of plant enzymes called *myrosinase* results in the formation of biologically active compounds, such as indoles and isothiocyanates.[3] Myrosinase is physically separated from glucosinolates in intact plant cells. However, when cruciferous vegetables are chopped or chewed, myrosinase comes in contact with glucosinolates and catalyzes their hydrolysis. Scientists are currently interested in the potential for high intakes of cruciferous vegetables as well as several glucosinolate hydrolysis products to prevent cancer (see Chapters 13 and 14).

Disease Prevention

Cancer

Like most other vegetables, cruciferous vegetables are good sources of a variety of nutrients and phytochemicals that may work synergistically to help prevent cancer.[4] One challenge in studying the relationships between cruciferous vegetable intake and cancer risk in humans is separating the benefits of diets that are generally rich in vegetables from those that are specifically rich in cruciferous vegetables.[5] One characteristic that sets cruciferous vegetables apart from other vegetables is their high glucosinolate content.[6] Glucosinolate hydrolysis products could help prevent cancer by enhancing the elimination of carcinogens before they can damage DNA, or by altering cell-signaling pathways in ways that help prevent normal cells from being transformed into cancerous cells.[7] Some glucosinolate hydrolysis products may alter the metabolism or activity of hormones like estrogen in ways that inhibit the development of hormone-sensitive cancers.[8]

An extensive review of epidemiological studies published prior to 1996 reported that the majority (67%) of 87 case–control studies found an inverse association between some type of cruciferous vegetable intake and cancer risk.[9] At that time, the inverse association appeared to be most consistent for cancers of the lung and digestive tract. The results of retrospective case–control studies are more likely to be distorted by bias in the selection of participants (cases and controls) and dietary recall than prospective cohort studies, which collect dietary information from participants before they are diagnosed with cancer.[10] In the past decade, results of prospective cohort studies and studies taking into account individual genetic variation suggest that the relationship between cruciferous vegetable intake and the risk of several types of cancer is more complex than previously thought.

Lung Cancer

When evaluating the effect of cruciferous vegetable consumption on lung cancer risk, it is important to remember that the benefit of increasing cruciferous vegetable intake is likely to be small compared with the benefit of smoking cessation.[11,12] Although several case–control studies found that people diagnosed with lung cancer had significantly lower intakes of cruciferous vegetables than people in cancer-free control groups,[9] the findings of more recent prospective cohort studies have been mixed. Prospective studies of Dutch men and women,[13] US women,[14] and Finnish men[15] found that higher intakes of cruciferous vegetables (more than three weekly servings) were associated with significant reductions in lung cancer risk, but prospective studies of US men[14] and European men and women[11] found no inverse association. The results of several studies suggest that genetic factors affecting the metabolism of glucosinolate hydrolysis products may influence the effects of cruciferous vegetable consumption on lung cancer risk[16–23] (see the Genetic Influences section below).

Colorectal Cancer

A small clinical trial found that the consumption of 250 g/day (9 oz/day) of broccoli and 250 g/day of Brussels sprouts significantly increased the urinary excretion of a potential carcinogen found in well-done meat, suggesting that high intakes of cruciferous vegetables might decrease colorectal cancer risk by enhancing the elimination of some dietary carcinogens.[22] Although several case–control studies conducted prior to 1990 found that people diagnosed with colorectal cancer were more likely to have lower intakes of various cruciferous vegetables than people without colorectal cancer,[23–26] most prospective cohort studies have not found significant inverse associations between cruciferous vegetable intake and the risk of developing colorectal cancer over time.[27–32] One exception was a prospective study of Dutch adults, which found that men and women with the highest intakes of cruciferous vegetables (averaging 58 g/day) were significantly less likely to develop colon cancer than those with the lowest intakes (averaging 11 g/day).[33] Surprisingly, higher intakes of cruciferous vegetables were associated with increased risk of rectal cancer in women in that study. As in lung cancer, the relationship between cruciferous vegetable consumption and colorectal cancer risk may be complicated by genetic factors. The results of several epidemiological studies suggest that the protective effects of cruciferous vegetable consumption may be influenced by inherited differences in the capacity of individuals to metabolize and eliminate glucosinolate hydrolysis products[34–37] (see the Genetic Influences section below).

Breast Cancer

The endogenous estrogen 17β-estradiol can be irreversibly metabolized to 16α-hydroxyestrone (16αOHE1) or 2-hydroxyestrone (2OHE1). In contrast to 2OHE1, 16αOHE1 is highly estrogenic and has been found to enhance the proliferation of estrogen-sensitive breast cancer cells in culture.[38,39] It has been hypothesized that shifting the metabolism of 17β-estradiol toward 2OHE1, and away from 16αOHE1, could decrease the risk of estrogen-sensitive cancers like breast cancer.[40] In a small clinical trial, increasing the cruciferous vegetable intake of healthy postmenopausal women for 4 weeks increased urinary 2OHE1:16αOHE1 ratios, suggesting that high intakes of cruciferous vegetables can shift estrogen metabolism. However, the relationship between urinary 2OHE1:16αOHE1 ratios and breast cancer risk is not clear. Several small case–control studies found that women with breast cancer had lower urinary ratios of 2OHE1:16αOHE1,[41–43] but larger case–control and prospective cohort studies did not find significant associations between urinary 2OHE1:16αOHE1 ratios and breast cancer risk.[44–46] The results of epidemiological studies of cruciferous vegetable intake and breast cancer risk are also inconsistent. Several case–control studies in the US, Sweden, and China found that measures of cruciferous vegetable intake were significantly lower in women diagnosed with breast cancer than in women in the cancer-free control groups,[47–49] but cruciferous vegetable intake was not associated with breast cancer risk in a pooled analysis of seven large prospective cohort studies.[50] In a prospective study in 285 526 women, total vegetable consumption was not related to risk of breast cancer; individual subcategories of vegetable type, including cabbages, root vegetables, and leafy vegetables, were not individually associated with breast cancer in this cohort.[51]

Prostate Cancer

Although glucosinolate hydrolysis products have been found to inhibit growth and promote programmed death (apoptosis) of cultured prostate cancer cells,[52,53] the results of epidemiological studies of cruciferous vegetable intake and prostate cancer risk are inconsistent. Four out of eight case–control studies published since 1990 found that some measure of cruciferous vegetable intake was significantly lower in men diagnosed with prostate cancer than men in a cancer-free control group.[54–57] Of the five prospective cohort studies that have examined associations between cruciferous vegetable intake and the risk of prostate cancer, none found statistically significant inverse associations overall.[58–62] However, the prospective study that included the longest follow-up period and the most cases of prostate cancer found a significant inverse association between cruciferous vegetable intake and the risk of prostate cancer when the analysis was limited to men who had a prostate-specific antigen (PSA) test.[58] Since men who have PSA screening are more likely to be diagnosed with prostate cancer, limiting the analysis in this way is one way to reduce detection bias.[63] Additionally, the most recent prospective study found that intake of cruciferous vegetables was inversely associated with metastatic prostate cancer—cancer that has spread beyond the prostate (i.e., late-stage prostate cancer).[62] At present, epidemiological studies provide only modest support for the hypothesis that high intakes of cruciferous vegetables reduce prostate cancer risk.[1]

Genetic Influences

There is increasing evidence that genetic differences in humans may influence the effects of cruciferous vegetable intake on cancer risk.[64] Isothiocyanates are glucosinolate hydrolysis products, which are thought to play a role in the cancer-preventive effects associated with cruciferous vegetable consumption. Glutathione S-transferases (GSTs) are a family of enzymes that metabolize a variety of compounds, including isothiocyanates, in a way that promotes their elimination from the body. Genetic variations (polymorphisms) that affect the activity of GST enzymes have been identified in humans. Null variants of the GSTM1 gene and GSTT1 gene contain large deletions, and individuals who inherit two copies of the GSTM1-null or GSTT1-null gene cannot produce the corresponding GST enzyme.[65] Lower GST activity in such individuals could result in slower elimination and longer exposure to isothiocyanates after consumption of cruciferous vegetables.[66] In support of this idea, several epidemiological studies have found that inverse associations between isothiocyanate intake from cruciferous vegetables and risk of lung cancer[16–19] or colon cancer[34–36] were more pronounced in GSTM1-null and/or GSTT1-null individuals. These findings suggest that the protective effects of high intakes of cruciferous vegetables may be enhanced in individuals who more slowly eliminate potentially protective compounds like isothiocyanates. Alternatively, these same GSTs play a major role in detoxication of carcinogens and individuals with the null gene would be expected to be more susceptible to cancer; thus, the cruciferous vegetables may exhibit significant protection

in this population if their protective effect is increasingly important at high carcinogen levels.[67]

Nutrient Interactions

Iodine and Thyroid Function

Very high intakes of cruciferous vegetables, such as cabbage and turnips, have been found to cause hypothyroidism (insufficient thyroid hormone) in animals.[68] There has been one case report of an 88-year-old woman developing severe hypothyroidism and coma following consumption of an estimated 1.0–1.5 kg/day of raw bok choy for several months.[69] Two mechanisms have been identified to explain this effect. The hydrolysis of some glucosinolates found in cruciferous vegetables (e.g., progoitrin) may yield a compound known as *goitrin*, which has been found to interfere with the synthesis of thyroid hormone. The hydrolysis of another class of glucosinolates, known as *indole glucosinolates*, results in the release of thiocyanate ions, which can compete with iodine for uptake by the thyroid gland. Increased exposure to thiocyanate ions from cruciferous vegetable consumption or, more commonly, from cigarette smoking, does not appear to increase the risk of hypothyroidism unless accompanied by iodine deficiency. One study in humans found that the consumption of 150 g/day (5 oz/day) of cooked Brussels sprouts for 4 weeks had no adverse effects on thyroid function.[70]

Intake Recommendations

Although many organizations, including the National Cancer Institute, recommend eating a variety of fruits and vegetables daily (the serving number depends on age, sex, and activity level);[71] separate recommendations for cruciferous vegetables have not been established. Much remains to be learned regarding cruciferous vegetable consumption and cancer prevention, but the results of some epidemiological studies suggest that adults should aim for at least five weekly servings of cruciferous vegetables.[14,58,71]

Summary

- Cruciferous vegetables are unique in that they are rich sources of sulfur-containing compounds known as *glucosinolates*.
- Chopping or chewing cruciferous vegetables results in the formation of bioactive glucosinolate hydrolysis products, such as isothiocyanates and indole-3-carbinol.
- High intakes of cruciferous vegetables have been associated with lower risk of lung and colorectal cancer in some epidemiological studies, but there is evidence that genetic differences may influence the effect of cruciferous vegetables on human cancer risk.
- Although glucosinolate hydrolysis products may alter the metabolism or activity of sex hormones in ways that could inhibit the development of hormone-sensitive cancers, evidence of an inverse association between cruciferous vegetable intake and breast or prostate cancer in humans is limited and inconsistent.
- Many organizations, including the National Cancer Institute, recommend eating a variety of fruits and vegetables daily; the recommended serving number depends on age, sex, and physical activity level. However, separate recommendations for cruciferous vegetables have not been established.

References

1. Kristal AR, Lampe JW. Brassica vegetables and prostate cancer risk: a review of the epidemiological evidence. Nutr Cancer 2002;42(1):1–9
2. Drewnowski A, Gomez-Carneros C. Bitter taste, phytonutrients, and the consumer: a review. Am J Clin Nutr 2000;72(6):1424–1435
3. Holst B, Williamson G. A critical review of the bioavailability of glucosinolates and related compounds. Nat Prod Rep 2004;21(3):425–447
4. Liu RH. Potential synergy of phytochemicals in cancer prevention: mechanism of action. J Nutr 2004;134(12, Suppl):3479S–3485S
5. McNaughton SA, Marks GC. Development of a food composition database for the estimation of dietary intakes of glucosinolates, the biologically active constituents of cruciferous vegetables. Br J Nutr 2003;90(3):687–697
6. van Poppel G, Verhoeven DT, Verhagen H, Goldbohm RA. Brassica vegetables and cancer prevention. Epidemiology and mechanisms. Adv Exp Med Biol 1999;472:159–168
7. Zhang Y. Cancer-preventive isothiocyanates: measurement of human exposure and mechanism of action. Mutat Res 2004;555(1–2):173–190
8. Auborn KJ, Fan S, Rosen EM, et al. Indole-3-carbinol is a negative regulator of estrogen. J Nutr 2003;133(7, Suppl):2470S–2475S
9. Verhoeven DT, Goldbohm RA, van Poppel G, Verhagen H, van den Brandt PA. Epidemiological studies on brassica vegetables and cancer risk. Cancer Epidemiol Biomarkers Prev 1996;5(9):733–748
10. Willett W. Nutritional Epidemiology. 2nd ed. New York: Oxford University Press; 1998.
11. Miller AB, Altenburg HP, Bueno-de-Mesquita B, et al. Fruits and vegetables and lung cancer: Findings from the European Prospective Investigation into Cancer and Nutrition. Int J Cancer 2004;108(2):269–276
12. Smith-Warner SA, Spiegelman D, Yaun SS, et al. Fruits, vegetables and lung cancer: a pooled analysis of cohort studies. Int J Cancer 2003;107(6):1001–1011
13. Voorrips LE, Goldbohm RA, Verhoeven DT, et al. Vegetable and fruit consumption and cancer risk in the Netherlands Cohort Study on diet and cancer. Cancer Causes Control 2000;11(2):101–115
14. Feskanich D, Ziegler RG, Michaud DS, et al. Prospective study of fruit and vegetable consumption and risk of lung cancer among men and women. J Natl Cancer Inst 2000;92(22):1812–1823
15. Neuhouser ML, Patterson RE, Thornquist MD, Omenn GS, King IB, Goodman GE. Fruits and vegetables are associated with lower lung cancer risk only in the placebo arm of the beta-carotene and retinol efficacy trial (CARET). Cancer Epidemiol Biomarkers Prev 2003;12(4):350–358
16. Spitz MR, Duphorne CM, Detry MA, et al. Dietary intake of isothiocyanates: evidence of a joint effect with glutathione S-transferase polymorphisms in lung cancer risk. Cancer Epidemiol Biomarkers Prev 2001;10(10):1105–1106
17. Lewis S, Brennan P, Nyberg F, et al. Re., Spitz MR, Duphorne CM, Detry MA, et al. Dietary intake of isothiocyanates: evidence of a joint effect with glutathione S-transferase polymorphisms in lung cancer risk. Cancer Epidemiol Biomarkers Prev 2000;9(10):1017–1020
18. London SJ, Yuan JM, Chung FL, et al. Isothiocyanates, glutathione S-transferase M1 and T1 polymorphisms, and lung-cancer risk: a prospective study of men in Shanghai, China. Lancet 2000;356(9231):724–729
19. Zhao B, Seow A, Lee EJ, et al. Dietary isothiocyanates, glutathione S-transferase -M1, -T1 polymorphisms and lung cancer risk among Chinese women in Singapore. Cancer Epidemiol Biomarkers Prev 2001;10(10):1063–1067
20. Brennan P, Hsu CC, Moullan N, et al. Effect of cruciferous vegetables on lung cancer in patients stratified by genetic status: a mendelian randomisation approach. Lancet 2005;366(9496):1558–1560
21. Wang LI, Giovannucci EL, Hunter D, Neuberg D, Su L, Christiani DC. Dietary intake of Cruciferous vegetables, Glutathione S-transferase (GST) polymorphisms and lung cancer risk in a Caucasian population. Cancer Causes Control 2004;15(10):977–985
22. Walters DG, Young PJ, Agus C, et al. Cruciferous vegetable consumption alters the metabolism of the dietary carcinogen 2-amino-1-methyl-6-phenylimidazo[4,5-b]pyridine (PhIP) in humans. Carcinogenesis 2004;25(9):1659–1669
23. Benito E, Obrador A, Stiggelbout A, et al. A population-based case-control study of colorectal cancer in Majorca. I. Dietary factors. Int J Cancer 1990;45(1):69–76

24. West DW, Slattery ML, Robison LM, et al. Dietary intake and colon cancer: sex- and anatomic site-specific associations. Am J Epidemiol 1989;130(5):883–894

25. Young TB, Wolf DA. Case-control study of proximal and distal colon cancer and diet in Wisconsin. Int J Cancer 1988;42(2):167–175

26. Graham S, Dayal H, Swanson M, Mittelman A, Wilkinson G. Diet in the epidemiology of cancer of the colon and rectum. J Natl Cancer Inst 1978;61(3):709–714

27. Kojima M, Wakai K, Tamakoshi K, et al; Japan Collaborative Cohort Study Group. Diet and colorectal cancer mortality: results from the Japan Collaborative Cohort Study. Nutr Cancer 2004;50(1):23–32

28. McCullough ML, Robertson AS, Chao A, et al. A prospective study of whole grains, fruits, vegetables and colon cancer risk. Cancer Causes Control 2003; 14(10):959–970

29. Michels KB, Edward Giovannucci, Joshipura KJ, et al. Prospective study of fruit and vegetable consumption and incidence of colon and rectal cancers. J Natl Cancer Inst 2000;92(21):1740–1752

30. Steinmetz KA, Kushi LH, Bostick RM, Folsom AR, Potter JD. Vegetables, fruit, and colon cancer in the Iowa Women's Health Study. Am J Epidemiol 1994;139(1):1–15

31. Hsing AW, McLaughlin JK, Chow WH, et al. Risk factors for colorectal cancer in a prospective study among U.S. white men. Int J Cancer 1998;77(4):549–553

32. Pietinen P, Malila N, Virtanen M, et al. Diet and risk of colorectal cancer in a cohort of Finnish men. Cancer Causes Control 1999;10(5):387–396

33. Voorrips LE, Goldbohm RA, van Poppel G, Sturmans F, Hermus RJ, van den Brandt PA. Vegetable and fruit consumption and risks of colon and rectal cancer in a prospective cohort study: The Netherlands Cohort Study on Diet and Cancer. Am J Epidemiol 2000;152(11):1081–1092

34. Turner F, Smith G, Sachse C, et al. Vegetable, fruit and meat consumption and potential risk modifying genes in relation to colorectal cancer. Int J Cancer 2004;112(2):259–264

35. Seow A, Yuan JM, Sun CL, Van Den Berg D, Lee HP, Yu MC. Dietary isothiocyanates, glutathione S-transferase polymorphisms and colorectal cancer risk in the Singapore Chinese Health Study. Carcinogenesis 2002;23(12):2055–2061

36. Slattery ML, Kampman E, Samowitz W, Caan BJ, Potter JD. Interplay between dietary inducers of GST and the GSTM-1 genotype in colon cancer. Int J Cancer 2000;87(5):728–733

37. Lin HJ, Probst-Hensch NM, Louie AD, et al. Glutathione transferase null genotype, broccoli, and lower prevalence of colorectal adenomas. Cancer Epidemiol Biomarkers Prev 1998;7(8):647–652

38. Telang NT, Suto A, Wong GY, Osborne MP, Bradlow HL. Induction by estrogen metabolite 16 alpha-hydroxyestrone of genotoxic damage and aberrant proliferation in mouse mammary epithelial cells. J Natl Cancer Inst 1992;84(8):634–638

39. Yuan F, Chen DZ, Liu K, Sepkovic DW, Bradlow HL, Auborn K. Anti-estrogenic activities of indole-3-carbinol in cervical cells: implication for prevention of cervical cancer. Anticancer Res 1999;19(3A):1673–1680

40. Bradlow HL, Telang NT, Sepkovic DW, Osborne MP. 2-hydroxyestrone: the 'good' estrogen. J Endocrinol 1996;150(Suppl):S259–S265

41. Ho GH, Luo XW, Ji CY, Foo SC, Ng EH. Urinary 2/16 alpha-hydroxyestrone ratio: correlation with serum insulin-like growth factor binding protein-3 and a potential biomarker of breast cancer risk. Ann Acad Med Singapore 1998;27(2):294–299

42. Kabat GC, Chang CJ, Sparano JA, et al. Urinary estrogen metabolites and breast cancer: a case-control study. Cancer Epidemiol Biomarkers Prev 1997;6(7):505–509

43. Schneider J, Kinne D, Fracchia A, et al. Abnormal oxidative metabolism of estradiol in women with breast cancer. Proc Natl Acad Sci U S A 1982;79(9):3047–3051

44. Cauley JA, Zmuda JM, Danielson ME, et al. Estrogen metabolites and the risk of breast cancer in older women. Epidemiology 2003;14(6):740–744

45. Meilahn EN, De Stavola B, Allen DS, et al. Do urinary oestrogen metabolites predict breast cancer? Guernsey III cohort follow-up. Br J Cancer 1998;78(9):1250–1255

46. Ursin G, London S, Stanczyk FZ, et al. Urinary 2-hydroxyestrone/16alpha-hydroxyestrone ratio and risk of breast cancer in postmenopausal women. J Natl Cancer Inst 1999;91(12):1067–1072

47. Ambrosone CB, McCann SE, Freudenheim JL, Marshall JR, Zhang Y, Shields PG. Breast cancer risk in premenopausal women is inversely associated with consumption of broccoli, a source of isothiocyanates, but is not modified by GST genotype. J Nutr 2004; 134(5):1134–1138

48. Fowke JH, Chung FL, Jin F, et al. Urinary isothiocyanate levels, brassica, and human breast cancer. Cancer Res 2003;63(14):3980–3986

49. Terry P, Wolk A, Persson I, Magnusson C. Brassica vegetables and breast cancer risk. JAMA 2001;285(23):2975–2977

50. Smith-Warner SA, Spiegelman D, Yaun SS, et al. Intake of fruits and vegetables and risk of breast cancer: a pooled analysis of cohort studies. JAMA 2001;285(6):769–776

51. van Gils CH, Peeters PH, Bueno-de-Mesquita HB, et al. Consumption of vegetables and fruits and risk of breast cancer. JAMA 2005;293(2):183–193

52. Singh AV, Xiao D, Lew KL, Dhir R, Singh SV. Sulforaphane induces caspase-mediated apoptosis in cultured PC-3 human prostate cancer cells and retards growth of PC-3 xenografts in vivo. Carcinogenesis 2004;25(1):83–90

53. Sarkar FH, Li Y. Indole-3-carbinol and prostate cancer. J Nutr 2004;134(12, Suppl):3493S–3498S

54. Cohen JH, Kristal AR, Stanford JL. Fruit and vegetable intakes and prostate cancer risk. J Natl Cancer Inst 2000;92(1):61–68

55. Jain MG, Hislop GT, Howe GR, Ghadirian P. Plant foods, antioxidants, and prostate cancer risk: findings from case-control studies in Canada. Nutr Cancer 1999;34(2):173–184

56. Joseph MA, Moysich KB, Freudenheim JL, et al. Cruciferous vegetables, genetic polymorphisms in glutathione S-transferases M1 and T1, and prostate cancer risk. Nutr Cancer 2004;50(2):206–213

57. Kolonel LN, Hankin JH, Whittemore AS, et al. Vegetables, fruits, legumes and prostate cancer: a multiethnic case-control study. Cancer Epidemiol Biomarkers Prev 2000;9(8):795–804

58. Giovannucci E, Rimm EB, Liu Y, Stampfer MJ, Willett WC. A prospective study of cruciferous vegetables and prostate cancer. Cancer Epidemiol Biomarkers Prev 2003;12(12):1403–1409

59. Hsing AW, McLaughlin JK, Schuman LM, et al. Diet, tobacco use, and fatal prostate cancer: results from the Lutheran Brotherhood Cohort Study. Cancer Res 1990;50(21):6836–6840

60. Key TJ, Allen N, Appleby P, et al; European Prospective Investigation into Cancer and Nutrition (EPIC). Fruits and vegetables and prostate cancer: no association among 1104 cases in a prospective study of 130544 men in the European Prospective Investigation into Cancer and Nutrition (EPIC). Int J Cancer 2004; 109(1):119–124

61. Schuurman AG, Goldbohm RA, Dorant E, van den Brandt PA. Vegetable and fruit consumption and prostate cancer risk: a cohort study in The Netherlands. Cancer Epidemiol Biomarkers Prev 1998;7(8): 673–680

62. Kirsh VA, Peters U, Mayne ST, et al; Prostate, Lung, Colorectal and Ovarian Cancer Screening Trial. Prospective study of fruit and vegetable intake and risk of prostate cancer. J Natl Cancer Inst 2007;99(15):1200–1209

63. Kristal AR, Stanford JL. Cruciferous vegetables and prostate cancer risk: confounding by PSA screening. Cancer Epidemiol Biomarkers Prev 2004;13(7):1265

64. Lampe JW, Peterson S. Brassica, biotransformation and cancer risk: genetic polymorphisms alter the preventive effects of cruciferous vegetables. J Nutr 2002;132(10):2991–2994

65. Coles BF, Kadlubar FF. Detoxification of electrophilic compounds by glutathione S-transferase catalysis: determinants of individual response to chemical carcinogens and chemotherapeutic drugs? Biofactors 2003;17(1–4):115–130

66. Seow A, Shi CY, Chung FL, et al. Urinary total isothiocyanate (ITC) in a population-based sample of middle-aged and older Chinese in Singapore: relationship with dietary total ITC and glutathione S-transferase M1/T1/P1 genotypes. Cancer Epidemiol Biomarkers Prev 1998;7(9):775–781

67. Perera FP, Mooney LA, Stampfer M, et al; Physicians' Health Cohort Study. Associations between carcinogen-DNA damage, glutathione S-transferase genotypes, and risk of lung cancer in the prospective Physicians' Health Cohort Study. Carcinogenesis 2002; 23(10):1641–1646

68. Fenwick GR, Heaney RK, Mullin WJ. Glucosinolates and their breakdown products in food and food plants. Crit Rev Food Sci Nutr 1983;18(2):123–201

69. Chu M, Seltzer TF. Myxedema coma induced by ingestion of raw bok choy. N Engl J Med 2010;362(20):1945–1946

70. McMillan M, Spinks EA, Fenwick GR. Preliminary observations on the effect of dietary brussels sprouts on thyroid function. Hum Toxicol 1986;5(1):15–19

71. National Cancer Institute. Eat a Variety of Fruits & Vegetables Every Day. Available at: http://www.fruitsandveggiesmatter.gov/. Accessed Sep 22, 2008

3 Legumes

Legumes are plants with seedpods that split into two halves. Edible seeds from plants in the legume family include beans, peas, lentils, soybeans, and peanuts. Since peanuts are nutritionally similar to tree nuts, information on the health benefits of peanuts is presented in Chapter 4 on Nuts. Although legumes are an important part of traditional diets around the world, they are often neglected in typical Western diets. Legumes are inexpensive, nutrient-dense sources of protein that can be substituted for dietary animal protein.[1] While sources of animal protein are often rich in saturated fats, the small quantities of fats in legumes are mostly unsaturated fats. Not only are legumes excellent sources of essential minerals, but they are also rich in dietary fiber and other phytochemicals that may affect health. Soybeans have attracted the most scientific interest, mainly because they are a unique source of phytoestrogens known as isoflavones.[2] Although most other legumes lack isoflavones, they also represent unique packages of nutrients and phytochemicals that may work synergistically to reduce the risk of chronic diseases. In this chapter, the health effects of diets rich in legumes and soy foods are summarized. Research on the health effects of soy isoflavones is discussed in Chapter 12.

Disease Prevention

Type 2 Diabetes Mellitus

The glycemic index is a measure of the potential for carbohydrates in different foods to raise blood glucose levels. In general, consuming foods with high-glycemic-index values causes blood glucose levels to rise more rapidly, which results in greater insulin secretion by the pancreas, than after consuming foods with low-glycemic-index values. Chronically elevated blood glucose levels and excessive insulin secretion are thought to play important roles in the development of type 2 diabetes mellitus (DM).[3] Because legumes generally have low-glycemic-index values, substituting legumes for high-glycemic-index foods like white rice or potatoes lowers the glycemic load of one's diet. In several large prospective studies, low-glycemic-load diets have been associated with reduced risk of developing type 2 DM.[4-7] Obesity is another important risk factor for type 2 DM. Numerous clinical trials have shown that the consumption of low-glycemic-index foods delays the return of hunger, decreases subsequent food intake, and increases the sensation of fullness compared with high-glycemic-index foods.[8,9] The results of several small, short-term trials (1–6 months) suggest that low-glycemic-load diets result in significantly more weight or fat loss than high-glycemic-load diets.[10-13] Thus, diets rich in legumes may decrease the risk of type 2 diabetes by improving blood glucose control, decreasing insulin secretion, and delaying the return of hunger after a meal. For more information on glycemic index values and glycemic load, see Appendix 1 on Glycemic Index and Glycemic Load.

One study in elderly men and women reported that consumption of legumes was protective against the development of glucose intolerance.[14] More recently, a prospective cohort study in 64 227 middle-aged Chinese women found that their total legume consumption, which included soybeans, peanuts, and other legumes, was associated with a 38% lower risk of developing type 2 DM.[15] Moreover, a prospective study that followed 10 449 individuals with diabetes for 9 years found that legume intake was inversely associated with cardiovascular-related mortality and all-cause mortality, but not with cancer-related mortality.[16]

Cardiovascular Disease

Beans, Peas, and Lentils

One prospective cohort study that examined the effect of legume intake on cardiovascular disease risk followed men and women for 19 years and found those who ate dry beans, peas, or peanuts at least four times weekly had a risk of coronary heart disease (CHD) that was 21% lower than for those who ate them less than once weekly.[17]

When compared with a typical Western diet, legume intake as part of a healthy dietary pattern that included higher intakes of vegetables, fruits, whole grains, fish, and poultry was associated with a risk of CHD that was 30% lower in men[18] and 24% lower in women.[19] The results of controlled clinical trials suggest that increasing bean consumption improves serum lipid and lipoprotein profiles. A meta-analysis that combined the results of 11 clinical trials found that increasing the consumption of dry beans resulted in modest (6%–7%) decreases in total cholesterol and low-density lipoprotein (LDL) cholesterol.[20] Several characteristics of beans may contribute to their cardioprotective effects. Beans are rich in soluble fiber, which is known to have a cholesterol-lowering effect. Elevated plasma homocysteine levels are associated with increased cardiovascular disease risk, and beans are good sources of folate, which helps to lower homocysteine levels. Beans are also good sources of magnesium and potassium, which may decrease cardiovascular disease risk by helping to lower blood pressure.[20] The low-glycemic-index values of beans means that they are less likely to raise blood glucose and insulin levels, which may also decrease cardiovascular disease risk. For more information on glycemic index, see Appendix 1.

Soy

In 1999, the US Food and Drug Administration approved the following health claim: "Diets low in saturated fat and cholesterol that include 25 grams of soy protein a day may reduce the risk of heart disease."[21] Most of the evidence to support this health claim was included in the Anderson et al. meta-analysis of 38 controlled clinical trials that was published in 1995. This meta-analysis found that an average intake of 47 g/day of soy protein decreased serum total cholesterol levels by an average of 9% and LDL cholesterol levels by an average of 13%.[22] Hypocholesterolemic effects were primarily noted in individuals with high baseline cholesterol levels.[22] A more recent meta-analysis of 33 studies published since 1995 confirmed the hypocholesterolemic effect of soy protein reported in the Anderson et al. publication.[23] Another meta-analysis of 30 studies in individuals with normal or mildly elevated cholesterol levels concluded that approximately 25 g/day of soy protein significantly lowers LDL cholesterol concentrations by about 6%.[24]

Yet, a recent science advisory from the Nutrition Committee of the American Heart Association concluded that earlier research indicating that soy protein consumption resulted in clinically important reductions in LDL cholesterol compared with other proteins has not been confirmed.[25] The consumption of isolated soy isoflavones (as supplements or extracts) does not appear to have favorable effects on serum lipid profiles.[26-29] In addition to possibly lowering cholesterol, many soy products may be beneficial for overall cardiovascular health due to their relatively high content of polyunsaturated fat, fiber, and phytosterols compared with animal products.[30]

Cancer

Beans, Peas, and Lentils

Although beans are rich in several compounds that could potentially reduce the risk of certain cancers, the results of epidemiological studies are too inconsistent to draw any firm conclusions regarding bean intake and cancer risk in general.[31,32]

Prostate cancer. There is limited evidence from observational studies that legume intake is inversely related to the risk of prostate cancer. In a 6-year prospective study of more than 14 000 Seventh Day Adventist men living in the United States, those with the highest intakes of legumes (beans, lentils, or split peas) had a significantly lower risk of prostate cancer.[33] More recently, a prospective study of more than 58 000 men in the Netherlands found that those with the highest intakes of legumes had a risk of prostate cancer that was 29% lower than those with the lowest intakes.[34] Similarly, in a case–control study of 1619 North American men diagnosed with prostate cancer and 1618 healthy men matched for age and ethnicity, those with the highest legume intakes had a risk of prostate cancer that was 38% lower than in those with the lowest intakes.[35] Excluding the intake of soy foods from the analysis did not weaken the inverse association between legume intake and prostate cancer, suggesting that soy was not the only legume that conferred protection against prostate cancer. A recent prospective study in a multi-ethnic cohort of 82 483 men examined the risk of prostate cancer in men who consumed legumes excluding soy products.

In this study, men who consumed the highest amount of non-soy legumes had a 10% lower risk of total prostate cancer and a 28% lower risk of nonlocalized or high-grade prostate cancer, compared with those who consumed the least amount of non-soy legumes.[36]

Soy

Prostate cancer. Although there is considerable scientific interest in the potential for soy products to prevent prostate cancer, evidence that higher intakes of soy foods can reduce the risk of prostate cancer in humans is limited. Only two out of six case–control studies found that higher intakes of soy products were associated with a significantly lower risk of prostate cancer. In the largest case–control study, North American men who consumed an average of at least 1.4 oz of soy foods daily were 38% less likely to have prostate cancer than men who did not consume soy foods.[35] A much smaller case–control study of Chinese men found that men who consumed at least 4 oz of soy foods daily were only half as likely to have prostate cancer as those who consumed less than 1 oz daily.[37] However, case–control studies conducted among North American,[38,39] Japanese,[40] and Taiwanese men[41] did not find that higher soy intakes were associated with significantly lower prostate cancer risk. A 6-year prospective cohort study of more than 12 000 Seventh Day Adventist men in the United States found that those who drank soy milk more than once daily had a risk of prostate cancer that was 70% lower than in those who never drank soy milk,[42] but a 23-year study of more than 5000 Japanese American men found no association between tofu consumption and prostate cancer risk.[43] More recently, a prospective study in a cohort of 43 509 Japanese men found that consumption of soy foods was associated with a decreased risk of localized prostate cancer in men who were older than 60 years.[44] Clinical trials are needed to determine whether consumption of soy foods affects the risk of prostate cancer.

Breast cancer. More than 25 epidemiological studies have assessed the relationship between soy food intake and the risk of breast cancer. A recent meta-analysis of prospective cohort studies and case–control studies reported differential effects based on the typical level of soy consumption.[45] In Asian populations, where soy intake is high, the authors found an inverse association between soy food intake and breast cancer; however, no association was observed in studies completed in Western populations, where soy food intake is much lower.[45] Age at exposure to soy foods may affect the subsequent risk of developing breast cancer. For instance, two case–control studies have found higher soy intake during adolescence may lower the risk of developing breast cancer later in life.[46,47] Soy intake later in life may not have as strong an effect on breast cancer as exposure during adolescence.[45]

Intake Recommendations

Substituting beans, peas, and lentils for foods that are high in saturated fat or refined carbohydrates is likely to help lower the risk of type 2 DM and cardiovascular disease. Soybeans and foods made from soybeans (soy foods) are excellent sources of protein. In fact, soy protein is complete protein, meaning it provides all of the essential amino acids in adequate amounts for human health.[2] Like beans, peas, and lentils, soy foods are also excellent substitutes for protein sources that are high in saturated fat like red meat or cheese. Although several health-related organizations recommend daily consumption of five to nine servings (2.5–4.5 cups) of fruits and vegetables daily (see Chapter 1), few make specific recommendations for legumes. In the 2010 Dietary Guidelines for Americans, an intake of 1.5 cups (three servings) of legumes (beans and peas, excluding green beans and green peas) weekly is recommended for people who consume 2000 kcal/day. A serving of legumes is equal to 0.5 cup of cooked dried beans or peas.[48]

Summary

- Foods from the legume family include beans, peas, lentils, peanuts, and soybeans.
- Legumes are excellent sources of protein, low-glycemic-index carbohydrates, essential micronutrients, and fiber.
- Substituting legumes for foods that are high in saturated fats or refined carbohydrates is likely to lower the risk of cardiovascular disease and type 2 diabetes mellitus.

- Although legumes are rich in several compounds that could potentially reduce the risk of certain cancers, the results of epidemiological studies are too inconsistent to draw any firm conclusions regarding legume intake and cancer risk in general.
- The 2010 Dietary Guidelines for Americans recommend a weekly intake of three servings (1.5 cups) of legumes, defined as beans and peas, not including green beans and green peas, for people who consume 2000 kcal/day.

References

1. Anderson JW, Smith BM, Washnock CS. Cardiovascular and renal benefits of dry bean and soybean intake. Am J Clin Nutr 1999; 70(3, Suppl):464S–474S
2. Messina MJ. Legumes and soybeans: overview of their nutritional profiles and health effects. Am J Clin Nutr 1999; 70(3, Suppl):439S–450S
3. Willett W, Manson J, Liu S. Glycemic index, glycemic load, and risk of type 2 diabetes. Am J Clin Nutr 2002;76(1):274S–280S
4. Salmerón J, Ascherio A, Rimm EB, et al. Dietary fiber, glycemic load, and risk of NIDDM in men. Diabetes Care 1997;20(4):545–550
5. Salmerón J, Manson JE, Stampfer MJ, Colditz GA, Wing AL, Willett WC. Dietary fiber, glycemic load, and risk of non-insulin-dependent diabetes mellitus in women. JAMA 1997;277(6):472–477
6. Patel AV, McCullough ML, Pavluck AL, Jacobs EJ, Thun MJ, Calle EE. Glycemic load, glycemic index, and carbohydrate intake in relation to pancreatic cancer risk in a large US cohort. Cancer Causes Control 2007;18(3):287–294
7. Krishnan S, Rosenberg L, Singer M, et al. Glycemic index, glycemic load, and cereal fiber intake and risk of type 2 diabetes in US black women. Arch Intern Med 2007;167(21):2304–2309
8. Ludwig DS. Dietary glycemic index and the regulation of body weight. Lipids 2003;38(2):117–121
9. Bornet FR, Jardy-Gennetier AE, Jacquet N, Stowell J. Glycaemic response to foods: impact on satiety and long-term weight regulation. Appetite 2007;49(3):535–553
10. Bouché C, Rizkalla SW, Luo J, et al. Five-week, low-glycemic index diet decreases total fat mass and improves plasma lipid profile in moderately overweight nondiabetic men. Diabetes Care 2002;25(5):822–828
11. Spieth LE, Harnish JD, Lenders CM, et al. A low-glycemic index diet in the treatment of pediatric obesity. Arch Pediatr Adolesc Med 2000;154(9):947–951
12. Slabber M, Barnard HC, Kuyl JM, Dannhauser A, Schall R. Effects of a low-insulin-response, energy-restricted diet on weight loss and plasma insulin concentrations in hyperinsulinemic obese females. Am J Clin Nutr 1994;60(1):48–53
13. Thomas DE, Elliott EJ, Baur L. Low glycaemic index or low glycaemic load diets for overweight and obesity. Cochrane Database Syst Rev 2007; (3):CD005105
14. Feskens EJ, Bowles CH, Kromhout D. Carbohydrate intake and body mass index in relation to the risk of glucose intolerance in an elderly population. Am J Clin Nutr 1991;54(1):136–140
15. Villegas R, Gao YT, Yang G, et al. Legume and soy food intake and the incidence of type 2 diabetes in the Shanghai Women's Health Study. Am J Clin Nutr 2008;87(1):162–167
16. Nöthlings U, Schulze MB, Weikert C, et al. Intake of vegetables, legumes, and fruit, and risk for all-cause, cardiovascular, and cancer mortality in a European diabetic population. J Nutr 2008;138(4):775–781
17. Bazzano LA, He J, Ogden LG, et al. Legume consumption and risk of coronary heart disease in US men and women: NHANES I Epidemiologic Follow-up Study. Arch Intern Med 2001;161(21):2573–2578
18. Hu FB, Rimm EB, Stampfer MJ, Ascherio A, Spiegelman D, Willett WC. Prospective study of major dietary patterns and risk of coronary heart disease in men. Am J Clin Nutr 2000;72(4):912–921
19. Fung TT, Willett WC, Stampfer MJ, Manson JE, Hu FB. Dietary patterns and the risk of coronary heart disease in women. Arch Intern Med 2001;161(15):1857–1862
20. Anderson JW, Major AW. Pulses and lipaemia, short-and long-term effect: potential in the prevention of cardiovascular disease. Br J Nutr 2002;88(Suppl 3): S263–S271
21. US Food and Drug Administration. Final Rule: Food Labeling: Health Claims; Soy Protein and Coronary Heart Disease. Fed Register 1999;64(206):57699–57733. Available at: http://www.fda.gov/Food/LabelingNutrition/LabelClaims/HealthClaimsMeetingSignificantScientificAgreementSSA/ucm074740.htm. Accessed May 1, 2012
22. Anderson JW, Johnstone BM, Cook-Newell ME. Meta-analysis of the effects of soy protein intake on serum lipids. N Engl J Med 1995;333(5):276–282
23. Sirtori CR, Eberini I, Arnoldi A. Hypocholesterolaemic effects of soya proteins: results of recent studies are predictable from the Anderson meta-analysis data. Br J Nutr 2007;97(5):816–822
24. Harland JI, Haffner TA. Systematic review, meta-analysis and regression of randomised controlled trials reporting an association between an intake of circa 25 g soya protein per day and blood cholesterol. Atherosclerosis 2008;200(1):13–27
25. Sacks FM, Lichtenstein A, Van Horn L, Harris W, Kris-Etherton P, Winston M; American Heart Association Nutrition Committee. Soy protein, isoflavones, and cardiovascular health: an American Heart Association Science Advisory for professionals from the Nutrition Committee. Circulation 2006;113(7):1034–1044
26. Lichtenstein AH, Jalbert SM, Adlercreutz H, et al. Lipoprotein response to diets high in soy or animal protein with and without isoflavones in moderately hypercholesterolemic subjects. Arterioscler Thromb Vasc Biol 2002;22(11):1852–1858
27. Nikander E, Tiitinen A, Laitinen K, Tikkanen M, Ylikorkala O. Effects of isolated isoflavonoids on lipids, lipoproteins, insulin sensitivity, and ghrelin in postmenopausal women. J Clin Endocrinol Metab 2004;89(7):3567–3572
28. Weggemans RM, Trautwein EA. Relation between soy-associated isoflavones and LDL and HDL cholesterol concentrations in humans: a meta-analysis. Eur J Clin Nutr 2003;57(8):940–946
29. Dewell A, Hollenbeck PL, Hollenbeck CB. Clinical review: a critical evaluation of the role of soy protein and isoflavone supplementation in the control of plasma cholesterol concentrations. J Clin Endocrinol Metab 2006;91(3):772–780

30. Kendall CW, Jenkins DJ. A dietary portfolio: maximal reduction of low-density lipoprotein cholesterol with diet. Curr Atheroscler Rep 2004;6(6):492–498

31. Mathers JC. Pulses and carcinogenesis: potential for the prevention of colon, breast and other cancers. Br J Nutr 2002;88(Suppl 3):S273–S279

32. World Cancer Research Fund. Food, Nutrition, and the Prevention of Cancer: A Global Perspective. Washington, DC: American Institute for Cancer Research; 1997

33. Mills PK, Beeson WL, Phillips RL, Fraser GE. Cohort study of diet, lifestyle, and prostate cancer in Adventist men. Cancer 1989;64(3):598–604

34. Schuurman AG, Goldbohm RA, Dorant E, van den Brandt PA. Vegetable and fruit consumption and prostate cancer risk: a cohort study in The Netherlands. Cancer Epidemiol Biomarkers Prev 1998;7(8):673–680

35. Kolonel LN, Hankin JH, Whittemore AS, et al. Vegetables, fruits, legumes and prostate cancer: a multiethnic case-control study. Cancer Epidemiol Biomarkers Prev 2000;9(8):795–804

36. Park SY, Murphy SP, Wilkens LR, Henderson BE, Kolonel LN; Multiethnic Cohort Study. Legume and isoflavone intake and prostate cancer risk: The Multiethnic Cohort Study. Int J Cancer 2008;123(4):927–932

37. Lee MM, Gomez SL, Chang JS, Wey M, Wang RT, Hsing AW. Soy and isoflavone consumption in relation to prostate cancer risk in China. Cancer Epidemiol Biomarkers Prev 2003;12(7):665–668

38. Strom SS, Yamamura Y, Duphorne CM, et al. Phytoestrogen intake and prostate cancer: a case-control study using a new database. Nutr Cancer 1999;33(1):20–25

39. Villeneuve PJ, Johnson KC, Kreiger N, Mao Y; The Canadian Cancer Registries Epidemiology Research Group. Risk factors for prostate cancer: results from the Canadian National Enhanced Cancer Surveillance System. Cancer Causes Control 1999;10(5):355–367

40. Oishi K, Okada K, Yoshida O, et al. A case-control study of prostatic cancer with reference to dietary habits. Prostate 1988;12(2):179–190

41. Sung JF, Lin RS, Pu YS, Chen YC, Chang HC, Lai MK. Risk factors for prostate carcinoma in Taiwan: a case-control study in a Chinese population. Cancer 1999; 86(3):484–491

42. Jacobsen BK, Knutsen SF, Fraser GE. Does high soy milk intake reduce prostate cancer incidence? The Adventist Health Study (United States). Cancer Causes Control 1998;9(6):553–557

43. Nomura AM, Hankin JH, Lee J, Stemmermann GN. Cohort study of tofu intake and prostate cancer: no apparent association. Cancer Epidemiol Biomarkers Prev 2004;13(12):2277–2279

44. Kurahashi N, Iwasaki M, Sasazuki S, Otani T, Inoue M, Tsugane S; Japan Public Health Center-Based Prospective Study Group. Soy product and isoflavone consumption in relation to prostate cancer in Japanese men. Cancer Epidemiol Biomarkers Prev 2007;16(3):538–545

45. Wu AH, Yu MC, Tseng CC, Pike MC. Epidemiology of soy exposures and breast cancer risk. Br J Cancer 2008;98(1):9–14

46. Shu XO, Jin F, Dai Q, et al. Soyfood intake during adolescence and subsequent risk of breast cancer among Chinese women. Cancer Epidemiol Biomarkers Prev 2001;10(5):483–488

47. Wu AH, Wan P, Hankin J, Tseng CC, Yu MC, Pike MC. Adolescent and adult soy intake and risk of breast cancer in Asian-Americans. Carcinogenesis 2002; 23(9):1491–1496

48. US Department of Health and Human Services, US Department of Agriculture. Dietary Guidelines for Americans. 2010. Available at: http://health.gov/dietaryguidelines/2010.asp. Accessed May 1, 2012

4 Nuts

In the not too distant past, nuts were considered unhealthy because of their relatively high fat content. In contrast, recent research suggests that regular nut consumption is an important part of a healthful diet.[1] Although the fat content of nuts is relatively high (14–19 g/oz or 49–67%), most of the fats in nuts are the healthier, monounsaturated and polyunsaturated fats (see **Table 4.1**)[2]. The term "nuts" includes almonds, Brazil nuts, cashews, hazelnuts, macadamia nuts, pecans, pistachios, walnuts, and peanuts. Despite their name, peanuts are actually legumes like peas and beans. However, they are nutritionally similar to tree nuts and have some of the same beneficial properties.

Disease Prevention

Cardiovascular Disease

Coronary Heart Disease

In large prospective cohort studies, regular nut consumption has been consistently associated with significant reductions in the risk of coronary heart disease (CHD).[3] One of the first studies to observe a protective effect of nut consumption was the Adventist Health Study, which followed more than 30 000 Seventh Day Adventists over 12 years.[4] In general, the dietary and lifestyle habits of Seventh Day Adventists are closer to those recommended for cardiovascular disease prevention than those of average Americans. Few of those who participated in the Adventist Health Study smoked, and most consumed a diet lower in saturated fat than the average American. In this healthy group, those who consumed nuts at least five times weekly had a 48% lower risk of death from CHD and a 51% lower risk of a nonfatal myocardial infarction (MI) compared with those who consumed nuts less than once weekly.[4] In Seventh Day Adventists who were older than 83 years of age, those who ate nuts at least five times weekly had a risk of death from CHD that was 39% lower than those who consumed nuts less than once weekly.[5] A smaller prospective study of more than 3 000 black men and women reported similar results.[6] Those who consumed nuts at least five times weekly had a risk of death from CHD that was 44% lower than those who consumed nuts less than once weekly.[6]

The cardioprotective effects of nuts are not limited to Seventh Day Adventists. In a 14-year study of more than 86 000 women participating

Table 4.1 Energy, fat, phytosterol, and fiber content in a one-ounce serving of selected nuts

Nut (1 oz)	Energy (kcal)	Total Fat (g)	Monounsaturated Fat (g)	Polyunsaturated Fat (g)	Phytosterols (mg)	Fiber (g)
Almonds	163	14.0	8.8	3.4	39	3.5
Brazil nuts	186	18.8	7.0	5.8	N/A[a]	2.1
Cashews	163	13.1	7.7	2.2	45	0.9
Hazelnuts	178	17.2	12.9	2.2	27	2.7
Macadamia nuts	204	21.5	16.7	0.4	33	2.4
Peanuts (legume)	161	14.0	6.9	4.4	62	2.4
Peanut butter, smooth (2 tbsp)	188	16.1	7.6	4.4	33	1.9
Pecans	196	20.4	11.6	6.1	29	2.7
Pine nuts (pignoli)	191	19.4	5.3	9.7	40	1.0
Pistachio nuts	158	12.6	6.6	3.8	61	2.9
Walnuts, black	175	16.7	4.3	9.9	31	1.9

[a] Not available.

in the Nurses' Health Study (NHS), those who consumed more than 5 oz of nuts weekly had a risk of CHD that was 35% lower than those who ate less than 1 oz of nuts monthly.[7] Similar decreases were observed for the risk of nonfatal MI and death from CHD. More recently, a 17-year study of more than 21 000 male physicians found that those who consumed nuts at least twice weekly had a risk of sudden cardiac death that was 53% lower than those who rarely or never consumed nuts, although there was no significant decrease in the risk of nonfatal MI or non-sudden CHD death.[8] A follow-up analysis in this cohort of male physicians found that nut consumption was not associated with incident heart failure.[9] The Iowa Women's Health Study, which followed more than 30 000 postmenopausal women for 12 years, is the only published prospective study that did not observe a significant inverse association between nut consumption and CHD mortality, although a slight but significant decrease in all-cause mortality was observed in those who consumed nuts twice weekly.[10] Overall, the results of most prospective cohort studies suggest that regular nut consumption is associated with a substantial decrease in the risk of death related to CHD. In fact, a recent pooled analysis of four of the US epidemiological studies mentioned above found those with the highest intake of nuts (around five times per week) had a 35% lower risk of CHD.[11]

Results of controlled clinical trials indicate that at least part of the cardioprotective effect of nuts is derived from beneficial effects on serum total and low-density lipoprotein (LDL) cholesterol concentrations.[3] At least 18 controlled clinical trials have found that adding nuts to a diet that is low in saturated fat results in significantly reductions in serum total cholesterol and LDL cholesterol concentrations in people with normal or elevated serum cholesterol. These effects have been observed for almonds,[12-15] hazelnuts,[16] macadamia nuts,[17-19] peanuts,[20,21] pecans,[22] pistachio nuts,[23,24] and walnuts.[25-30] More recently, a cross-sectional study found that frequent nut and seed consumption was associated with lower serum levels of inflammatory biomarkers in a multi-ethnic population.[31] Although the evidence is circumstantial, these findings suggest that compounds in nuts may lower the risk of cardiovascular disease by decreasing inflammation.

Cardioprotective Compounds in Nuts

Substituting dietary saturated fats with polyunsaturated and monounsaturated fats like those found in nuts can decrease serum total and LDL cholesterol concentrations.[3] However, in some clinical trials, the cholesterol-lowering effect of nut consumption was greater than would be predicted from the polyunsaturated and monounsaturated fat content of the nuts, suggesting there may be other protective factors in nuts.[32] Other bioactive compounds in nuts that may contribute to their cholesterol-lowering effects include fiber (Chapter 16) and phytosterols (Chapter 18).[33] See Table 4.1 for the unsaturated fat, fiber, and phytosterol content of selected nuts. Walnuts are especially rich in α-linolenic acid, an omega-3 fatty acid with several cardioprotective effects, including the prevention of cardiac arrhythmias that may lead to sudden cardiac death (Chapter 20). Other nutrients that may contribute to the cardioprotective effects of nuts include folate, vitamin E, and potassium.[3,33-35] The US Food and Drug Administration has acknowledged the emerging evidence for a relationship between nut consumption and cardiovascular disease risk, by approving the following qualified health claim for nuts[36]: "Scientific evidence suggests but does not prove that eating 1.5 oz/day of most nuts as part of a diet low in saturated fat and cholesterol may reduce the risk of heart disease."

Type 2 Diabetes Mellitus

Recent results from the NHS suggest that nut and peanut butter consumption may be inversely associated with the risk of type 2 diabetes mellitus (DM) in women.[37] In this cohort of more than 86 000 women followed over 16 years, those who consumed an ounce of nuts at least five times weekly had a risk of developing type 2 DM that was 27% lower than in those who rarely or never consumed nuts. Similarly those who consumed peanut butter at least five times weekly had a risk of developing type 2 DM that was 21% lower than in those who rarely or never consumed peanut butter. While these findings require confirmation in other studies, they provide additional evidence that nuts can be a component of a healthful diet. Compounds in nuts that could contribute to the observed decrease in type 2 DM include unsaturated fats, fiber, and magnesium.

Body Weight

A major concern is that increased consumption of nuts may cause weight gain and obesity. However, several cross-sectional analyses of large cohort studies, including the Adventist Health Study[5] and the NHS,[7] have shown that individuals who consume nuts regularly tend to weigh less than those who rarely consume them. Recently, a 28-month prospective study conducted in Spain found that participants who consumed higher amount of nuts had lower risk of weight gain than those who rarely ate nuts.[38] A similar association was observed in the NHS II.[39] These epidemiologic data indicate that in free-living subjects, higher nut consumption does not cause greater weight gain; rather, incorporating nuts into diets may be beneficial for weight control. It is possible that higher amounts of protein and fiber in nuts enhance satiety and suppress hunger.

Safety

Nut Allergies

Allergies to peanuts and tree nuts (almonds, cashews, hazelnuts, pecans, pistachios, and walnuts) are among the most common food allergies, affecting at least 1% of the US population.[40] Although all food allergies have the potential to induce severe reactions, peanuts and tree nuts are among the foods most commonly associated with anaphylaxis, a life-threatening allergic reaction.[41] People with severe peanut or tree nut allergies need to take special precautions to avoid inadvertently consuming peanuts or tree nuts, by checking labels and avoiding unlabeled snacks, candies, and desserts.

Adverse Effects

Brazil nuts grown in areas of Brazil with selenium-rich soil may provide more than 100 µg of selenium in one nut, while those grown in selenium-poor soil may provide 10 times less.[42]

Intake Recommendations

Regular nut consumption, equivalent to an ounce of nuts five times weekly, has been consistently associated with significant reductions in CHD risk in epidemiological studies. Consuming 1–2 oz of nuts daily as part of a diet that is low in saturated fat has been found to lower serum total and LDL cholesterol in several controlled clinical trials. Since an ounce of most nuts provides at least 669 kJ (160 kcal), simply adding an ounce of nuts daily to one's habitual diet without eliminating other foods may result in weight gain. Substituting unsalted nuts for other less healthful snacks, or for meat in main dishes, are two ways to make nuts part of a healthful diet.

Summary

- Nuts are good sources of fiber, phytosterols, and unsaturated fat.
- The results of most prospective cohort studies suggest that regular nut consumption (equivalent to 1 oz at least five times weekly) is associated with a significantly lower risk of cardiovascular disease.
- One prospective cohort study has found that regular nut consumption is associated with significantly lower risk of developing type 2 diabetes.
- Most prospective studies have shown that people who consume nuts regularly weigh less than those who rarely consume nuts. Nonetheless, since an ounce of most nuts provides approximately 669 kJ (160 kcal), substituting nuts for other less healthful snacks is a good strategy for avoiding weight gain when increasing nut intake.

References

1. Hu FB, Stampfer MJ. Nut consumption and risk of coronary heart disease: a review of epidemiologic evidence. Curr Atheroscler Rep 1999;1(3):204–209
2. Kris-Etherton PM, Yu-Poth S, Sabaté J, Ratcliffe HE, Zhao G, Etherton TD. Nuts and their bioactive constituents: effects on serum lipids and other factors that affect disease risk. Am J Clin Nutr 1999; 70(3, Suppl):504S–511S
3. Kris-Etherton PM, Zhao G, Binkoski AE, Coval SM, Etherton TD. The effects of nuts on coronary heart disease risk. Nutr Rev 2001;59(4):103–111
4. Fraser GE, Sabaté J, Beeson WL, Strahan TM. A possible protective effect of nut consumption on risk of coronary heart disease. The Adventist Health Study. Arch Intern Med 1992;152(7):1416–1424
5. Fraser GE, Shavlik DJ. Risk factors for all-cause and coronary heart disease mortality in the oldest-old. The Adventist Health Study. Arch Intern Med 1997;157(19):2249–2258
6. Fraser GE, Sumbureru D, Pribis P, Neil RL, Frankson MA. Association among health habits, risk factors, and all-cause mortality in a black California population. Epidemiology 1997;8(2):168–174
7. Hu FB, Stampfer MJ, Manson JE, et al. Frequent nut consumption and risk of coronary heart disease in women: prospective cohort study. BMJ 1998;317 (7169):1341–1345
8. Albert CM, Gaziano JM, Willett WC, Manson JE. Nut consumption and decreased risk of sudden cardiac death in the Physicians' Health Study. Arch Intern Med 2002;162(12):1382–1387
9. Djoussé L, Rudich T, Gaziano JM. Nut consumption and risk of heart failure in the Physicians' Health Study I. Am J Clin Nutr 2008;88(4):930–933
10. Ellsworth JL, Kushi LH, Folsom AR. Frequent nut intake and risk of death from coronary heart disease and all causes in postmenopausal women: the Iowa Women's Health Study. Nutr Metab Cardiovasc Dis 2001;11(6):372–377
11. Kris-Etherton PM, Hu FB, Ros E, Sabaté J. The role of tree nuts and peanuts in the prevention of coronary heart disease: multiple potential mechanisms. J Nutr 2008;138(9):1746S–1751S
12. Hyson DA, Schneeman BO, Davis PA. Almonds and almond oil have similar effects on plasma lipids and LDL oxidation in healthy men and women. J Nutr 2002;132(4):703–707
13. Jenkins DJ, Kendall CW, Marchie A, et al. Dose response of almonds on coronary heart disease risk factors: blood lipids, oxidized low-density lipoproteins, lipoprotein(a), homocysteine, and pulmonary nitric oxide: a randomized, controlled, crossover trial. Circulation 2002;106(11):1327–1332
14. Sabaté J, Haddad E, Tanzman JS, Jambazian P, Rajaram S. Serum lipid response to the graduated enrichment of a Step I diet with almonds: a randomized feeding trial. Am J Clin Nutr 2003;77(6):1379–1384
15. Spiller GA, Jenkins DA, Bosello O, Gates JE, Cragen LN, Bruce B. Nuts and plasma lipids: an almond-based diet lowers LDL-C while preserving HDL-C. J Am Coll Nutr 1998;17(3):285–290
16. Durak I, Köksal I, Kaçmaz M, Büyükkoçak S, Cimen BM, Oztürk HS. Hazelnut supplementation enhances plasma antioxidant potential and lowers plasma cholesterol levels. Clin Chim Acta 1999;284(1):113–115
17. Curb JD, Wergowske G, Dobbs JC, Abbott RD, Huang B. Serum lipid effects of a high-monounsaturated fat diet based on macadamia nuts. Arch Intern Med 2000;160(8):1154–1158
18. Garg ML, Blake RJ, Wills RB. Macadamia nut consumption lowers plasma total and LDL cholesterol levels in hypercholesterolemic men. J Nutr 2003; 133(4):1060–1063
19. Griel AE, Cao Y, Bagshaw DD, Cifelli AM, Holub B, Kris-Etherton PM. A macadamia nut-rich diet reduces total and LDL-cholesterol in mildly hypercholesterolemic men and women. J Nutr 2008;138(4):761–767
20. Kris-Etherton PM, Pearson TA, Wan Y, et al. High-monounsaturated fatty acid diets lower both plasma cholesterol and triacylglycerol concentrations. Am J Clin Nutr 1999;70(6):1009–1015
21. O'Byrne DJ, Knauft DA, Shireman RB. Low fat-monounsaturated rich diets containing high-oleic peanuts improve serum lipoprotein profiles. Lipids 1997; 32(7):687–695
22. Morgan WA, Clayshulte BJ. Pecans lower low-density lipoprotein cholesterol in people with normal lipid levels. J Am Diet Assoc 2000;100(3):312–318
23. Edwards K, Kwaw I, Matud J, Kurtz I. Effect of pistachio nuts on serum lipid levels in patients with moderate hypercholesterolemia. J Am Coll Nutr 1999; 18(3):229–232
24. Sheridan MJ, Cooper JN, Erario M, Cheifetz CE. Pistachio nut consumption and serum lipid levels. J Am Coll Nutr 2007;26(2):141–148
25. Abbey M, Noakes M, Belling GB, Nestel PJ. Partial replacement of saturated fatty acids with almonds or walnuts lowers total plasma cholesterol and low-density-lipoprotein cholesterol. Am J Clin Nutr 1994;59(5):995–999
26. Almario RU, Vonghavaravat V, Wong R, Kasim-Karakas SE. Effects of walnut consumption on plasma fatty acids and lipoproteins in combined hyperlipidemia. Am J Clin Nutr 2001;74(1):72–79
27. Chisholm A, Mann J, Skeaff M, et al. A diet rich in walnuts favourably influences plasma fatty acid profile in moderately hyperlipidaemic subjects. Eur J Clin Nutr 1998;52(1):12–16
28. Morgan JM, Horton K, Reese D, Carey C, Walker K, Capuzzi DM. Effects of walnut consumption as part of a low-fat, low-cholesterol diet on serum cardiovascular risk factors. Int J Vitam Nutr Res 2002;72(5):341–347
29. Sabaté J, Fraser GE, Burke K, Knutsen SF, Bennett H, Lindsted KD. Effects of walnuts on serum lipid levels and blood pressure in normal men. N Engl J Med 1993;328(9):603–607
30. Zambón D, Sabaté J, Muñoz S, et al. Substituting walnuts for monounsaturated fat improves the serum lipid profile of hypercholesterolemic men and women. A randomized crossover trial. Ann Intern Med 2000;132(7):538–546
31. Jiang R, Jacobs DR Jr, Mayer-Davis E, et al. Nut and seed consumption and inflammatory markers in the multi-ethnic study of atherosclerosis. Am J Epidemiol 2006;163(3):222–231
32. Coulston AM. Do Nuts Have a Place in a Healthful Diet? Nutr Today 2003;38(3):95–99
33. Segura R, Javierre C, Lizarraga MA, Ros E. Other relevant components of nuts: phytosterols, folate and minerals. Br J Nutr 2006;96(Suppl 2):S36–S44
34. Willett WC. Eat, Drink, and be Healthy: The Harvard Medical School Guide to Healthy Eating. New York: Simon & Schuster; 2001.

35. Coates AM, Howe PR. Edible nuts and metabolic health. Curr Opin Lipidol 2007;18(1):25–30

36. US Food and Drug Administration, Center for Food Safety and Nutrition. Summary of Qualified Health Claims Subject to Enforcement Discretion. 2003. Available at: http://www.fda.gov/Food/LabelingNutrition/LabelClaims/QualifiedHealthClaims/ucm073992.htm#nuts. Accessed May 1, 2012

37. Jiang R, Manson JE, Stampfer MJ, Liu S, Willett WC, Hu FB. Nut and peanut butter consumption and risk of type 2 diabetes in women. JAMA 2002;288(20):2554–2560

38. Bes-Rastrollo M, Sabaté J, Gómez-Gracia E, Alonso A, Martínez JA, Martínez-González MA. Nut consumption and weight gain in a Mediterranean cohort: The SUN study. Obesity (Silver Spring) 2007;15(1):107–116

39. Bes-Rastrollo M, Wedick NM, Martinez-Gonzalez MA, Li TY, Sampson L, Hu FB. Prospective study of nut consumption, long-term weight change, and obesity risk in women. Am J Clin Nutr 2009;89(6):1913–1919

40. Sicherer SH, Muñoz-Furlong A, Burks AW, Sampson HA. Prevalence of peanut and tree nut allergy in the US determined by a random digit dial telephone survey. J Allergy Clin Immunol 1999;103(4):559–562

41. Al-Muhsen S, Clarke AE, Kagan RS. Peanut allergy: an overview. CMAJ 2003;168(10):1279–1285

42. Chang JC, Gutenmann WH, Reid CM, Lisk DJ. Selenium content of Brazil nuts from two geographic locations in Brazil. Chemosphere 1995;30(4):801–802

5 Whole Grains

Grains are seeds of plants belonging to the grass family. Species that produce edible grains include wheat, rice, maize (corn), barley, oats, and rye.[1] An intact grain has an outer layer of bran, a carbohydrate-rich middle layer called the *endosperm*, and an inner germ layer. Although not always intact, whole-grain foods contain the entire grain, including the bran, the endosperm, and the germ. Whole grains are rich in potentially beneficial compounds, including vitamins, minerals, and phytochemicals, such as lignans (Chapter 15), phytosterols (Chapter 18), and fiber (Chapter 16). Most of these compounds are located in the bran or the germ of the grain, both of which are lost during the refining process, leaving only the starchy endosperm.[2] Compared with diets that are high in refined grains, diets rich in whole grains are associated with reduced risks of several chronic diseases. The health benefits of whole grains are not entirely explained by the individual contributions of the nutrients and phytochemicals they contain. Whole grains represent a unique package of energy, micronutrients, and phytochemicals that work synergistically to promote health and prevent disease.

Disease Prevention

Type 2 Diabetes Mellitus

At least seven large prospective studies have found that higher whole-grain intakes are associated with significant reductions in the risk of developing type 2 diabetes mellitus (DM) over time.[3–8] In the studies conducted in the United States, those who consumed an average of approximately three daily servings of whole-grain foods had a risk of type 2 DM that was 21%–30% lower than those who rarely or never consumed whole grains.[3–5] In Finland, the quarter of the population with the highest whole-grain intake had a risk of type 2 DM that was 35% lower than the quarter with the lowest intakes.[6] A recent systematic review of six prospective cohort studies, including more than 286 000 participants, found that increasing daily intake of whole grains by two servings resulted in a 21% reduction in risk for type 2 DM.[7] Insulin resistance is a condition of decreased insulin sensitivity that increases the risk of developing type 2 DM. In observational studies, higher whole-grain intakes have been associated with decreased insulin resistance[9] and increased insulin sensitivity[10] in people who do not have type 2 DM. In a controlled clinical trial that compared the effects of a diet rich in whole grains with a diet high in refined grains in overweight and obese adults, several clinical measures of insulin resistance were significantly lower after 6 weeks on the whole-grain diet compared with the refined-grain diet.[11] Well-designed, long-term randomized controlled trials are necessary to determine whether whole grains are protective against the development of type 2 DM.[12]

The refining process makes the carbohydrate in the endosperm of the grain easier to digest. Immediately after a meal, carbohydrate from refined grains elicits a higher and more rapid elevation in blood glucose, as well as greater demand for insulin.[13] Over time, elevated blood glucose levels and compensatory increases in insulin secretion may lead to the development of type 2 diabetes. The glycemic index is a way of ranking the glucose-raising potential of carbohydrate in different foods. Foods made from whole grains generally have lower glycemic-index values than foods made from refined grains.[14] Substituting whole-grain foods for refined grain foods decreases dietary glycemic load, which has been associated with decreased risk of type 2 DM[15,16] and improved control of blood glucose levels in people who have diabetes.[17] Thus, substituting low-glycemic-index, whole-grain foods for high-glycemic-index, refined-grain foods may substantially decrease the risk of developing type 2 diabetes. For more information on glycemic index and glycemic load, see Appendix 1.

Cardiovascular Disease

At least seven large prospective cohort studies have found that higher intakes of whole grains are associated with significant reductions in coronary heart disease (CHD) risk when compared with lower intakes.[18–24] In general, those with the highest intakes of whole grains (approx. three servings daily) had a risk of CHD that was 20%–30% lower than in those with the lowest intakes, even after adjusting the risk estimates for other heart disease risk factors. Whole-grain foods consumed in these studies included dark bread, whole-grain breakfast cereals, popcorn, cooked oatmeal, brown rice, bran, barley, and other grains like bulgar and kasha. A study that followed more than 85 000 male physicians for 5 years found that those who consumed at least one serving of whole-grain breakfast cereal daily had a 20% lower risk of death from cardiovascular disease than those who rarely or never consumed whole-grain cereal.[23] A recent study in a multiethnic cohort found that whole-grain intake was inversely associated with intimal medial thickness of the common carotid artery, a marker for atherosclerosis.[25] Higher intakes of whole grains have also been associated with a decreased risk of ischemic stroke (a stroke caused by the obstruction of a blood vessel that supplies the brain). A study that followed more than 75 000 women participating in the Nurses' Health Study for 12 years found that women who consumed an average of almost three servings of whole grains daily had a risk of ischemic stroke that was more than 30% lower than in women who rarely consumed whole grains.[26] Moreover, a recent meta-analysis of seven prospective cohort studies found that those with higher whole-grain intakes (average of 2.5 servings daily) had a 21% lower risk of cardiovascular disease events when compared with those with much lower whole-grain intakes (average of 0.2 servings daily).[27]

There are several possible explanations for the cardioprotective effects associated with higher intakes of whole grains and lower intakes of refined grains. Compared with refined grains, whole grains are richer in nutrients associated with cardiovascular risk reduction, including folate, magnesium, and potassium. Although wheat fiber has not been found to lower serum cholesterol levels, numerous clinical studies have demonstrated that increasing oat fiber intake results in modest reductions in total and low-density lipoprotein (LDL) cholesterol.[1] In light of these findings, the US Food and Drug Administration (FDA) approved the following health claim: "Diets low in saturated fat and cholesterol that provide 3 g or more per day of soluble fiber from oat bran, rolled oats (oatmeal), or whole oat flour may reduce the risk of heart disease."[28] Barley intake can also lower serum total and LDL cholesterol,[29,30] and the FDA health claim was recently amended to include soluble fiber from barley.[31] Whole grains are also sources of phytosterols, compounds that decrease serum cholesterol by interfering with the intestinal absorption of cholesterol.[32] The relatively low glycemic-index values of whole grains compared with refined grains may also play a role in decreasing the risk of heart disease. Substituting whole-grain products for refined-grain products in one's diet decreases dietary glycemic load. Recent results from large prospective studies suggest that low-glycemic-load diets are associated with lower coronary heart disease risk than high-glycemic-load diets;[33] for more information on glycemic index and glycemic load, see Appendix 1. Further, whole-grain intake was recently associated with a reduced risk of hypertension, a risk factor for cardiovascular disease.[34,35]

Cancer

Although the protective effects of whole grains against various types of cancer are not as well established as those against diabetes and cardiovascular disease, numerous case–control studies have found inverse associations between various measures of whole-grain intake and cancer risk.[36–38] A meta-analysis of 40 case–control studies examining 20 different types of cancer found that people with higher whole-grain intakes had an overall risk of cancer that was 34% lower than in those with lower whole-grain intakes.[36] These studies generally used some measure of whole-grain bread intake to assess intake of whole grains, although a series of Italian case–control studies also assessed the intake of whole-grain pasta.[37] Higher intakes of whole grains were most consistently associated with decreased risk of gastrointestinal tract cancers, including cancers of the mouth, throat, stomach, colon, and rectum. A prospective cohort study that followed more than 61 000 Swedish women

Table 5.1 Examples of one serving of whole-grain food

Whole-Grain Food	Amount in One Serving
Whole-grain bread	1 slice
Whole-grain English muffin, bagel, or bun	1 half
Whole-grain cereal, ready to eat	1 oz
Oatmeal, brown rice, or whole-wheat pasta, cooked	½ cup
Whole-wheat tortilla	1 tortilla, (7 in [17.7 cm] diameter)
Whole-grain crackers	5–6 crackers
Popped popcorn	3 cups

for 15 years found that those who consumed more than 4.5 servings of whole grains daily had a risk of colon cancer that was 35% lower than those who consumed less than 1.5 servings of whole grains daily.[39] A much larger prospective study in a cohort of 291 988 men and 197 623 women found that whole-grain intake was inversely associated with risk of colorectal cancer, especially rectal cancer.[40] Specifically, compared with those in the lowest quintile of whole-grain intake, those in the highest quintile had a 21% and 36% lower risk of developing colorectal or rectal cancer, respectively.[40] Intake of whole-grain foods was related to a 41% lower risk for cancer of the small intestine in this cohort, but the trend did not reach statistical significance.[41] However, not all cohort studies have reported that whole grains are protective against intestinal cancers.[42,43]

In contrast to refined-grain products, whole grains are rich in numerous compounds that may be protective against cancer, particularly cancers of the gastrointestinal tract.[44] Higher fiber intakes are known to speed up the passage of stool through the colon, allowing less time for potentially carcinogenic compounds to stay in contact with cells that line the inner surface of the colon. Lignans in whole grains are phytoestrogens, which may affect the development of hormone-dependent cancers. Phenolic compounds in whole grains may modify signal-transduction pathways that promote the development of cancer or bind potentially damaging free metal ions in the gastrointestinal tract.

Intestinal Health

Diets rich in whole grains and fiber help prevent constipation by softening and adding bulk to stool and by speeding its passage through the colon.[45] Such diets are also associated with decreased risk of diverticulosis, a condition characterized by the formation of small pouches (diverticula) in the colon. Although most people with diverticulosis experience no symptoms, around 15%–20% may develop pain or inflammation, known as *diverticulitis*. Diverticulitis was virtually unheard of before the practice of milling (refining) flour began in industrialized countries, and the role of a low-fiber diet in the development of diverticular disease is well established.[46] Although high-fiber diets are recommended for people with constipation and diverticulosis, people with diverticulosis are sometimes advised to avoid eating small seeds and husks, to prevent them from becoming lodged in diverticula and causing diverticulitis. However, it should be noted that no study has ever shown that avoiding seeds or popcorn reduces the risk of diverticulitis in an individual with diverticulosis.[46]

Intake Recommendations

Whole-grain intakes approaching three servings daily are associated with significant reductions in chronic disease risk in populations with relatively low whole-grain intakes. One of the objectives of the US Department of Health and Human Services' disease-prevention agenda, Healthy People 2010, was to increase the proportion of people in the United States of America who consume three servings of whole grains daily. However, most Americans consume less than one serving daily.[2] **Table 5.1** provides some examples of a serving of whole grains. The 2010 Dietary Guidelines for Americans recommend consuming at least half of total grains as whole grains.[47] In view of the potential health benefits of increasing whole-grain intake, three daily servings of whole-grain foods should be seen as a minimum, and whole-grain foods should be substituted for refined carbohydrates whenever possible.

Increasing Whole-Grain Intake

Finding Whole-Grain Foods

Whole grains include amaranth, barley, brown rice, buckwheat (kasha), flaxseed, millet, oats, popcorn, quinoa, rye, spelt, triticale, whole wheat (wheat berries), and wild rice.[48] Unfortunately, it is not always clear from the label whether a product is made mostly from whole grains or refined grains. Some strategies to use when shopping for whole-grain foods include:

- Looking for products that list whole grain(s) as the first ingredient(s)
- Looking for whole-grain products that contain at least 2 g of fiber per serving, since whole-grain foods are rich in fiber
- Looking for products that display this health claim, "Diets rich in whole-grain foods and other plant foods and low in total fat, saturated fat and cholesterol may help reduce the risk of heart disease and certain cancers." Products displaying this health claim must contain at least 51% whole grain by weight.[49]
- Looking for whole-wheat pasta that lists whole-wheat flour as the first ingredient. Most pasta is made from refined semolina or durum wheat flour.

Some Strategies for Increasing Whole-Grain Intake

- Eat whole-grain breakfast cereals, such as wheat flakes, shredded wheat, muesli, and oatmeal. Bran cereals are not actually whole-grain cereals, but their high fiber content also makes them a good breakfast choice.
- Substitute whole-grain breads, rolls, tortillas, and crackers for those made from refined grains.
- Substitute whole-wheat pasta or pasta made from 50% whole-wheat and 50% white flour for conventional pastas.
- Substitute brown rice for white rice.
- Add barley to soups and stews.
- When baking, substitute whole-wheat flour for white or unbleached flour.

Summary

- Whole-grain foods contain the entire grain, including the bran, the endosperm, and the germ.
- Epidemiological studies have found that diets rich in whole grains are associated with reduced risks of cardiovascular disease and type 2 diabetes compared with diets high in refined grains.
- Although the protective effects of whole grains against cancer are not as well established as those against cardiovascular disease and type 2 diabetes, some epidemiological studies have found whole-grain intake to be associated with decreased cancer risk.
- Diets rich in whole grains and fiber help prevent constipation and are also associated with decreased risk of diverticulosis.
- The 2010 Dietary Guidelines for Americans recommend consuming at least half of total grains as whole grains.

References

1. Truswell AS. Cereal grains and coronary heart disease. Eur J Clin Nutr 2002;56(1):1–14
2. Slavin JL, Jacobs D, Marquart L, Wiemer K. The role of whole grains in disease prevention. J Am Diet Assoc 2001;101(7):780–785
3. Meyer KA, Kushi LH, Jacobs DR Jr, Slavin J, Sellers TA, Folsom AR. Carbohydrates, dietary fiber, and incident type 2 diabetes in older women. Am J Clin Nutr 2000;71(4):921–930
4. Liu S, Manson JE, Stampfer MJ, et al. A prospective study of whole-grain intake and risk of type 2 diabetes mellitus in US women. Am J Public Health 2000;90(9):1409–1415
5. Fung TT, Hu FB, Pereira MA, et al. Whole-grain intake and the risk of type 2 diabetes: a prospective study in men. Am J Clin Nutr 2002;76(3):535–540
6. Montonen J, Knekt P, Järvinen R, Aromaa A, Reunanen A. Whole-grain and fiber intake and the incidence of type 2 diabetes. Am J Clin Nutr 2003;77(3):622–629
7. de Munter JS, Hu FB, Spiegelman D, Franz M, van Dam RM. Whole grain, bran, and germ intake and risk of type 2 diabetes: a prospective cohort study and systematic review. PLoS Med 2007;4(8):e261
8. van Dam RM, Hu FB, Rosenberg L, Krishnan S, Palmer JR. Dietary calcium and magnesium, major food sources, and risk of type 2 diabetes in U.S. black women. Diabetes Care 2006;29(10):2238–2243
9. McKeown NM, Meigs JB, Liu S, Wilson PW, Jacques PF. Whole-grain intake is favorably associated with metabolic risk factors for type 2 diabetes and cardiovascular disease in the Framingham Offspring Study. Am J Clin Nutr 2002;76(2):390–398
10. Liese AD, Roach AK, Sparks KC, Marquart L, D'Agostino RB Jr, Mayer-Davis EJ. Whole-grain intake and insulin sensitivity: the Insulin Resistance Atherosclerosis Study. Am J Clin Nutr 2003;78(5):965–971

11. Pereira MA, Jacobs DR Jr, Pins JJ, et al. Effect of whole grains on insulin sensitivity in overweight hyperinsulinemic adults. Am J Clin Nutr 2002;75(5):848–855

12. Priebe MG, van Binsbergen JJ, de Vos R, Vonk RJ. Whole grain foods for the prevention of type 2 diabetes mellitus. Cochrane Database Syst Rev 2008; (1):CD006061

13. Liu S. Intake of refined carbohydrates and whole grain foods in relation to risk of type 2 diabetes mellitus and coronary heart disease. J Am Coll Nutr 2002;21(4):298–306

14. Hallfrisch J, Facn, Behall KM. Mechanisms of the effects of grains on insulin and glucose responses. J Am Coll Nutr 2000; 19(3, Suppl):320S–325S

15. Salmerón J, Ascherio A, Rimm EB, et al. Dietary fiber, glycemic load, and risk of NIDDM in men. Diabetes Care 1997;20(4):545–550

16. Salmerón J, Manson JE, Stampfer MJ, Colditz GA, Wing AL, Willett WC. Dietary fiber, glycemic load, and risk of non-insulin-dependent diabetes mellitus in women. JAMA 1997;277(6):472–477

17. Brand-Miller J, Hayne S, Petocz P, Colagiuri S. Low-glycemic index diets in the management of diabetes: a meta-analysis of randomized controlled trials. Diabetes Care 2003;26(8):2261–2267

18. Fraser GE, Sabaté J, Beeson WL, Strahan TM. A possible protective effect of nut consumption on risk of coronary heart disease. The Adventist Health Study. Arch Intern Med 1992;152(7):1416–1424

19. Pietinen P, Rimm EB, Korhonen P, et al. Intake of dietary fiber and risk of coronary heart disease in a cohort of Finnish men. The Alpha-Tocopherol, Beta-Carotene Cancer Prevention Study. Circulation 1996;94(11):2720–2727

20. Jacobs DR Jr, Meyer KA, Kushi LH, Folsom AR. Whole-grain intake may reduce the risk of ischemic heart disease death in postmenopausal women: the Iowa Women's Health Study. Am J Clin Nutr 1998;68(2):248–257

21. Liu S, Stampfer MJ, Hu FB, et al. Whole-grain consumption and risk of coronary heart disease: results from the Nurses' Health Study. Am J Clin Nutr 1999;70(3):412–419

22. Jacobs DR Jr, Meyer HE, Solvoll K. Reduced mortality among whole grain bread eaters in men and women in the Norwegian County Study. Eur J Clin Nutr 2001;55(2):137–143

23. Liu S, Sesso HD, Manson JE, Willett WC, Buring JE. Is intake of breakfast cereals related to total and cause-specific mortality in men? Am J Clin Nutr 2003; 77(3):594–599

24. Jensen MK, Koh-Banerjee P, Hu FB, et al. Intakes of whole grains, bran, and germ and the risk of coronary heart disease in men. Am J Clin Nutr 2004;80(6):1492–1499

25. Mellen PB, Liese AD, Tooze JA, Vitolins MZ, Wagenknecht LE, Herrington DM. Whole-grain intake and carotid artery atherosclerosis in a multiethnic cohort: the Insulin Resistance Atherosclerosis Study. Am J Clin Nutr 2007;85(6):1495–1502

26. Liu S, Manson JE, Stampfer MJ, et al. Whole grain consumption and risk of ischemic stroke in women: A prospective study. JAMA 2000;284(12):1534–1540

27. Mellen PB, Walsh TF, Herrington DM. Whole grain intake and cardiovascular disease: a meta-analysis. Nutr Metab Cardiovasc Dis 2008;18(4):283–290

28. Food and Drug Administration, HHS. Food labeling: health claims; soluble dietary fiber from certain foods and coronary heart disease. Final rule. Fed Regist 2003;68(144):44207–44209

29. Behall KM, Scholfield DJ, Hallfrisch J. Lipids significantly reduced by diets containing barley in moderately hypercholesterolemic men. J Am Coll Nutr 2004;23(1):55–62

30. Ames NP, Rhymer CR. Issues surrounding health claims for barley. J Nutr 2008;138(6):1237S–1243S

31. US Food and Drug Administration. Food Labeling: Health Claims; Soluble Fiber from Certain Foods and Risk of Coronary Heart Disease. Final Rule. Fed Regist 2008;73(159):47828–47829. Available at: http://www.fda.gov/Food/LabelingNutrition/LabelClaims/HealthClaimsMeetingSignificantScientificAgreementSSA/ucm074245.htm. Accessed July 26, 2012

32. Slavin J. Why whole grains are protective: biological mechanisms. Proc Nutr Soc 2003;62(1):129–134

33. Liu S, Willett WC. Dietary glycemic load and atherothrombotic risk. Curr Atheroscler Rep 2002;4(6):454–461

34. Wang L, Gaziano JM, Liu S, Manson JE, Buring JE, Sesso HD. Whole- and refined-grain intakes and the risk of hypertension in women. Am J Clin Nutr 2007; 86(2):472–479

35. Flint AJ, Hu FB, Glynn RJ, et al. Whole grains and incident hypertension in men. Am J Clin Nutr 2009; 90(3):493–498

36. Jacobs DR Jr, Marquart L, Slavin J, Kushi LH. Whole-grain intake and cancer: an expanded review and meta-analysis. Nutr Cancer 1998;30(2):85–96

37. La Vecchia C, Chatenoud L, Negri E, Franceschi S. Session: whole cereal grains, fibre and human cancer wholegrain cereals and cancer in Italy. Proc Nutr Soc 2003;62(1):45–49

38. Chan JM, Wang F, Holly EA. Whole grains and risk of pancreatic cancer in a large population-based case-control study in the San Francisco Bay Area, California. Am J Epidemiol 2007;166(10):1174–1185

39. Larsson SC, Giovannucci E, Bergkvist L, Wolk A. Whole grain consumption and risk of colorectal cancer: a population-based cohort of 60,000 women. Br J Cancer 2005;92(9):1803–1807

40. Schatzkin A, Mouw T, Park Y, et al. Dietary fiber and whole-grain consumption in relation to colorectal cancer in the NIH-AARP Diet and Health Study. Am J Clin Nutr 2007;85(5):1353–1360

41. Schatzkin A, Park Y, Leitzmann MF, Hollenbeck AR, Cross AJ. Prospective study of dietary fiber, whole grain foods, and small intestinal cancer. Gastroenterology 2008;135(4):1163–1167

42. McCullough ML, Robertson AS, Chao A, et al. A prospective study of whole grains, fruits, vegetables, and colon cancer risk. Cancer Causes Control 2003; 14(10):959–970

43. Pietinen P, Malila N, Virtanen M, et al. Diet and risk of colorectal cancer in a cohort of Finnish men. Cancer Causes Control 1999;10(5):387–396

44. Slavin JL. Mechanisms for the impact of whole grain foods on cancer risk. J Am Coll Nutr 2000; 19(3, Suppl):300S–307S

45. Marlett JA, McBurney MI, Slavin JL; American Dietetic Association. Position of the American Dietetic Association: health implications of dietary fiber. J Am Diet Assoc 2002;102(7):993–1000

46. Farrell RJ, Farrell JJ, Morrin MM. Diverticular disease in the elderly. Gastroenterol Clin North Am 2001;30(2):475–496

47. US Department of Health and Human Services, US Department of Agriculture. Dietary Guidelines for

Americans. 2010. Available at: http://health.gov/dietaryguidelines/2010.asp. Accessed May 1, 2012

48. Willett WC. Eat, Drink, and be Healthy: The Harvard Medical School Guide to Healthy Eating. New York: Simon & Schuster; 2001

49. US Food and Drug Administration. Health Claim Notification for Whole Grain Foods. 1999. Available at: http://www.fda.gov/Food/LabelingNutrition/LabelClaims/FDAModernizationActFDAMAClaims/ucm073639.htm. Accessed May 1, 2012

6 Coffee

Coffee, an infusion of ground, roasted coffee beans, is among the most widely consumed beverages in the world. Although caffeine has received the most attention from scientists, coffee is a complex mixture of many chemicals, including carbohydrates, lipids (fats), amino acids, vitamins, minerals, alkaloids, and phenolic compounds.[1]

Some Bioactive Compounds in Coffee

Chlorogenic Acid

Chlorogenic acids are actually a family of esters formed between quinic acid and phenolic compounds known as *cinnamic acids*.[2] The most abundant chlorogenic acid in coffee is 5-O-caffeoylquinic acid, an ester formed between quinic acid and caffeic acid (Fig. 6.1). Coffee represents one of the richest dietary sources of chlorogenic acid. The chlorogenic acid content of a 200 mL (7 oz) cup of coffee has been reported to range from 70 mg to 350 mg, which would provide approximately 35–175 mg of caffeic acid. Although chlorogenic acid and caffeic acid have antioxidant activity in vitro,[3] it is unclear how much antioxidant activity they contribute in vivo because they are extensively metabolized, and the metabolites often have lower antioxidant activity than the parent compounds.[4]

Caffeine

Caffeine is a purine alkaloid that occurs naturally in coffee beans (Fig. 6.2). At intake levels associated with coffee consumption, caffeine appears to exert most of its biological effects through an-

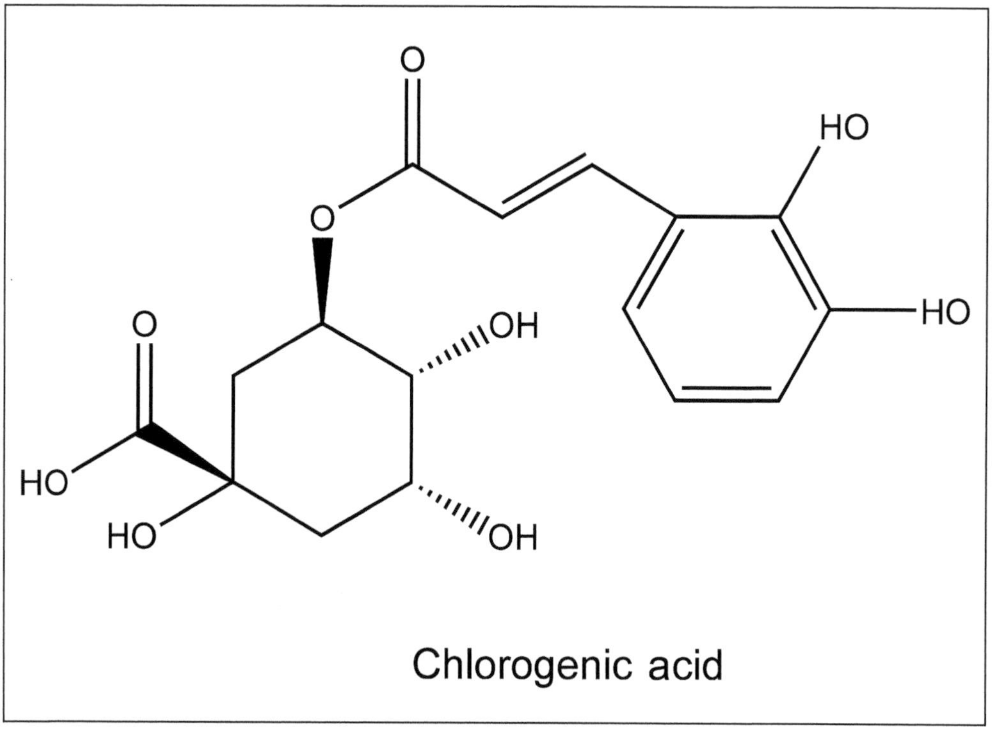

Fig. 6.1 Chemical structure of 5-O-caffeoylquinic acid (chlorogenic acid).

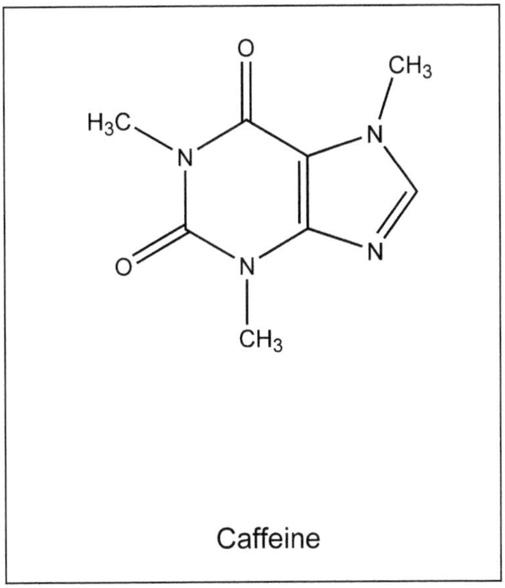

Fig. 6.2 Chemical structure of caffeine.

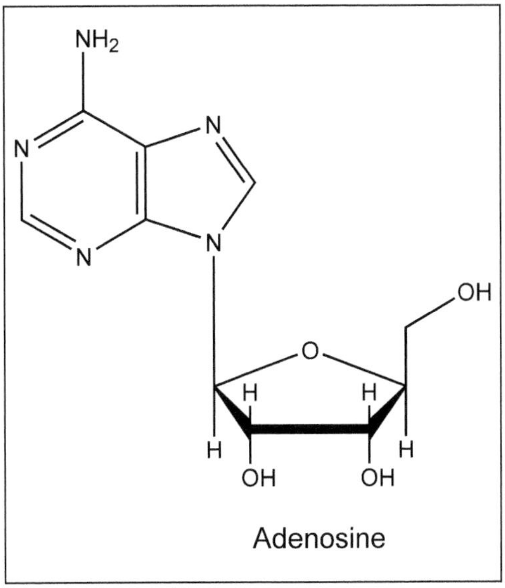

Fig. 6.3 Chemical structure of adenosine.

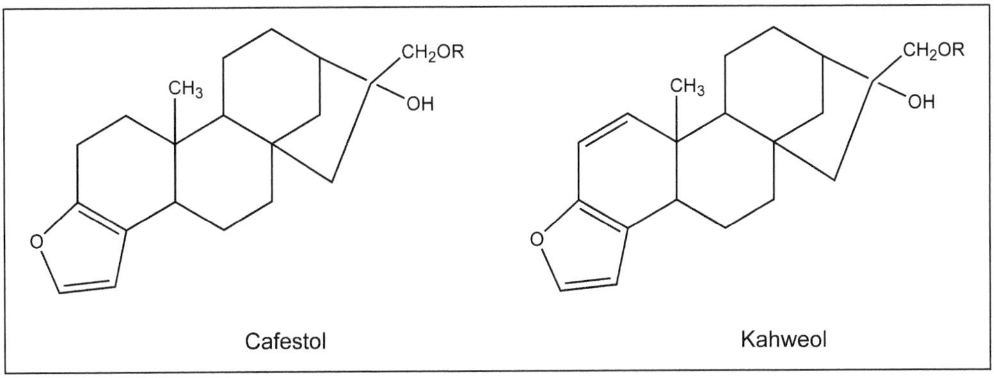

Fig. 6.4 Chemical structures of cafestol and kahweol, diterpenes in coffee with cholesterol-raising effects. R=H: free diterpene; R=fatty acid: diterpene ester.

tagonism of the adenosine A_1 and A_{2A} subtypes of the adenosine receptor.[5] Adenosine (Fig. 6.3) is an endogenous compound that modulates the response of neurons to neurotransmitters. Adenosine has mostly inhibitory effects in the central nervous system, so the effects of adenosine antagonism by caffeine are generally stimulatory. Caffeine is rapidly and almost completely absorbed in the stomach and small intestine and then distributed to all tissues, including the brain. Caffeine concentrations in coffee beverages can be quite variable. A standard cup of coffee is often assumed to provide 100 mg of caffeine, but an analysis of 14 different specialty coffees purchased at coffee shops in the United States

found that the amount of caffeine in 8 oz (approx. 240 mL) of brewed coffee ranged from 72 mg to 130 mg.[6] Caffeine in espresso coffees ranged from 58 mg to 76 mg in a single shot. In countries other than the United States, coffee is often stronger but the volume per cup is smaller, making 100 mg of caffeine/cup a reasonable estimate.

Diterpenes

Cafestol and kahweol are fat-soluble compounds known as *diterpenes* (Fig. 6.4), which have been found to raise serum total and low-density lipoprotein (LDL) cholesterol concentrations in humans.[7] Some cafestol and kahweol are extracted from ground coffee during brewing, but are largely removed from coffee by paper filters. Scandinavian boiled coffee, Turkish coffee, and French press (cafetiere) coffee contain relatively high levels of cafestol and kahweol (6–12 mg/cup), while filtered coffee, percolated coffee, and instant coffee contain low levels of cafestol and kahweol (0.2–0.6 mg/cup).[8,9] Although diterpene concentrations are relatively high in espresso coffee, the small serving size makes it an intermediate source of cafestol and kahweol (4 mg/cup). Since coffee beans are high in cafestol and kahweol, ingestion of coffee beans or grounds on a regular basis may also raise serum and LDL cholesterol.

Disease Prevention

Type 2 Diabetes Mellitus

Several cohort studies have found higher coffee intakes to be associated with significant reductions in the risk of type 2 diabetes mellitus (DM).[10–18] A systematic review of nine prospective cohort studies, including more than 193 000 men and women, found that the risk of type 2 DM was 35% lower in those who consumed at least six cups of coffee daily and 28% lower in those who consumed between four and six cups per day compared with those who consumed fewer than two cups per day.[16] The three prospective cohort studies in the United States to examine the relationship between caffeinated coffee consumption and type 2 DM were the Health Professional's Follow-up Study (HPFS) (41 934 men), the Nurses' Health Study (NHS) (84 276 women), and the NHS II (88 259 women). Men who drank at least six cups of coffee daily had a risk of developing type 2 DM that was 54% lower than in men who did not drink coffee. In one cohort, women who drank at least six cups of coffee daily had a risk of type 2 DM that was 29% lower than in women who did not drink coffee.[13] In the other cohort, women who consumed four or more cups of coffee daily had a 39% lower risk of developing type 2 DM; similar results were found in women who drank two to three cups of coffee daily.[18] In all three cohorts, higher caffeine intakes were also associated with significant reductions in the risk of type 2 DM. In general, consumption of decaffeinated coffee was associated with a more modest decrease in the risk of type 2

DM, suggesting that compounds other than caffeine may contribute to the reduction in risk. Interestingly, decaffeinated coffee was the only type of coffee that was significantly associated with a lower risk of type 2 DM in a cohort of 28 812 postmenopausal women.[19] The mechanism explaining the significant reductions in the risk for type 2 DM observed in the majority of prospective studies is unclear, since short-term clinical trials have found that caffeine administration impairs glucose tolerance and decreases insulin sensitivity.[20,21] Until the relationship between the long-term coffee consumption and type 2 DM risk is better understood, it is premature to recommend coffee consumption as a means of preventing type 2 DM.[13,16]

Parkinson Disease

Several large prospective cohort studies have found higher coffee and caffeine intakes to be associated with significant reductions in the risk for Parkinson disease in men.[22–24] In a prospective study of 47 000 men, those who regularly consumed at least one cup of coffee daily had a 40% lower risk of developing Parkinson disease over the next 10 years than men who did not drink coffee.[23] Caffeine consumption from other sources was also inversely associated with risk of Parkinson disease, in a dose-dependent manner. More recently, a prospective study in 29 335 Finnish men and women found that consumption of one or more cups of coffee daily decreased the risk of Parkinson disease by 60%.[25] In this study, consumption of three or more cups of tea also decreased the risk for Parkinson disease,[25] suggesting that caffeine might be the protective component. Studies in animal models of Parkinson disease suggest that caffeine may protect dopaminergic neurons by acting as an adenosine A_{2A}-receptor antagonist in the brain.[26]

In contrast to the results of prospective studies in men, inverse associations between coffee or caffeine consumption and the risk for Parkinson disease have generally not been observed in women.[22,23] The failure of prospective studies to find inverse associations between coffee or caffeine consumption and Parkinson disease in women may be due to the modifying effect of estrogen-replacement therapy. Further analysis of a prospective study of more than 77 000 female nurses revealed that coffee consumption was inversely associated with Parkinson disease risk in women who had never used postmenopausal estrogen, but a significant increase in Parkinson disease risk was observed in postmenopausal estrogen users who drank at least six cups of coffee daily.[27] In a prospective cohort study that included more than 238000 women, a significant inverse association between coffee consumption and Parkinson disease mortality was also observed in women who had never used postmenopausal estrogen but not in those who had used postmenopausal estrogen.[22] It is not known how estrogen modifies the effect of caffeine on the risk for Parkinson disease.[28] Although the results of epidemiological and animal studies suggest that caffeine may reduce the risk of developing Parkinson disease, it is not yet known whether caffeine consumption can prevent Parkinson disease, particularly in women taking estrogen.

Colorectal Cancer

Some studies have shown that coffee drinking protects against development of colorectal cancer. In general, coffee consumption has been inversely associated with the risk of colon cancer in case–control studies, but not in prospective cohort studies.[29,30] A meta-analysis that combined the results of 12 case–control studies and five prospective cohort studies found that those who drank four or more cups of coffee daily had a 24% lower risk of colorectal cancer than that of nondrinkers.[30] However, coffee consumption was not associated with colorectal cancer risk when the results of only the prospective cohort studies were combined. Although case–control studies usually include more cancer cases than prospective cohort studies, they may be subject to recall bias with respect to coffee consumption and selection bias with respect to the control group. A more recent review of epidemiological studies also found evidence of an inverse association between coffee consumption and colon cancer risk from case–control studies but no evidence of such an association from prospective cohort studies.[29] No overall associations between coffee and rectal cancer emerged in this review. In contrast, the two largest prospective cohort studies to examine the relationship between coffee and colorectal cancer to date found that American men and women who regularly consumed two or more cups of decaffeinated coffee daily had a risk of rectal cancer that was 48% lower than that of those who never consumed coffee.[31] Consumption of caffeinated coffee, tea, or total caffeine was not associated with either colon or rectal cancer risk in either study. More recently, prospective studies conducted in Sweden[32] and Japan[33–35] have generally not found consumption of caffeinated coffee to be associated with colon, rectal, or colorectal cancer in men or women; however, examination of two cohorts revealed an inverse association in women with respect to colon cancer[33] and invasive colon cancer.[34] Despite promising findings in case–control studies, it is unclear whether coffee consumption decreases the risk of colon or rectal cancer in humans. Coffee drinking has not been found to increase the risk of colon or rectal cancer.

Cirrhosis and Liver Cancer

Liver injury resulting from chronic inflammation may result in cirrhosis. In cirrhosis, the formation of fibrotic scar tissue results in progressive deterioration of liver function and other complications, including liver cancer (hepatocellular carcinoma).[36] The most common causes of cirrhosis in developed countries are alcohol abuse and viral hepatitis B and C infection. Coffee consumption was inversely associated with the risk of cirrhosis in several case–control studies[37–39] and with mortality from alcoholic cirrhosis in two prospective cohort studies.[40,41] An 8-year study of more than 120000 men and women in the United States found that the risk of death from alcoholic cirrhosis was 22% lower per cup of coffee consumed daily.[42] A 17-year study of more than 51000 men and women in Norway found that those who consumed at least two cups of coffee daily had a 40% lower risk of death from cirrhosis than those who never consumed coffee.[41] A recent prospective cohort study in 125580 US adults found that coffee drinking was protective against alcoholic cirrhosis but not nonalcoholic cirrhosis.[43] Specifically, the risk of developing alcoholic cirrhosis was 40% lower in those who drank one to three cups of coffee daily and 80% lower in those who drank four or more cups daily.[43] Several case–control studies in Europe[44–46] and Japan[47,48] have found significant inverse associations between coffee consumption and the risk of hepatocellular carcinoma. Results of three prospective cohort studies in Japan[49–51] and one in Finland[52] have supported the findings of case–control studies. In two of the prospective cohort studies, coffee consumption was associated with significant reductions in the risk of hepatocellular carcinoma in Japanese men and women with liver disease or hepatitis C infection.[49,50] In those high-risk individuals, consumption of at least one cup of coffee daily was associated with a 50% reduction in the risk of hepatocellular carcinoma compared with those who never drank coffee. Similarly, one of the prospective studies found that drinking at least one cup of coffee daily resulted in a 50% reduction in risk for death caused by hepatocellular cancer, but the association was not statistically significant in subjects without a history of liver diseases.[51] Further, two meta-analyses have found inverse associations between coffee consumption and liver cancer.[53,54]

Mortality

A prospective cohort study in US adults (41 736 men and 86 214 women) participating in the HPFS and the NHS examined whether coffee drinking was associated with all-cause, cardiovascular disease, or cancer mortality. In both men and women, caffeinated coffee consumption was inversely associated with all-cause and cardiovascular-related mortality but not with cancer mortality.[55] Other smaller cohort studies have reported habitual consumption of caffeinated coffee reduces all-cause mortality[56–59] and cardiovascular-related mortality,[57] but the associations have not always been consistent among women and men. Yet, other studies have found that coffee is not related to or may increase all-cause or cause-specific mortality (reviewed in [55]).

Safety

Health Risks Associated with Coffee Consumption

Cardiovascular Disease

Coronary Heart Disease. Although limited by the potential for selection and recall bias, the results of most case–control studies suggest that people who consume five or more cups of coffee daily may be at increased risk of coronary heart disease (CHD).[60,61] In contrast, the majority of prospective cohort studies have not found significant associations between coffee intake and CHD risk. One exception was a prospective study in Norway that found that high intakes of unfiltered boiled coffee were associated with an increased risk of death from CHD before that population switched to filtered coffee.[62] The results of two separate meta-analyses that combined the results of more than 10 prospective cohort studies did not support an association between coffee consumption and the risk of CHD.[60,63] Similarly, most of the prospective cohort studies published since the last meta-analysis have not found significant associations between coffee consumption and CHD risk, including studies of large cohorts in the United States,[64–66] Scotland,[67] and Finland.[68]

Hypertension. Hypertension is a well-recognized risk factor for cardiovascular disease. It has been well established that caffeine consumption acutely raises blood pressure, particularly in individuals with hypertension.[5] Although habitual consumption has been found to result in a degree of tolerance to the blood-pressure-raising effect of caffeine, the results of several clinical trials suggest that this tolerance is not always complete, even in those who consume caffeine daily.[69–71] Two meta-analyses have examined the results of randomized controlled trials of the effect on blood pressure of coffee consumption for more than one week. A meta-analysis that included 11 randomized controlled trials, in which the median duration of coffee consumption was 56 days and the median intake was five cups per day, found that coffee consumption significantly increased systolic and diastolic blood pressure by 2.4 mmHg and 1.2 mmHg, respectively.[72] More recently, a meta-analysis that included 18 randomized controlled trials, with a median duration of 43 days and a median intake of 725 mL/day (approx. three cups daily), found that coffee consumption significantly increased systolic blood pressure by 1.2 mmHg.[73] Although the increases in systolic blood pressure seem modest by individual standards, it has been estimated that an average systolic blood pressure reduction of 2 mmHg in a population may result in 10% lower mortality from stroke and 7% lower mortality from CHD.[74] The most recent meta-analysis found that caffeine in the form of a pill elevated blood pressure more than caffeine consumed as coffee,[73] suggesting that other compounds in coffee may counteract caffeine's blood-pressure-raising effect. Moreover, a recent prospective study conducted in the NHS I and II cohorts (a total of 140 544 women) reported that caffeinated cola intake, but not habitual coffee intake, was linked to an increased risk for hypertension.[75] However, the available evidence from short-term randomized controlled trials suggests that chronic coffee and caffeine consumption modestly raises systolic blood pressure, which, given the widespread consumption of caffeine and coffee, may result in increased risk of stroke and CHD in the population, particularly in those with hypertension.

Low-density lipoprotein cholesterol. A meta-analysis of 14 randomized controlled trials found that the consumption of unfiltered, boiled coffee dose-dependently increased serum total and LDL cholesterol concentrations, while the consumption of filtered coffee resulted in very little change.[76] Overall, the consumption of boiled coffee increased serum total cholesterol by 23 mg/dL and LDL cholesterol by 14 mg/dL, while the consumption of filtered coffee raised total cholesterol by only 3 mg/dL and did not affect LDL cholesterol. The cholesterol-raising factors in unfiltered coffee have been identified as cafestol and kahweol, two diterpenes that are largely removed from coffee by paper filters (see the Diterpenes section above).[7]

Homocysteine. An elevated plasma total homocysteine (tHcy) concentration is associated with increased risk of cardiovascular disease, including CHD, stroke, and peripheral vascular disease, but it is unclear whether the relationship is causal.[77] Higher coffee intakes have been associated with increased plasma tHcy concentrations, in cross-sectional studies conducted in Europe, Scandinavia, and the United States.[78-82] Controlled clinical trials have confirmed the homocysteine-raising effect of coffee at intakes of approximately four cups per day.[83-85]

Cardiac arrhythmias. Clinical trials have not found coffee or caffeine intake equivalent to five to six cups per day to increase the frequency or severity of cardiac arrhythmias in healthy people

or in people with CHD.[86,87] A large prospective study in the United States that followed more than 128 000 people for 7 years found no association between coffee consumption and sudden cardiac death. More recently, two prospective studies in Scandinavia found no association between coffee consumption and the risk of developing atrial fibrillation, a common supraventricular arrhythmia.[88,89]

Cancer

Numerous epidemiological studies have examined relationships between coffee and caffeine intake and cancer risk in humans. In general, there is little evidence that coffee consumption increases the risk of cancer, especially when the analyses are adjusted for cigarette smoking (reviewed in [90]).

Pregnancy

Miscarriage. The results of epidemiological studies that have examined the relationship between maternal coffee or caffeine intake and the risk of miscarriage (spontaneous abortion) have been conflicting. While some studies have observed significant associations between high caffeine intakes, particularly from coffee, and the risk of spontaneous abortion,[91-95] other studies have not.[96-98] Most studies that observed significant associations between self-reported coffee or caffeine consumption and the risk of spontaneous abortion did so at intake levels of at least 300 mg/day of caffeine.[90] The only study that assessed caffeine intake by measuring serum concentrations of paraxanthine, a caffeine metabolite, found that the risk of spontaneous abortion was only elevated in women with paraxanthine concentrations that suggested caffeine intakes of at least 600 mg/day.[99] It has been proposed that an association between caffeine consumption and the risk of spontaneous abortion could be explained by the relationship between nausea and fetal viability.[100] Nausea is more common in women with viable pregnancies than nonviable pregnancies, suggesting that women with viable pregnancies are more likely to avoid or limit caffeine consumption due to nausea. However, at least one study found that the significant increase in risk of spontaneous abortion observed in women with caffeine intakes higher than 300 mg/day was independent of nausea in pregnancy.[92] Additionally, two other studies found that caffeine consumption was associated with increased risk of spontaneous abortion in women who experienced nausea or aversion to coffee during pregnancy.[91,94] Although the topic remains controversial, the available epidemiological evidence suggests that maternal consumption of less than 300 mg/day of caffeine is unlikely to increase the risk of spontaneous abortion.

Fetal growth. Epidemiological studies examining the effects of maternal caffeine and coffee consumption on fetal growth have assessed mean birth weight, incidence of low birth weight (less than 2500 g), and fetal growth retardation (less than the 10th percentile of birth weight for gestational age). Several studies found that maternal caffeine intakes ranging from 200 to 400 mg/day were associated with decreases in mean birth weight of approximately 100 g (3.5 oz).[101–103] However, a large prospective study found that caffeine-associated decreases in birth weight were unlikely to be clinically important in women with caffeine intakes of less than 600 mg/day.[104] The results of epidemiological studies examining the association between maternal caffeine consumption and the risk of low birth weight or fetal growth retardation have been mixed (reviewed in [90]). Moreover, some of the available epidemiological studies have been criticized for inadequately controlling for important risk factors for low birth weight and fetal growth retardation, particularly smoking.[100] More recently, a double-blind, intervention trial randomized women to drink decaffeinated (median caffeine intake of 117 mg/day) or caffeinated coffee (median caffeine intake of 317 mg/day) throughout the second half of their pregnancy.[105] No differences in length of gestation or infant birth weight were found between the two groups.[105] Although the relationship between maternal caffeine consumption and fetal growth requires further clarification, it appears unlikely that caffeine intakes below 300 mg/day would adversely affect fetal growth in nonsmoking women.

Birth defects. At present, there is no convincing evidence from epidemiological studies that maternal caffeine consumption ranging from 300 mg/day to 1000 mg/day increases the risk of congenital malformations in humans (reviewed in [90,106,107]).

Lactation

The American Academy of Pediatrics categorizes caffeine as a maternal medication that is usually compatible with breast-feeding.[108] Although high maternal caffeine intakes have been reported to cause irritability and poor sleeping patterns in infants, no adverse effects have been reported with moderate maternal intake of caffeinated beverages equivalent to two to three cups of coffee daily.

Adverse Effects

Most adverse effects attributed to coffee consumption are related to caffeine. Adverse reactions to caffeine may include tachycardia (rapid heart rate), palpitations, insomnia, restlessness, nervousness, tremor, headache, abdominal pain, nausea, vomiting, diarrhea, and diuresis (increased urination).[109] Very high caffeine intakes, not usually from coffee, may induce hypokalemia (abnormally low serum potassium).[110] Sudden cessation of caffeine consumption after long-term use may result in caffeine-withdrawal symptoms.[111] Commonly reported caffeine-withdrawal symptoms include headache, fatigue, drowsiness, irritability, difficulty concentrating, and depressed mood. Significant withdrawal symptoms have been observed at long-term intakes as low as 100 mg/day, although they are more common with higher intakes. Gradual withdrawal from caffeine appears less likely to result in withdrawal symptoms than abrupt withdrawal.[112]

Drug Interactions

Habitual caffeine consumption increases hepatic cytochrome P450 (CYP) 1A2 activity, which has implications for the metabolism of several medications.[113] Additionally, drugs that inhibit the activity of CYP1A2 interfere with the metabolism and elimination of caffeine, thereby increasing the risk of adverse effects.[114]

Drugs that Alter Caffeine Metabolism

The following medications may impair the hepatic metabolism of caffeine, decreasing its elimination and potentially increasing the risk of caffeine-related side effects: cimetidine (Tagamet), disulfiram (Antabuse), estrogens, fluconazole (Diflucan), fluvoxamine (Luvox, Faverin), mexiletine (Mexitil), quinolone class antibiotics, and terbinafine (Lamisil).[113] Use of the drug phenytoin (Dilantin, Epanutin) or cigarette smoking increases the hepatic metabolism of caffeine, resulting in increased elimination and decreased plasma caffeine concentrations.[109]

Caffeine Effects on Other Drugs

Caffeine and other methylxanthines may enhance the effects and side effects of β-adrenergic-stimulating agents, such as epinephrine and albuterol.[109,113] Caffeine may inhibit the hepatic metabolism of the antipsychotic medication, clozapine, potentially elevating serum clozapine levels and increasing the risk of toxicity. Caffeine consumption can decrease the elimination of theophylline, potentially increasing serum theophylline levels. Caffeine has been found to decrease the systemic elimination of acetaminophen (paracetamol) and to increase the bioavailability of aspirin, which may partially explain its efficacy in enhancing their analgesic effects. This is important because many pain-relievers on the market today combine caffeine with aspirin and/ or acetaminophen. Further, caffeine may decrease serum lithium concentrations by enhancing its elimination.

Nutrient Interactions

Calcium and Osteoporosis

The results of controlled studies in humans indicate that coffee and caffeine consumption decrease the efficiency of calcium absorption, resulting in a loss of approximately 4–6 mg of calcium per cup of coffee.[115,116] Most studies have found no association between caffeine consumption and change in bone mineral density (BMD) over time (reviewed in [117]). However, one study found that caffeine consumption was associated with accelerated loss of BMD only in women with calcium intakes below 744 mg/day,[118] while another study found that consumption of more than 300 mg/day of caffeine was associated with accelerated bone loss in elderly women.[119] At least six prospective cohort studies have examined associations between caffeine (mainly from coffee) or coffee consumption and the risk of hip fracture in women. Two studies, one in Finland and one in Japan, found no association.[120,121] Another study in Norway found that women who consumed at least nine cups of coffee daily tend-

ed to have an increased risk of hip fracture, but only 7% of women consumed this much coffee.[122] However, three prospective cohort studies in the United States found that coffee or caffeine consumption was positively associated with the risk of hip fracture in women.[123–125] In the Framingham cohort, women who consumed more than two cups of coffee daily had a 69% higher risk of hip fracture over the next 12 years than women who did not consume caffeinated beverages.[123] In the NHS cohort, women who consumed four or more cups of coffee daily had a risk of hip fracture over the next six years that was three times that of those who did not drink coffee.[124] A prospective cohort study of women aged 65 years and older found that daily consumption of caffeine equivalent to what is found in two cups of coffee (approx. 200 mg) increased the risk of osteoporotic hip fracture.[125] Most recently, a prospective study in a cohort of 31 527 older Swedish women found that those who consumed four or more cups of coffee daily had an increased risk for any type of osteoporotic fracture, but the association was only significant in women with low calcium intakes (<700 mg/day).[126] Given the multifactorial etiology of osteoporosis, the impact of coffee or caffeine consumption on the risk of osteoporosis is not clear. However, currently available evidence suggests that ensuring adequate calcium and vitamin D intake and limiting coffee consumption to three cups per day or fewer may help reduce the risk of osteoporosis and osteoporotic fracture, particularly in older adults.

Nonheme Iron

Phenolic compounds in coffee can bind nonheme iron and inhibit its intestinal absorption.[127] Drinking 150–250 mL of coffee with a test meal has been found to inhibit the absorption of iron by 24%–73%.[128,129] To maximize iron absorption from a meal or iron supplements, concomitant intake of coffee should be avoided.

Summary

- Coffee is a complex mixture of chemicals that provides significant amounts of chlorogenic acid and caffeine.
- Unfiltered coffee is a significant source of cafestol and kahweol, diterpenes that have been found to raise serum total and low-density li-

poprotein cholesterol concentrations in humans.

- The results of epidemiological studies suggest that coffee consumption is associated with decreased risk of type 2 diabetes, Parkinson disease, and liver disease. However, it is premature to recommend coffee consumption for disease prevention based on this evidence.
- At present, there is little evidence that coffee consumption increases the risk of cancer.
- Despite evidence from clinical trials that caffeine in coffee can increase blood pressure, most prospective cohort studies have not found moderate coffee consumption to be associated with increased risk of cardiovascular disease.
- Overall, there is little evidence of health risk and some evidence of health benefits for adults consuming moderate amounts of filtered coffee (three to four cups daily, providing 300–400 mg/day of caffeine).
- Some people may be more vulnerable to the adverse effects of caffeine in coffee:
  - Caffeine consumption comparable to the amount in two to three cups of coffee may raise blood pressure, especially in people with borderline or high blood pressure.
  - Until the effects of caffeine on the risk of miscarriage and fetal growth are clarified, women who are pregnant or planning to become pregnant should limit coffee consumption to three cups per day, providing no more than 300 mg/day of caffeine.
  - Ensuring adequate calcium and vitamin D intake and limiting coffee consumption to three cups per day (300 mg/day of caffeine) may help reduce the risk of osteoporosis and osteoporotic fracture, particularly in older adults.

References

1. Spiller MA. The Chemical Components of Coffee. In: Spiller GA, ed. Caffeine. Boca Raton, FL: CRC Press; 1998:97–161
2. Clifford MN. Chlorogenic acids and other cinnamates–nature occurrence and dietary burden. J Sci Food Agric 1999;79(3):362–372
3. Iwai K, Kishimoto N, Kakino Y, Mochida K, Fujita T. In vitro antioxidative effects and tyrosinase inhibitory activities of seven hydroxycinnamoyl derivatives in green coffee beans. J Agric Food Chem 2004; 52(15): 4893–4898
4. Olthof MR, Hollman PC, Buijsman MN, van Amelsvoort JM, Katan MB. Chlorogenic acid, quercetin-3-rutinoside and black tea phenols are extensively metabolized in humans. J Nutr 2003;133(6):1806–1814
5. James JE. Critical review of dietary caffeine and blood pressure: a relationship that should be taken more seriously. Psychosom Med 2004;66(1):63–71
6. McCusker RR, Goldberger BA, Cone EJ. Caffeine content of specialty coffees. J Anal Toxicol 2003; 27(7):520–522
7. Urgert R, Katan MB. The cholesterol-raising factor from coffee beans. Annu Rev Nutr 1997;17:305–324
8. Gross G, Jaccaud E, Huggett AC. Analysis of the content of the diterpenes cafestol and kahweol in coffee brews. Food Chem Toxicol 1997;35(6):547–554
9. Urgert R, van der Weg G, Kosmeijer-Schuil TG, van de Bovenkamp P, Hovenier R, Katan MB. Levels of the cholesterol-elevating diterpenes cafestol and kahweol in various coffee brews. J Agric Food Chem 1995;43(8):2167–2172
10. Hu G, Jousilahti P, Peltonen M, Bidel S, Tuomilehto J. Joint association of coffee consumption and other factors to the risk of type 2 diabetes: a prospective study in Finland. Int J Obes (Lond) 2006;30(12):1742–1749
11. Carlsson S, Hammar N, Grill V, Kaprio J. Coffee consumption and risk of type 2 diabetes in Finnish twins. Int J Epidemiol 2004;33(3):616–617
12. Rosengren A, Dotevall A, Wilhelmsen L, Thelle D, Johansson S. Coffee and incidence of diabetes in Swedish women: a prospective 18-year follow-up study. J Intern Med 2004;255(1):89–95
13. Salazar-Martinez E, Willett WC, Ascherio A, et al. Coffee consumption and risk for type 2 diabetes mellitus. Ann Intern Med 2004;140(1):1–8
14. Tuomilehto J, Hu G, Bidel S, Lindström J, Jousilahti P. Coffee consumption and risk of type 2 diabetes mellitus among middle-aged Finnish men and women. JAMA 2004;291(10):1213–1219
15. van Dam RM, Feskens EJ. Coffee consumption and risk of type 2 diabetes mellitus. Lancet 2002;360(9344): 1477–1478
16. van Dam RM, Hu FB. Coffee consumption and risk of type 2 diabetes: a systematic review. JAMA 2005; 294(1):97–104
17. Greenberg JA, Axen KV, Schnoll R, Boozer CN. Coffee, tea and diabetes: the role of weight loss and caffeine. Int J Obes (Lond) 2005;29(9):1121–1129
18. van Dam RM, Willett WC, Manson JE, Hu FB. Coffee, caffeine, and risk of type 2 diabetes: a prospective cohort study in younger and middle-aged U.S. women. Diabetes Care 2006;29(2):398–403
19. Pereira MA, Parker ED, Folsom AR. Coffee consumption and risk of type 2 diabetes mellitus: an 11-year prospective study of 28 812 postmenopausal women. Arch Intern Med 2006;166(12):1311–1316
20. Keijzers GB, De Galan BE, Tack CJ, Smits P. Caffeine can decrease insulin sensitivity in humans. Diabetes Care 2002;25(2):364–369
21. Petrie HJ, Chown SE, Belfie LM, et al. Caffeine ingestion increases the insulin response to an oral-glucose-tolerance test in obese men before and after weight loss. Am J Clin Nutr 2004;80(1):22–28
22. Ascherio A, Weisskopf MG, O'Reilly EJ, et al. Coffee consumption, gender, and Parkinson's disease mortality in the cancer prevention study II cohort: the modifying effects of estrogen. Am J Epidemiol 2004;160(10):977–984
23. Ascherio A, Zhang SM, Hernán MA, et al. Prospective study of caffeine consumption and risk of Parkinson's disease in men and women. Ann Neurol 2001; 50(1):56–63

24. Ross GW, Abbott RD, Petrovitch H, et al. Association of coffee and caffeine intake with the risk of Parkinson's disease. JAMA 2000;283(20):2674–2679

25. Hu G, Bidel S, Jousilahti P, Antikainen R, Tuomilehto J. Coffee and tea consumption and the risk of Parkinson's disease. Mov Disord 2007;22(15):2242–2248

26. Schwarzschild MA, Chen JF, Ascherio A. Caffeinated clues and the promise of adenosine A(2A) antagonists in PD. Neurology 2002;58(8):1154–1160

27. Ascherio A, Chen H, Schwarzschild MA, Zhang SM, Colditz GA, Speizer FE. Caffeine, postmenopausal estrogen, and risk of Parkinson's disease. Neurology 2003;60(5):790–795

28. Pollock BG, Wylie M, Stack JA, et al. Inhibition of caffeine metabolism by estrogen replacement therapy in postmenopausal women. J Clin Pharmacol 1999; 39(9):936–940

29. Tavani A, La Vecchia C. Coffee, decaffeinated coffee, tea and cancer of the colon and rectum: a review of epidemiological studies, 1990-2003. Cancer Causes Control 2004;15(8):743–757

30. Giovannucci E. Meta-analysis of coffee consumption and risk of colorectal cancer. Am J Epidemiol 1998;147(11):1043–1052

31. Michels KB, Willett WC, Fuchs CS, Giovannucci E. Coffee, tea, and caffeine consumption and incidence of colon and rectal cancer. J Natl Cancer Inst 2005; 97(4):282–292

32. Larsson SC, Bergkvist L, Giovannucci E, Wolk A. Coffee consumption and incidence of colorectal cancer in two prospective cohort studies of Swedish women and men. Am J Epidemiol 2006;163(7):638–644

33. Oba S, Shimizu N, Nagata C, et al. The relationship between the consumption of meat, fat, and coffee and the risk of colon cancer: a prospective study in Japan. Cancer Lett 2006;244(2):260–267

34. Lee KJ, Inoue M, Otani T, Iwasaki M, Sasazuki S, Tsugane S; JPHC Study Group. Coffee consumption and risk of colorectal cancer in a population-based prospective cohort of Japanese men and women. Int J Cancer 2007;121(6):1312–1318

35. Naganuma T, Kuriyama S, Akhter M, et al. Coffee consumption and the risk of colorectal cancer: a prospective cohort study in Japan. Int J Cancer 2007; 120(7):1542–1547

36. Friedman SL, Schiano TD. Cirrhosis and its sequelae. In: Goldman L, Ausiello D, eds. Cecil Textbook of Medicine. 22nd ed. St. Louis: WB Saunders; 2004:940–944

37. Corrao G, Lepore AR, Torchio P, et al; Provincial Group for the Study of Chronic Liver Disease. The effect of drinking coffee and smoking cigarettes on the risk of cirrhosis associated with alcohol consumption. A case-control study. Eur J Epidemiol 1994;10(6):657–664

38. Corrao G, Zambon A, Bagnardi V, D'Amicis A, Klatsky A; Collaborative SIDECIR Group. Coffee, caffeine, and the risk of liver cirrhosis. Ann Epidemiol 2001; 11(7):458–465

39. Gallus S, Tavani A, Negri E, La Vecchia C. Does coffee protect against liver cirrhosis? Ann Epidemiol 2002;12(3):202–205

40. Klatsky AL, Armstrong MA. Alcohol, smoking, coffee, and cirrhosis. Am J Epidemiol 1992;136(10):1248–1257

41. Tverdal A, Skurtveit S. Coffee intake and mortality from liver cirrhosis. Ann Epidemiol 2003;13(6):419–423

42. Klatsky AL, Armstrong MA, Friedman GD. Coffee, tea, and mortality. Ann Epidemiol 1993;3(4):375–381

43. Klatsky AL, Morton C, Udaltsova N, Friedman GD. Coffee, cirrhosis, and transaminase enzymes. Arch Intern Med 2006;166(11):1190–1195

44. Gallus S, Bertuzzi M, Tavani A, et al. Does coffee protect against hepatocellular carcinoma? Br J Cancer 2002;87(9):956–959

45. Gelatti U, Covolo L, Franceschini M, et al; Brescia HCC Study Group. Coffee consumption reduces the risk of hepatocellular carcinoma independently of its aetiology: a case-control study. J Hepatol 2005;42(4):528–534

46. Montella M, Polesel J, La Vecchia C, et al. Coffee and tea consumption and risk of hepatocellular carcinoma in Italy. Int J Cancer 2007;120(7):1555–1559

47. Tanaka K, Hara M, Sakamoto T, et al. Inverse association between coffee drinking and the risk of hepatocellular carcinoma: a case-control study in Japan. Cancer Sci 2007;98(2):214–218

48. Ohfuji S, Fukushima W, Tanaka T, et al. Coffee consumption and reduced risk of hepatocellular carcinoma among patients with chronic type C liver disease: A case-control study. Hepatol Res 2006;36(3):201–208

49. Shimazu T, Tsubono Y, Kuriyama S, et al. Coffee consumption and the risk of primary liver cancer: pooled analysis of two prospective studies in Japan. Int J Cancer 2005;116(1):150–154

50. Inoue M, Yoshimi I, Sobue T, Tsugane S; JPHC Study Group. Influence of coffee drinking on subsequent risk of hepatocellular carcinoma: a prospective study in Japan. J Natl Cancer Inst 2005;97(4):293–300

51. Kurozawa Y, Ogimoto I, Shibata A, et al; JACC Study Group. Coffee and risk of death from hepatocellular carcinoma in a large cohort study in Japan. Br J Cancer 2005;93(5):607–610

52. Hu G, Tuomilehto J, Pukkala E, et al. Joint effects of coffee consumption and serum gamma-glutamyltransferase on the risk of liver cancer. Hepatology 2008;48(1):129–136

53. Bravi F, Bosetti C, Tavani A, et al. Coffee drinking and hepatocellular carcinoma risk: a meta-analysis. Hepatology 2007;46(2):430–435

54. Larsson SC, Wolk A. Coffee consumption and risk of liver cancer: a meta-analysis. Gastroenterology 2007;132(5):1740–1745

55. Lopez-Garcia E, van Dam RM, Li TY, Rodriguez-Artalejo F, Hu FB. The relationship of coffee consumption with mortality. Ann Intern Med 2008;148(12):904–914

56. Iwai N, Ohshiro H, Kurozawa Y, et al. Relationship between coffee and green tea consumption and all-cause mortality in a cohort of a rural Japanese population. J Epidemiol 2002;12(3):191–198

57. Murray SS, Bjelke E, Gibson RW, Schuman LM. Coffee consumption and mortality from ischemic heart disease and other causes: results from the Lutheran Brotherhood study, 1966-1978. Am J Epidemiol 1981;113(6):661–667

58. Jazbec A, Simić D, Corović N, Duraković Z, Pavlović M. Impact of coffee and other selected factors on general mortality and mortality due to cardiovascular disease in Croatia. J Health Popul Nutr 2003;21(4):332–340

59. Rosengren A, Wilhelmsen L. Coffee, coronary heart disease and mortality in middle-aged Swedish men: findings from the Primary Prevention Study. J Intern Med 1991;230(1):67–71

60. Kawachi I, Colditz GA, Stone CB. Does coffee drinking increase the risk of coronary heart disease? Results from a meta-analysis. Br Heart J 1994;72(3):269–275

61. Greenland S. A meta-analysis of coffee, myocardial infarction, and coronary death. Epidemiology 1993;4(4):366–374

62. Tverdal A, Stensvold I, Solvoll K, Foss OP, Lund-Larsen P, Bjartveit K. Coffee consumption and death from coronary heart disease in middle aged Norwegian men and women. BMJ 1990;300(6724):566–569

63. Myers MG, Basinski A. Coffee and coronary heart disease. Arch Intern Med 1992;152(9):1767–1772

64. Willett WC, Stampfer MJ, Manson JE, et al. Coffee consumption and coronary heart disease in women. A ten-year follow-up. JAMA 1996;275(6):458–462

65. Lopez-Garcia E, van Dam RM, Willett WC, et al. Coffee consumption and coronary heart disease in men and women: a prospective cohort study. Circulation 2006;113(17):2045–2053

66. Andersen LF, Jacobs DR Jr, Carlsen MH, Blomhoff R. Consumption of coffee is associated with reduced risk of death attributed to inflammatory and cardiovascular diseases in the Iowa Women's Health Study. Am J Clin Nutr 2006;83(5):1039–1046

67. Woodward M, Tunstall-Pedoe H. Coffee and tea consumption in the Scottish Heart Health Study follow up: conflicting relations with coronary risk factors, coronary disease, and all cause mortality. J Epidemiol Community Health 1999;53(8):481–487

68. Bidel S, Hu G, Qiao Q, Jousilahti P, Antikainen R, Tuomilehto J. Coffee consumption and risk of total and cardiovascular mortality among patients with type 2 diabetes. Diabetologia 2006;49(11):2618–2626

69. Denaro CP, Brown CR, Jacob P III, Benowitz NL. Effects of caffeine with repeated dosing. Eur J Clin Pharmacol 1991;40(3):273–278

70. James JE. Chronic effects of habitual caffeine consumption on laboratory and ambulatory blood pressure levels. J Cardiovasc Risk 1994;1(2):159–164

71. Lovallo WR, Wilson MF, Vincent AS, Sung BH, McKey BS, Whitsett TL. Blood pressure response to caffeine shows incomplete tolerance after short-term regular consumption. Hypertension 2004;43(4):760–765

72. Jee SH, He J, Whelton PK, Suh I, Klag MJ. The effect of chronic coffee drinking on blood pressure: a meta-analysis of controlled clinical trials. Hypertension 1999;33(2):647–652

73. Noordzij M, Uiterwaal CS, Arends LR, Kok FJ, Grobbee DE, Geleijnse JM. Blood pressure response to chronic intake of coffee and caffeine: a meta-analysis of randomized controlled trials. J Hypertens 2005;23(5): 921–928

74. Lewington S, Clarke R, Qizilbash N, Peto R, Collins R; Prospective Studies Collaboration. Age-specific relevance of usual blood pressure to vascular mortality: a meta-analysis of individual data for one million adults in 61 prospective studies. Lancet 2002;360 (9349):1903–1913

75. Winkelmayer WC, Stampfer MJ, Willett WC, Curhan GC. Habitual caffeine intake and the risk of hypertension in women. JAMA 2005;294(18):2330–2335

76. Jee SH, He J, Appel LJ, Whelton PK, Suh I, Klag MJ. Coffee consumption and serum lipids: a meta-analysis of randomized controlled clinical trials. Am J Epidemiol 2001;153(4):353–362

77. Splaver A, Lamas GA, Hennekens CH. Homocysteine and cardiovascular disease: biological mechanisms, observational epidemiology, and the need for randomized trials. Am Heart J 2004;148(1):34–40

78. Husemoen LL, Thomsen TF, Fenger M, Jørgensen T. Effect of lifestyle factors on plasma total homocysteine concentrations in relation to MTHFR(C677T) genotype. Inter99 (7). Eur J Clin Nutr 2004;58(8):1142–1150

79. Mennen LI, de Courcy GP, Guilland JC, et al. Homocysteine, cardiovascular disease risk factors, and habitual diet in the French Supplementation with Antioxidant Vitamins and Minerals Study. Am J Clin Nutr 2002;76(6):1279–1289

80. de Bree A, Verschuren WM, Blom HJ, Kromhout D. Lifestyle factors and plasma homocysteine concentrations in a general population sample. Am J Epidemiol 2001;154(2):150–154

81. Stolzenberg-Solomon RZ, Miller ER III, Maguire MG, Selhub J, Appel LJ. Association of dietary protein intake and coffee consumption with serum homocysteine concentrations in an older population. Am J Clin Nutr 1999;69(3):467–475

82. Nygård O, Refsum H, Ueland PM, et al. Coffee consumption and plasma total homocysteine: The Hordaland Homocysteine Study. Am J Clin Nutr 1997;65(1):136–143

83. Christensen B, Mosdol A, Retterstol L, Landaas S, Thelle DS. Abstention from filtered coffee reduces concentrations of plasma homocysteine and serum cholesterol—a randomized controlled trial. Am J Clin Nutr 2001;74(3):302–307

84. Urgert R, van Vliet T, Zock PL, Katan MB. Heavy coffee consumption and plasma homocysteine: a randomized controlled trial in healthy volunteers. Am J Clin Nutr 2000;72(5):1107–1110

85. Grubben MJ, Boers GH, Blom HJ, et al. Unfiltered coffee increases plasma homocysteine concentrations in healthy volunteers: a randomized trial. Am J Clin Nutr 2000;71(2):480–484

86. Chelsky LB, Cutler JE, Griffith K, Kron J, McClelland JH, McAnulty JH. Caffeine and ventricular arrhythmias. An electrophysiological approach. JAMA 1990;264 (17):2236–2240

87. Myers MG. Caffeine and cardiac arrhythmias. Ann Intern Med 1991;114(2):147–150

88. Frost L, Vestergaard P. Caffeine and risk of atrial fibrillation or flutter: the Danish Diet, Cancer, and Health Study. Am J Clin Nutr 2005;81(3):578–582

89. Wilhelmsen L, Rosengren A, Lappas G. Hospitalizations for atrial fibrillation in the general male population: morbidity and risk factors. J Intern Med 2001;250(5):382–389

90. Nawrot P, Jordan S, Eastwood J, Rotstein J, Hugenholtz A, Feeley M. Effects of caffeine on human health. Food Addit Contam 2003;20(1):1–30

91. Cnattingius S, Signorello LB, Annerén G, et al. Caffeine intake and the risk of first-trimester spontaneous abortion. N Engl J Med 2000;343(25):1839–1845

92. Giannelli M, Doyle P, Roman E, Pelerin M, Hermon C. The effect of caffeine consumption and nausea on the risk of miscarriage. Paediatr Perinat Epidemiol 2003;17(4):316–323

93. Rasch V. Cigarette, alcohol, and caffeine consumption: risk factors for spontaneous abortion. Acta Obstet Gynecol Scand 2003;82(2):182–188

94. Wen W, Shu XO, Jacobs DR Jr, Brown JE. The associations of maternal caffeine consumption and nausea with spontaneous abortion. Epidemiology 2001; 12(1):38–42

95. Weng X, Odouli R, Li DK. Maternal caffeine consumption during pregnancy and the risk of miscarriage: a prospective cohort study. Am J Obstet Gynecol 2008;198(3):279.e1–8

96. Fenster L, Hubbard AE, Swan SH, et al. Caffeinated beverages, decaffeinated coffee, and spontaneous abortion. Epidemiology 1997;8(5):515–523

97. Mills JL, Holmes LB, Aarons JH, et al. Moderate caffeine use and the risk of spontaneous abortion and intrauterine growth retardation. JAMA 1993;269(5): 593–597

98. Savitz DA, Chan RL, Herring AH, Howards PP, Hartmann KE. Caffeine and miscarriage risk. Epidemiology 2008;19(1):55–62

99. Klebanoff MA, Levine RJ, DerSimonian R, Clemens JD, Wilkins DG. Maternal serum paraxanthine, a caffeine metabolite, and the risk of spontaneous abortion. N Engl J Med 1999;341(22):1639–1644

100. Leviton A, Cowan L. A review of the literature relating caffeine consumption by women to their risk of reproductive hazards. Food Chem Toxicol 2002; 40(9):1271–1310

101. Bracken MB, Triche E, Grosso L, Hellenbrand K, Belanger K, Leaderer BP. Heterogeneity in assessing self-reports of caffeine exposure: implications for studies of health effects. Epidemiology 2002; 13(2):165–171

102. Martin TR, Bracken MB. The association between low birth weight and caffeine consumption during pregnancy. Am J Epidemiol 1987;126(5):813–821

103. Peacock JL, Bland JM, Anderson HR. Effects on birthweight of alcohol and caffeine consumption in smoking women. J Epidemiol Community Health 1991;45(2):159–163

104. Bracken MB, Triche EW, Belanger K, Hellenbrand K, Leaderer BP. Association of maternal caffeine consumption with decrements in fetal growth. Am J Epidemiol 2003;157(5):456–466

105. Bech BH, Obel C, Henriksen TB, Olsen J. Effect of reducing caffeine intake on birth weight and length of gestation: randomised controlled trial. BMJ 2007; 334(7590):409

106. Christian MS, Brent RL. Teratogen update: evaluation of the reproductive and developmental risks of caffeine. Teratology 2001;64(1):51–78

107. Browne ML. Maternal exposure to caffeine and risk of congenital anomalies: a systematic review. Epidemiology 2006;17(3):324–331

108. American Academy of Pediatrics Committee on Drugs. Transfer of drugs and other chemicals into human milk. Pediatrics 2001;108(3):776–789

109. Novak K, ed. Drug Facts and Comparisons. St. Louis: Wolters Kluwer Health; 2005

110. Engebretsen KM, Harris CR. Caffeine and Related Nonprescription Sympathomimetics. In: Ford MD, et al., eds. Clinical Toxicology. Philadelphia: WB Saunders; 2001:310–315

111. Juliano LM, Griffiths RR. A critical review of caffeine withdrawal: empirical validation of symptoms and signs, incidence, severity, and associated features. Psychopharmacology (Berl) 2004;176(1):1–29

112. Dews PB, Curtis GL, Hanford KJ, O'Brien CP. The frequency of caffeine withdrawal in a population-based survey and in a controlled, blinded pilot experiment. J Clin Pharmacol 1999;39(12):1221–1232

113. Carrillo JA, Benitez J. Clinically significant pharmaco-kinetic interactions between dietary caffeine and medications. Clin Pharmacokinet 2000;39(2):127–153

114. Faber MS, Fuhr U. Time response of cytochrome P450 1A2 activity on cessation of heavy smoking. Clin Pharmacol Ther 2004;76(2):178–184

115. Barger-Lux MJ, Heaney RP. Caffeine and the calcium economy revisited. Osteoporos Int 1995;5(2):97–102

116. Hasling C, Søndergaard K, Charles P, Mosekilde L. Calcium metabolism in postmenopausal osteoporotic women is determined by dietary calcium and coffee intake. J Nutr 1992;122(5):1119–1126

117. Heaney RP. Effects of caffeine on bone and the calcium economy. Food Chem Toxicol 2002;40(9):1263–1270

118. Harris SS, Dawson-Hughes B. Caffeine and bone loss in healthy postmenopausal women. Am J Clin Nutr 1994;60(4):573–578

119. Rapuri PB, Gallagher JC, Kinyamu HK, Ryschon KL. Caffeine intake increases the rate of bone loss in elderly women and interacts with vitamin D receptor genotypes. Am J Clin Nutr 2001;74(5):694–700

120. Fujiwara S, Kasagi F, Yamada M, Kodama K. Risk factors for hip fracture in a Japanese cohort. J Bone Miner Res 1997;12(7):998–1004

121. Huopio J, Kröger H, Honkanen R, Saarikoski S, Alhava E. Risk factors for perimenopausal fractures: a prospective study. Osteoporos Int 2000;11(3):219–227

122. Meyer HE, Pedersen JI, Løken EB, Tverdal A. Dietary factors and the incidence of hip fracture in middle-aged Norwegians. A prospective study. Am J Epidemiol 1997;145(2):117–123

123. Kiel DP, Felson DT, Hannan MT, Anderson JJ, Wilson PW. Caffeine and the risk of hip fracture: the Framingham Study. Am J Epidemiol 1990;132(4):675–684

124. Hernandez-Avila M, Colditz GA, Stampfer MJ, Rosner B, Speizer FE, Willett WC. Caffeine, moderate alcohol intake, and risk of fractures of the hip and forearm in middle-aged women. Am J Clin Nutr 1991;54(1):157–163

125. Cummings SR, Nevitt MC, Browner WS, et al; Study of Osteoporotic Fractures Research Group. Risk factors for hip fracture in white women. N Engl J Med 1995;332(12):767–773

126. Hallström H, Wolk A, Glynn A, Michaëlsson K. Coffee, tea and caffeine consumption in relation to osteoporotic fracture risk in a cohort of Swedish women. Osteoporos Int 2006;17(7):1055–1064

127. Fairweather-Tait SJ. Iron nutrition in the UK: getting the balance right. Proc Nutr Soc 2004;63(4):519–528

128. Morck TA, Lynch SR, Cook JD. Inhibition of food iron absorption by coffee. Am J Clin Nutr 1983;37(3):416–420

129. Hallberg L, Rossander L. Effect of different drinks on the absorption of non-heme iron from composite meals. Hum Nutr Appl Nutr 1982;36(2):116–123

7 Tea

Tea is an infusion of the leaves of the *Camellia sinensis* plant and is the most widely consumed beverage in the world, aside from water.[1] Herbal teas are infusions of herbs or plants other than *Camellia sinensis* and will not be discussed in this article. Although tea contains several bioactive chemicals, including caffeine and fluoride, scientists are particularly interested in the potential health benefits of a class of compounds in tea known as *flavonoids*. In many cultures, tea is an important source of dietary flavonoids.

Definitions

Types of Tea

All teas are derived from the leaves of *Camellia sinensis*, but different processing methods produce different types of tea. Fresh tea leaves are rich in flavonoids known as *catechins* (**Fig. 7.1**). Tea leaves also contain polyphenol oxidase enzymes in separate compartments from catechins. When tea leaves are intentionally broken or rolled during processing, contact with polyphenol oxidase causes catechins to join together, forming dimers and polymers known as *theaflavins* (**Fig. 7.2**) and *thearubigins*, respectively. This

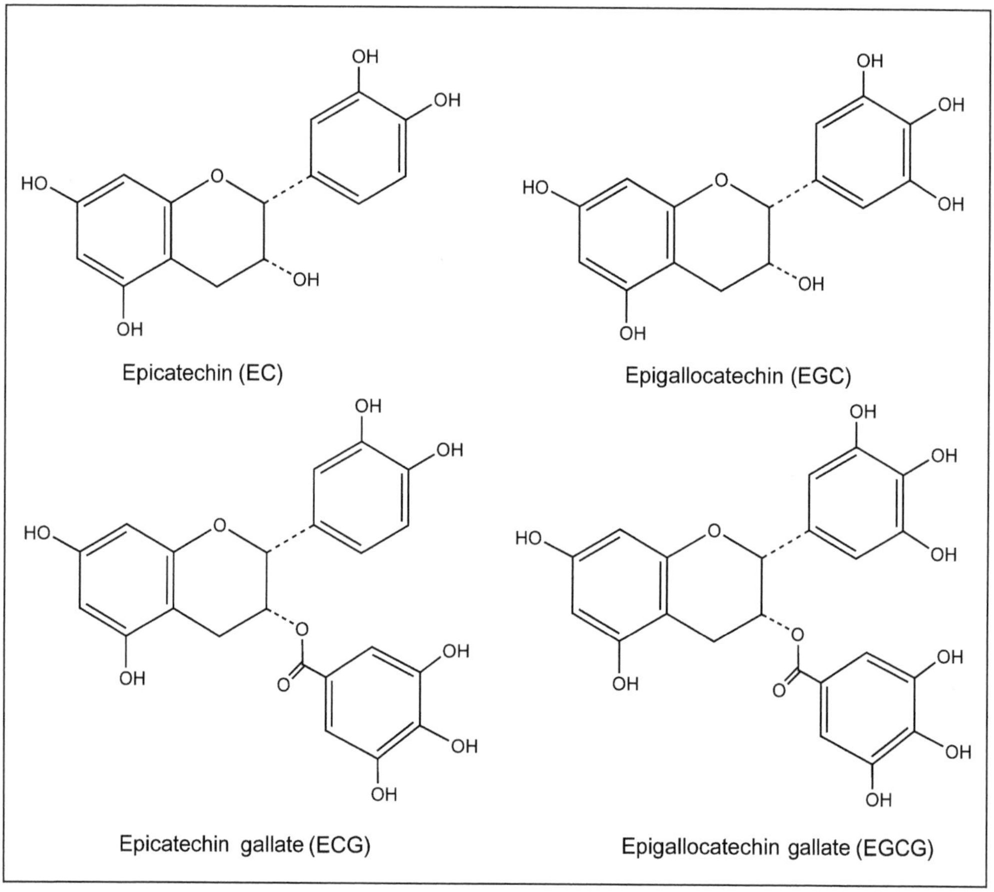

Epicatechin (EC)

Epigallocatechin (EGC)

Epicatechin gallate (ECG)

Epigallocatechin gallate (EGCG)

Fig. 7.1 Chemical structures of the principal catechins in tea.

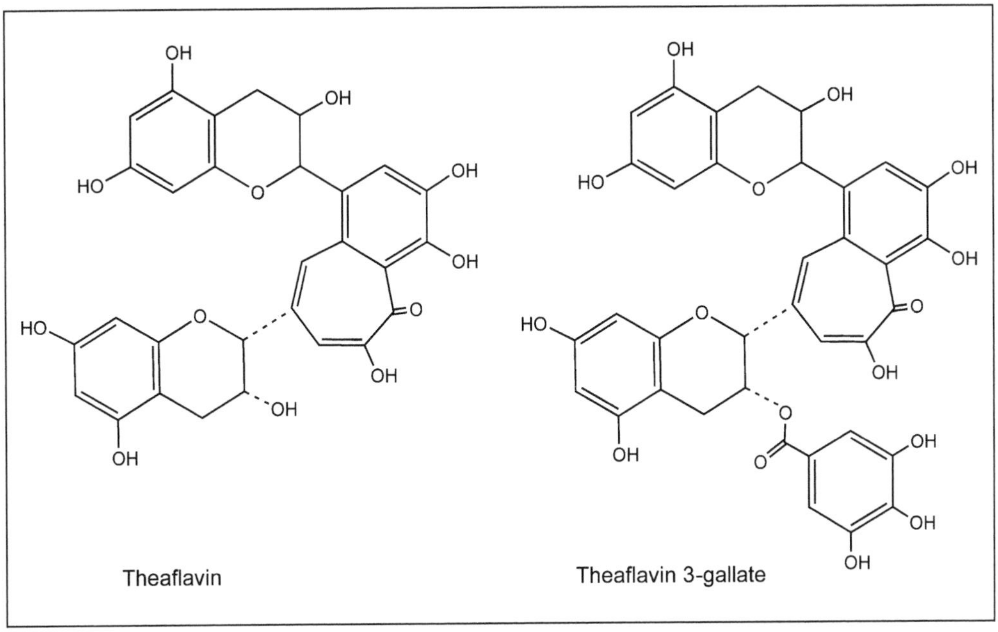

Fig. 7.2 Chemical structures of some theaflavins in tea.

oxidation process is known (incorrectly) in the tea industry as "fermentation." Steaming or firing tea leaves inactivates polyphenol oxidase and stops the oxidation process.[2] Although there are thousands of tea varieties, teas may be divided into three groups based on the amount of oxidation they undergo during processing.

Unfermented Teas (White and Green Teas)

White tea is made from buds and young leaves, which are steamed or fired to inactivate polyphenol oxidase, and then dried. Thus, due to minimal oxidation, white tea retains the high concentrations of catechins present in fresh tea leaves. Green tea is made from more mature tea leaves than white tea, and tea leaves may be withered prior to steaming or firing. Although they are also rich in catechins, green teas may have catechin profiles that are different from those of white teas, with slightly higher levels of oxidation products.[3]

Semifermented Teas (Oolong Teas)

Tea leaves destined to become oolong teas are "bruised" to allow the release of some of the polyphenol oxidase present in the leaves. Oolong teas are allowed to oxidize to a greater extent than white or green teas, but for less time than

black teas, before they are heated and dried. Consequently, the catechin, theaflavin, and thearubigin levels in oolong teas are generally between those of green/white teas and completely oxidized black teas.[2]

Fully Fermented Teas (Black Teas)

Tea leaves that are destined to become black tea are fully rolled or broken to maximize the interaction between catechins and polyphenol oxidase. Because they are allowed to oxidize completely before drying, most black teas are rich in theaflavins and thearubigins, but relatively low in monomeric catechins, such as epigallocatechin gallate (EGCG).[4]

Cup Sizes

The definition of a cup of tea varies in different countries or regions. In Japan, a typical cup of green tea may contain only 100 mL (3.5 oz). A traditional European teacup holds approximately 125–150 mL (5 oz), while a mug of tea may contain 235 mL (8 oz) or more.

Table 7.1 Caffeine content of teas and coffee[5,6]

Type of Tea/Coffee	Caffeine (mg/L)	Caffeine (mg/8 oz)
Green	40–211	9–50
Black	177–303	42–72
Coffee, brewed	306–553	72–130

Table 7.2 Fluoride content of teas[12]

Type of Tea	Fluoride (mg/L)[a]	Fluoride (mg/8 oz)
Green	1.2–1.7	0.3–0.4
Oolong	0.6–1.0	0.1–0.2
Black	1.0–1.9	0.2–0.5
Brick tea	2.2–7.3	0.5–1.7

[a] Fluoride in 1% w/v tea prepared by continuous infusion from 5 to 360 minutes.

Bioactive Compounds in Tea

Flavonoids

Flavanols are the most abundant class of flavonoids in all types of tea. Flavanol monomers are also known as *catechins*. The principal catechins found in white and green tea are epicatechin (EC), epigallocatechin (EGC), epicatechin gallate (ECG), and epigallocatechin gallate (EGCG) (**Fig. 7.1**).[2] In oolong and black teas, theaflavins (**Fig. 7.2**) and thearubigins are more abundant. Tea is also a good source of another class of flavonoids called *flavonols*. Flavonols found in tea include kaempferol, quercetin, and myricetin. The flavonol content of tea is minimally affected by processing, and flavonols are present in comparable quantities in all teas. Unlike flavanols, flavonols are usually present in tea as glycosides (bound to a sugar molecule).

Caffeine

All teas contain caffeine, unless they are deliberately decaffeinated during processing. The caffeine content of different varieties of tea may vary considerably and is influenced by factors like brewing time, the amount of tea and water used for brewing, and whether the tea is loose or in teabags. In general, a mug of tea contains about half as much caffeine as a mug of coffee.[4] The caffeine contents of more than 20 green and black teas prepared according to package directions are presented in **Table 7.1**.[5] The caffeine content of oolong teas is comparable to green teas.[3] There is little information on the caffeine content of white teas, since they are often grouped together with green teas. Buds and young tea leaves have been found to contain higher levels of caffeine than older leaves,[8] suggesting that the caffeine content of some white teas may be slightly higher than that of green teas.[3] See Chapter 6 on Coffee for more information on caffeine.

Fluoride

Tea plants accumulate fluoride in their leaves. In general, the oldest tea leaves contain the most fluoride.[9] Most high-quality teas are made from the bud or the first two to four leaves—the youngest leaves on the plant. Brick tea, a lower quality tea, is made from the oldest tea leaves and is often very high in fluoride. Symptoms of fluoride excess (i.e., dental and skeletal fluorosis) have been observed in Tibetan children and adults who consume large amounts of brick tea.[10,11] Unlike brick tea, fluoride levels in green, oolong, and black teas are generally comparable to those recommended for the prevention of dental caries (cavities). Thus, daily consumption of up to 1 L of green, oolong, or black tea would be unlikely to result in fluoride intakes higher than those recommended for dental health.[12,13] The fluoride content of white tea is likely to be less than that of other teas, since white teas are made from the buds and youngest leaves of the tea plant. The fluoride contents of 17 brands of green, oolong, and black teas are presented in **Table 7.2**.[12] These values do not include the fluoride content of the water used to make the tea.

Disease Prevention

Cardiovascular Disease

Epidemiological Studies

Many epidemiological studies have examined associations between tea consumption and manifestations of cardiovascular disease, including myocardial infarction (MI) and stroke. A meta-analysis that combined the results of ten prospective cohort studies and seven case–control studies found that a 24-oz increase in daily tea consumption was associated with an 11% decrease in the risk of MI.[14] However, caution was urged in the interpretation of these results because of bias toward the publication of studies suggesting a protective effect. Since then, the results of several other prospective cohort studies have been mixed. A 6-year study of Dutch men and women found that those who drank at least three cups (approx. 13 oz) daily had a significantly lower risk of MI than those who did not drink tea.[15] A 7-year study of US women found that the risk of important vascular events (MI, stroke, or death from cardiovascular disease) was significantly lower in a small number of women who drank at least four cups of black tea daily.[16] However, the sample size in this group was very limited and thus the significance of this finding is unclear. A 15-year study of US men found no association between tea consumption and cardiovascular disease risk, but tea consumption in this population was relatively low, averaging one cup per day.[17] Overall, the available research suggests that consumption of at least three cups per day of black tea may be associated with a modest decrease in the risk of MI. A recent prospective cohort study in 40 530 Japanese adults reported that green tea consumption was associated with reductions in all-cause mortality and cardiovascular-related mortality.[18] Specifically, when compared with drinking less than one cup per day, consumption of up to five cups of green tea daily was associated with a 16% reduction in mortality from all causes and a 26% reduction in mortality from cardiovascular diseases. Both relationships were stronger in women than in men, and among types of cardiovascular diseases, the inverse association was strongest for stroke mortality.[18] Thus, green tea may also protect against the development of cardiovascular diseases, but more research is necessary to draw any firm conclusions.

Endothelial Function

Vascular endothelial cells play an important role in maintaining cardiovascular health by producing nitric oxide, a compound that promotes arterial relaxation (vasodilation).[19] Arterial vasodilation resulting from endothelial production of nitric oxide is termed *endothelium-dependent vasodilation*. Two controlled clinical trials found that the daily consumption of four to five cups (900–1250 mL) of black tea for four weeks significantly improved endothelium-dependent vasodilation

in patients with coronary artery disease[20] and in patients with mildly elevated serum cholesterol levels[21] compared with the equivalent amount of hot water. One of these studies noted that caffeine, provided at an equivalent dose to that of tea, had no short-term effects on endothelium-dependent vasodilation, suggesting that non-caffeine components of black tea may be responsible for the reported short-term vasodilatory effects. Indeed, flavonoids contained in tea may exert such effects.[22] See Chapter 11 for more information on Flavonoids. Several small studies have suggested that green tea, or its major catechin, EGCG, may have similar vasodilatory effects.[23-25] The beneficial effect of tea consumption on vascular endothelial function could help explain the modest reduction in cardiovascular disease risk observed in some epidemiological studies.

Cancer

Animal Studies

Green and black tea have been found to have cancer-preventive activity in a variety of animal models of cancer, including cancer of the skin, lung, mouth, esophagus, stomach, colon, pancreas, bladder, and prostate.[26,27] Additionally, white tea and green tea were shown to suppress intestinal polyps in mice. In most cases, flavonoids appear to contribute substantially to the cancer-preventing effects of tea, but caffeine has also been found to have cancer-preventing activity in some animal models of skin,[28] lung,[29] and colon[30] cancer. Although the beneficial effects of tea flavonoids were often attributed to their antioxidant activity, the overall contribution of tea flavonoids to plasma and tissue antioxidant activity in humans is now thought to be relatively minor.[31] Currently, scientists are focusing their attention on the potential for tea flavonoids to modulate cell-signaling pathways that promote the transformation of healthy cells to cancerous cells.[32,33] See Chapter 11 for more information on flavonoids.

Epidemiological Studies

Despite promising results from animal studies, it is not clear whether increasing tea consumption will help prevent cancers in humans. The results of numerous epidemiological studies, focusing on many different types of cancers, do not provide any consistent evidence that consumption of green or black tea is associated with significant reductions in cancer risk.[34] A recent prospective cohort study in 40530 Japanese adults participating in the Ohsaki National Health Insurance Cohort Study reported that green tea consumption was not associated with total cancer mortality, or mortality from gastric, lung, or colorectal cancers.[18] Because tea comes into direct contact with the gastrointestinal tract, scientists have been particularly interested in whether increased tea consumption may prevent cancers of the stomach and colon. Although a few case–control studies suggested that higher intakes of green tea were associated with decreased stomach cancer risk[35-37], prospective cohort studies do not support an inverse association between green tea consumption and stomach cancer risk in Japanese men and women.[38-42] Despite promising findings in animal models of colon cancer,[43] the majority of epidemiological studies have not found tea consumption to be associated with lower risk for colorectal cancer.[44,45] A meta-analysis of case–control and prospective studies concluded that currently available data do not suggest that either green or black tea is protective against colorectal cancer.[46] More recently, a systematic review of 51 studies, including more than 1.6 million participants, concluded that there is no convincing evidence that green tea consumption prevents various types of cancer.[47]

There are several possible reasons for the discrepancies between findings from animal models of cancer and epidemiological studies in humans. Aside from potential species differences, it may be difficult for humans drinking tea to reach sufficient plasma and tissue levels of tea flavonoids to realize a protective effect. In general, flavonoids are rapidly metabolized and eliminated from the body, but there is considerable variation among individuals in this respect.[48] Catechol-O-methyltransferase (COMT) is one of the enzymes involved in flavonoid metabolism. There are two forms of the gene for COMT—a low-activity form and a high-activity form. A case–control study found that higher intakes of green tea were as-sociated with lower breast cancer risk only in women who had inherited at least one copy of the low-activity form of COMT, suggesting that those who are less efficient at eliminating green tea flavonoids may be more likely to benefit from their consumption.[49] Relationships between tea consumption and cancer risk are likely to be complex, and further study is needed before specific recommendations can be made regarding tea consumption and cancer prevention.

Osteoporosis

Many factors can affect the development of osteoporosis, including nutrition, physical activity, and genetic factors. Components in tea, including caffeine, fluoride, and flavonoids, may influence bone mineral density (BMD).[50] Although one cross-sectional study found that black tea consumption was associated with slightly lower BMD in US women,[51] three other cross-sectional studies found that habitual tea consumption was associated with higher BMD in British[52] and Canadian women[53] and in Taiwanese men and women.[50] A prospective study in 164 elderly women found that consumption of tea blunted the age-related loss in total-hip BMD.[54] Hip fracture is one of the most serious consequences of osteoporosis. A large case–control study in Mediterranean countries found that low tea consumption was associated with higher risk of hip fracture in men[55] and women.[56] However, two large prospective cohort studies of US women found no relationship between tea consumption and the risk of hip or wrist fracture over 4–6 years of follow-up.[57,58] The most recent of these two studies found that higher tea intakes were associated with slightly higher BMD in postmenopausal women, but this finding did not translate into a lower risk of hip or wrist fracture.[57] Further study is required to determine whether tea consumption affects the development of osteoporosis or the risk of osteoporotic fracture in a meaningful way.

Dental Caries

Fluoride concentrations in tea are comparable to those recommended for US water supplies to prevent dental caries (cavities).[59] Green, black, and oolong tea extracts have been found to inhibit the growth and acid production of cavity-producing bacteria in the test tube.[60–62] Although tea extracts reportedly prevent or decrease dental caries in animal models,[63] few published studies have examined the effect of tea consumption on dental caries in humans. A cross-sectional study of more than 6000 14-year old children in the United Kingdom found that those who drank tea had significantly fewer dental caries than nondrinkers; results were independent of whether sugar was added to tea.[64]

Kidney Stones

Two large prospective studies found that the risk of developing symptomatic kidney stones decreased by 8% in women[65] and 14% in men[66] for each 8-oz (235 mL) mug of tea consumed daily. A study in rats concluded that the antioxidants in green tea may be involved in inhibiting calcium oxalate precipitation and thus kidney stone formation.[67] The implications of these findings for individuals with a previous history of calcium oxalate stone formation are unclear. High fluid intake, including tea intake, is generally considered the most effective and economical means of preventing kidney stones.[68] However, tea consumption has been found to increase urinary oxalate levels in healthy individuals,[69] and some experts continue to advise people with a history of calcium oxalate stones to limit tea consumption.[70]

Weight Loss

Weight reduction can be achieved by long-term decreases in energy intake and/or increases in energy expenditure. Several small short-term trials have reported modest 3%–4% increases in energy expenditure after the consumption of oolong tea[71,72] or green tea extract.[73] However, none of these studies was specifically designed to assess weight loss. More recently, a clinical trial in overweight men and women, who had lost an average of 7.5% of their body weight by adhering to a very low-calorie diet for 4 weeks, found that green tea capsules (containing 573 mg/day of catechins and 104 mg/day of caffeine) were no better than placebo in preventing weight regain over the next 8 weeks.[74] A follow-up study by the same group of investigators reported that supplementation with green tea extract prevented weight regain after weight loss in subjects with low habitual caffeine intake (<300 mg/day) but not in those with high habitual caffeine intake (>300 mg/day).[75] A recent 12-week intervention trial in 35 overweight men reported that those given oolong tea enriched with green tea extract (690 mg catechins/day) experienced significant reductions in body weight, body mass index (BMI), waist circumference, body fat mass, and subcutaneous fat area compared with those administered oolong tea (33 mg catechins/day).[76] Large-scale intervention trials that control for energy intake and physical activity are needed to determine if tea or tea extracts promote weight loss or improve maintenance in humans. Interestingly, animal model studies showed a lowering of tissue fat levels in mice drinking green tea, black tea, or a caffeine-containing solution.[28]

Safety

Adverse Effects

Tea

Tea is generally considered to be safe, even in large amounts. However, two cases of hypokalemia (abnormally low serum potassium levels) in the elderly have been attributed to excessive consumption of black and oolong tea (3–14 L/day).[77,78] Hypokalemia is a potentially life-threatening condition that has been associated with caffeine toxicity.

Tea Extracts

In clinical trials employing caffeinated green tea extracts, cancer patients who took 6 g/day, in three to six divided doses, experienced mild to moderate gastrointestinal side effects, including nausea, vomiting, abdominal pain, and diarrhea.[79,80] Central nervous system symptoms, including agitation, restlessness, insomnia, tremors, dizziness, and confusion, have also been reported. In one case, confusion was severe enough to require hospitalization.[79] These side effects were likely related to the caffeine in the green tea extract.[80] In a 4-week clinical trial that assessed the safety of decaffeinated green tea extracts (800 mg/day of EGCG) in healthy individuals, a few of the participants reported mild nausea, stomach upset, dizziness, or muscle pain.[81]

Pregnancy and Lactation

The safety of tea extracts or supplements for pregnant or breast-feeding women has not been established. Some organizations advise pregnant women to limit their caffeine consumption to 300 mg/day, because higher caffeine intakes have been associated with increased risk of miscarriage and lower birth weight in some epidemiological studies. See Chapter 6 on coffee.

Drug Interactions

Green Tea

Excessive green tea consumption may decrease the therapeutic effects of the anticoagulant, warfarin (Coumadin). Such an effect was documented in one patient who began drinking one half gallon to one gallon of green tea daily.[82] It is probably not necessary for people on warfarin therapy to avoid green tea entirely; however, large quantities of green tea may decrease warfarin's effectiveness.[83]

Caffeine

Several drugs can impair the metabolism of caffeine, increasing the potential for adverse effects from caffeine.[84] Such drugs include cimetidine (Tagamet), disulfiram (Antabuse), estrogens, fluoroquinolone antibiotics (e.g., ciprofloxacin, enoxacin, norfloxacin), fluconazole (Diflucan), fluvoxamine (Luvox), mexiletine (Mexitil), riluzol (Rilutek), terbinafine (Lamisil), and verapamil (Calan). High caffeine intakes may increase the risk of toxicity of some drugs, including albuterol (Alupent), clozapine (Clozaril), ephedrine, epinephrine, monoamine oxidase inhibitors, phenylpropanolamine, and theophylline. Abrupt caffeine withdrawal has been found to increase serum lithium levels in people taking lithium, potentially increasing the risk of lithium toxicity. See Chapter 6 for more information on caffeine–drug interactions.

Nutrient Interactions

Nonheme Iron

Flavonoids in tea can bind nonheme iron, inhibiting its intestinal absorption. Nonheme iron is the principal form of iron in plant foods, dairy products, and iron supplements. The consumption of one cup of tea with a meal has been found to decrease the absorption of nonheme iron in that meal by approximately 70%.[85,86] To maximize iron absorption from a meal or iron supplements, tea should not be consumed at the same time.

Summary

- Tea is an infusion of the leaves of the *Camellia sinensis* plant, which is not to be confused with so-called herbal teas.
- Some biologically active chemicals in tea include flavonoids, caffeine, and fluoride.
- Overall, observational studies in humans suggest that daily consumption of at least three cups of tea may be associated with a modest (11%) decrease in the risk of myocardial infarction (heart attack).
- Despite promising results from animal studies, it is not clear whether increasing tea consumption will help prevent cancers in humans.
- Although tea consumption has been positively associated with bone density in some studies, it is not clear whether tea consumption reduces the risk of fractures due to osteoporosis.
- Limited research suggests that tea consumption may be associated with fewer cavities and a slightly lower risk of kidney stones, but more research is needed to confirm these findings.
- It is currently unclear whether tea or tea extracts promote weight loss. Large-scale clinical trials that control for energy intake and expenditure are needed to answer this question.

References

1. Graham HN. Green tea composition, consumption, and polyphenol chemistry. Prev Med 1992;21(3):334–350
2. Balentine DA, Paetau-Robinson I. Tea as a source of dietary antioxidants with a potential role in prevention of chronic diseases. In: Mazza G, Oomah BD, eds. Herbs, Botanicals, & Teas. Lancaster: Technomic Publishing Co., Inc.; 2000:265–287
3. Santana-Rios G, Orner GA, Amantana A, Provost C, Wu SY, Dashwood RH. Potent antimutagenic activity of white tea in comparison with green tea in the Salmonella assay. Mutat Res 2001;495(1–2):61–74
4. Lakenbrink C, Lapczynski S, Maiwald B, Engelhardt UH. Flavonoids and other polyphenols in consumer brews of tea and other caffeinated beverages. J Agric Food Chem 2000;48(7):2848–2852
5. Astill C, Birch MR, Dacombe C, Humphrey PG, Martin PT. Factors affecting the caffeine and polyphenol contents of black and green tea infusions. J Agric Food Chem 2001;49(11):5340–5347

6. McCusker RR, Goldberger BA, Cone EJ. Caffeine content of specialty coffees. J Anal Toxicol 2003;27(7): 520–522

7. Lin JK, Lin CL, Liang YC, Lin-Shiau SY, Juan IM. Survey of catechins, gallic acid, and methylxanthines in green, oolong, pu-erh, and black teas. J Agric Food Chem 1998;46(9):3635–3642

8. Lin YS, Tsai YJ, Tsay JS, Lin JK. Factors affecting the levels of tea polyphenols and caffeine in tea leaves. J Agric Food Chem 2003;51(7):1864–1873

9. Wong MH, Fung KF, Carr HP. Aluminium and fluoride contents of tea, with emphasis on brick tea and their health implications. Toxicol Lett 2003;137(1–2):111–120

10. Cao J, Bai X, Zhao Y, et al. The relationship of fluorosis and brick tea drinking in Chinese Tibetans. Environ Health Perspect 1996;104(12):1340–1343

11. Cao J, Zhao Y, Liu J, et al. Brick tea fluoride as a main source of adult fluorosis. Food Chem Toxicol 2003;41(4):535–542

12. Fung KF, Zhang ZQ, Wong JWC, Wong MH. Fluoride contents in tea and soil from tea plantations and the release of fluoride into tea liquor during infusion. Environ Pollut 1999;104(2):197–205

13. Cao J, Luo SF, Liu JW, Li YH. Safety evaluation on fluoride content in black tea. Food Chem 2004;88(2):233–236

14. Peters U, Poole C, Arab L. Does tea affect cardiovascular disease? A meta-analysis. Am J Epidemiol 2001;154(6):495–503

15. Geleijnse JM, Launer LJ, Van der Kuip DA, Hofman A, Witteman JC. Inverse association of tea and flavonoid intakes with incident myocardial infarction: the Rotterdam Study. Am J Clin Nutr 2002;75(5):880–886

16. Sesso HD, Gaziano JM, Liu S, Buring JE. Flavonoid intake and the risk of cardiovascular disease in women. Am J Clin Nutr 2003;77(6):1400–1408

17. Sesso HD, Paffenbarger RS Jr, Oguma Y, Lee IM. Lack of association between tea and cardiovascular disease in college alumni. Int J Epidemiol 2003;32(4):527–533

18. Kuriyama S, Shimazu T, Ohmori K, et al. Green tea consumption and mortality due to cardiovascular disease, cancer, and all causes in Japan: the Ohsaki study. JAMA 2006;296(10):1255–1265

19. Vita JA. Tea consumption and cardiovascular disease: effects on endothelial function. J Nutr 2003; 133(10):3293S–3297S

20. Duffy SJ, Keaney JF Jr, Holbrook M, et al. Short- and long-term black tea consumption reverses endothelial dysfunction in patients with coronary artery disease. Circulation 2001;104(2):151–156

21. Hodgson JM, Puddey IB, Burke V, Watts GF, Beilin LJ. Regular ingestion of black tea improves brachial artery vasodilator function. Clin Sci (Lond) 2002; 102(2):195–201

22. Vita JA. Polyphenols and cardiovascular disease: effects on endothelial and platelet function. Am J Clin Nutr 2005; 81(1, Suppl):292S–297S

23. Nagaya N, Yamamoto H, Uematsu M, et al. Green tea reverses endothelial dysfunction in healthy smokers. Heart 2004;90(12):1485–1486

24. Kim W, Jeong MH, Cho SH, et al. Effect of green tea consumption on endothelial function and circulating endothelial progenitor cells in chronic smokers. Circ J 2006;70(8):1052–1057

25. Widlansky ME, Hamburg NM, Anter E, et al. Acute EGCG supplementation reverses endothelial dysfunction in patients with coronary artery disease. J Am Coll Nutr 2007;26(2):95–102

26. Lambert JD, Yang CS. Mechanisms of cancer prevention by tea constituents. J Nutr 2003;133(10):3262S–3267S

27. Yang CS, Maliakal P, Meng X. Inhibition of carcinogenesis by tea. Annu Rev Pharmacol Toxicol 2002;42:25–54

28. Lu YP, Lou YR, Lin Y, et al. Inhibitory effects of orally administered green tea, black tea, and caffeine on skin carcinogenesis in mice previously treated with ultraviolet B light (high-risk mice): relationship to decreased tissue fat. Cancer Res 2001;61(13):5002–5009

29. Chung FL, Wang M, Rivenson A, et al. Inhibition of lung carcinogenesis by black tea in Fischer rats treated with a tobacco-specific carcinogen: caffeine as an important constituent. Cancer Res 1998;58(18):4096–4101

30. Carter O, Dashwood RH, Wang R, et al. Comparison of white tea, green tea, epigallocatechin-3-gallate, and caffeine as inhibitors of PhIP-induced colonic aberrant crypts. Nutr Cancer 2007;58(1):60–65

31. Williams RJ, Spencer JP, Rice-Evans C. Flavonoids: antioxidants or signalling molecules? Free Radic Biol Med 2004;36(7):838–849

32. Hou Z, Lambert JD, Chin KV, Yang CS. Effects of tea polyphenols on signal transduction pathways related to cancer chemoprevention. Mutat Res 2004;555(1–2):3–19

33. Khan N, Afaq F, Saleem M, Ahmad N, Mukhtar H. Targeting multiple signaling pathways by green tea polyphenol (-)-epigallocatechin-3-gallate. Cancer Res 2006;66(5):2500–2505

34. Higdon JV, Frei B. Tea catechins and polyphenols: health effects, metabolism, and antioxidant functions. Crit Rev Food Sci Nutr 2003;43(1):89–143

35. Kono S, Ikeda M, Tokudome S, Kuratsme M. A case control study of gastric cancer and diet in northern Kyushu, Japan. Jpn J Cancer Res 1988;79:1067–1074

36. Setiawan VW, Zhang Zf, Yu GP, et al. Protective effect of green tea on the risks of chronic gastritis and stomach cancer. Int J Cancer 2001; 92:600–604

37. Yu GP, Hsieh CC, Wang LY, Yu St, Li XL, Jin TH. Green tea consumption and risk of stomach cancer: a population-based case control study in Shanghai, China. Cancer Causes Control 1995;6:532–538

38. Hoshiyama Y, Kawaguchi T, Miura Y, et al; Japan Collaborative Cohort Study Group. A nested case-control study of stomach cancer in relation to green tea consumption in Japan. Br J Cancer 2004;90(1):135–138

39. Koizumi Y, Tsubono Y, Nakaya N, et al. No association between green tea and the risk of gastric cancer: pooled analysis of two prospective studies in Japan. Cancer Epidemiol Biomarkers Prev 2003;12(5):472–473

40. Hoshiyama Y, Kawaguchi T, Miura Y, et al; Japan Collaborative Cohort Study Group. A prospective study of stomach cancer death in relation to green tea consumption in Japan. Br J Cancer 2002;87(3):309–313

41. Tsubono Y, Nishino Y, Komatsu S, et al. Green tea and the risk of gastric cancer in Japan. N Engl J Med 2001;344(9):632–636

42. Hoshiyama Y, Kawaguchi T, Miura Y, et al; JACC Study Group. Green tea and stomach cancer—a short review of prospective studies. J Epidemiol 2005;15(Suppl 2):S109–S112

43. Orner GA, Dashwood WM, Blum CA, Díaz GD, Li Q, Dashwood RH. Suppression of tumorigenesis in the Apc(min) mouse: down-regulation of beta-catenin signaling by a combination of tea plus sulindac. Carcinogenesis 2003;24(2):263–267

44. Arab L, Il'yasova D. The epidemiology of tea consumption and colorectal cancer incidence. J Nutr 2003; 133(10):3310S–3318S
45. Tavani A, La Vecchia C. Coffee, decaffeinated coffee, tea and cancer of the colon and rectum: a review of epidemiological studies, 1990–2003. Cancer Causes Control 2004;15(8):743–757
46. Sun CL, Yuan JM, Koh WP, Yu MC. Green tea, black tea and colorectal cancer risk: a meta-analysis of epidemiologic studies. Carcinogenesis 2006;27(7):1301–1309
47. Boehm K, Borrelli F, Ernst E, et al. Green tea (Camellia sinensis) for the prevention of cancer. Cochrane Database Syst Rev 2009; (3):CD005004
48. Manach C, Scalbert A, Morand C, Rémésy C, Jiménez L. Polyphenols: food sources and bioavailability. Am J Clin Nutr 2004;79(5):727–747
49. Wu AH, Tseng CC, Van Den Berg D, Yu MC. Tea intake, COMT genotype, and breast cancer in Asian-American women. Cancer Res 2003;63(21):7526–7529
50. Wu CH, Yang YC, Yao WJ, Lu FH, Wu JS, Chang CJ. Epidemiological evidence of increased bone mineral density in habitual tea drinkers. Arch Intern Med 2002;162(9):1001–1006
51. Hernández-Avila M, Stampfer MJ, Ravnikar VA, et al. Caffeine and other predictors of bone density among pre- and perimenopausal women. Epidemiology 1993;4(2):128–134
52. Hegarty VM, May HM, Khaw KT. Tea drinking and bone mineral density in older women. Am J Clin Nutr 2000;71(4):1003–1007
53. Hoover PA, Webber CE, Beaumont LF, Blake JM. Postmenopausal bone mineral density: relationship to calcium intake, calcium absorption, residual estrogen, body composition, and physical activity. Can J Physiol Pharmacol 1996;74(8):911–917
54. Devine A, Hodgson JM, Dick IM, Prince RL. Tea drinking is associated with benefits on bone density in older women. Am J Clin Nutr 2007;86(4):1243–1247
55. Kanis J, Johnell O, Gullberg B, et al. Risk factors for hip fracture in men from southern Europe: the MEDOS study. Mediterranean Osteoporosis Study. Osteoporos Int 1999;9(1):45–54
56. Johnell O, Gullberg B, Kanis JA, et al. Risk factors for hip fracture in European women: the MEDOS Study. Mediterranean Osteoporosis Study. J Bone Miner Res 1995;10(11):1802–1815
57. Chen Z, Pettinger MB, Ritenbaugh C, et al. Habitual tea consumption and risk of osteoporosis: a prospective study in the women's health initiative observational cohort. Am J Epidemiol 2003;158(8):772–781
58. Hernandez-Avila M, Colditz GA, Stampfer MJ, Rosner B, Speizer FE, Willett WC. Caffeine, moderate alcohol intake, and risk of fractures of the hip and forearm in middle-aged women. Am J Clin Nutr 1991;54(1):157–163
59. Trevisanato SI, Kim YI. Tea and health. Nutr Rev 2000;58(1):1–10
60. Rasheed A, Haider M. Antibacterial activity of Camellia sinensis extracts against dental caries. Arch Pharm Res 1998;21(3):348–352
61. Matsumoto M, Minami T, Sasaki H, Sobue S, Hamada S, Ooshima T. Inhibitory effects of oolong tea extract on caries-inducing properties of mutans streptococci. Caries Res 1999;33(6):441–445
62. Hirasawa M, Takada K, Otake S. Inhibition of acid production in dental plaque bacteria by green tea catechins. Caries Res 2006;40(3):265–270
63. Linke HA, LeGeros RZ. Black tea extract and dental caries formation in hamsters. Int J Food Sci Nutr 2003;54(1):89–95
64. Jones C, Woods K, Whittle G, Worthington H, Taylor G. Sugar, drinks, deprivation and dental caries in 14-year-old children in the north west of England in 1995. Community Dent Health 1999;16(2):68–71
65. Curhan GC, Willett WC, Speizer FE, Stampfer MJ. Beverage use and risk for kidney stones in women. Ann Intern Med 1998;128(7):534–540
66. Curhan GC, Willett WC, Rimm EB, Spiegelman D, Stampfer MJ. Prospective study of beverage use and the risk of kidney stones. Am J Epidemiol 1996; 143(3):240–247
67. Itoh Y, Yasui T, Okada A, Tozawa K, Hayashi Y, Kohri K. Preventive effects of green tea on renal stone formation and the role of oxidative stress in nephrolithiasis. J Urol 2005;173(1):271–275
68. Borghi L, Meschi T, Schianchi T, et al. Urine volume: stone risk factor and preventive measure. Nephron 1999;81(Suppl 1):31–37
69. Massey LK, Roman-Smith H, Sutton RA. Effect of dietary oxalate and calcium on urinary oxalate and risk of formation of calcium oxalate kidney stones. J Am Diet Assoc 1993;93(8):901–906
70. Massey LK. Tea oxalate. Nutr Rev 2000;58(3 Pt 1):88–89
71. Komatsu T, Nakamori M, Komatsu K, et al. Oolong tea increases energy metabolism in Japanese females. J Med Invest 2003;50(3–4):170–175
72. Rumpler W, Seale J, Clevidence B, et al. Oolong tea increases metabolic rate and fat oxidation in men. J Nutr 2001;131(11):2848–2852
73. Dulloo AG, Duret C, Rohrer D, et al. Efficacy of a green tea extract rich in catechin polyphenols and caffeine in increasing 24-h energy expenditure and fat oxidation in humans. Am J Clin Nutr 1999;70(6):1040–1045
74. Kovacs EM, Lejeune MP, Nijs I, Westerterp-Plantenga MS. Effects of green tea on weight maintenance after body-weight loss. Br J Nutr 2004;91(3):431–437
75. Westerterp-Plantenga MS, Lejeune MP, Kovacs EM. Body weight loss and weight maintenance in relation to habitual caffeine intake and green tea supplementation. Obes Res 2005;13(7):1195–1204
76. Nagao T, Komine Y, Soga S, et al. Ingestion of a tea rich in catechins leads to a reduction in body fat and malondialdehyde-modified LDL in men. Am J Clin Nutr 2005;81(1):122–129
77. Aizaki T, Osaka M, Hara H, et al. Hypokalemia with syncope caused by habitual drinking of oolong tea. Intern Med 1999;38(3):252–256
78. Trewby PN, Rutter MD, Earl UM, Sattar MA. Teapot myositis. Lancet 1998;351(9111):1248
79. Jatoi A, Ellison N, Burch PA, et al. A phase II trial of green tea in the treatment of patients with androgen independent metastatic prostate carcinoma. Cancer 2003;97(6):1442–1446
80. Pisters KM, Newman RA, Coldman B, et al. Phase I trial of oral green tea extract in adult patients with solid tumors. J Clin Oncol 2001;19(6):1830–1838
81. Chow HH, Cai Y, Hakim IA, et al. Pharmacokinetics and safety of green tea polyphenols after multiple-dose administration of epigallocatechin gallate and polyphenon E in healthy individuals. Clin Cancer Res 2003;9(9):3312–3319
82. Taylor JR, Wilt VM. Probable antagonism of warfarin by green tea. Ann Pharmacother 1999;33(4):426–428

83. Heck AM, DeWitt BA, Lukes AL. Potential interactions between alternative therapies and warfarin. Am J Health Syst Pharm 2000;57(13):1221–1227, quiz 1228–1230

84. Carrillo JA, Benitez J. Clinically significant pharmacokinetic interactions between dietary caffeine and medications. Clin Pharmacokinet 2000;39(2):127–153

85. Hurrell RF, Reddy M, Cook JD. Inhibition of non-haem iron absorption in man by polyphenolic-containing beverages. Br J Nutr 1999;81(4):289–295

86. Zijp IM, Korver O, Tijburg LB. Effect of tea and other dietary factors on iron absorption. Crit Rev Food Sci Nutr 2000;40(5):371–398

8 Carotenoids

Carotenoids are a class of more than 600 naturally occurring pigments synthesized by plants, algae, and photosynthetic bacteria. These richly colored molecules are the sources of the yellow, orange, and red colors of many plants.[1] Fruits and vegetables provide most of the carotenoids in the human diet. Alpha-carotene, β-carotene, β-cryptoxanthin, lutein, lycopene, and zeaxanthin are the most common dietary carotenoids. Alpha-carotene, β-carotene and β-cryptoxanthin are provitamin A carotenoids, meaning they can be converted by the body to retinol (**Fig. 8.1**). Lutein, lycopene, and zeaxanthin cannot be converted to retinol, so they have no vitamin A activity (**Fig. 8.2**). Carotenoids can be broadly classified into two classes, carotenes (α-carotene, β-carotene, and lycopene) and xanthophylls (β-cryptoxanthin, lutein, and zeaxanthin).

Bioavailability and Metabolism

For dietary carotenoids to be absorbed intestinally, they must be released from the food matrix and incorporated into mixed micelles (mixtures of bile salts and several types of lipids).[2] Therefore, carotenoid absorption requires the presence of fat in a meal. As little as 3–5 g of fat in a meal appears sufficient to ensure carotenoid absorption.[3,4] Because they do not need to be released from the plant matrix, carotenoid supplements (in oil) are more efficiently absorbed than carotenoids in foods.[4] Within the cells that line the intestine (enterocytes), carotenoids are incorporated into triglyceride-rich lipoproteins called *chylomicrons* and released into the circulation.[2] Triglycerides are depleted from circulating chylomicrons through the activity of an enzyme called

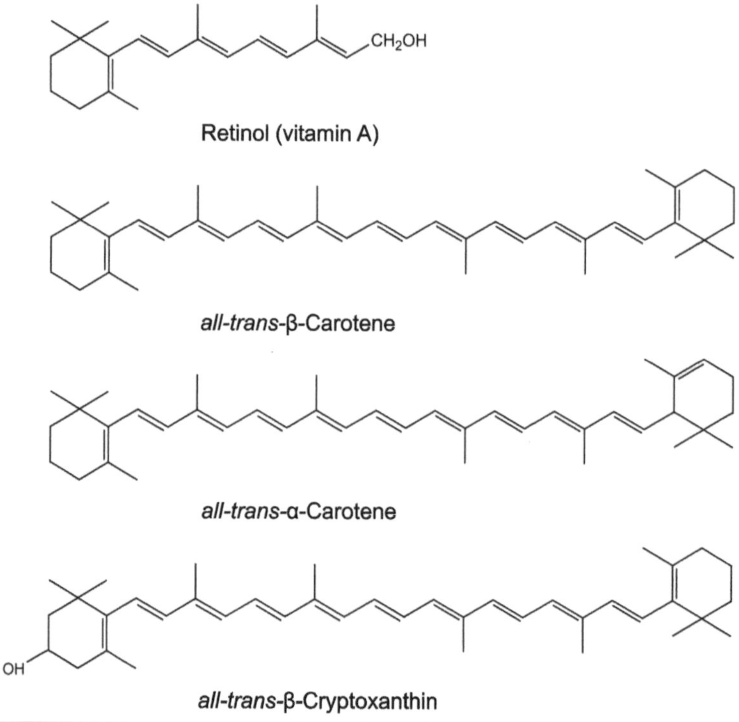

Fig. 8.1 The chemical structures of retinol (vitamin A) and the provitamin A carotenoids, β-carotene, α-carotene, and β-cryptoxanthin.

lipoprotein lipase, resulting in the formation of chylomicron remnants. Chylomicron remnants are taken up by the liver, where carotenoids are incorporated into lipoproteins and secreted back into the circulation. In the intestine and the liver, provitamin A carotenoids may be cleaved to produce retinal, a form of vitamin A. The conversion of provitamin A carotenoids to vitamin A is influenced by the vitamin A status of the individual.[5] Although the regulatory mechanism is not yet clear in humans, cleavage of provitamin A carotenoids appears to be inhibited when vitamin A stores are high.

Biological Activities

Vitamin A Activity

Vitamin A is essential for normal growth and development, immune system function, and vision. Currently, the only essential function of carotenoids recognized in humans is that of provitamin A carotenoids (α-carotene, β-carotene and β-cryptoxanthin) to serve as a source of vitamin A.[6] The vitamin A activity of β-carotene in foods is $1/12$ that of retinol (preformed vitamin A), while the vitamin A activities of α-carotene and β-cryptoxanthin are both $1/24$ that of retinol.[6]

Antioxidant Activity

In plants, carotenoids have the important antioxidant function of quenching (deactivating) singlet oxygen, an oxidant formed during photosynthesis.[7] Test tube studies indicate that lycopene is one of the most effective quenchers of singlet oxygen among carotenoids.[8] Although important for plants, the relevance of singlet oxygen quenching to human health is less clear. Test tube studies indicate that carotenoids can also inhibit the oxidation of fats (i.e., lipid peroxidation) under certain conditions, but their actions in humans appear to be more complex.[9] At present, it is unclear whether the biological effects of carotenoids in humans are a result of their antioxidant activity or other non-antioxidant mechanisms.

Light Filtering

The long system of alternating double and single bonds common to all carotenoids allows them to absorb light in the visible range of the spectrum.[7]

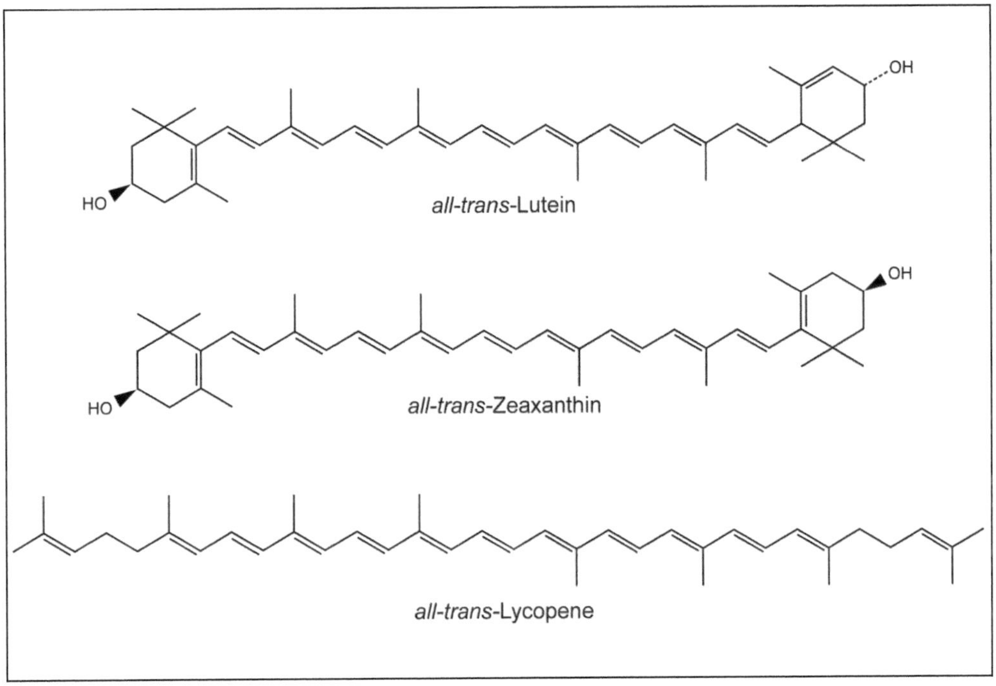

Fig. 8.2 The chemical structures of lutein, zeaxanthin, and lycopene.

This feature has particular relevance to the eye, where lutein and zeaxanthin efficiently absorb blue light. Reducing the amount of blue light that reaches the critical visual structures of the eye may protect them from light-induced oxidative damage.[10]

Intercellular Communication

Carotenoids can facilitate communication between neighboring cells grown in culture by stimulating the synthesis of connexin proteins.[11] Connexins form pores (gap junctions) in cell membranes, allowing cells to communicate through the exchange of small molecules. This type of intercellular communication is important for maintaining cells in a differentiated state and is often lost in cancer cells. Carotenoids facilitate intercellular communication by increasing the expression of the gene encoding a connexin protein, an effect that appears unrelated to the vitamin A or antioxidant activities of various carotenoids.[12]

Immune System Function

Because vitamin A is essential for normal immune system function, it is difficult to determine whether the effects of provitamin A carotenoids are related to their vitamin A activity or other activities of carotenoids. Although some clinical trials have found that β-carotene supplementation improves several biomarkers of immune function,[13–15] increasing the intakes of lycopene and lutein—carotenoids without vitamin A activity—has not resulted in similar improvements in biomarkers of immune function.[16–18]

Deficiency

Although consumption of provitamin A carotenoids (α-carotene, β-carotene, and β-cryptoxanthin) can prevent vitamin A deficiency, no overt deficiency symptoms have been identified in people consuming low-carotenoid diets if they consume adequate vitamin A.[6] After reviewing the published scientific research in 2000, the Food and Nutrition Board of the Institute of Medicine concluded that the existing evidence was insufficient to establish a recommended dietary allowance (RDA) or adequate intake (AI) for ca-

rotenoids. The Board has set an RDA for vitamin A. Recommendations by the National Cancer Institute, American Cancer Society, and American Heart Association to consume a variety of fruits and vegetables daily are aimed, in part, at increasing intakes of carotenoids.

Disease Prevention

Lung Cancer

Dietary Carotenoids

Beta-carotene was the first carotenoid to be measured in foods and human blood. The results of early observational studies suggested an inverse relationship between lung cancer risk and β-carotene intake, often assessed by measuring blood levels of β-carotene.[19,20] More recently, the development of databases for other carotenoids in foods has allowed scientists to estimate dietary intakes of total and individual dietary carotenoids more accurately. In contrast to early retrospective studies, more recent prospective cohort studies have not consistently found inverse associations between β-carotene intake and lung cancer risk. Analysis of dietary carotenoid intake and lung cancer risk in two large prospective cohort studies in the United States that followed more than 120 000 men and women for at least 10 years revealed no significant association between dietary β-carotene intake and lung cancer risk.[21] However, men and women with the highest intakes of total carotenoids, α-carotene, and lycopene were at significantly lower risk of developing lung cancer than those with the lowest intakes. Dietary intakes of total carotenoids, lycopene, β-cryptoxanthin, lutein, and zeaxanthin, but not β-carotene, were associated with significant reductions in risk of lung cancer in a 14-year study of more than 27 000 Finnish male smokers,[22] while only dietary intakes of β-cryptoxanthin, lutein, and zeaxanthin were inversely associated with lung cancer risk in a 6-year study of more than 58 000 Dutch men.[23] An analysis of the pooled results of six prospective cohort studies in North America and Europe also found no relationship between dietary β-carotene intake and lung cancer risk, although those with the highest β-cryptoxanthin intakes had a risk of lung cancer that was 24% lower than in those with the lowest intakes.[24] While smoking remains the strongest risk factor for lung cancer, results of recent prospective studies using accurate estimates of dietary carotenoid intake suggest that diets rich in several carotenoids— not only β-carotene—may be associated with reduced lung cancer risk. However, a recent systematic review of prospective cohort studies concluded that any protective effect of dietary carotenoids against the development of lung cancer is likely small and not statistically significant.[25]

Beta-Carotene Supplements

The effect of β-carotene supplementation on the risk of developing lung cancer has been examined in three large randomized, placebo-controlled trials. In Finland, the Alpha-Tocopherol Beta-Carotene (ATBC) cancer-prevention trial evaluated the effects of 20 mg/day of β-carotene and/or 50 mg/day of α-tocopherol on more than 29 000 male smokers,[26] and in the United States, the β-Carotene and Retinol Efficacy Trial (CARET) evaluated the effects of a combination of 30 mg/day of β-carotene and 25 000 international units (IU)/day of retinol (vitamin A) in more than 18 000 men and women who were smokers or former smokers, or had a history of occupational asbestos exposure.[27] Unexpectedly, the risk of lung cancer in the groups taking β-carotene supplements was increased by 16% after 6 years in the ATBC participants and increased by 28% after 4 years in the CARET participants. The Physicians' Health Study examined the effect of β-carotene supplementation (50 mg every other day) on cancer risk in more than 22 000 male physicians in the United States, of whom only 11% were current smokers.[28] In that lower-risk population, β-carotene supplementation for more than 12 years was not associated with an increased risk of lung cancer. Although the reasons for the increase in lung cancer risk are not yet clear, several mechanisms have been proposed[29]; many experts feel that the risks of high-dose β-carotene supplementation outweigh any potential benefits for cancer prevention, especially in smokers or other high-risk populations.[30,31] Beta-carotene is sold as individual supplements and also found in supplements marketed to promote visual health.[32]

Prostate Cancer

Dietary Lycopene

The results of several prospective cohort studies suggest that lycopene-rich diets are associated with significant reductions in the risk of prostate cancer, particularly more aggressive forms.[33] In a prospective study of more than 47 000 health professionals followed for 8 years, those with the highest lycopene intake had a risk of prostate cancer that was 21% lower than in those with the lowest lycopene intake.[34] Those with the highest intakes of tomatoes and tomato products (accounting for 82% of total lycopene intake) had a risk of prostate cancer that was 35% lower and a risk of aggressive prostate cancer that was 53% lower than in those with the lowest intakes. Similarly, a prospective study of Seventh Day Adventist men found those who reported the highest tomato intakes were at significantly lower risk of prostate cancer,[35] and a prospective study of US physicians found those with the highest plasma lycopene levels were at significantly lower risk of developing aggressive prostate cancer.[36] However, dietary lycopene intake was not related to prostate cancer risk in a prospective study of more than 58 000 Dutch men.[37] A meta-analysis that combined the results of 11 case–control and 10 prospective studies found men with the highest intakes of dietary lycopene or tomatoes had modest, 11%–19% reductions in prostate cancer risk.[38] Most recently, a prospective study in a cohort of 29 361 men followed for 4.2 years found no association between dietary lycopene intake and prostate cancer risk.[39] Additionally, a recent large prospective study found no association between plasma concentrations of lycopene, or plasma concentrations of total carotenoids, and overall risk of prostate cancer.[40] While there is considerable scientific interest in the potential for lycopene to help prevent prostate cancer, it is not yet clear whether the prostate cancer risk reduction observed in some epidemiological studies is related to lycopene itself, other compounds in tomatoes, or other factors associated with lycopene-rich diets. To date, results of short-term, dietary intervention studies using lycopene in patients with prostate cancer have been promising.[41] Yet, the safety and efficacy of long-term use of lycopene supplements for prevention or treatment of prostate cancer is not known.[41] Large-scale, controlled clinical trials would be needed to address these issues.

Cardiovascular Disease

Dietary Carotenoids

Because they are very soluble in fat and very insoluble in water, carotenoids circulate in lipoproteins along with cholesterol and other fats. Evidence that low-density lipoprotein (LDL) oxidation plays a role in the development of atherosclerosis led scientists to investigate the role of antioxidant compounds like carotenoids in the prevention of cardiovascular disease.[42] The thickness of the inner layers of the carotid arteries can be measured noninvasively using ultrasound technology. This measurement of carotid intima–media thickness is considered a reliable marker of atherosclerosis.[43] Several case–control and cross-sectional studies have found higher blood levels of carotenoids to be associated with significantly lower measures of carotid artery intima–media thickness.[44–49] Higher plasma carotenoids at baseline have been associated with significant reductions in risk of cardiovascular disease in some prospective studies[50–54] but not in others.[55–58] While the results of several prospective studies indicate that people with higher intakes of carotenoid-rich fruits and vegetables are at lower risk of cardiovascular disease,[58–61] it is not yet clear whether this effect is a result of carotenoids or of other factors associated with diets high in carotenoid-rich fruits and vegetables.

Beta-Carotene Supplements

In contrast to the results of epidemiological studies suggesting that high dietary intakes of carotenoid-rich fruits and vegetables may decrease cardiovascular disease risk, four randomized controlled trials found no evidence that β-carotene supplements in doses ranging from 20 to 50 mg/day were effective in preventing cardiovascular diseases.[26,28,62,63] Based on the results of these randomized controlled trials, the US Preventive Health Services Task Force concluded that there was good evidence that β-carotene supplements provided no benefit in the prevention of cardiovascular disease in middle-aged and older adults.[31,64] Thus, although diets rich in β-carotene have generally been associated with reduced cardiovascular disease risk in observa-

tional studies, there is no evidence that β-carotene supplementation reduces cardiovascular disease risk.[65]

Age-Related Macular Degeneration

In Western countries, degeneration of the macula, the center of the eye's retina, is the leading cause of blindness in older adults. Unlike cataracts, in which the diseased lens can be replaced, there is no cure for age-related macular degeneration (AMD). Therefore, efforts are aimed at disease prevention or delaying the progression of AMD.

Dietary Lutein and Zeaxanthin

The only carotenoids found in the retina are lutein and zeaxanthin. Lutein and zeaxanthin are present at high concentrations in the macula, where they are efficient absorbers of blue light. By preventing a substantial amount of the blue light entering the eye from reaching the underlying structures involved in vision, lutein and zeaxanthin may protect against light-induced oxidative damage, which is thought to play a role in the pathology of AMD.[10] It is also possible, though not proven, that lutein and zeaxanthin act directly to neutralize oxidants formed in the retina. Epidemiological studies provide some evidence that higher intakes of lutein and zeaxanthin are associated with lower risk of AMD.[66] However, the relationship is by no means clear-cut. While cross-sectional and retrospective case–control studies found that higher levels of lutein and zeaxanthin in the diet,[67–69] blood,[70,71] and retina[72,73] were associated with a lower incidence of AMD, several prospective cohort studies found no relationship between baseline dietary intakes or serum levels of lutein and zeaxanthin and the risk of developing AMD over time.[74–77] Although scientists are very interested in the potential for increased lutein and zeaxanthin intakes to reduce the risk of macular degeneration, it is premature to recommend supplements without more data from randomized controlled trials.[78] A clinical trial, the Age-Related Eye Disease Study 2 (AREDS2), is currently under way to evaluate the effect of supplemental lutein and zeaxanthin on the progression of advanced AMD.[79] To date, the available scientific evidence suggests that consuming at least 6 mg/day of dietary lutein and zeaxanthin from fruits and vegetables may decrease the risk of AMD.[67–69]

Lutein Supplements

A randomized controlled trial in patients with atrophic AMD found that supplementation with 10 mg/day of lutein slightly improved visual acuity after 1 year compared with a placebo.[80] However, the investigators concluded that further research was needed to assess the effects of long-term lutein supplementation on atrophic AMD.

Beta-Carotene Supplements

The first randomized controlled trial (AREDS1) designed to examine the effect of a carotenoid supplement on AMD used β-carotene in combination with vitamin C, vitamin E, and zinc because lutein and zeaxanthin were not commercially available as supplements at the time the trial began.[81] Although the combination of antioxidants and zinc lowered the risk of developing advanced macular degeneration in individuals with signs of moderate to severe macular degeneration in at least one eye, it is unlikely that the benefit was related to β-carotene, since it is not present in the retina. Supplementation of male smokers in Finland with 20 mg/day of β-carotene for 6 years did not decrease the risk of AMD compared with placebo.[82] A placebo-controlled trial in a cohort of 22 071 healthy US men found that β-carotene supplementation (50 mg every other day) had no effect on the incidence of age-related maculopathy—an early stage of AMD.[83] Recent systematic reviews of randomized controlled trials have concluded that there is no evidence that β-carotene supplementation prevents or delays the onset of AMD.[84,85]

Cataracts

Ultraviolet light and oxidants can damage proteins in the eye's lens, causing structural changes that result in the formation of opacities known as *cataracts*. As people age, cumulative damage to lens proteins often results in cataracts that are large enough to interfere with vision.[7]

Dietary Lutein and Zeaxanthin

The observation that lutein and zeaxanthin are the only carotenoids in the human lens has stimulated interest in the potential for increased intakes of lutein and zeaxanthin to prevent or slow

the progression of cataracts.[10] Four large prospective studies found that men and women with the highest intakes of foods rich in lutein and zeaxanthin, particularly spinach, kale, and broccoli, were 18%–50% less likely to require cataract extraction[86,87] or develop cataracts.[88–90] Additional research is required to determine whether these findings are related specifically to lutein and zeaxanthin intake or to other factors associated with diets high in carotenoid-rich foods.[66]

Beta-Carotene Supplements

Evidence from epidemiological studies that cataracts were less prevalent in people with high dietary intakes and blood levels of carotenoids led to the inclusion of β-carotene supplements in several large randomized controlled trials of antioxidants. The results of those trials have been somewhat conflicting. Beta-carotene supplementation (20 mg/day) for more than 6 years did not affect the prevalence of cataracts or the frequency of cataract surgery in male smokers living in Finland.[82] In contrast, a 12-year study of male physicians in the United States found that β-carotene supplementation (50 mg every other day) decreased the risk of cataracts in smokers but not in nonsmokers.[91] Three randomized controlled trials examined the effect of an antioxidant combination that included β-carotene, vitamin C, and vitamin E on the progression of cataracts. Two trials found no benefit after supplementation for 5 years[92] or more than 6 years,[93] but one trial found a small decrease in the progression of cataracts after 3 years of supplementation.[94] Overall, the results of randomized controlled trials suggest that the benefit of β-carotene supplementation in slowing the progression of age-related cataracts does not outweigh the potential risks.

Sources

Food Sources

The most prevalent carotenoids in North American diets are α-carotene, β-carotene, β-cryptoxanthin, lycopene, lutein, and zeaxanthin.[6] Carotenoids in foods are mainly in the *all-trans* form (**Figs. 8.1 and 8.2**), although cooking may result in the formation of other isomers. The relatively low bioavailability of carotenoids from most foods compared with supplements is partly due

Table 8.1   Alpha-carotene content of selected foods

Food	Serving	α-Carotene (mg)
Pumpkin, canned	1 cup	11.7
Carrot juice, canned	1 cup (8 fl oz)	10.2
Carrots, cooked	1 cup	5.9
Carrots, raw	1 medium	2.1
Mixed vegetables, frozen, cooked	1 cup	1.8
Winter squash, baked	1 cup	1.4
Plantains, raw	1 medium	0.8
Collards, frozen, cooked	1 cup	0.2
Tomatoes, raw	1 medium	0.1
Tangerines, raw	1 medium	0.09
Peas, edible-podded, frozen, cooked	1 cup	0.09

Table 8.2   Beta-carotene content of selected foods

Food	Serving	β-Carotene (mg)
Carrot juice, canned	1 cup (8 fl oz)	22.0
Pumpkin, canned	1 cup	17.0
Spinach, frozen, cooked	1 cup	13.8
Sweet potato, baked	1 medium	13.1
Carrots, cooked	1 cup	13.0
Collards, frozen, cooked	1 cup	11.6
Kale, frozen, cooked	1 cup	11.5
Turnip greens, frozen, cooked	1 cup	10.6
Pumpkin pie	1 piece	7.4
Winter squash, cooked	1 cup	5.7
Carrots, raw	1 medium	5.1
Dandelion greens, cooked	1 cup	4.1
Cantaloupe, raw	1 cup	3.2

to the fact that they are associated with proteins in the plant matrix.[2] Chopping, homogenizing, and cooking disrupt the plant matrix, increasing the bioavailability of carotenoids.[4] The bioavailability of lycopene from tomatoes is substantially improved by heating tomatoes in oil.[95,96]

Alpha-Carotene and Beta-Carotene

Alpha-carotene and β-carotene are provitamin A carotenoids, meaning they can be converted in the body to vitamin A. The vitamin A activity of β-carotene in foods is $1/12$ that of retinol (preformed vitamin A). Thus, it would take 12 µg of β-carotene from foods to provide the equivalent of 1 µg (0.001 mg) of retinol. The vitamin A activity of α-carotene from foods is $1/24$ that of retinol, so it would take 24 µg of α-carotene from foods to provide the equivalent of 1 µg of retinol. Orange and yellow vegetables like carrots and winter squash are rich sources of α- and β-carotene. Spinach is also a rich source of β-carotene, although the chlorophyll in spinach leaves hides the yellow–orange pigment. Some foods that are good sources of α-carotene and β-carotene are listed in **Tables 8.1** and **8.2**, respectively.[97]

Beta-Cryptoxanthin

Like α- and β-carotene, β-cryptoxanthin is a provitamin A carotenoid. The vitamin A activity of β-cryptoxanthin from foods is $1/24$ that of retinol, so it would take 24 µg of β-cryptoxanthin from food to provide the equivalent of 1 µg of retinol. Orange and red fruits and vegetables like sweet red peppers and oranges are particularly rich sources of β-cryptoxanthin. Some foods that are good sources of β-cryptoxanthin are listed in **Table 8.3**.[97]

Lycopene

Lycopene gives tomatoes, pink grapefruit, watermelon, and guava their red color. It has been estimated that 80% of the lycopene in the US diet comes from tomatoes and tomato products like tomato sauce, tomato paste, and catsup (ketchup).[98] Lycopene is not a provitamin A carotenoid, meaning the body cannot convert lycopene to vitamin A. Some foods that are good sources of lycopene are listed in **Table 8.4**.[97]

Lutein and Zeaxanthin

Although lutein and zeaxanthin are different compounds, they are both from the class of carotenoids known as *xanthophylls*. They are not provitamin A carotenoids. Some methods used to quantify lutein and zeaxanthin in foods do not separate the two compounds, so they are typically reported as lutein and zeaxanthin or lutein + zeaxanthin. Lutein and zeaxanthin are present in a variety of fruits and vegetables. Dark green leafy vegetables like spinach and kale are particularly rich sources of lutein and zeaxanthin. One study found that the bioavailability of lutein from lutein-enriched eggs (from chickens fed a lutein-enriched diet) was significantly higher than from spinach or lutein supplements.[99] Some foods that are good sources lutein and zeaxanthin are listed in Table 8.5.[97]

Supplements

Dietary supplements providing purified carotenoids and combinations of carotenoids are commercially available in the United States without a prescription. Carotenoids are best absorbed when taken with a meal containing fat.

Beta-Carotene

Because it is has vitamin A activity, β-carotene may be used to provide all or part of the vitamin A in multivitamin supplements. The vitamin A activity of β-carotene from supplements is much higher than that of β-carotene from foods. It takes only 2 µg (0.002 mg) of β-carotene from supplements to provide 1 µg of retinol (preformed vitamin A). The β-carotene content of supplements is often listed in IU rather than µg; 3000 µg (3 mg) of β-carotene provides 5000 IU of vitamin A. Most commercial supplements contain 5000–25 000 IU of β-carotene.[100]

Lycopene

Lycopene has no vitamin A activity. Synthetic lycopene and lycopene from natural sources, mainly tomatoes, are available as nutritional supplements. Many commercial supplements provide 5–20 mg of lycopene.[100]

Lutein and Zeaxanthin

Lutein and zeaxanthin have no vitamin A activity. Lutein and zeaxanthin supplements are available as free carotenoids or as esters (esterified to

Table 8.3 Beta-cryptoxanthin content of selected foods

Food	Serving	β-Cryptoxanthin (mg)
Pumpkin, cooked	1 cup	3.6
Papayas, raw	1 medium	2.3
Sweet red peppers, cooked	1 cup	0.6
Sweet red peppers, raw	1 medium	0.6
Orange juice, fresh	1 cup (8 fl oz)	0.4
Tangerines, raw	1 medium	0.4
Carrots, frozen, cooked	1 cup	0.3
Yellow corn, frozen, cooked	1 cup	0.2
Watermelon, raw	1 wedge (1/16 of a melon 15 in long × 7.5 in diameter [38×19 cm])	0.2
Paprika, dried	1 tsp	0.2
Oranges, raw	1 medium	0.2
Nectarines, raw	1 medium	0.1

Table 8.4 Lycopene content of selected foods

Food	Serving	Lycopene (mg)
Tomato paste, canned	1 cup	75.4
Tomato purée, canned	1 cup	54.4
Tomato soup, canned, condensed	1 cup	26.4
Vegetable juice cocktail, canned	1 cup	23.3
Tomato juice, canned	1 cup	22.0
Watermelon, raw	1 wedge (1/16 of a melon 15 in long × 7.5 in diameter [38×19 cm])	13.0
Tomatoes, raw	1 cup	4.6
Catsup (ketchup)	1 tablespoon	2.5
Pink grapefruit, raw	½ grapefruit	1.7
Baked beans, canned	1 cup	1.3

Table 8.5   Lutein + zeaxanthin content of selected foods

Food	Serving	Lutein + Zeaxanthin (mg)
Spinach, frozen, cooked	1 cup	29.8
Kale, frozen, cooked	1 cup	25.6
Turnip greens, frozen, cooked	1 cup	19.5
Collards, frozen, cooked	1 cup	18.5
Dandelion greens, cooked	1 cup	9.6
Mustard greens, cooked	1 cup	8.3
Summer squash, cooked	1 cup	4.0
Peas, frozen, cooked	1 cup	3.8
Winter squash, baked	1 cup	2.9
Pumpkin, cooked	1 cup	2.5
Brussels sprouts, frozen, cooked	1 cup	2.4
Broccoli, frozen, cooked	1 cup	2.0
Sweet yellow corn, boiled	1 cup	1.5

fatty acids). One study found that free lutein and lutein esters had comparable bioavailability,[99] while another found that lutein esters were more bioavailable than free lutein.[101] Many commercially available lutein and zeaxanthin supplements have much higher amounts of lutein than zeaxanthin.[102] Such supplements typically contain 4–20 mg of lutein and 0.2–1 mg of zeaxanthin, although other dosages are available.[100] Supplements containing only lutein or only zeaxanthin are also available.

Safety

Toxicity

Beta-Carotene

Although β-carotene can be converted to vitamin A, the conversion of β-carotene to vitamin A decreases when body stores of vitamin A are high. This may explain why high doses of β-carotene have never been found to cause vitamin A toxicity.[103] High doses of β-carotene (up to 180 mg/day) have been used to treat erythropoietic protoporphyria, a photosensitivity disorder, without toxic side effects.[6]

Lycopene, Lutein, and Zeaxanthin

No toxicities have been reported.[104]

Adverse Effects

Beta-Carotene

Increased lung cancer risk. Two randomized controlled trials in smokers and former asbestos workers found that supplementation with 20–30 mg/day of β-carotene for 4–6 years was associated with significant 16%–28% increases in the risk of lung cancer compared with placebo. Although the reasons for these findings are not yet clear, many experts feel that the risks of high-dose β-carotene supplementation outweigh any potential benefits for chronic disease prevention, especially in smokers or other high-risk populations.[30,31]

Carotenodermia. High doses of β-carotene supplements (30 mg/day or more) and the consumption of large amounts of carotene-rich foods have resulted in a yellow discoloration of the skin known as *carotenodermia*. Carotenodermia is not associated with any underlying health problems and resolves when β-carotene supplements are discontinued or dietary carotene intake is reduced.

Lycopene

Lycopenodermia. High intakes of lycopene-rich foods or supplements may result in a deep orange discoloration of the skin known as *lycopenodermia*. Because lycopene is more intensely colored than the carotenes, lycopenodermia may occur at lower doses than carotenodermia.[6]

Lutein and Zeaxanthin

Adverse effects of lutein and zeaxanthin have not been reported.[102]

Safety in Pregnancy and Lactation

Beta-Carotene

Unlike vitamin A, high doses of β-carotene taken by pregnant women have not been associated with increased risk of birth defects.[6] However, the safety of high-dose β-carotene supplements in pregnancy and lactation has not been well studied. Although there is no reason to limit dietary β-carotene intake, pregnant and breastfeeding women should avoid consuming more than 3 mg/day (5000 IU/day) of β-carotene from supplements, unless they are prescribed under medical supervision.[102,103]

Other Carotenoids

The safety of carotenoid supplements other than β-carotene in pregnancy and lactation has not been established, so pregnant and breast-feeding women should obtain carotenoids from foods rather than supplements. There is no reason to limit the consumption of carotenoid-rich fruits and vegetables during pregnancy.[102,105]

Drug Interactions

The cholesterol-lowering agents, cholestyramine (Questran) and colestipol (Colestid), can reduce absorption of fat-soluble vitamins and carotenoids, as can mineral oil and orlistat (Xenical), a drug used to treat obesity.[102] Colchicine, a drug used to treat gout, can cause intestinal malabsorption. However, long-term use of 1–2 mg/day of colchicine did not affect serum β-carotene levels in one study.[106] Increasing gastric pH through the use of proton pump inhibitors, such as omeprazole (Prilosec, Losec), lansoprazole (Prevacid), rabeprazole (Aciphex), and pantoprazole (Protonix, Pantoloc), decreased the absorption of a single dose of a β-carotene supplement, but it is not known if the absorption of dietary carotenoids is affected.[107]

Antioxidant Supplements and HMG-CoA Reductase Inhibitors (Statins)

A 3-year randomized controlled trial in 160 patients with documented coronary heart disease and low serum high-density lipoprotein (HDL) concentrations found that a combination of simvastatin (Zocor) and niacin increased HDL2 levels, inhibited the progression of coronary artery stenosis, and decreased the frequency of cardiovascular events, including myocardial infarction (MI) and stroke.[108] Surprisingly, when an antioxidant combination (1000 mg of vitamin C, 800 IU of α-tocopherol, 100 μg of selenium, and 25 mg of β-carotene daily) was taken with the simvastatin–niacin combination, these protective effects were diminished. Since the antioxidants were taken together in this trial, the individual contribution of β-carotene cannot be determined. In contrast, a much larger randomized controlled trial of simvastatin and an antioxidant

combination (600 mg of vitamin E, 250 mg of vitamin C, and 20 mg of β-carotene daily) in more than 20 000 men and women with coronary artery disease or diabetes found that the antioxidant combination did not diminish the cardioprotective effects of simvastatin therapy over a 5-year period,[109] suggesting that the antioxidant combination may have interfered with the HDL-raising effect of niacin in the former trial. Further research is needed to determine potential interactions between antioxidant supplements and cholesterol-lowering agents, such as niacin and HMG-CoA reductase inhibitors (statins).

Interactions with Foods

Olestra

In a controlled feeding study, consumption of 18 g/day of the fat substitute Olestra (sucrose polyester) resulted in a 27% decrease in serum carotenoid concentrations after 3 weeks.[110] Studies in people before and after the introduction of Olestra-containing snacks to the marketplace found that total serum carotenoid concentrations decreased by 15% in those who reported consuming at least 2 g/day of Olestra.[111] One study in adults found that those who consumed more than 4.4 g of Olestra weekly experienced a 9.7% decline in total serum carotenoids compared with those not consuming Olestra.[112]

Plant Sterol- or Stanol-Containing Foods

Some studies found that the regular use of plant sterol-containing spreads resulted in modest, 10%–20% decreases in the plasma concentrations of some carotenoids, particularly α-carotene, β-carotene, and lycopene[113,114] (see Chapter 18 on Phytosterols). However, advising people who use plant sterol- or stanol-containing margarines to consume an extra serving of carotenoid-rich fruits or vegetables daily prevented decreases in plasma carotenoid concentrations.[115,116]

Alcohol. The relationships between alcohol consumption and carotenoid metabolism are not well understood. There is some evidence that regular alcohol consumption inhibits the conversion of β-carotene to retinol.[117] Increases in lung cancer risk associated with high-dose β-carotene supplementation in two randomized controlled trials were enhanced in those with higher alcohol intakes.[27,118]

Interactions Among Carotenoids

The results of metabolic studies suggest that high doses of β-carotene compete for absorption with lutein and lycopene when consumed at the same time.[119–121] However, the consumption of high-dose β-carotene supplements did not adversely affect serum carotenoid concentrations in long-term clinical trials.[122–125]

Summary

- Carotenoids are yellow, orange, and red pigments synthesized by plants. The most common carotenoids in North American diets are α-carotene, β-carotene, β-cryptoxanthin, lutein, zeaxanthin, and lycopene.
- Alpha-carotene, β-carotene, and β-cryptoxanthin are provitamin A carotenoids, meaning they can be converted by the body to retinol (vitamin A). Lutein, zeaxanthin, and lycopene have no vitamin A activity.
- At present, it is unclear whether the biological effects of carotenoids in humans are related to their antioxidant activity or other non-antioxidant activities.
- Although the results of epidemiological studies suggest that diets high in carotenoid-rich fruits and vegetables are associated with reduced risk of cardiovascular disease and some cancers, high-dose β-carotene supplements did not reduce the risk of cardiovascular diseases or cancers in large randomized controlled trials.
- Two randomized controlled trials found that high-dose β-carotene supplements increased the risk of lung cancer in smokers and former asbestos workers.
- Several epidemiological studies found that men with high intakes of lycopene from tomatoes and tomato products were less likely to develop prostate cancer than men with low intakes, but it is not known whether lycopene supplements will decrease the incidence or severity of prostate cancer.
- Lutein and zeaxanthin are the only carotenoids found in the retina and lens of the eye. The results of epidemiological studies suggest that diets rich in lutein and zeaxanthin may help slow the development of age-related macular degeneration and cataracts, but it is not known whether lutein and zeaxanthin supplements will slow the development of these age-related eye diseases.
- Carotenoids are best absorbed with fat in a meal. Chopping, puréeing, and cooking carotenoid-containing vegetables in oil generally increases the bioavailability of the carotenoids they contain.

References

1. International Agency for Research on Cancer. IARC Handbooks of Cancer Prevention: Carotenoids. Lyon, France: International Agency for Research on Cancer; 1998
2. Yeum KJ, Russell RM. Carotenoid bioavailability and bioconversion. Annu Rev Nutr 2002;22:483–504
3. Jalal F, Nesheim MC, Agus Z, Sanjur D, Habicht JP. Serum retinol concentrations in children are affected by food sources of beta-carotene, fat intake, and anthelmintic drug treatment. Am J Clin Nutr 1998;68(3):623–629
4. van Het Hof KH, West CE, Weststrate JA, Hautvast JG. Dietary factors that affect the bioavailability of carotenoids. J Nutr 2000;130(3):503–506
5. During A, Harrison EH. Intestinal absorption and metabolism of carotenoids: insights from cell culture. Arch Biochem Biophys 2004;430(1):77–88
6. Institute of Medicine, Food and Nutrition Board. Beta-carotene and other Carotenoids. Dietary Reference Intakes for Vitamin C, Vitamin E, Selenium, and Carotenoids. Washington, DC: National Academy Press; 2000:325–400
7. Halliwell B, Gutteridge JMC. Free Radicals in Biology and Medicine. 3rd ed. New York, NY: Oxford University Press; 1999
8. Di Mascio P, Kaiser S, Sies H. Lycopene as the most efficient biological carotenoid singlet oxygen quencher. Arch Biochem Biophys 1989;274(2):532–538
9. Young AJ, Lowe GM. Antioxidant and prooxidant properties of carotenoids. Arch Biochem Biophys 2001;385(1):20–27
10. Krinsky NI, Landrum JT, Bone RA. Biologic mechanisms of the protective role of lutein and zeaxanthin in the eye. Annu Rev Nutr 2003;23:171–201
11. Bertram JS. Carotenoids and gene regulation. Nutr Rev 1999;57(6):182–191
12. Stahl W, Nicolai S, Briviba K, et al. Biological activities of natural and synthetic carotenoids: induction of gap junctional communication and singlet oxygen quenching. Carcinogenesis 1997;18(1):89–92
13. van Poppel G, Spanhaak S, Ockhuizen T. Effect of beta-carotene on immunological indexes in healthy male smokers. Am J Clin Nutr 1993;57(3):402–407
14. Hughes DA, Wright AJ, Finglas PM, et al. The effect of beta-carotene supplementation on the immune function of blood monocytes from healthy male nonsmokers. J Lab Clin Med 1997;129(3):309–317
15. Santos MS, Gaziano JM, Leka LS, Beharka AA, Hennekens CH, Meydani SN. Beta-carotene-induced enhancement of natural killer cell activity in elderly men: an investigation of the role of cytokines. Am J Clin Nutr 1998;68(1):164–170
16. Hughes DA, Wright AJ, Finglas PM, et al. Effects of lycopene and lutein supplementation on the expression of functionally associated surface molecules on

blood monocytes from healthy male nonsmokers. J Infect Dis 2000;182(Suppl 1):S11–S15

17. Watzl B, Bub A, Blockhaus M, et al. Prolonged tomato juice consumption has no effect on cell-mediated immunity of well-nourished elderly men and women. J Nutr 2000;130(7):1719–1723

18. Corridan BM, O'Donoghue M, Hughes DA, Morrissey PA. Low-dose supplementation with lycopene or beta-carotene does not enhance cell-mediated immunity in healthy free-living elderly humans. Eur J Clin Nutr 2001;55(8):627–635

19. Peto R, Doll R, Buckley JD, Sporn MB. Can dietary beta-carotene materially reduce human cancer rates? Nature 1981;290(5803):201–208

20. Ziegler RG. A review of epidemiologic evidence that carotenoids reduce the risk of cancer. J Nutr 1989;119(1):116–122

21. Michaud DS, Feskanich D, Rimm EB, et al. Intake of specific carotenoids and risk of lung cancer in 2 prospective US cohorts. Am J Clin Nutr 2000;72(4):990–997

22. Holick CN, Michaud DS, Stolzenberg-Solomon R, et al. Dietary carotenoids, serum beta-carotene, and retinol and risk of lung cancer in the alpha-tocopherol, beta-carotene cohort study. Am J Epidemiol 2002; 156(6):536–547

23. Voorrips LE, Goldbohm RA, Brants HA, et al. A prospective cohort study on antioxidant and folate intake and male lung cancer risk. Cancer Epidemiol Biomarkers Prev 2000;9(4):357–365

24. Männistö S, Smith-Warner SA, Spiegelman D, et al. Dietary carotenoids and risk of lung cancer in a pooled analysis of seven cohort studies. Cancer Epidemiol Biomarkers Prev 2004;13(1):40–48

25. Gallicchio L, Boyd K, Matanoski G, et al. Carotenoids and the risk of developing lung cancer: a systematic review. Am J Clin Nutr 2008;88(2):372–383

26. The effect of vitamin E and beta carotene on the incidence of lung cancer and other cancers in male smokers. The Alpha-Tocopherol, Beta Carotene Cancer Prevention Study Group. N Engl J Med 1994;330(15): 1029–1035

27. Omenn GS, Goodman GE, Thornquist MD, et al. Risk factors for lung cancer and for intervention effects in CARET, the Beta-Carotene and Retinol Efficacy Trial. J Natl Cancer Inst 1996;88(21):1550–1559

28. Hennekens CH, Buring JE, Manson JE, et al. Lack of effect of long-term supplementation with beta carotene on the incidence of malignant neoplasms and cardiovascular disease. N Engl J Med 1996;334(18): 1145–1149

29. Palozza P, Simone R, Mele MC. Interplay of carotenoids with cigarette smoking: implications in lung cancer. Curr Med Chem 2008;15(9):844–854

30. Vainio H, Rautalahti M. An international evaluation of the cancer preventive potential of carotenoids. Cancer Epidemiol Biomarkers Prev 1998;7(8):725–728

31. US Preventive Services Task Force. Routine vitamin supplementation to prevent cancer and cardiovascular disease: recommendations and rationale. Ann Intern Med 2003;139(1):51–55

32. Tanvetyanon T, Bepler G. Beta-carotene in multivitamins and the possible risk of lung cancer among smokers versus former smokers: a meta-analysis and evaluation of national brands. Cancer 2008;113(1): 150–157

33. Giovannucci E. A review of epidemiologic studies of tomatoes, lycopene, and prostate cancer. Exp Biol Med (Maywood) 2002;227(10):852–859

34. Giovannucci E, Ascherio A, Rimm EB, Stampfer MJ, Colditz GA, Willett WC. Intake of carotenoids and retinol in relation to risk of prostate cancer. J Natl Cancer Inst 1995;87(23):1767–1776

35. Mills PK, Beeson WL, Phillips RL, Fraser GE. Cohort study of diet, lifestyle, and prostate cancer in Adventist men. Cancer 1989;64(3):598–604

36. Gann PH, Ma J, Giovannucci E, et al. Lower prostate cancer risk in men with elevated plasma lycopene levels: results of a prospective analysis. Cancer Res 1999;59(6):1225–1230

37. Schuurman AG, Goldbohm RA, Brants HA, van den Brandt PA. A prospective cohort study on intake of retinol, vitamins C and E, and carotenoids and prostate cancer risk (Netherlands). Cancer Causes Control 2002;13(6):573–582

38. Etminan M, Takkouche B, Caamaño-Isorna F. The role of tomato products and lycopene in the prevention of prostate cancer: a meta-analysis of observational studies. Cancer Epidemiol Biomarkers Prev 2004; 13(3):340–345

39. Kirsh VA, Mayne ST, Peters U, et al. A prospective study of lycopene and tomato product intake and risk of prostate cancer. Cancer Epidemiol Biomarkers Prev 2006;15(1):92–98

40. Key TJ, Appleby PN, Allen NE, et al. Plasma carotenoids, retinol, and tocopherols and the risk of prostate cancer in the European Prospective Investigation into Cancer and Nutrition study. Am J Clin Nutr 2007;86(3):672–681

41. Dahan K, Fennal M, Kumar NB. Lycopene in the prevention of prostate cancer. J Soc Integr Oncol 2008; 6(1):29–36

42. Kritchevsky SB. beta-Carotene, carotenoids and the prevention of coronary heart disease. J Nutr 1999; 129(1):5–8

43. Bots ML, Grobbee DE. Intima media thickness as a surrogate marker for generalised atherosclerosis. Cardiovasc Drugs Ther 2002;16(4):341–351

44. Rissanen TH, Voutilainen S, Nyyssönen K, Salonen R, Kaplan GA, Salonen JT. Serum lycopene concentrations and carotid atherosclerosis: the Kuopio Ischaemic Heart Disease Risk Factor Study. Am J Clin Nutr 2003;77(1):133–138

45. Dwyer JH, Paul-Labrador MJ, Fan J, Shircore AM, Merz CN, Dwyer KM. Progression of carotid intima-media thickness and plasma antioxidants: the Los Angeles Atherosclerosis Study. Arterioscler Thromb Vasc Biol 2004;24(2):313–319

46. McQuillan BM, Hung J, Beilby JP, Nidorf M, Thompson PL. Antioxidant vitamins and the risk of carotid atherosclerosis. The Perth Carotid Ultrasound Disease Assessment study (CUDAS). J Am Coll Cardiol 2001;38(7):1788–1794

47. Rissanen T, Voutilainen S, Nyyssönen K, Salonen R, Salonen JT. Low plasma lycopene concentration is associated with increased intima-media thickness of the carotid artery wall. Arterioscler Thromb Vasc Biol 2000;20(12):2677–2681

48. D'Odorico A, Martines D, Kiechl S, et al. High plasma levels of alpha- and beta-carotene are associated with a lower risk of atherosclerosis: results from the Bruneck study. Atherosclerosis 2000;153(1):231–239

49. Iribarren C, Folsom AR, Jacobs DR Jr, Gross MD, Belcher JD, Eckfeldt JH. Association of serum vitamin levels, LDL susceptibility to oxidation, and autoantibodies against MDA-LDL with carotid atherosclerosis. A case-control study. The ARIC Study Investigators.

Atherosclerosis Risk in Communities. Arterioscler Thromb Vasc Biol 1997;17(6):1171–1177

50. Sesso HD, Buring JE, Norkus EP, Gaziano JM. Plasma lycopene, other carotenoids, and retinol and the risk of cardiovascular disease in women. Am J Clin Nutr 2004;79(1):47–53

51. Rissanen TH, Voutilainen S, Nyyssönen K, et al. Low serum lycopene concentration is associated with an excess incidence of acute coronary events and stroke: the Kuopio Ischaemic Heart Disease Risk Factor Study. Br J Nutr 2001;85(6):749–754

52. Street DA, Comstock GW, Salkeld RM, Schüep W, Klag MJ. Serum antioxidants and myocardial infarction. Are low levels of carotenoids and alpha-tocopherol risk factors for myocardial infarction? Circulation 1994;90(3):1154–1161

53. Ito Y, Kurata M, Suzuki K, Hamajima N, Hishida H, Aoki K. Cardiovascular disease mortality and serum carotenoid levels: a Japanese population-based follow-up study. J Epidemiol 2006;16(4):154–160

54. Buijsse B, Feskens EJ, Kwape L, Kok FJ, Kromhout D. Both alpha- and beta-carotene, but not tocopherols and vitamin C, are inversely related to 15-year cardiovascular mortality in Dutch elderly men. J Nutr 2008;138(2):344–350

55. Sesso HD, Buring JE, Norkus EP, Gaziano JM. Plasma lycopene, other carotenoids, and retinol and the risk of cardiovascular disease in men. Am J Clin Nutr 2005;81(5):990–997

56. Hak AE, Stampfer MJ, Campos H, et al. Plasma carotenoids and tocopherols and risk of myocardial infarction in a low-risk population of US male physicians. Circulation 2003;108(7):802–807

57. Evans RW, Shaten BJ, Day BW, Kuller LH. Prospective association between lipid soluble antioxidants and coronary heart disease in men. The Multiple Risk Factor Intervention Trial. Am J Epidemiol 1998;147(2):180–186

58. Sahyoun NR, Jacques PF, Russell RM. Carotenoids, vitamins C and E, and mortality in an elderly population. Am J Epidemiol 1996;144(5):501–511

59. Rimm EB, Stampfer MJ, Ascherio A, Giovannucci E, Colditz GA, Willett WC. Vitamin E consumption and the risk of coronary heart disease in men. N Engl J Med 1993;328(20):1450–1456

60. Gaziano JM, Manson JE, Branch LG, Colditz GA, Willett WC, Buring JE. A prospective study of consumption of carotenoids in fruits and vegetables and decreased cardiovascular mortality in the elderly. Ann Epidemiol 1995;5(4):255–260

61. Osganian SK, Stampfer MJ, Rimm E, Spiegelman D, Manson JE, Willett WC. Dietary carotenoids and risk of coronary artery disease in women. Am J Clin Nutr 2003;77(6):1390–1399

62. Greenberg ER, Baron JA, Karagas MR, et al. Mortality associated with low plasma concentration of beta carotene and the effect of oral supplementation. JAMA 1996;275(9):699–703

63. Omenn GS, Goodman GE, Thornquist MD, et al. Effects of a combination of beta carotene and vitamin A on lung cancer and cardiovascular disease. N Engl J Med 1996;334(18):1150–1155

64. Morris CD, Carson S. Routine vitamin supplementation to prevent cardiovascular disease: a summary of the evidence for the U.S. Preventive Services Task Force. Ann Intern Med 2003;139(1):56–70

65. Voutilainen S, Nurmi T, Mursu J, Rissanen TH. Carotenoids and cardiovascular health. Am J Clin Nutr 2006;83(6):1265–1271

66. Mares-Perlman JA, Millen AE, Ficek TL, Hankinson SE. The body of evidence to support a protective role for lutein and zeaxanthin in delaying chronic disease. Overview. J Nutr 2002;132(3):518S–524S

67. Snellen EL, Verbeek AL, Van Den Hoogen GW, Cruysberg JR, Hoyng CB. Neovascular age-related macular degeneration and its relationship to antioxidant intake. Acta Ophthalmol Scand 2002;80(4):368–371

68. Mares-Perlman JA, Fisher AI, Klein R, et al. Lutein and zeaxanthin in the diet and serum and their relation to age-related maculopathy in the third national health and nutrition examination survey. Am J Epidemiol 2001;153(5):424–432

69. Seddon JM, Ajani UA, Sperduto RD, et al; Eye Disease Case-Control Study Group. Dietary carotenoids, vitamins A, C, and E, and advanced age-related macular degeneration. JAMA 1994;272(18):1413–1420

70. Gale CR, Hall NF, Phillips DI, Martyn CN. Lutein and zeaxanthin status and risk of age-related macular degeneration. Invest Ophthalmol Vis Sci 2003;44(6):2461–2465

71. Eye Disease Case-Control Study Group. Antioxidant status and neovascular age-related macular degeneration. Arch Ophthalmol 1993;111(1):104–109

72. Bone RA, Landrum JT, Mayne ST, Gomez CM, Tibor SE, Twaroska EE. Macular pigment in donor eyes with and without AMD: a case-control study. Invest Ophthalmol Vis Sci 2001;42(1):235–240

73. Beatty S, Murray IJ, Henson DB, Carden D, Koh H, Boulton ME. Macular pigment and risk for age-related macular degeneration in subjects from a Northern European population. Invest Ophthalmol Vis Sci 2001;42(2):439–446

74. Cho E, Seddon JM, Rosner B, Willett WC, Hankinson SE. Prospective study of intake of fruits, vegetables, vitamins, and carotenoids and risk of age-related maculopathy. Arch Ophthalmol 2004;122(6):883–892

75. Flood V, Smith W, Wang JJ, Manzi F, Webb K, Mitchell P. Dietary antioxidant intake and incidence of early age-related maculopathy: the Blue Mountains Eye Study. Ophthalmology 2002;109(12):2272–2278

76. Mares-Perlman JA, Klein R, Klein BE, et al. Association of zinc and antioxidant nutrients with age-related maculopathy. Arch Ophthalmol 1996;114(8):991–997

77. Mares-Perlman JA, Brady WE, Klein R, et al. Serum antioxidants and age-related macular degeneration in a population-based case-control study. Arch Ophthalmol 1995;113(12):1518–1523

78. Mares-Perlman JA. Too soon for lutein supplements. Am J Clin Nutr 1999;70(4):431–432

79. Coleman H, Chew E. Nutritional supplementation in age-related macular degeneration. Curr Opin Ophthalmol 2007;18(3):220–223

80. Richer S, Stiles W, Statkute L, et al. Double-masked, placebo-controlled, randomized trial of lutein and antioxidant supplementation in the intervention of atrophic age-related macular degeneration: the Veterans LAST study (Lutein Antioxidant Supplementation Trial). Optometry 2004;75(4):216–230

81. Age-Related Eye Disease Study Research Group. A randomized, placebo-controlled, clinical trial of high-dose supplementation with vitamins C and E, beta carotene, and zinc for age-related macular degeneration and vision loss: AREDS report no. 8. Arch Ophthalmol 2001;119(10):1417–1436

82. Teikari JM, Laatikainen L, Virtamo J, et al. Six-year supplementation with alpha-tocopherol and beta-

carotene and age-related maculopathy. Acta Ophthalmol Scand 1998;76(2):224–229

83. Christen WG, Manson JE, Glynn RJ, et al. Beta carotene supplementation and age-related maculopathy in a randomized trial of US physicians. Arch Ophthalmol 2007;125(3):333–339

84. Evans JR, Henshaw K. Antioxidant vitamin and mineral supplements for preventing age-related macular degeneration. Cochrane Database Syst Rev 2008;(1):CD000253

85. Evans J. Antioxidant supplements to prevent or slow down the progression of AMD: a systematic review and meta-analysis. Eye (Lond) 2008;22(6):751–760

86. Brown L, Rimm EB, Seddon JM, et al. A prospective study of carotenoid intake and risk of cataract extraction in US men. Am J Clin Nutr 1999;70(4):517–524

87. Chasan-Taber L, Willett WC, Seddon JM, et al. A prospective study of carotenoid and vitamin A intakes and risk of cataract extraction in US women. Am J Clin Nutr 1999;70(4):509–516

88. Lyle BJ, Mares-Perlman JA, Klein BE, Klein R, Greger JL. Antioxidant intake and risk of incident age-related nuclear cataracts in the Beaver Dam Eye Study. Am J Epidemiol 1999;149(9):801–809

89. Christen WG, Manson JE, Glynn RJ, et al. A randomized trial of beta carotene and age-related cataract in US physicians. Arch Ophthalmol 2003;121(3):372–378

90. Moeller SM, Voland R, Tinker L, et al; CAREDS Study Group; Women's Helath Initiative. Associations between age-related nuclear cataract and lutein and zeaxanthin in the diet and serum in the Carotenoids in the Age-Related Eye Disease Study, an Ancillary Study of the Women's Health Initiative. Arch Ophthalmol 2008;126(3):354–364

91. Christen WG, Manson JE, Glynn RJ, et al. A randomized trial of beta carotene and age-related cataract in US physicians. Arch Ophthalmol 2003;121(3):372–378

92. Gritz DC, Srinivasan M, Smith SD, et al. The Antioxidants in Prevention of Cataracts Study: effects of antioxidant supplements on cataract progression in South India. Br J Ophthalmol 2006;90(7):847–851

93. Age-Related Eye Disease Study Research Group. A randomized, placebo-controlled, clinical trial of high-dose supplementation with vitamins C and E and beta carotene for age-related cataract and vision loss: AREDS report no. 9. Arch Ophthalmol 2001;119(10):1439–1452

94. Chylack LT Jr, Brown NP, Bron A, et al. The Roche European American Cataract Trial (REACT): a randomized clinical trial to investigate the efficacy of an oral antioxidant micronutrient mixture to slow progression of age-related cataract. Ophthalmic Epidemiol 2002;9(1):49–80

95. Gärtner C, Stahl W, Sies H. Lycopene is more bioavailable from tomato paste than from fresh tomatoes. Am J Clin Nutr 1997;66(1):116–122

96. Stahl W, Sies H. Uptake of lycopene and its geometrical isomers is greater from heat-processed than from unprocessed tomato juice in humans. J Nutr 1992;122(11):2161–2166

97. US Department of Agriculture, Agricultural Research Service. USDA Nutrient Database for Standard Reference, Release 21. 2008. Available at: http://www.nal.usda.gov/fnic/foodcomp/search/. Accessed May 2, 2012

98. Clinton SK. Lycopene: chemistry, biology, and implications for human health and disease. Nutr Rev 1998;56(2 Pt 1):35–51

99. Chung HY, Rasmussen HM, Johnson EJ. Lutein bioavailability is higher from lutein-enriched eggs than from supplements and spinach in men. J Nutr 2004;134(8):1887–1893

100. Natural Medicines Comprehensive Database [Web site]. Available at: http://www.naturaldatabase.com. Accessed May 2, 2012

101. Bowen PE, Herbst-Espinosa SM, Hussain EA, Stacewicz-Sapuntzakis M. Esterification does not impair lutein bioavailability in humans. J Nutr 2002;132(12):3668–3673

102. Hendler SS, Rorvik DR, eds. PDR for Nutritional Supplements. Montvale, NJ: Medical Economics Company, Inc; 2001

103. Beta-Carotene. Natural Medicines Comprehensive Database [Web site]. Available at: http://www.naturaldatabase.com/monograph.asp?mono_id=999&brand_id=. Accessed May 2, 2012

104. Solomons NW. Vitamin A and carotenoids. In: Bowman BA, Russell RM, eds. Present Knowledge in Nutrition. 8th ed. Washington, DC: ILSI Press; 2001:127–145

105. Lutein. Natural Medicines Comprehensive Database [Web site]. Available at: http://www.naturaldatabase.com/monograph.asp?mono_id=754&brand_id=. Accessed May 2, 2012

106. Ehrenfeld M, Levy M, Sharon P, Rachmilewitz D, Eliakim M. Gastrointestinal effects of long-term colchicine therapy in patients with recurrent polyserositis (familial mediterranean fever). Dig Dis Sci 1982;27(8):723–727

107. Tang G, Serfaty-Lacrosniere C, Camilo ME, Russell RM. Gastric acidity influences the blood response to a beta-carotene dose in humans. Am J Clin Nutr 1996;64(4):622–626

108. Brown BG, Zhao XQ, Chait A, et al. Simvastatin and niacin, antioxidant vitamins, or the combination for the prevention of coronary disease. N Engl J Med 2001;345(22):1583–1592

109. Collins R, Peto R, Armitage J. The MRC/BHF Heart Protection Study: preliminary results. Int J Clin Pract 2002;56(1):53–56

110. Koonsvitsky BP, Berry DA, Jones MB, et al. Olestra affects serum concentrations of alpha-tocopherol and carotenoids but not vitamin D or vitamin K status in free-living subjects. J Nutr 1997;127(8,Suppl):1636S–1645S

111. Thornquist MD, Kristal AR, Patterson RE, et al. Olestra consumption does not predict serum concentrations of carotenoids and fat-soluble vitamins in free-living humans: early results from the sentinel site of the olestra post-marketing surveillance study. J Nutr 2000;130(7):1711–1718

112. Neuhouser ML, Rock CL, Kristal AR, et al. Olestra is associated with slight reductions in serum carotenoids but does not markedly influence serum fat-soluble vitamin concentrations. Am J Clin Nutr 2006;83(3):624–631

113. Katan MB, Grundy SM, Jones P, Law M, Miettinen T, Paoletti R; Stresa Workshop Participants. Efficacy and safety of plant stanols and sterols in the management of blood cholesterol levels. Mayo Clin Proc 2003;78(8):965–978

114. Weststrate JA, Meijer GW. Plant sterol-enriched margarines and reduction of plasma total- and LDL-cholesterol concentrations in normocholesterolae-

mic and mildly hypercholesterolaemic subjects. Eur J Clin Nutr 1998;52(5):334–343

115. Ntanios FY, Duchateau GS. A healthy diet rich in carotenoids is effective in maintaining normal blood carotenoid levels during the daily use of plant sterol-enriched spreads. Int J Vitam Nutr Res 2002; 72(1):32–39

116. Noakes M, Clifton P, Ntanios F, Shrapnel W, Record I, McInerney J. An increase in dietary carotenoids when consuming plant sterols or stanols is effective in maintaining plasma carotenoid concentrations. Am J Clin Nutr 2002;75(1):79–86

117. Leo MA, Lieber CS. Alcohol, vitamin A, and beta-carotene: adverse interactions, including hepatotoxicity and carcinogenicity. Am J Clin Nutr 1999;69(6):1071–1085

118. Albanes D, Heinonen OP, Taylor PR, et al. Alpha-Tocopherol and beta-carotene supplements and lung cancer incidence in the alpha-tocopherol, beta-carotene cancer prevention study: effects of base-line characteristics and study compliance. J Natl Cancer Inst 1996;88(21):1560–1570

119. van den Berg H. Carotenoid interactions. Nutr Rev 1999;57(1):1–10

120. Micozzi MS, Brown ED, Edwards BK, et al. Plasma carotenoid response to chronic intake of selected foods and beta-carotene supplements in men. Am J Clin Nutr 1992;55(6):1120–1125

121. Kostic D, White WS, Olson JA. Intestinal absorption, serum clearance, and interactions between lutein and beta-carotene when administered to human adults in separate or combined oral doses. Am J Clin Nutr 1995;62(3):604–610

122. Albanes D, Virtamo J, Taylor PR, Rautalahti M, Pietinen P, Heinonen OP. Effects of supplemental beta-carotene, cigarette smoking, and alcohol consumption on serum carotenoids in the Alpha-Tocopherol, Beta-Carotene Cancer Prevention Study. Am J Clin Nutr 1997;66(2):366–372

123. Nierenberg DW, Dain BJ, Mott LA, Baron JA, Greenberg ER. Effects of 4 y of oral supplementation with beta-carotene on serum concentrations of retinol, tocopherol, and five carotenoids. Am J Clin Nutr 1997;66(2):315–319

124. Wahlqvist ML, Wattanapenpaiboon N, Macrae FA, Lambert JR, MacLennan R, Hsu-Hage BH; Australian Polyp Prevention Project Investigators. Changes in serum carotenoids in subjects with colorectal adenomas after 24 mo of beta-carotene supplementation. Am J Clin Nutr 1994;60(6):936–943

125. Mayne ST, Cartmel B, Silva F, et al. Effect of supplemental beta-carotene on plasma concentrations of carotenoids, retinol, and alpha-tocopherol in humans. Am J Clin Nutr 1998;68(3):642–647

9 Chlorophyll and Chlorophyllin

Chlorophyll is the pigment that gives plants and algae their green color. Plants use chlorophyll to trap light needed for photosynthesis.[1] The basic structure of chlorophyll is a porphyrin ring similar to that of heme in hemoglobin, although the central atom in chlorophyll is magnesium instead of iron. The long hydrocarbon (phytol) tail attached to the porphyrin ring makes chlorophyll fat soluble and insoluble in water. Two different types of chlorophyll (chlorophyll a and chlorophyll b) are found in plants (**Fig. 9.1**). The small difference in chemical structure allows each type of chlorophyll to absorb light at slightly different wavelengths. Chlorophyllin is a semi-synthetic mixture of sodium copper salts derived from chlorophyll.[2,3] During the synthesis of chlorophyllin, the magnesium atom at the center of the ring is replaced with copper and the phytol tail is lost. Unlike natural chlorophyll, chlorophyllin is water soluble. Although the content of different chlorophyllin mixtures may vary, two compounds commonly found in commercial chlorophyllin mixtures are trisodium copper chlorin e_6 and disodium copper chlorin e_4 (**Fig. 9.2**).

Bioavailability and Metabolism

Little is known about the bioavailability and metabolism of chlorophyll or chlorophyllin. The lack of toxicity attributed to chlorophyllin led to the belief that it was poorly absorbed.[4] However, significant amounts of copper chlorin e_4 were measured in the plasma of humans taking chlorophyllin tablets in a controlled clinical trial, indicating that it is absorbed. More research is needed to understand the bioavailability and metabolism of natural chlorophylls and chlorin compounds in synthetic chlorophyllin.

Biological Activities

Complex Formation with Other Molecules

Chlorophyll and chlorophyllin are able to form tight molecular complexes with certain chemicals known or suspected to cause cancer, including polycyclic aromatic hydrocarbons found in tobacco smoke,[5] some heterocyclic amines found in cooked meat,[6] and aflatoxin-B_1.[7] The tight binding of chlorophyll or chlorophyllin to these potential carcinogens may interfere with gastro-

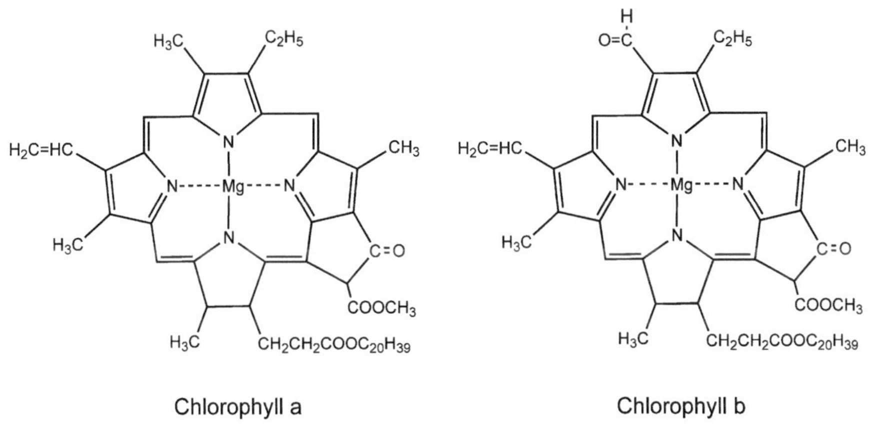

Fig. 9.1 Chemical structures of natural chlorophylls, chlorophyll a, and chlorophyll b.

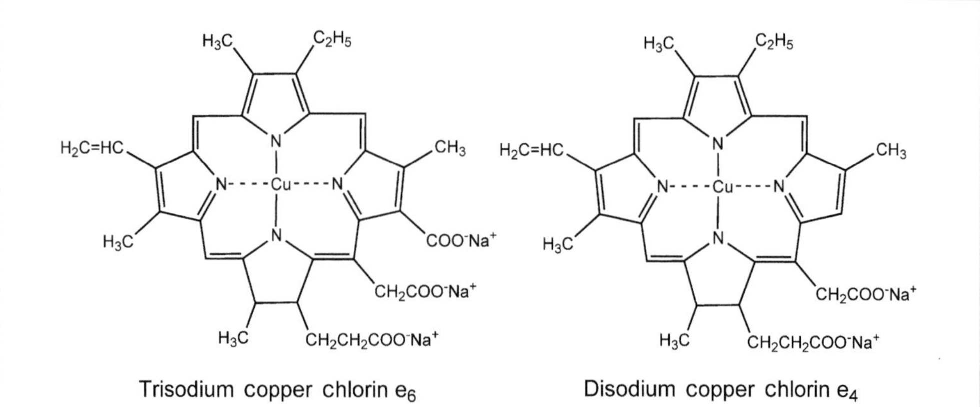

Fig. 9.2   Chemical structures of some compounds found in commercial sodium copper chlorophyllin—trisodium copper chlorin e_6 and disodium copper chlorin e_4.

intestinal absorption of potential carcinogens, reducing the amount that reaches susceptible tissues.[8]

Antioxidant Effects

Chlorophyllin can neutralize several physically relevant oxidants in vitro,[9,10] and limited data from animal studies suggest that chlorophyllin supplementation may decrease oxidative damage induced by chemical carcinogens and radiation.[11,12]

Modification of the Metabolism and Detoxification of Carcinogens

To initiate the development of cancer, some chemicals (procarcinogens) must first be metabolized to active carcinogens that are capable of damaging DNA or other critical molecules in susceptible tissues. Since enzymes in the cytochrome P450 (CYP) family are required for the activation of some procarcinogens, inhibition of CYP enzymes may decrease the risk of some types of chemically induced cancers. In vitro studies indicate that chlorophyllin may decrease the activity of CYP enzymes.[5,13] Phase II biotransformation enzymes promote the elimination of potentially harmful toxins and carcinogens from the body. Limited data from animal studies indicate that chlorophyllin may increase the activity of the phase II enzyme, quinone reductase.[14]

Therapeutic Effects

A recent study showed that human colon cancer cells undergo cell-cycle arrest after treatment with chlorophyllin.[15] The mechanism involved inhibition of ribonucleotide reductase activity. Ribonucleotide reductase plays a pivotal role in DNA synthesis and repair, and is a target of currently used cancer therapeutic agents, such as hydroxyurea.[15] This provides a potential new avenue for chlorophyllin in the clinical setting, sensitizing cancer cells to agents that damage DNA.

Disease Prevention

Aflatoxin-Associated Liver Cancer

Aflatoxin-B_1 (AFB$_1$), a liver carcinogen produced by certain species of fungus, is found in moldy grains and legumes, such as corn, peanuts, and soybeans.[2,8] In hot, humid regions of Africa and Asia with improper grain storage facilities, high levels of dietary AFB$_1$ are associated with increased risk of hepatocellular carcinoma. Moreover, the combination of hepatitis B infection and high dietary AFB$_1$ exposure increases the risk of hepatocellular carcinoma still further. In the liver, AFB$_1$ is metabolized to a carcinogen capable of binding DNA and causing mutations. In animal models of AFB$_1$-induced liver cancer, administration of chlorophyllin at the same time as dietary AFB$_1$ exposure significantly reduces AFB$_1$-induced DNA damage in the livers of rainbow trout and rats,[16–18] and dose-dependently inhibits the development of liver cancer in trout.[19] One rat study found that chlorophyllin did not protect against aflatoxin-induced liver damage when given after tumor initiation.[20] In addition, a recent study reported that natural chlorophyll inhibited AFB_1-induced liver cancer in the rat.[18]

Because of the long time period between AFB_1 exposure and the development of cancer in humans, an intervention trial might require as long as 20 years to determine whether chlorophyllin supplementation can reduce the incidence of hepatocellular carcinoma in people exposed to high levels of dietary AFB_1. However, a biomarker of AFB_1-induced DNA damage (AFB_1-N^7-guanine) can be measured in the urine, and high urinary levels of AFB_1-N^7-guanine have been associated with significantly increased risk of developing hepatocellular carcinoma.[21] To determine whether chlorophyllin could decrease AFB_1-induced DNA damage in humans, a randomized, placebo-controlled intervention trial was conducted in 180 adults residing in a region in China where the risk of hepatocellular carcinoma is very high, due to unavoidable dietary AFB_1 exposure and a high prevalence of chronic hepatitis B infection.[22] Participants took either 100 mg of chlorophyllin or a placebo before meals three times daily. After 16 weeks of treatment, urinary levels of AFB_1-N^7-guanine were 55% lower in those taking chlorophyllin than in those taking the placebo, suggesting that chlorophyllin supplementation before meals can substantially decrease AFB_1-induced DNA damage. Although a reduction in hepatocellular carcinoma has not yet been demonstrated in humans taking chlorophyllin, scientists are hopeful that chlorophyllin supplementation will provide some protection to high-risk populations with unavoidable dietary AFB_1 exposure.[8]

It is not known whether chlorophyllin will be useful in the prevention of cancers in people who are not exposed to significant levels of dietary AFB_1, as is the case for most people living in the United States. Many questions remain to be answered regarding the exact mechanisms of cancer prevention by chlorophyllin, the implications for the prevention of other types of cancer, and the potential for natural chlorophylls in the diet to provide cancer protection.

Disease Treatment

Internal Deodorant

Observations in the 1940s and 1950s that topical chlorophyllin had deodorizing effects on foul-smelling wounds led clinicians to administer chlorophyllin orally to patients with colostomies and ileostomies to control fecal odor.[23] While early case reports indicated that chlorophyllin doses of 100–200 mg/day were effective in reducing fecal odor in ostomy patients,[24,25] at least one placebo-controlled trial found that 75 mg of oral chlorophyllin three times daily was no more effective than placebo in decreasing fecal odor assessed by colostomy patients.[26] Several case reports have been published indicating that oral chlorophyllin (100–300 mg/day) decreased subjective assessments of urinary and fecal odor in incontinent patients.[23,27] Trimethylaminuria is a hereditary disorder characterized by the excretion of trimethylamine, a compound with a "fishy" or foul odor. A study in a small number of Japanese patients with trimethylaminuria found that oral chlorophyllin (60 mg three times a day) for 3 weeks significantly decreased urinary trimethylamine concentrations.[28]

Wound Healing

Research in the 1940s indicating that chlorophyllin slowed the growth of certain anaerobic bacteria in the test tube and accelerated the healing of experimental wounds in animals led to the use of topical chlorophyllin solutions and ointments in the treatment of persistent open wounds in humans.[29] During the late 1940s and 1950s, a series of largely uncontrolled studies in patients with slow-healing wounds, such as vascular ulcers and pressure (decubitus) ulcers, reported that the application of topical chlorophyllin promoted healing more effectively than other commonly used treatments.[30,31] In the late 1950s, chlorophyllin was added to papain- and urea-containing ointments used for the chemical debridement of wounds to reduce local inflammation, promote healing, and control odor.[23] Chlorophyllin-containing papain/urea ointments are still available in the United States by prescription.[32] Several studies have reported that such ointments are effective in wound healing.[33] Recently, a spray formulation of the papain/urea/chlorophyllin therapy has become available.[34]

Sources

Food Sources

Chlorophylls are the most abundant pigments in plants. Dark green, leafy vegetables like spinach are rich sources of natural chlorophylls. The chlorophyll contents of selected vegetables are presented in **Table 9.1**.[35]

Supplements

Chlorophyll

Green algae like chlorella are often marketed as supplemental sources of chlorophyll. Because natural chlorophyll is not as stable as chlorophyllin and is much more expensive, most over-the-counter chlorophyll supplements actually contain chlorophyllin.

Chlorophyllin

Oral preparations of sodium copper chlorophyllin (also called *chlorophyllin copper complex*) are available in supplements and as an over-the-counter drug (Derifil) used to reduce odor from colostomies or ileostomies or to reduce fecal odor due to incontinence.[36] Sodium copper chlorophyllin may also be used as a color additive in foods, drugs, and cosmetics.[37] Oral doses of 100–300 mg/day in three divided doses have been used to control fecal and urinary odor (see Disease Treatment section above).

Safety

Natural chlorophylls are not known to be toxic, and no toxic effects have been attributed to chlorophyllin despite more than 50 years of clinical use in humans.[8,23,29] When taken orally, chlorophyllin may cause green discoloration of urine or feces, or yellow or black discoloration of the tongue.[38] There have also been occasional reports of diarrhea related to oral chlorophyllin use. When applied topically to wounds, chlorophyllin has been reported to cause mild burning or itching in some cases.[39] Oral chlorophyllin may result in false-positive results on guaiac card tests for occult blood.[40] Since the safety of chlorophyll or chlorophyllin supplements has not been tested in pregnant or lactating women, they should be avoided during pregnancy and lactation.

Table 9.1 Chlorophyll content of selected raw vegetables[30]

Food	Serving	Chlorophyll (mg)
Spinach	1 cup	23.7
Parsley	½ cup	19.0
Cress, garden	1 cup	15.6
Green beans	1 cup	8.3
Arugula (rocket)	1 cup	8.2
Leeks	1 cup	7.7
Endive	1 cup	5.2
Sugar peas	1 cup	4.8
Chinese cabbage	1 cup	4.1

Summary

- Chlorophyll a and chlorophyll b are natural, fat-soluble chlorophylls found in plants.
- Chlorophyllin is a semi-synthetic mixture of water-soluble sodium copper salts derived from chlorophyll.
- Chlorophyllin has been used orally as an internal deodorant and topically in the treatment of slow-healing wounds for more than 50 years without any serious side effects.
- Chlorophylls and chlorophyllin form molecular complexes with some chemicals known or suspected to cause cancer, and, in doing so, may block carcinogenic effects. Carefully controlled studies have not been undertaken to determine whether a similar mechanism might limit the uptake of required nutrients.
- Supplementation with chlorophyllin before meals substantially decreased a urinary biomarker of aflatoxin-induced DNA damage in a Chinese population at high risk of liver cancer due to unavoidable, dietary aflatoxin exposure from moldy grains and legumes.
- Scientists are hopeful that chlorophyllin supplementation will be helpful in decreasing the risk of liver cancer in high-risk populations with unavoidable dietary aflatoxin exposure. However, it is not yet known whether chlorophyllin or natural chlorophylls will be useful in the prevention of cancers in people who are not exposed to significant levels of dietary aflatoxin.

References

1. Matthews CK, van Holde KE. Biochemistry. 2nd ed. Menlo Park, CA: The Benjamin/Cummings Publishing Company; 1996
2. Sudakin DL. Dietary aflatoxin exposure and chemo-prevention of cancer: a clinical review. J Toxicol Clin Toxicol 2003;41(2):195–204
3. Dashwood RH. The importance of using pure chemicals in (anti) mutagenicity studies: chlorophyllin as a case in point. Mutat Res 1997;381(2):283–286
4. Egner PA, Stansbury KH, Snyder EP, Rogers ME, Hintz PA, Kensler TW. Identification and characterization of chlorin e(4) ethyl ester in sera of individuals partici-pating in the chlorophyllin chemoprevention trial. Chem Res Toxicol 2000;13(9):900–906
5. Tachino N, Guo D, Dashwood WM, Yamane S, Larsen R, Dashwood R. Mechanisms of the in vitro antimuta-genic action of chlorophyllin against benzo[a]pyrene: studies of enzyme inhibition, molecular complex for-mation and degradation of the ultimate carcinogen. Mutat Res 1994;308(2):191–203
6. Dashwood R, Yamane S, Larsen R. Study of the forces of stabilizing complexes between chlorophylls and heterocyclic amine mutagens. Environ Mol Mutagen 1996;27(3):211–218
7. Breinholt V, Schimerlik M, Dashwood R, Bailey G. Mechanisms of chlorophyllin anticarcinogenesis against aflatoxin B1: complex formation with the car-cinogen. Chem Res Toxicol 1995;8(4):506–514
8. Egner PA, Muñoz A, Kensler TW. Chemoprevention with chlorophyllin in individuals exposed to dietary aflatoxin. Mutat Res 2003;523-524:209–216
9. Kumar SS, Devasagayam TP, Bhushan B, Verma NC. Scavenging of reactive oxygen species by chlorophyl-lin: an ESR study. Free Radic Res 2001;35(5):563–574
10. Kamat JP, Boloor KK, Devasagayam TP. Chlorophyllin as an effective antioxidant against membrane dam-age in vitro and ex vivo. Biochim Biophys Acta 2000;1487(2-3):113–127
11. Park KK, Park JH, Jung YJ, Chung WY. Inhibitory ef-fects of chlorophyllin, hemin and tetrakis(4-benzoic acid)porphyrin on oxidative DNA damage and mouse skin inflammation induced by 12-O-tetradec-anoylphorbol-13-acetate as a possible anti-tumor promoting mechanism. Mutat Res 2003;542(1-2):89–97
12. Kumar SS, Shankar B, Sainis KB. Effect of chlorophyl-lin against oxidative stress in splenic lymphocytes in vitro and in vivo. Biochim Biophys Acta 2004;1672(2):100–111
13. Yun CH, Jeong HG, Jhoun JW, Guengerich FP. Non-specific inhibition of cytochrome P450 activities by chlorophyllin in human and rat liver microsomes. Carcinogenesis 1995;16(6):1437–1440
14. Dingley KH, Ubick EA, Chiarappa-Zucca ML, et al. Ef-fect of dietary constituents with chemopreventive potential on adduct formation of a low dose of the heterocyclic amines PhIP and IQ and phase II hepatic enzymes. Nutr Cancer 2003;46(2):212–221
15. Chimploy K, Díaz GD, Li Q, et al. E2F4 and ribonucleo-tide reductase mediate S-phase arrest in colon cancer cells treated with chlorophyllin. Int J Cancer 2009;125(9):2086–2094
16. Dashwood RH, Breinholt V, Bailey GS. Chemopreven-tive properties of chlorophyllin: inhibition of aflatox-in B1 (AFB1)-DNA binding in vivo and anti-mutagenic activity against AFB1 and two heterocyclic amines in the Salmonella mutagenicity assay. Carcinogenesis 1991;12(5):939–942
17. Kensler TW, Groopman JD, Roebuck BD. Use of afla-toxin adducts as intermediate endpoints to assess the efficacy of chemopreventive interventions in animals and man. Mutat Res 1998;402(1-2):165–172
18. Simonich MT, Egner PA, Roebuck BD, et al. Natural chlorophyll inhibits aflatoxin B1-induced multi-or-gan carcinogenesis in the rat. Carcinogenesis 2007;28(6):1294–1302
19. Breinholt V, Hendricks J, Pereira C, Arbogast D, Bailey G. Dietary chlorophyllin is a potent inhibitor of afla-toxin B1 hepatocarcinogenesis in rainbow trout. Can-cer Res 1995;55(1):57–62
20. Orner GA, Roebuck BD, Dashwood RH, Bailey GS. Post-initiation chlorophyllin exposure does not modulate aflatoxin-induced foci in the liver and colon of rats. J Carcinog 2006;5:6
21. Qian GS, Ross RK, Yu MC, et al. A follow-up study of urinary markers of aflatoxin exposure and liver can-cer risk in Shanghai, People's Republic of China. Can-cer Epidemiol Biomarkers Prev 1994;3(1):3–10
22. Egner PA, Wang JB, Zhu YR, et al. Chlorophyllin inter-vention reduces aflatoxin-DNA adducts in individuals at high risk for liver cancer. Proc Natl Acad Sci U S A 2001;98(25):14601–14606
23. Chernomorsky SA, Segelman AB. Biological activities of chlorophyll derivatives. N J Med 1988;85(8):669–673
24. Siegel LH. The control of ileostomy and colostomy odors. Gastroenterology 1960;38:634–636
25. Weingarten M, Payson B. Deodorization of colosto-mies with chlorophyll. Rev Gastroenterol 1951;18(8):602–604
26. Christiansen SB, Byel SR, Strømsted H, Stenderup JK, Eickhoff JH. [in Danish]. Can chlorophyll reduce fecal odor in colostomy patients? Ugeskr Laeger 1989;151(27):1753–1754
27. Young RW, Beregi JS Jr. Use of chlorophyllin in the care of geriatric patients. J Am Geriatr Soc 1980;28(1):46–47
28. Yamazaki H, Fujieda M, Togashi M, et al. Effects of the dietary supplements, activated charcoal and copper chlorophyllin, on urinary excretion of trimethyl-amine in Japanese trimethylaminuria patients. Life Sci 2004;74(22):2739–2747
29. Kephart JC. Chlorophyll derivatives – their chemistry, commercial preparation and uses. Econ Bot 1955;9(1):3–38
30. Bowers WF. Chlorophyll in wound healing and sup-purative disease. Am J Surg 1947;73(1):37–50
31. Carpenter EB. Clinical experiences with chlorophyll preparations with particular reference to chronic os-teomyelitis and chronic ulcers. Am J Surg 1949;77(2):167–171
32. 2004 Physicians' Desk Reference. 58th ed. Stamford: Thomson Health Care, Inc.; 2003
33. Smith RG. Enzymatic debriding agents: an evaluation of the medical literature. Ostomy Wound Manage 2008;54(8):16–34
34. Weir D, Farley KL. Relative delivery efficiency and convenience of spray and ointment formulations of papain/urea/chlorophyllin enzymatic wound thera-pies. J Wound Ostomy Continence Nurs 2006;33(5):482–490
35. Bohn T, Walczyk S, Leisibach S, Hurrell RF. Chloro-phyll-bound magnesium in commonly consumed vegetables and fruits: relevance to magnesium nutri-tion. J Food Sci 2004;69(9):S347–S350

36. Access GPO. Electronic Code of Federal Regulations: Miscellaneous Internal Drug Products for Over the Counter Use. Available at: http://ecfr.gpoaccess.gov/cgi/t/text/text-idx?c=ecfr&sid=6bb427d78a48e3983 e0456d15a058c40&rgn=div6&view=text&node= 21:5.0.1.1.27.5&idno=21. Accessed May 2, 2012

37. Access GPO. Electronic Code of Federal Regulations: Listing of Color Additives Exempt from Certification. Available at: http://ecfr.gpoaccess.gov/cgi/t/text/text-idx?c=ecfr&sid=090fc8b3dcd5f08075f3d2d0c265407 3&rgn=div8&view=text&node= 21:1.0.1.1.26.3.31.7&idno=21. Accessed May 2, 2012

38. Hendler SS, Rorvik DR, eds. PDR for Nutritional Supplements. 2nd ed. Montvale, NJ: Physicians' Desk Reference, Inc; 2008

39. Smith LW. The present status of topical chlorophyll therapy. N Y State J Med 1955;55(14):2041–2050

40. Gogel HK, Tandberg D, Strickland RG. Substances that interfere with guaiac card tests: implications for gastric aspirate testing. Am J Emerg Med 1989;7(5):474–480

10   Curcumin

Turmeric is a spice derived from the rhizomes of *Curcuma longa*, which is a member of the ginger family (*Zingiberaceae*). Rhizomes are horizontal underground stems that send out shoots as well as roots. The bright yellow color of turmeric comes mainly from fat-soluble, polyphenolic pigments known as *curcuminoids* (**Fig. 10.1**). Curcumin, the principal curcuminoid found in turmeric, is generally considered its most active constituent.[1] Other curcuminoids found in turmeric include demethoxycurcumin and bisdemethoxycurcumin. In addition to its use as a spice and pigment, turmeric has been used in India for medicinal purposes for centuries. More recently, evidence that curcumin may have anti-inflammatory and anticancer activities has renewed scientific interest in its potential to prevent and treat disease.

Bioavailability and Metabolism

Clinical trials in humans indicate that the systemic bioavailability of orally administered curcumin is relatively low and that mostly metabolites of curcumin, instead of curcumin itself, are detected in plasma or serum following oral consumption.[3,4] In the intestine and liver, curcumin

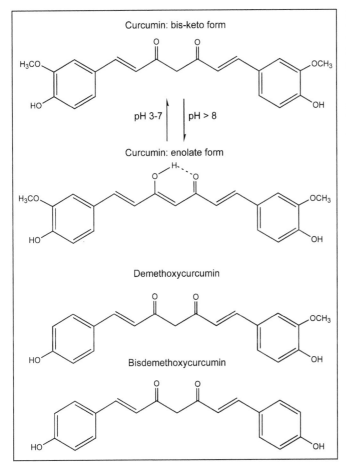

Curcumin: bis-keto form

pH 3-7 | pH > 8

Curcumin: enolate form

Demethoxycurcumin

Bisdemethoxycurcumin

Fig. 10.1 Chemical structures of the curcuminoids, curcumin, demethoxycurcumin, and bisdemethoxycurcumin. Curcumin exists in equilibrium between its bis-keto and enolate form.[2] The bis-keto form predominates at acidic and neutral pH, whereas the enolate form predominates at pH values above 8.

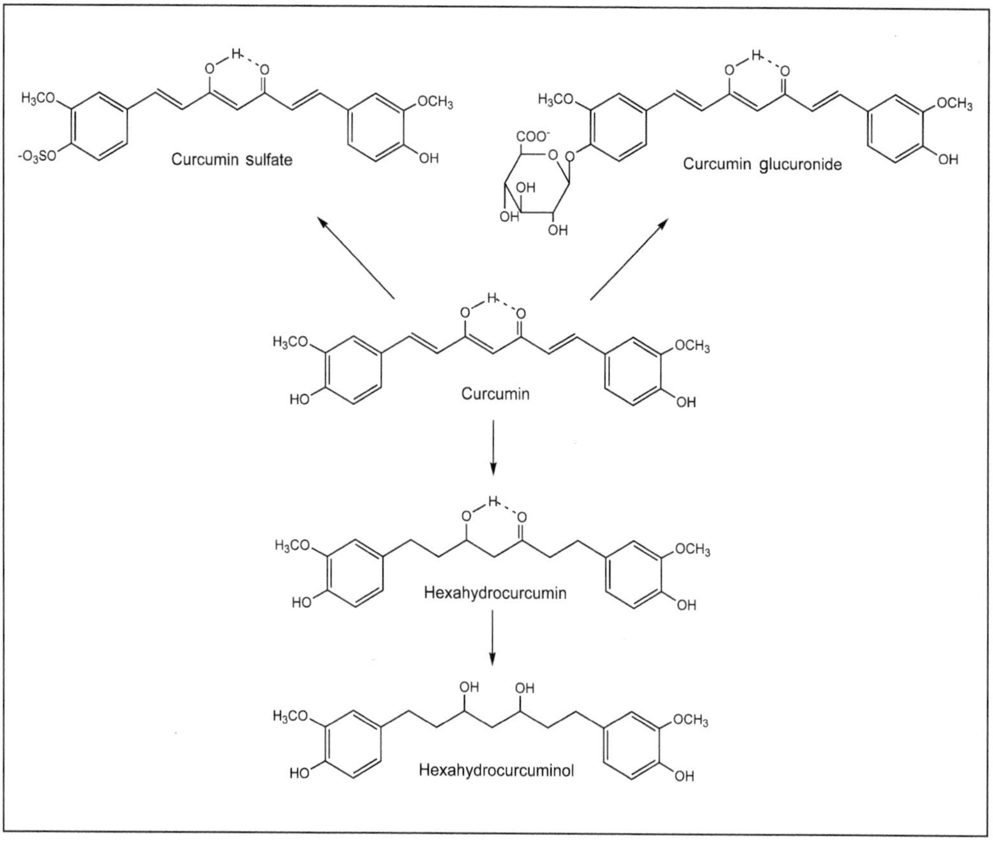

Fig. 10.2 Chemical structures of curcumin metabolites, including O-conjugation products, curcumin glucuronide and curcumin sulfate, as well as curcumin bioreduction products, hexahydrocurcumin and hexahydrocurcuminol.[5]

is readily conjugated to form curcumin glucuronides and curcumin sulfates or, alternately, reduced to hexahydrocurcumin (**Fig. 10.2**).[6] Curcumin metabolites may not have the same biological activity as the parent compound. In one study, conjugated or reduced metabolites of curcumin were less effective inhibitors of inflammatory enzyme expression in cultured human colon cells than curcumin itself.[7] In a clinical trial conducted in Taiwan, serum curcumin concentrations peaked 1–2 h after an oral dose; peak serum concentrations of curcumin were 0.5, 0.6, and 1.8 μmol/L following doses of 4, 6, and 8 g of curcumin, respectively.[8] Curcumin could not be detected in serum at doses lower than 4 g/day. More recently, a clinical trial conducted in the United Kingdom found that plasma concentrations of curcumin, curcumin sulfate, and curcumin glucuronide were in the range of 10 nmol/L (0.01 μmol/L) 1 h after a 3.6 g oral dose

of curcumin.[9] Curcumin and its metabolites could not be detected in plasma at doses lower than 3.6 g/day. Curcumin and its glucuronidated and sulfated metabolites were also measured in urine after a dose of 3.6 g/day. There is some evidence that orally administered curcumin accumulates in gastrointestinal tissues. For instance, when colorectal cancer patients took 3.6 g/day of curcumin orally for 7 days prior to surgery, curcumin was detected in malignant and normal colorectal tissue.[10] In contrast, curcumin was not detected in the liver tissue of patients with liver metastases of colorectal cancer after the same oral dose of curcumin,[11] suggesting that administration of oral curcumin may not effectively deliver curcumin to tissues outside the gastrointestinal tract.

Biological Activities

Antioxidant Activity

Curcumin is an effective scavenger of reactive oxygen species and reactive nitrogen species in the test tube (in vitro).[12,13] However, it is not clear whether curcumin acts directly as an antioxidant in vivo. Due to its limited oral bioavailability in humans (see the Bioavailability and Metabolism section above), plasma and tissue curcumin concentrations are likely to be much lower than those of other fat-soluble antioxidants, such as α-tocopherol (vitamin E). However, the finding that oral curcumin supplementation (3.6 g/day) for 7 days decreased the number of oxidative DNA adducts in malignant colorectal tissue suggests that curcumin taken orally may reach sufficient concentrations in the gastrointestinal tract to inhibit oxidative DNA damage.[11] In addition to direct antioxidant activity, curcumin may function indirectly as an antioxidant, by inhibiting the activity of inflammatory enzymes or by enhancing the synthesis of glutathione, an important intracellular antioxidant (see the section on Glutathione Synthesis below).

Anti-inflammatory Activity

The metabolism of arachidonic acid in cell membranes plays an important role in the inflammatory response by generating potent chemical messengers known as *eicosanoids*.[14] Membrane phospholipids are hydrolyzed by phospholipase A_2 (PLA_2), releasing arachidonic acid, which may be metabolized by cyclooxygenases (COXs) to form prostaglandins and thromboxanes, or by lipoxygenases (LOXs) to form leukotrienes. Curcumin has been found to inhibit PLA_2, COX-2, and 5-LOX activities in cultured cells.[15] Although curcumin inhibited the catalytic activity of 5-LOX directly, it inhibited PLA_2 by preventing its phosphorylation and COX-2 mainly by inhibiting its transcription. Nuclear factor kappa B (NF-κB) is a transcription factor that binds DNA and enhances the transcription of the *COX-2* gene, as well as other pro-inflammatory genes, such as inducible nitric oxide synthase (iNOS). In inflammatory cells, such as macrophages, iNOS catalyzes the synthesis of nitric oxide, which can react with superoxide to form peroxynitrite, a reactive nitrogen species that can damage proteins and DNA. Curcumin has been found to inhibit NF-κB-dependent gene transcription[16] and the induction of COX-2 and iNOS in cell culture and animal studies.[17,18]

Glutathione Synthesis

Glutathione is an important intracellular antioxidant that plays a critical role in cellular adaptation to stress.[19] Stress-related increases in cellular glutathione levels result from increased expression of γ-glutamyl-cysteine ligase (GCL), the rate-limiting enzyme in glutathione synthesis. Studies in cell culture suggest that curcumin can increase cellular glutathione levels by enhancing the transcription of genes that encode GCL.[20,21]

Effects on Biotransformation Enzymes Involved in Carcinogen Metabolism

Biotransformation enzymes play important roles in the metabolism and elimination of a variety of biologically active compounds, including drugs and carcinogens. In general, phase I biotransformation enzymes, including those of the cytochrome P450 (CYP) family, catalyze reactions that increase the reactivity of hydrophobic (fat-soluble) compounds, preparing them for reactions catalyzed by phase II biotransformation enzymes. Reactions catalyzed by phase II enzymes generally increase water solubility and promote the elimination of these compounds.[22] Although increasing biotransformation enzyme activity may enhance the elimination of potential carcinogens, some carcinogen precursors (procarcinogens) are metabolized to active carcinogens by phase I enzymes.[23] CYP1A1 is involved in the metabolic activation of several chemical carcinogens. In cell culture and animal studies, curcumin has been found to inhibit procarcinogen bioactivation or measures of CYP1A1 activity.[24-27] Increasing phase II biotransformation enzyme activity is generally thought to enhance the elimination of potential carcinogens. Several studies in animals have found that dietary curcumin increased the activity of phase II enzymes, such as glutathione *S*-transferases (GSTs).[26,28,29] However, curcumin intakes ranging from 0.45 to 3.6 g/day for up to 4 months did not increase leukocyte GST activity in humans.[9]

Induction of Cell-Cycle Arrest and Apoptosis

After a cell divides, it passes through a sequence of stages—collectively known as the *cell cycle*—before it can divide again. Following DNA damage, the cell cycle can be transiently arrested to allow for DNA repair or, if the damage cannot be repaired, for activation of pathways leading to cell death (apoptosis).[30] Defective cell-cycle regulation may result in the propagation of mutations that contribute to the development of cancer. Curcumin has been found to induce cell-cycle arrest and apoptosis in a variety of cancer cell lines grown in culture.[1,31–35] The mechanisms by which curcumin induces apoptosis are varied but may include inhibitory effects on several cell-signaling pathways. However, not all studies have found that curcumin induces apoptosis in cancer cells. Curcumin inhibited apoptosis induced by the tumor suppressor protein p53 in cultured human colon cancer cells,[36,37] and one study found that curcumin inhibited apoptosis induced by several chemotherapeutic agents in cultured breast cancer cells at concentrations of 1–10 μmol/L.[38]

Inhibition of Tumor Invasion and Angiogenesis

Cancerous cells invade normal tissue with the aid of enzymes called *matrix metalloproteinases*. Curcumin has been found to inhibit the activity of several matrix metalloproteinases in cell culture studies.[39–43] To fuel their rapid growth, invasive tumors must also develop new blood vessels by a process known as *angiogenesis*. Curcumin has been found to inhibit angiogenesis in cultured vascular endothelial cells[44,45] and in an animal model.[46]

Note:

It is important to keep in mind that many of the biological activities discussed above were observed in cells cultured in the presence of curcumin at higher concentrations than are likely to be achieved in cells of humans consuming curcumin orally (see the Bioavailability and Metabolism section at the beginning of this chapter).

Disease Prevention

Cancer

The ability of curcumin to induce apoptosis in cultured cancer cells by several different mechanisms has generated scientific interest in the potential for curcumin to prevent some types of cancer.[1] Oral curcumin administration has been found to inhibit the development of chemically induced cancer in animal models of oral,[47,48] stomach,[49,50] liver,[51] and colon[52–54] cancer. $APC^{Min/+}$ mice have a mutation in the *APC* (adenomatous polyposis coli) gene similar to that in humans with familial adenomatous polyposis, a genetic condition characterized by the development of numerous colorectal adenomas (polyps) and a high risk for colorectal cancer. Oral curcumin administration has been found to inhibit the development of intestinal adenomas in $APC^{Min/+}$ mice.[55,56] In contrast, oral curcumin administration has not consistently been found to inhibit the development of mammary (breast) cancer in animal models.[52,57,58]

Although the results of animal studies are promising, particularly with respect to colorectal cancer, there is currently little evidence that high intakes of curcumin or turmeric are associated with decreased cancer risk in humans. A phase I clinical trial in Taiwan examined the effects of oral curcumin supplementation up to 8 g/day for 3 months in patients with precancerous lesions of the mouth (oral leukoplakia), cervix (high-grade cervical intraepithelial neoplasia), skin (squamous carcinoma in situ), or stomach (intestinal metaplasia).[8] Histologic improvement on biopsy was observed in two out of seven patients with oral leukoplakia, one out of four patients with cervical intraepithelial neoplasia, two out of six patients with squamous carcinoma in situ, and one out of six patients with intestinal metaplasia. However, cancer developed in one out of seven patients with oral leukoplakia and one out of four patients with cervical intraepithelial neoplasia by the end of the treatment period. This study was designed mainly to examine the bioavailability and safety of oral curcumin, and interpretation of its results is limited by the lack of a control group for comparison. As a result of the promising findings in animal studies, several controlled clinical trials in humans designed to evaluate the effect of oral curcumin supplementation on precancerous colorectal lesions, such as adenomas, are under way.[59]

Disease Treatment

Cancer

The ability of curcumin to induce apoptosis in a variety of cancer cell lines, and its low toxicity, have led to scientific interest in its potential for cancer therapy as well as cancer prevention.[60] To date, most of the controlled clinical trials of curcumin supplementation in cancer patients have been phase I trials. Phase I trials are clinical trials in small groups of people, which are aimed at determining the bioavailability, safety, and early evidence of the efficacy of a new therapy.[61] A phase I clinical trial in patients with advanced colorectal cancer found that doses up to 3.6 g/day for 4 months were well tolerated, although the systemic bioavailability of oral curcumin was low.[62] When colorectal cancer patients with liver metastases took 3.6 g/day of curcumin orally for 7 days, trace levels of curcumin metabolites were measured in liver tissue, but curcumin itself was not detected.[11] In contrast, curcumin was measurable in normal and malignant colorectal tissue after patients with advanced colorectal cancer took 3.6 g/day of curcumin orally for 7 days.[10] These findings suggest that oral curcumin is more likely to be effective as a therapeutic agent in cancers of the gastrointestinal tract than other tissues. Phase II trials are clinical trials designed to investigate the effectiveness of a new therapy in larger numbers of people and to further evaluate short-term side effects and safety of the new therapy. Phase II clinical trials of curcumin in patients with colorectal cancer are currently under way.[59] A phase II clinical trial in patients with advanced pancreatic cancer found that curcumin exhibited some anticancer activity in two out of 21 patients; however, the bioavailability of curcumin was extremely poor.[63] Due to low systemic bioavailability and the fact that curcumin is hydrophobic, the authors proposed that intravenous administration of liposome-encapsulated curcumin be used in future clinical trials.[63]

Inflammatory Diseases

Although the anti-inflammatory activity of curcumin has been demonstrated in cell culture and animal studies, few controlled clinical trials have examined the efficacy of curcumin in the treatment of inflammatory conditions. A preliminary intervention trial that compared curcumin with a nonsteroidal anti-inflammatory drug (NSAID) in 18 rheumatoid arthritis patients found that improvements in morning stiffness, walking time, and joint swelling after two weeks of curcumin supplementation (1200 mg/day) were comparable to those experienced after two weeks of phenylbutazone (NSAID) therapy (300 mg/day).[64] A placebo-controlled trial in 40 men who had surgery to repair an inguinal hernia or hydrocele found that oral curcumin supplementation (1200 mg/day) for 5 days was more effective than placebo in reducing postsurgical edema, tenderness and pain, and was comparable to phenylbutazone therapy (300 mg/day).[65] Two uncontrolled studies found that oral curcumin (1125 mg/day) for 12 weeks or longer improved anterior uveitis and idiopathic inflammatory orbital pseudotumor, two inflammatory conditions of the eye.[66,67] However, without a control group, it is difficult to draw conclusions regarding the anti-inflammatory effects of curcumin in these conditions. Larger randomized controlled trials are needed to determine whether oral curcumin supplementation is effective in the treatment of inflammatory diseases, such as rheumatoid arthritis.

Cystic Fibrosis

Cystic fibrosis is a hereditary disease caused by mutations in the cystic fibrosis transmembrane conductance regulator (*CFTR*) gene.[62] CFTR is a transmembrane protein that acts as a chloride channel and plays a critical role in ion and fluid transport. In the lungs, CFTR mutations ultimately result in increased mucus concentration and decreased mucus clearance, which leads to progressive lung disease. The most common *CFTR* mutation contributing to the development of cystic fibrosis is the ΔF508 mutation, which results in CFTR protein misfolding and degradation before the protein can be targeted to the cell membrane. However, the mutated protein retains some ability to function as a chloride channel if it can be inserted in the cell membrane. In 2004, a study in mice with the ΔF508 mutation found that oral curcumin administration corrected abnormal ion transport and improved the survival of these mice.[68] However, unlike humans, mice with the ΔF508 mutation experience only the digestive complications of cystic fibrosis without the lung complications, and treatment benefits in the mouse model are not always realized in humans.[62] More recently, another group of scientists was unable to duplicate the beneficial effects of curcumin in the same mouse model given the same dose of curcumin.[69] It is unclear whether curcumin supplementation will be of benefit to humans with cystic fibrosis. In a phase I clinical trial funded by the Cystic Fibrosis Foundation, curcumin did not correct the function of the defective CFTR protein; a follow-up study using higher curcumin dosages is currently under way.[70] Until the safety and efficacy of curcumin in individuals with cystic fibrosis has been evaluated in clinical trials, the Cystic Fibrosis Foundation does not recommend the use of curcumin as a therapy for cystic fibrosis.[71]

Alzheimer Disease

In Alzheimer disease, a peptide called *amyloid β* forms aggregates (oligomers), which accumulate in the brain and form deposits known as *amyloid plaques*.[72] Inflammation and oxidative damage are also associated with the progression of Alzheimer disease.[73] Curcumin has been found to inhibit amyloid β oligomer formation in vitro.[74] When injected peripherally, curcumin was found to cross the blood–brain barrier in an animal model of Alzheimer disease.[74] In animal models of Alzheimer disease, dietary curcumin has decreased biomarkers of inflammation and oxidative damage, amyloid plaque burden in the brain, and amyloid β-induced memory deficits.[74–77] It is not known whether curcumin taken orally can cross the blood–brain barrier or inhibit the progression of Alzheimer disease in humans. As a result of the promising findings in animal models, clinical trials of oral curcumin supplementation in patients with early Alzheimer disease are under way.[59,78] The results of a 6-month trial in 27 patients with Alzheimer disease found that oral supplementation with up to 4 g/day of curcumin was safe.[4] Larger controlled trials are needed to determine whether or not oral curcumin supplementation is efficacious in Alzheimer disease.

Sources

Food Sources

Turmeric is the dried ground rhizome of *Curcuma longa*.[79] It is used as a spice in Indian, Southeast Asian, and Middle Eastern cuisines. Curcuminoids comprise approximately 2%–9% of turmeric.[80] Curcumin is the most abundant curcuminoid in turmeric, providing approximately 75% of the total curcuminoids, while demethoxycurcumin provides 10%–20% and bisdemethoxycurcumin generally provides less than 5%. Curry powder contains turmeric along with other spices, but the amount of curcumin in curry powders is variable and often relatively low.[81] Curcumin extracts are also used as food-coloring agents.[82]

Supplements

Curcumin extracts are available as dietary supplements without a prescription in the United States. The labels of several of these extracts state that they are standardized to contain 95% curcuminoids, although such claims are not strictly regulated by the US Food and Drug Administration (FDA). Some curcumin preparations also contain piperine, which may increase the bioavailability of curcumin by inhibiting its metabolism. However, piperine may also affect the metabolism of drugs (see the Drug Interactions section below). Optimal doses of curcumin for cancer chemoprevention or therapeutic uses have not been established. It is unclear whether doses below 3.6 g/day are biologically active in humans (see the section on Bioavailability and Metabolism at the beginning of this chapter).

Safety

Adverse Effects

In the United States, turmeric is generally recognized as safe (GRAS) by the FDA as a food additive.[82] Serious adverse effects have not been reported in humans taking high doses of curcumin. A dose-escalation trial in 24 adults found that single oral dosages up to 12 g were safe, and adverse effects were not dose related.[5] In a phase I trial in Taiwan, curcumin supplementation up to 8 g/day for 3 months was reported to be well tolerated in patients with precancerous conditions or noninvasive cancer.[8] In another clinical trial in the United Kingdom, curcumin supplementation ranging from 0.45 to 3.6 g/day for 4 months was generally well tolerated by people with advanced colorectal cancer, although two participants experienced diarrhea and another reported nausea.[9] Increases in serum alkaline phosphatase and lactate dehydrogenase were also observed in several participants, but it was not clear whether these increases were related to curcumin supplementation or cancer progression.[1] Curcumin supplementation of 20–40 mg has been reported to increase gallbladder contractions in healthy people.[83,84] Although increasing gallbladder contractions could decrease the risk of gallstone formation by promoting gallbladder emptying, it could potentially increase the risk of symptoms in people who already have gallstones.

Pregnancy and Lactation

Although there is no evidence that dietary consumption of turmeric as a spice adversely affects pregnancy or lactation, the safety of curcumin supplements in pregnancy and lactation has not been established.

Drug Interactions

Curcumin has been found to inhibit platelet aggregation in vitro,[85,86] suggesting a potential for curcumin supplementation to increase the risk of bleeding in people taking anticoagulant or antiplatelet medications, such as aspirin, clopidogrel (Plavix), dalteparin (Fragmin), enoxaparin (Lovenox), heparin, ticlopidine (Ticlid), and warfarin (Coumadin). In cultured breast cancer cells, curcumin inhibited apoptosis induced by the chemotherapeutic agents, camptothecin, mechlorethamine, and doxorubicin at concentrations of 1–10 μmol/L.[38] In an animal model of breast cancer, dietary curcumin inhibited cyclophosphamide-induced tumor regression. Although it is not known whether oral curcumin administration will result in breast tissue concentrations that are high enough to inhibit cancer chemotherapeutic agents in humans,[11] it may be advisable for women undergoing chemotherapy for breast cancer to avoid curcumin supplements.[38] Some curcumin supplements also contain piperine, for the purpose of increasing the bioavailability of curcumin. However, piperine may also increase the bioavailability and slow the elimina-

tion of several drugs, including phenytoin (Dilantin), propranolol (Inderal), and theophylline.[87,88]

Summary

- Turmeric is a spice derived from the rhizomes of *Curcuma longa*, a member of the ginger family. Curcuminoids are polyphenolic compounds that give turmeric its yellow color; curcumin is the principal curcuminoid in turmeric.
- The results of phase I clinical trials in patients with colorectal cancer suggest that biologically active levels of curcumin can be achieved in the gastrointestinal tract through oral curcumin supplementation. Such trials provide support for further clinical evaluation in people at risk for gastrointestinal cancers.
- Until the safety and efficacy of curcumin in individuals with cystic fibrosis has been evaluated in clinical trials, the Cystic Fibrosis Foundation does not recommend the use of curcumin as a therapy for cystic fibrosis.
- Although a few preliminary trials suggest that curcumin may have anti-inflammatory activity in humans, larger randomized controlled trials are needed to determine whether oral curcumin supplementation is effective in the treatment of inflammatory diseases.
- As a result of promising findings in animal models of Alzheimer disease, clinical trials of curcumin supplementation in patients with early Alzheimer disease are under way.

References

1. Sharma RA, Gescher AJ, Steward WP. Curcumin: the story so far. Eur J Cancer 2005;41(13):1955–1968
2. Anand P, Kunnumakkara AB, Newman RA, Aggarwal BB. Bioavailability of curcumin: problems and promises. Mol Pharm 2007;4(6):807–818
3. Baum L, Lam CW, Cheung SK, et al. Six-month randomized, placebo-controlled, double-blind, pilot clinical trial of curcumin in patients with Alzheimer disease. J Clin Psychopharmacol 2008;28(1):110–113
4. Lao CD, Ruffin MT IV, Normolle D, et al. Dose escalation of a curcuminoid formulation. BMC Complement Altern Med 2006;6:10
5. Maheshwari RK, Singh AK, Gaddipati J, Srimal RC. Multiple biological activities of curcumin: a short review. Life Sci 2006;78(18):2081–2087
6. Ireson CR, Jones DJ, Orr S, et al. Metabolism of the cancer chemopreventive agent curcumin in human and rat intestine. Cancer Epidemiol Biomarkers Prev 2002;11(1):105–111

7. Ireson C, Orr S, Jones DJ, et al. Characterization of metabolites of the chemopreventive agent curcumin in human and rat hepatocytes and in the rat in vivo, and evaluation of their ability to inhibit phorbol ester-induced prostaglandin E2 production. Cancer Res 2001;61(3):1058–1064

8. Cheng AL, Hsu CH, Lin JK, et al. Phase I clinical trial of curcumin, a chemopreventive agent, in patients with high-risk or pre-malignant lesions. Anticancer Res 2001;21(4B):2895–2900

9. Sharma RA, Euden SA, Platton SL, et al. Phase I clinical trial of oral curcumin: biomarkers of systemic activity and compliance. Clin Cancer Res 2004;10(20):6847–6854

10. Garcea G, Berry DP, Jones DJ, et al. Consumption of the putative chemopreventive agent curcumin by cancer patients: assessment of curcumin levels in the colorectum and their pharmacodynamic consequences. Cancer Epidemiol Biomarkers Prev 2005;14(1):120–125

11. Garcea G, Jones DJ, Singh R, et al. Detection of curcumin and its metabolites in hepatic tissue and portal blood of patients following oral administration. Br J Cancer 2004;90(5):1011–1015

12. Sreejayan, Rao MN. Nitric oxide scavenging by curcuminoids. J Pharm Pharmacol 1997;49(1):105–107

13. Sreejayan N, Rao MN. Free radical scavenging activity of curcuminoids. Arzneimittelforschung 1996;46(2):169–171

14. Steele VE, Hawk ET, Viner JL, Lubet RA. Mechanisms and applications of non-steroidal anti-inflammatory drugs in the chemoprevention of cancer. Mutat Res 2003;523–524:137–144

15. Hong J, Bose M, Ju J, et al. Modulation of arachidonic acid metabolism by curcumin and related beta-diketone derivatives: effects on cytosolic phospholipase A(2), cyclooxygenases and 5-lipoxygenase. Carcinogenesis 2004;25(9):1671–1679

16. Plummer SM, Holloway KA, Manson MM, et al. Inhibition of cyclo-oxygenase 2 expression in colon cells by the chemopreventive agent curcumin involves inhibition of NF-kappaB activation via the NIK/IKK signalling complex. Oncogene 1999;18(44):6013–6020

17. Brouet I, Ohshima H. Curcumin, an anti-tumour promoter and anti-inflammatory agent, inhibits induction of nitric oxide synthase in activated macrophages. Biochem Biophys Res Commun 1995;206(2):533–540

18. Nanji AA, Jokelainen K, Tipoe GL, Rahemtulla A, Thomas P, Dannenberg AJ. Curcumin prevents alcohol-induced liver disease in rats by inhibiting the expression of NF-kappa B-dependent genes. Am J Physiol Gastrointest Liver Physiol 2003;284(2):G321–G327

19. Dickinson DA, Levonen AL, Moellering DR, et al. Human glutamate cysteine ligase gene regulation through the electrophile response element. Free Radic Biol Med 2004;37(8):1152–1159

20. Dickinson DA, Iles KE, Zhang H, Blank V, Forman HJ. Curcumin alters EpRE and AP-1 binding complexes and elevates glutamate-cysteine ligase gene expression. FASEB J 2003;17(3):473–475

21. Zheng S, Yumei F, Chen A. De novo synthesis of glutathione is a prerequisite for curcumin to inhibit hepatic stellate cell (HSC) activation. Free Radic Biol Med 2007;43(3):444–453

22. Lampe JW, Peterson S. Brassica, biotransformation and cancer risk: genetic polymorphisms alter the preventive effects of cruciferous vegetables. J Nutr 2002;132(10):2991–2994

23. Baird WM, Hooven LA, Mahadevan B. Carcinogenic polycyclic aromatic hydrocarbon-DNA adducts and mechanism of action. Environ Mol Mutagen 2005;45(2–3):106–114

24. Ciolino HP, Daschner PJ, Wang TT, Yeh GC. Effect of curcumin on the aryl hydrocarbon receptor and cytochrome P450 1A1 in MCF-7 human breast carcinoma cells. Biochem Pharmacol 1998;56(2):197–206

25. Rinaldi AL, Morse MA, Fields HW, et al. Curcumin activates the aryl hydrocarbon receptor yet significantly inhibits (-)-benzo(a)pyrene-7R-trans-7,8-dihydrodiol bioactivation in oral squamous cell carcinoma cells and oral mucosa. Cancer Res 2002;62(19):5451–5456

26. Singh SV, Hu X, Srivastava SK, et al. Mechanism of inhibition of benzo[a]pyrene-induced forestomach cancer in mice by dietary curcumin. Carcinogenesis 1998;19(8):1357–1360

27. Thapliyal R, Maru GB. Inhibition of cytochrome P450 isozymes by curcumins in vitro and in vivo. Food Chem Toxicol 2001;39(6):541–547

28. Iqbal M, Sharma SD, Okazaki Y, Fujisawa M, Okada S. Dietary supplementation of curcumin enhances antioxidant and phase II metabolizing enzymes in ddY male mice: possible role in protection against chemical carcinogenesis and toxicity. Pharmacol Toxicol 2003;92(1):33–38

29. Susan M, Rao MN. Induction of glutathione S-transferase activity by curcumin in mice. Arzneimittelforschung 1992;42(7):962–964

30. Stewart ZA, Westfall MD, Pietenpol JA. Cell-cycle dysregulation and anticancer therapy. Trends Pharmacol Sci 2003;24(3):139–145

31. Duvoix A, Blasius R, Delhalle S, et al. Chemopreventive and therapeutic effects of curcumin. Cancer Lett 2005;223(2):181–190

32. Surh YJ, Chun KS. Cancer chemopreventive effects of curcumin. Adv Exp Med Biol 2007;595:149–172

33. Singh S, Khar A. Biological effects of curcumin and its role in cancer chemoprevention and therapy. Anticancer Agents Med Chem 2006;6(3):259–270

34. Kuttan G, Kumar KB, Guruvayoorappan C, Kuttan R. Antitumor, anti-invasion, and antimetastatic effects of curcumin. Adv Exp Med Biol 2007;595:173–184

35. Kunnumakkara AB, Anand P, Aggarwal BB. Curcumin inhibits proliferation, invasion, angiogenesis and metastasis of different cancers through interaction with multiple cell signaling proteins. Cancer Lett 2008;269(2):199–225

36. Moos PJ, Edes K, Mullally JE, Fitzpatrick FA. Curcumin impairs tumor suppressor p53 function in colon cancer cells. Carcinogenesis 2004;25(9):1611–1617

37. Tsvetkov P, Asher G, Reiss V, Shaul Y, Sachs L, Lotem J. Inhibition of NAD(P)H:quinone oxidoreductase 1 activity and induction of p53 degradation by the natural phenolic compound curcumin. Proc Natl Acad Sci U S A 2005;102(15):5535–5540

38. Somasundaram S, Edmund NA, Moore DT, Small GW, Shi YY, Orlowski RZ. Dietary curcumin inhibits chemotherapy-induced apoptosis in models of human breast cancer. Cancer Res 2002;62(13):3868–3875

39. Banerji A, Chakrabarti J, Mitra A, Chatterjee A. Effect of curcumin on gelatinase A (MMP-2) activity in B16F10 melanoma cells. Cancer Lett 2004;211(2):235–242

40. Ohashi Y, Tsuchiya Y, Koizumi K, Sakurai H, Saiki I. Prevention of intrahepatic metastasis by curcumin in an orthotopic implantation model. Oncology 2003;65(3):250–258

41. Menon LG, Kuttan R, Kuttan G. Anti-metastatic activity of curcumin and catechin. Cancer Lett 1999;141(1–2):159–165

42. Mitra A, Chakrabarti J, Banerji A, Chatterjee A, Das BR. Curcumin, a potential inhibitor of MMP-2 in human laryngeal squamous carcinoma cells HEp2. J Environ Pathol Toxicol Oncol 2006;25(4):679–690

43. Hong JH, Ahn KS, Bae E, Jeon SS, Choi HY. The effects of curcumin on the invasiveness of prostate cancer in vitro and in vivo. Prostate Cancer Prostatic Dis 2006;9(2):147–152

44. Thaloor D, Singh AK, Sidhu GS, Prasad PV, Kleinman HK, Maheshwari RK. Inhibition of angiogenic differentiation of human umbilical vein endothelial cells by curcumin. Cell Growth Differ 1998;9(4):305–312

45. Bhandarkar SS, Arbiser JL. Curcumin as an inhibitor of angiogenesis. Adv Exp Med Biol 2007;595:185–195

46. Arbiser JL, Klauber N, Rohan R, et al. Curcumin is an in vivo inhibitor of angiogenesis. Mol Med 1998;4(6):376–383

47. Krishnaswamy K, Goud VK, Sesikeran B, Mukundan MA, Krishna TP. Retardation of experimental tumorigenesis and reduction in DNA adducts by turmeric and curcumin. Nutr Cancer 1998;30(2):163–166

48. Li N, Chen X, Liao J, et al. Inhibition of 7,12-dimethylbenz[a]anthracene (DMBA)-induced oral carcinogenesis in hamsters by tea and curcumin. Carcinogenesis 2002;23(8):1307–1313

49. Ikezaki S, Nishikawa A, Furukawa F, et al. Chemopreventive effects of curcumin on glandular stomach carcinogenesis induced by N-methyl-N'-nitro-N-nitrosoguanidine and sodium chloride in rats. Anticancer Res 2001;21(5):3407–3411

50. Huang MT, Lou YR, Ma W, Newmark HL, Reuhl KR, Conney AH. Inhibitory effects of dietary curcumin on forestomach, duodenal, and colon carcinogenesis in mice. Cancer Res 1994;54(22):5841–5847

51. Chuang SE, Kuo ML, Hsu CH, et al. Curcumin-containing diet inhibits diethylnitrosamine-induced murine hepatocarcinogenesis. Carcinogenesis 2000;21(2):331–335

52. Pereira MA, Grubbs CJ, Barnes LH, et al. Effects of the phytochemicals, curcumin and quercetin, upon azoxymethane-induced colon cancer and 7,12-dimethylbenz[a]anthracene-induced mammary cancer in rats. Carcinogenesis 1996;17(6):1305–1311

53. Rao CV, Rivenson A, Simi B, Reddy BS. Chemoprevention of colon carcinogenesis by dietary curcumin, a naturally occurring plant phenolic compound. Cancer Res 1995;55(2):259–266

54. Kawamori T, Lubet R, Steele VE, et al. Chemopreventive effect of curcumin, a naturally occurring anti-inflammatory agent, during the promotion/progression stages of colon cancer. Cancer Res 1999;59(3):597–601

55. Mahmoud NN, Carothers AM, Grunberger D, et al. Plant phenolics decrease intestinal tumors in an animal model of familial adenomatous polyposis. Carcinogenesis 2000;21(5):921–927

56. Perkins S, Verschoyle RD, Hill K, et al. Chemopreventive efficacy and pharmacokinetics of curcumin in the min/+ mouse, a model of familial adenomatous polyposis. Cancer Epidemiol Biomarkers Prev 2002;11(6):535–540

57. Huang MT, Lou YR, Xie JG, et al. Effect of dietary curcumin and dibenzoylmethane on formation of 7,12-dimethylbenz[a]anthracene-induced mammary tumors and lymphomas/leukemias in Sencar mice. Carcinogenesis 1998;19(9):1697–1700

58. Singletary K, MacDonald C, Iovinelli M, Fisher C, Wallig M. Effect of the beta-diketones diferuloylmethane (curcumin) and dibenzoylmethane on rat mammary DNA adducts and tumors induced by 7,12-dimethylbenz[a]anthracene. Carcinogenesis 1998;19(6):1039–1043

59. National Institutes of Health. Clinical Trials.gov. 2005. Available at: http://clinicaltrials.gov/. Accessed Jan 13, 2009

60. Karunagaran D, Rashmi R, Kumar TR. Induction of apoptosis by curcumin and its implications for cancer therapy. Curr Cancer Drug Targets 2005;5(2):117–129

61. National Institutes of Health. An Introduction to Clinical Trials. 2005. Available at: http://clinicaltrials.gov/ct/info/whatis. Accessed May 3, 2012

62. Mall M, Kunzelmann K. Correction of the CF defect by curcumin: hypes and disappointments. Bioessays 2005;27(1):9–13

63. Dhillon N, Aggarwal BB, Newman RA, et al. Phase II trial of curcumin in patients with advanced pancreatic cancer. Clin Cancer Res 2008;14(14):4491–4499

64. Deodhar SD, Sethi R, Srimal RC. Preliminary study on antirheumatic activity of curcumin (diferuloyl methane). Indian J Med Res 1980;71:632–634

65. Satoskar RR, Shah SJ, Shenoy SG. Evaluation of anti-inflammatory property of curcumin (diferuloyl methane) in patients with postoperative inflammation. Int J Clin Pharmacol Ther Toxicol 1986;24(12):651–654

66. Lal B, Kapoor AK, Agrawal PK, Asthana OP, Srimal RC. Role of curcumin in idiopathic inflammatory orbital pseudotumours. Phytother Res 2000;14(6):443–447

67. Lal B, Kapoor AK, Asthana OP, et al. Efficacy of curcumin in the management of chronic anterior uveitis. Phytother Res 1999;13(4):318–322

68. Egan ME, Pearson M, Weiner SA, et al. Curcumin, a major constituent of turmeric, corrects cystic fibrosis defects. Science 2004;304(5670):600–602

69. Song Y, Sonawane ND, Salinas D, et al. Evidence against the rescue of defective DeltaF508-CFTR cellular processing by curcumin in cell culture and mouse models. J Biol Chem 2004;279(39):40629–40633

70. Cystic Fibrosis Foundation. Drug Development Pipeline. Available at: http://www.cff.org/research/DrugDevelopmentPipeline/. Accessed May 3, 2012

71. Cystic Fibrosis Foundation. Curcumin: Information for Patients and Families. 2004. Available at: http://www.cff.org/images/customcontent/CurcuminQAFinal.pdf. Accessed May 3, 2012

72. Gandy S. The role of cerebral amyloid beta accumulation in common forms of Alzheimer disease. J Clin Invest 2005;115(5):1121–1129

73. Cole GM, Morihara T, Lim GP, Yang F, Begum A, Frautschy SA. NSAID and antioxidant prevention of Alzheimer's disease: lessons from in vitro and animal models. Ann N Y Acad Sci 2004;1035:68–84

74. Yang F, Lim GP, Begum AN, et al. Curcumin inhibits formation of amyloid beta oligomers and fibrils, binds plaques, and reduces amyloid in vivo. J Biol Chem 2005;280(7):5892–5901

75. Lim GP, Chu T, Yang F, Beech W, Frautschy SA, Cole GM. The curry spice curcumin reduces oxidative damage and amyloid pathology in an Alzheimer transgenic mouse. J Neurosci 2001;21(21):8370–8377

76. Frautschy SA, Hu W, Kim P, et al. Phenolic anti-inflammatory antioxidant reversal of Abeta-induced cogni-

tive deficits and neuropathology. Neurobiol Aging 2001;22(6):993–1005

77. Pan R, Qiu S, Lu DX, Dong J. Curcumin improves learning and memory ability and its neuroprotective mechanism in mice. Chin Med J (Engl) 2008; 121(9):832–839

78. Kelley BJ, Knopman DS. Alternative medicine and Alzheimer disease. Neurologist 2008;14(5):299–306

79. Joe B, Vijaykumar M, Lokesh BR. Biological properties of curcumin-cellular and molecular mechanisms of action. Crit Rev Food Sci Nutr 2004;44(2):97–111

80. Lechtenberg M, Quandt B, Nahrstedt A. Quantitative determination of curcuminoids in Curcuma rhizomes and rapid differentiation of Curcuma domestica Val. and Curcuma xanthorrhiza Roxb. by capillary electrophoresis. Phytochem Anal 2004;15(3):152–158

81. Tayyem Rf, Heath DD, Al-Delaimy WK, Lock Ch. Curcumin content of turmeric and curry powders. Nutr Cancer 2006;55(2):126–131

82. US Food and Drug Administration. Color Additive Status List. Available at: http://www.fda.gov/forindustry/coloradditives/coloradditive inventories/ucm1066260.htm. Accessed July 26, 2012

83. Rasyid A, Lelo A. The effect of curcumin and placebo on human gall-bladder function: an ultrasound study. Aliment Pharmacol Ther 1999;13(2):245–249

84. Rasyid A, Rahman AR, Jaalam K, Lelo A. Effect of different curcumin dosages on human gall bladder. Asia Pac J Clin Nutr 2002;11(4):314–318

85. Shah BH, Nawaz Z, Pertani SA, et al. Inhibitory effect of curcumin, a food spice from turmeric, on platelet-activating factor- and arachidonic acid-mediated platelet aggregation through inhibition of thromboxane formation and Ca2+ signaling. Biochem Pharmacol 1999;58(7):1167–1172

86. Srivastava KC, Bordia A, Verma SK. Curcumin, a major component of food spice turmeric (Curcuma longa) inhibits aggregation and alters eicosanoid metabolism in human blood platelets. Prostaglandins Leukot Essent Fatty Acids 1995;52(4):223–227

87. Bano G, Raina RK, Zutshi U, Bedi KL, Johri RK, Sharma SC. Effect of piperine on bioavailability and pharmacokinetics of propranolol and theophylline in healthy volunteers. Eur J Clin Pharmacol 1991;41(6):615–617

88. Velpandian T, Jasuja R, Bhardwaj RK, Jaiswal J, Gupta SK. Piperine in food: interference in the pharmacokinetics of phenytoin. Eur J Drug Metab Pharmacokinet 2001;26(4):241–247

11 Flavonoids

Flavonoids are a large family of compounds synthesized by plants that have a common chemical structure.[1] Flavonoids may be further divided into subclasses based on their chemical structure (**Fig. 11.1**). Over the past decade, scientists have become increasingly interested in the potential for various dietary flavonoids to explain some of the health benefits associated with diets that are rich in fruit and vegetables. The scientific evidence for the hypothesis that dietary flavonoids promote health and prevent disease in humans is reviewed in this chapter. See Chapter 12 for more

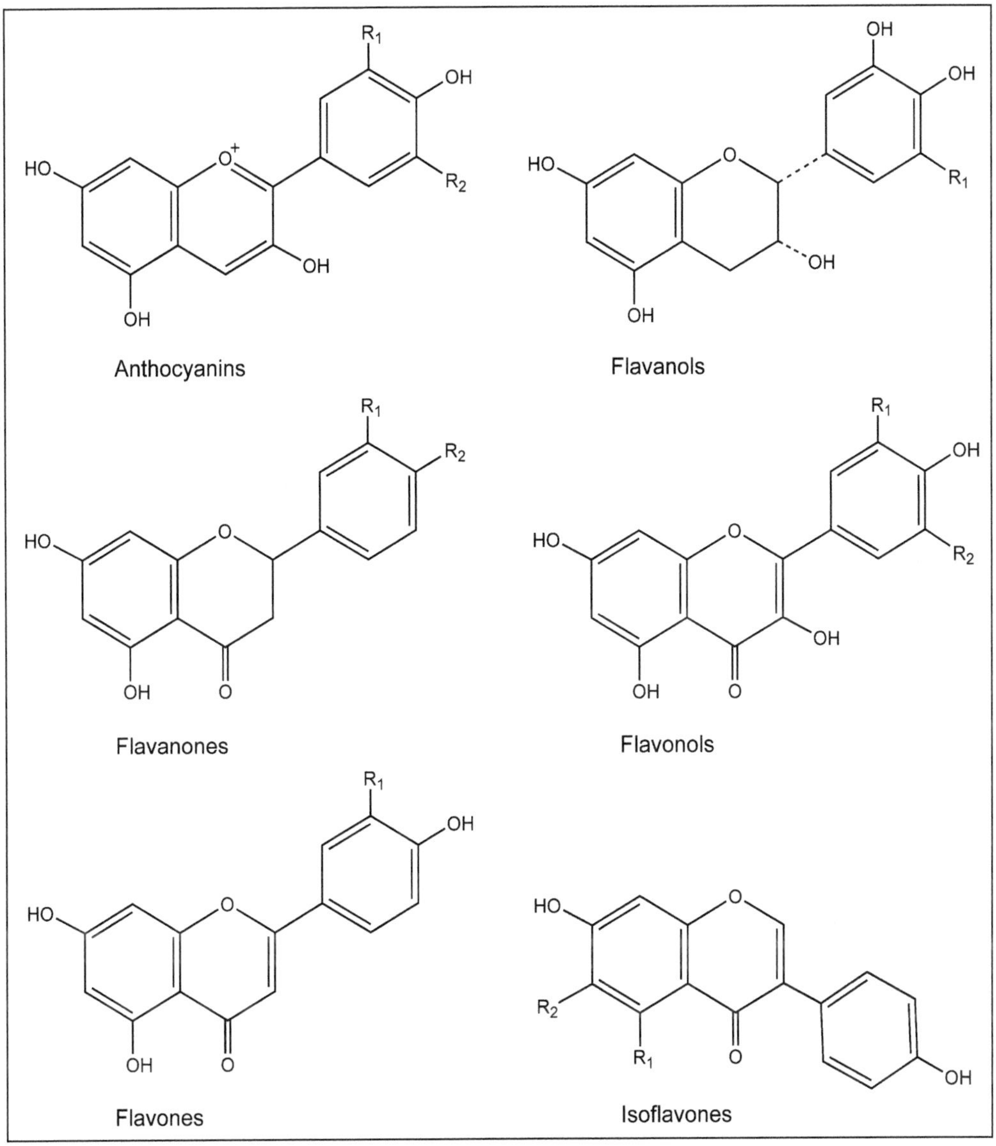

Fig. 11.1 Basic chemical structures of the flavonoid subclasses.

detailed information on the health effects of iso-flavones, a subclass of flavonoids with estrogenic activity.

Bioavailability and Metabolism

Absorption and Metabolism

Flavonoids connected to one or more sugar molecules are known as *flavonoid glycosides*, while those that are not connected to a sugar molecule are called *aglycones*. With the exception of flavanols (catechins and proanthocyanidins), flavonoids occur in plants and most foods as glycosides.[2] Even after cooking, most flavonoid glycosides reach the small intestine intact. Only flavonoid aglycones and flavonoid glucosides (bound to glucose) are absorbed in the small intestine, where they are rapidly metabolized to form methylated, glucuronidated, or sulfated metabolites.[3] Bacteria that normally colonize the colon also play an important role in flavonoid absorption and metabolism. Flavonoids or flavonoid metabolites that reach the colon may be further metabolized by bacterial enzymes, and then absorbed. A person's ability to produce specific flavonoid metabolites may vary and depends on the milieu of the colonic microflora.[4,5] In general, the bioavailability of flavonoids is relatively low, due to limited absorption and rapid elimination. Bioavailability differs for the various flavonoids: isoflavones are the most bioavailable group of flavonoids, while flavanols (proanthocyanidins and tea catechins) and anthocyanins are very poorly absorbed.[6] Since flavonoids are rapidly and extensively metabolized, the biological activities of flavonoid metabolites are not always the same as those of the parent compound (reviewed in [7]). When evaluating the data from flavonoid research in cultured cells, it is important to consider whether the flavonoid concentrations and metabolites used are physiologically relevant.[8] In humans, peak plasma concentrations of soy isoflavones and citrus flavanones have not been found to exceed 10 µmol/L after oral consumption. Peak plasma concentrations measured after the consumption of anthocyanins, flavanols, and flavonols (including those from tea) are generally less than 1 µmol/L.[3]

Biological Activities

Direct Antioxidant Activity

Flavonoids are effective scavengers of free radicals in the test tube (in vitro).[9,10] However, even with very high flavonoid intakes, plasma and intracellular flavonoid concentrations in humans are likely to be 100 to 1000 times lower than concentrations of other antioxidants, such as ascorbate (vitamin C), uric acid, or glutathione. Moreover, most circulating flavonoids are actually flavonoid metabolites, some of which have lower antioxidant activity than the parent flavonoid. For these reasons, the relative contribution of dietary flavonoids to plasma and tissue antioxidant function in vivo is likely to be very small or negligible.[7,11,12]

Metal Chelation

Metal ions, such as iron and copper, can catalyze the production of free radicals. The ability of flavonoids to chelate (bind) metal ions appears to contribute to their antioxidant activity in vitro.[13,14] In living organisms, most iron and copper are bound to proteins, limiting their participation in reactions that produce free radicals. Although the metal-chelating activities of flavonoids may be beneficial in pathological conditions of iron or copper excess, it is not known whether flavonoids or their metabolites function as effective metal chelators in vivo.[11]

Effects on Cell-Signaling Pathways

Cells are capable of responding to a variety of different stresses or signals by increasing or decreasing the availability of specific proteins. The complex cascades of events that lead to changes in the expression of specific genes are known as *cell-signaling pathways* or *signal transduction pathways*. These pathways regulate numerous cell processes, including growth, proliferation, and death (apoptosis). Although it was initially hypothesized that the biological effects of flavonoids would be related to their antioxidant activity, available evidence from cell culture experiments suggests that many of the biological effects of flavonoids are related to their ability to modulate cell-signaling pathways.[7] Intracellular concentrations of flavonoids required to affect cell-signaling pathways are considerably lower than those required to affect cellular antioxidant capacity. Flavonoid metabolites may retain their ability to interact with cell-signaling proteins even if their antioxidant activity is diminished.[15,16] Effective signal transduction requires proteins known as *kinases* that catalyze the phosphorylation of target proteins at specific sites. Cascades involving specific phosphorylations or dephosphorylations of signal transduction proteins ultimately affect the activity of transcription factors—proteins that bind to specific response elements on DNA and promote or inhibit the transcription of various genes. The results of numerous studies in cell culture suggest that flavonoids may affect chronic disease by selectively inhibiting kinases.[7,17] Cell growth and proliferation are also regulated by growth factors that initiate cell-signaling cascades by binding to specific receptors in cell membranes. Flavonoids may alter growth factor signaling by inhibiting receptor phosphorylation or blocking receptor binding by growth factors.[18]

Biological Activities Related to Cancer Prevention

Stimulating Phase II Detoxification Enzyme Activity[19,20]

Phase II detoxification enzymes catalyze reactions that promote the excretion of potentially toxic or carcinogenic chemicals.

Preserving Normal Cell-Cycle Regulation[21,22]

Once a cell divides, it passes through a sequence of stages collectively known as *the cell cycle* before it divides again. Following DNA damage, the cell cycle can be transiently arrested at damage checkpoints, which allows for DNA repair or activation of pathways leading to cell death (apoptosis) if the damage is irreparable.[23] Defective cell-cycle regulation may result in the propagation of mutations that contribute to the development of cancer.

Inhibiting Proliferation and Inducing Apoptosis[24–26]

Unlike normal cells, cancer cells proliferate rapidly and lose the ability to respond to cell death signals that initiate apoptosis.

Inhibiting Tumor Invasion and Angiogenesis[27,28]

Cancerous cells invade normal tissue, aided by enzymes called *matrix metalloproteinases*. To fuel their rapid growth, invasive tumors must develop new blood vessels by a process known as *angiogenesis*.

Decreasing Inflammation[29–31]

Inflammation can result in locally increased production of free radicals by inflammatory enzymes, as well as the release of inflammatory mediators that promote cell proliferation and angiogenesis and inhibit apoptosis.[32]

Biological Activities Related to Cardiovascular Disease Prevention

Decreasing Inflammation[29–31]

Atherosclerosis is now recognized as an inflammatory disease, and several measures of inflammation are associated with increased risk of myocardial infarction (MI) (heart attack).[33]

Decreasing Vascular Cell Adhesion Molecule Expression[34,35]

One of the earliest events in the development of atherosclerosis is the recruitment of inflammatory white blood cells from the blood to the arterial wall. This event is dependent on the expression of adhesion molecules by the vascular endothelial cells that line the inner walls of blood vessels.[36]

Increasing Endothelial Nitric Oxide Synthase (eNOS) Activity[37]

eNOS is the enzyme that catalyzes the formation of nitric oxide by vascular endothelial cells. Nitric oxide is needed to maintain arterial relaxation (vasodilation). Impaired nitric-oxide-dependent vasodilation is associated with increased risk of cardiovascular disease.[38]

Decreasing Platelet Aggregation[39,40]

Platelet aggregation is one of the first steps in the formation of a blood clot that can occlude a coronary or cerebral artery, resulting in MI or stroke, respectively. Inhibiting platelet aggregation is considered an important strategy in the primary and secondary prevention of cardiovascular disease.[41]

Disease Prevention

Cardiovascular Disease

Epidemiological Evidence

Several prospective cohort studies conducted in the United States and Europe have examined the relationship between some measure of dietary flavonoid intake and coronary heart disease (CHD) risk.[42–49] Some studies have found higher flavonoid intakes to be associated with significant reductions in CHD risk,[42–46,50] while others have reported no significant relationship.[47–49,51] In general, the foods that contributed most to total flavonoid intake in these cohorts were black tea, apples, and onions. One study in the Netherlands also found cocoa to be a significant source of dietary flavonoids. Of seven prospective cohort studies that examined relationships between dietary flavonoid intake and the risk of stroke, only two studies found that higher flavonoid intakes were associated with significant reductions in the risk of stroke,[45,52] while five found no relationship.[46,49,50,53,54] Although data from prospective cohort studies suggest that higher intakes of flavonoid-rich foods may help protect against CHD, it cannot be determined whether such protection is conferred by flavonoids, other nutrients and phytochemicals in flavonoid-rich foods, or the whole foods themselves.[55]

Clinical Trials Assessing Vascular Endothelial Function

Vascular endothelial cells play an important role in maintaining cardiovascular health by producing nitric oxide, a compound that promotes arterial relaxation (vasodilation).[56] Arterial vasodilation resulting from endothelial production of nitric oxide is termed endothelium-dependent vasodilation. Several clinical trials have examined the effect of flavonoid-rich foods and beverages on endothelium-dependent vasodilation. Two controlled clinical trials found that daily consumption of 4–5 cups (900–1250 mL) of black tea for 4 weeks significantly improved endothelium-dependent vasodilation in patients with coronary artery disease[57] and in patients with mildly elevated serum cholesterol levels[58] compared with the equivalent amount of caffeine alone or hot water. Other small clinical trials found similar improvements in endothelium-dependent vasodilation in response to daily consumption of around 3 cups (640 mL) of purple grape juice[59] or a high-flavonoid dark chocolate bar for 2 weeks.[60] More recently, a 6-week cocoa intervention trial in 32 postmenopausal women with high cholesterol levels found significant improvements in endothelial function with daily cocoa supplementation.[61] Improvements in endothelial function were also noted in conventionally medicated individuals with type 2 diabetes, following flavanol-rich cocoa supplementation for 30 days.[62] The flavanol epicatechin appears to be one of the compounds in flavanol-rich cocoa responsible for its vasodilatory effects.[63] Interestingly, a recent randomized controlled trial in 44 older adults found that low doses of flavonoid-rich dark chocolate (6.3 g/day for 18 weeks; equivalent to 30 calories) increased levels of plasma S-nitrosoglutathione, an indicator of nitric oxide production, compared with flavonoid-devoid white chocolate.[64]

Platelet Aggregation

Endothelial nitric oxide production also inhibits the adhesion and aggregation of platelets, one of the first steps in blood clot formation.[56] Several clinical trials have examined the potential for high flavonoid intakes to decrease various measures of platelet aggregation outside of the body (ex vivo); such trials have reported mixed results. In general, increasing flavonoid intakes by increasing fruit and/or vegetable intake did not significantly affect ex-vivo platelet aggregation,[41,65,66] nor did increasing black tea consumption.[67,68] However, several small clinical trials in healthy adults have reported significant decreases in ex-vivo measures of platelet aggregation after consumption of grape juice (approx. 500 mL/day) for 7–14 days.[69–71] Similar inhibition of platelet aggregation has been reported following acute or short-term consumption of dark chocolate[72] and following acute consumption of a flavonoid-rich cocoa beverage.[73,74] In addition, a placebo-controlled trial in 32 healthy adults found that 4-week supplementation with flavanols and procyanidins from cocoa inhibited platelet aggregation and function.[75] The results of some controlled clinical trials suggest that relatively high intakes of some flavonoid-rich foods and beverages, including black tea, purple grape juice, and cocoa, may improve vascular endothelial function, but it is not known whether these short-term improvements will result in long-term reductions in cardiovascular disease risk.

Cancer

Although various flavonoids have been found to inhibit the development of chemically induced cancers in animal models of lung,[76] oral,[77] esophageal,[78] stomach,[79] colon,[80] skin,[81] prostate,[82,83] and mammary (breast) cancer,[84] epidemiological studies do not provide convincing evidence that high intakes of dietary flavonoids are associated with substantial reductions in human cancer risk. Most prospective cohort studies that have assessed dietary flavonoid intake using food frequency questionnaires have not found flavonoid intake to be inversely associated with cancer risk.[85] Two prospective cohort studies in Europe found no relationship between the risk of various cancers and dietary intakes of flavones and flavonols,[86] catechins,[87] or tea.[88] In a cohort of postmenopausal women in the United States, catechin intake from tea, but not fruits and vegetables, was inversely associated with the risk of rectal cancer, but not other cancers.[89] Two prospective cohort studies in Finland, where average flavonoid intakes are relatively low, found that men with the highest dietary intakes of flavonols and flavones had a significantly lower risk of developing lung cancer than those with the lowest intakes.[44,45] When individual dietary flavonoids were analyzed, dietary quercetin intake, mainly from apples, was inversely associated with the risk of lung cancer; myricetin intake was inversely associated with the risk of prostate cancer.[45] Tea is an important source of flavonoids (flavanols and flavonols) in some populations, but most prospective cohort studies have not found tea consumption to be inversely associated with cancer risk (reviewed in [90]). The results of case–control studies, which are more likely to be influenced by recall bias, are mixed. While some studies have observed lower flavonoid intakes in people diagnosed with lung,[91] stomach,[92,93] and breast[94] cancer, many others have found no significant differences in flavonoid intake between cancer cases and controls.[95,96] There is limited evidence that low intakes of flavonoids from food are associated with increased risk of certain cancers, but it is not clear whether these findings are related to insufficient intakes of flavonoids or other nutrients and phytochemicals found in flavonoid-rich foods. Clinical trials will be necessary to determine if specific flavonoids are beneficial in the prevention or treatment of cancer; a few clinical trials are currently under way.

Neurodegenerative Disease

Inflammation, oxidative stress, and transition metal accumulation appear to play a role in the pathology of several neurodegenerative diseases, including Parkinson disease and Alzheimer disease.[97] Because flavonoids have anti-inflammatory, antioxidant, and metal-chelating properties, scientists are interested in the neuroprotective potential of flavonoid-rich diets or individual flavonoids. At present, the extent to which various dietary flavonoids and flavonoid metabolites cross the blood–brain barrier in humans is not known.[98,99] Although flavonoid-rich diets and flavonoid administration have been found to prevent cognitive impairment associated with aging and inflammation in some animal studies,[100–103] prospective cohort studies have not found consistent inverse associations between flavonoid intake and the risk of dementia or neurodegenerative disease in humans.[104–108] In a cohort of Japanese-American men followed for 25–30 years, flavonoid intake from tea during mid-life was not associated with the risk of Alzheimer or other types of dementia in late life.[104] Surprisingly, higher intakes of isoflavone-rich tofu during mid-life were associated with cognitive impairment and brain atrophy in late life (see Chapter 12 on Soy Isoflavones).[105] A prospective study of Dutch adults found that total dietary flavonoid intake was not associated with the risk of developing Parkinson disease[106] or Alzheimer disease,[107] except in current smokers whose risk of Alzheimer disease decreased by 50% for every 12 mg increase in daily flavonoid intake. In contrast, a study of elderly French men and women found that those with the lowest flavonoid intakes had a risk of developing dementia over the next 5 years that was 50% higher than for those with the highest intakes.[108] More recently, a study in 1640 elderly men and women found that those with higher dietary flavonoid intake (>13.6 mg/day) had better cognitive performance at baseline and experienced significantly less age-related cognitive decline over a 10-year period than those with a lower flavonoid intake (0–10.4 mg/day).[109] Additionally, a randomized,

Table 11.1   Subclasses of common dietary flavonoids and some common food sources[3]

Flavonoid Subclass	Dietary Flavonoids	Some Common Food Sources
Anthocyanins	Cyanidin, delphinidin, malvidin, pelargonidin, peonidin, petunidin	Red, blue, and purple berries; red and purple grapes; red wine
Flavanols		
Monomers	Catechin, epicatechin, epigallocatechin, epicatechin gallate, epigallocatechin gallate	Teas (green and white), chocolate, grapes, berries, apples
Dimers and polymers	Theaflavins, thearubigins, proanthocyanidins	Teas (black and oolong), chocolate, apples, berries, red grapes, red wine
Flavanones	Hesperetin, naringenin, eriodictyol	Citrus fruits and juices
Flavonols	Quercetin, kaempferol, myricetin, isorhamnetin	Yellow onions, scallions, kale, broccoli, apples, berries, teas
Flavones	Apigenin, luteolin	Parsley, thyme, celery, hot peppers
Isoflavones	Daidzein, genistein, glycitein	Soybeans, soy foods, legumes

double-blind, placebo-controlled clinical trial in 202 postmenopausal women reported that daily supplementation with 25.6 g of soy protein (containing 99 mg of isoflavones) for 1 year did not improve cognitive function.[110] However, a randomized, double-blind, placebo-controlled, crossover trial in 77 postmenopausal women found that 6-month supplementation with 60 mg/day of isoflavones improved some measures of cognitive performance.[111] Although scientists are interested in the potential of flavonoids to protect the aging brain, it is not yet clear how flavonoid consumption affects the risk of neurodegenerative disease in humans.

Sources

Food Sources

Although some subclasses of dietary flavonoids like flavonols are found in many different fruits and vegetables, others are not as widely distributed (see **Table 11.1**).[3] Anthocyanins are most abundant in red, purple, and blue berries, and flavanones are limited to citrus fruits. Flavones are most commonly found in foods used as spices, such as parsley or chillies, while the principal dietary source of isoflavones is soybeans. Flavanols occur in foods as monomers, which are also called *catechins*, or as dimers and polymers. Tea is a rich source of flavanols. Unfermented teas, such as green and white teas, are rich in catechins. Black and oolong teas are fermented during processing, which results in the formation of

catechin dimers and polymers known as *theaflavins* and *thearubigins*, respectively. See Chapter 7 for more information on tea and tea processing. Proanthocyanidins, also known as *condensed tannins*, are a family of flavanol polymers of varying lengths.[112] Research suggests that proanthocyanidins account for a substantial portion of the total flavonoids consumed in typical Western diets. Individual flavonoid intakes may vary considerably, depending on whether tea, red wine, soy products, or fruits and vegetables are commonly consumed.[3] Although individual flavonoid intakes may vary, total flavonoid intakes in Western populations appear to average approximately 150–200 mg/day.[3,112] Information on the flavonoid content of some flavonoid-rich foods is presented in **Table 11.2**. These values should be considered approximate, since several factors may affect the flavonoid content of foods, including agricultural practices, environmental factors, ripening, processing, storing, and cooking.

Supplements

Anthocyanins

Bilberry, elderberry, blackcurrant, blueberry, red grape, and mixed berry extracts that are rich in anthocyanins are available as dietary supplements without a prescription in the United States. The anthocyanin content of these products may vary considerably. Standardized extracts that list the amount of anthocyanins per dose are available.

Table 11.2 Flavonoid content of 100 g or 100 mL of selected foods by flavonoid subclass[3,113–120]

100 g or 100 mL[a]	Anthocya-nins (mg)	Flavanols (mg)	Proanthocy-anidins (mg)	Flavones (mg)	Flavonols (mg)	Flavanones (mg)
Blackberry	89–211	13–19	6–47	–	0–2	–
Blueberry	67–183	1	88–261	–	2–16	–
Grapes, red	25–92	2	44–76	–	3–4	–
Strawberry	15–75	–	97–183	–	1–4	–
Red wine	1–35	1–55	24–70	0	2–30	–
Plum	2–25	1–6	106–334	0	1–2	–
Onion, red	13–25	–	–	0	4–100	–
Onion, yellow	–	0	–	0	3–120	–
Green tea	–	24–216	–	0–1	3–9	–
Black tea	–	5–158	4	0	1–7	–
Chocolate, dark	–	43–63	90–322	–	–	–
Parsley, fresh	–	–	–	24–634	8–10	0
Grapefruit juice	–	–	–	0	0	10–104

[a] Per 100 g (fresh weight) or 100 mL (liquids); 100 g is equivalent to 3.5 oz; 100 mL is equivalent to 3.5 fl oz.

Flavanols

Numerous tea extracts are available in the United States as dietary supplements and may be labeled as tea catechins or tea polyphenols. Green tea extracts are the most commonly marketed, but black and oolong tea extracts are also available. Green tea extracts generally have higher levels of catechins (flavanol monomers), while black tea extracts are richer in theaflavins and thearubigins (flavanol polymers found in tea). Oolong tea extracts fall somewhere in between green and black tea extracts with respect to their flavanol content. Some tea extracts contain caffeine, while others are decaffeinated. Flavanol and caffeine content vary considerably among different products, so it is important to check the label or consult the manufacturer to determine the amounts of flavanols and caffeine that would be consumed daily with each supplement.

Flavanones

Citrus bioflavonoid supplements may contain glycosides of hesperetin (hesperidin), naringenin (naringin), and eriodictyol (eriocitrin). Hesperidin is also available in hesperidin-complex supplements.[120]

Flavones

The peels of citrus fruits are rich in polymethoxylated flavones: tangeretin, nobiletin, and si-nensetin.[3] Although dietary intakes of these naturally occurring flavones are generally low, they are often present in citrus bioflavonoid supplements.

Flavonols

The flavonol aglycone, quercetin, and its glycoside rutin are available as dietary supplements without a prescription in the United States. Other names for rutin include rutinoside, quercetin-3-rutinoside, and sophorin.[120] Citrus bioflavonoid supplements may also contain quercetin or rutin.

Safety

Adverse Effects

No adverse effects have been associated with high dietary intakes of flavonoids from plant-based foods. This lack of adverse effects may be explained by the relatively low bioavailability and rapid metabolism and elimination of most flavonoids.

Quercetin

Some men taking quercetin supplements (1000 mg/day for 1 month) reported nausea, headache, or tingling of the extremities.[121] Some cancer patients given intravenous quercetin in a phase I clinical trial reported nausea, vomiting, sweating, flushing, and dyspnea (difficulty breathing).[122] Intravenous administration of quercetin at doses of 945 mg/m^2 or more was associated with renal (kidney) toxicity in that trial.

Tea Extracts

There have been several reports of hepatotoxicity (liver toxicity) following consumption of supplements containing tea (*Camellia sinensis*) extracts.[123,124] In clinical trials of caffeinated green tea extracts, cancer patients who took 6 g/day in 3–6 divided doses have reported mild to moderate gastrointestinal side effects, including nausea, vomiting, abdominal pain, and diarrhea.[125,126] Central nervous system symptoms, including agitation, restlessness, insomnia, tremors, dizziness, and confusion, have also been reported. In one case, confusion was severe enough to require hospitalization.[125] These side effects were likely related to the caffeine in the green tea extract.[126] In a 4-week clinical trial that assessed the safety of decaffeinated green tea extracts (800 mg/day of epigallocatechin gallate [EGCG]) in healthy individuals, a few of the participants reported mild nausea, stomach upset, dizziness, or muscle pain.[127]

Pregnancy and Lactation

The safety of flavonoid supplements in pregnancy and lactation has not been established.[120]

Drug Interactions

Inhibition of Cytochrome P450 3A4 by Grapefruit Juice and Flavonoids

As little as 200 mL (7 fl oz) of grapefruit juice has been found to irreversibly inhibit the intestinal drug-metabolizing enzyme, cytochrome P450 (CYP) 3A4.[128] Although the most potent inhibitors of CYP3A4 in grapefruit are thought to be furanocoumarins, particularly dihydroxybergamottin, the flavonoids naringenin and quercetin have also been found to inhibit CYP3A4 in vitro. Inhibition of intestinal CYP3A4 can increase the bioavailability and the risk of toxicity of several drugs, including but not limited to HMG-CoA reductase inhibitors (atorvastatin, lovastatin, and simvastatin), calcium channel antagonists (felodipine, nicardipine, nisoldipine, nitrendipine, and verapamil), antiarrhythmic agents (amiodarone), HIV protease inhibitors (saquinavir), im-

munosuppressants (ciclosporin), antihistamines (terfenadine), gastrointestinal stimulants (cisapride), benzodiazepines (diazepam, midazolam, and triazolam), anticonvulsants (carbamazepine), anxiolytics (buspirone) serotonin-specific reuptake inhibitors (sertraline), and drugs used to treat erectile dysfunction (sildenafil).[129] Grapefruit juice may reduce the therapeutic effect of the angiotensin II receptor antagonist, losartan. Because of the potential for adverse drug interactions, some clinicians recommend that people taking medications that undergo extensive presystemic metabolism by CYP3A4 avoid consuming grapefruit juice altogether, to avoid potential toxicities.[129]

Inhibition of P-glycoprotein by Grapefruit Juice and Flavonoids

P-glycoprotein is an efflux transporter that decreases the absorption of several drugs. There is some evidence that the consumption of grapefruit juice inhibits the activity of P-glycoprotein.[129] Quercetin, naringenin, and the green tea flavanol, EGCG, have been found to inhibit the efflux activity of P-glycoprotein in cultured cells.[130] Thus, very high or supplemental intakes of these flavonoids could potentially increase flavonoid bioavailability, potentially increasing the toxicity of drugs that are substrates of P-glycoprotein. Drugs known to be substrates of P-glycoprotein include digoxin, antihypertensive agents, antiarrhythmic agents, chemotherapeutic agents, antifungal agents, HIV protease inhibitors, immunosuppressive agents, H$_2$ receptor antagonists, and some antibiotics.[131]

Anticoagulant and Antiplatelet Drugs

High intakes of flavonoids from purple grape juice (500 mL/day) and dark chocolate (235 mg/day of flavanols) have been found to inhibit platelet aggregation in ex-vivo assays.[69–71,75] Theoretically, high intakes of flavonoids (e.g., from supplements) could increase the risk of bleeding when taken with anticoagulant drugs, such as warfarin (Coumadin), and antiplatelet drugs, such as clopidogrel (Plavix), dipyridamole (Persantin), nonsteroidal anti-inflamatory drugs, and aspirin.

Nutrient Interactions

Iron

Flavonoids can bind nonheme iron, inhibiting its intestinal absorption. Nonheme iron is the principal form of iron in plant foods, dairy products, and iron supplements. The consumption of one cup of tea or cocoa with a meal has been found to decrease the absorption of nonheme iron in that meal by approximately 70%.[132,133] To maximize iron absorption from a meal or iron supplements, flavonoid-rich beverages or flavonoid supplements should not be taken at the same time.

Vitamin C

Studies in cell culture indicate that several flavonoids inhibit the transport of vitamin C into cells, and supplementation of rats with quercetin and vitamin C decreased the intestinal absorption of vitamin C.[134] More research is needed to determine the significance of these findings in humans.

Summary

- Flavonoids are a large family of polyphenolic compounds synthesized by plants.
- Scientists are interested in the potential health benefits of flavonoids associated with diets that are rich in fruit and vegetables.
- Many of the biological effects of flavonoids appear to be related to their ability to modulate cell-signaling pathways, rather than their antioxidant activity.
- Although higher intakes of flavonoid-rich foods are associated with reductions in cardiovascular disease risk, it is not yet known whether flavonoids themselves are cardioprotective.
- Despite promising results in animal studies, it is not clear whether high flavonoid intakes can help prevent cancer in humans.
- It is not yet clear how flavonoid consumption affects the risk of neurodegenerative disease in humans.
- Higher intakes of flavonoid-rich foods have been associated with reduced risk of chronic disease in some studies, but it is not known whether isolated flavonoid supplements or extracts will confer the same benefits as flavonoid-rich foods.

References

1. Beecher GR. Overview of dietary flavonoids: nomenclature, occurrence and intake. J Nutr 2003; 133(10):3248S–3254S
2. Williamson G. Common features in the pathways of absorption and metabolism of flavonoids. In: Meskin MS et al. eds. Phytochemicals: Mechanisms of Action. Boca Raton, FL: CRC Press; 2004:21–33
3. Manach C, Scalbert A, Morand C, Rémésy C, Jiménez L. Polyphenols: food sources and bioavailability. Am J Clin Nutr 2004;79(5):727–747
4. Setchell KD, Brown NM, Lydeking-Olsen E. The clinical importance of the metabolite equol–a clue to the effectiveness of soy and its isoflavones. J Nutr 2002;132(12):3577–3584
5. Yuan JP, Wang JH, Liu X. Metabolism of dietary soy isoflavones to equol by human intestinal microflora—implications for health. Mol Nutr Food Res 2007; 51(7):765–781
6. Manach C, Williamson G, Morand C, Scalbert A, Rémésy C. Bioavailability and bioefficacy of polyphenols in humans. I. Review of 97 bioavailability studies. Am J Clin Nutr 2005; 81(1, Suppl):230S–242S
7. Williams RJ, Spencer JP, Rice-Evans C. Flavonoids: antioxidants or signalling molecules? Free Radic Biol Med 2004;36(7):838–849
8. Kroon PA, Clifford MN, Crozier A, et al. How should we assess the effects of exposure to dietary polyphenols in vitro? Am J Clin Nutr 2004;80(1):15–21
9. Heijnen CG, Haenen GR, van Acker FA, van der Vijgh WJ, Bast A. Flavonoids as peroxynitrite scavengers: the role of the hydroxyl groups. Toxicol In Vitro 2001;15(1):3–6
10. Chun OK, Kim DO, Lee CY. Superoxide radical scavenging activity of the major polyphenols in fresh plums. J Agric Food Chem 2003;51(27):8067–8072
11. Frei B, Higdon JV. Antioxidant activity of tea polyphenols in vivo: evidence from animal studies. J Nutr 2003;133(10):3275S–3284S
12. Lotito SB, Frei B. Consumption of flavonoid-rich foods and increased plasma antioxidant capacity in humans: cause, consequence, or epiphenomenon? Free Radic Biol Med 2006;41(12):1727–1746
13. Mira L, Fernandez MT, Santos M, Rocha R, Florêncio MH, Jennings KR. Interactions of flavonoids with iron and copper ions: a mechanism for their antioxidant activity. Free Radic Res 2002;36(11):1199–1208
14. Cheng IF, Breen K. On the ability of four flavonoids, baicilein, luteolin, naringenin, and quercetin, to suppress the Fenton reaction of the iron-ATP complex. Biometals 2000;13(1):77–83
15. Spencer JP, Rice-Evans C, Williams RJ. Modulation of pro-survival Akt/protein kinase B and ERK1/2 signaling cascades by quercetin and its in vivo metabolites underlie their action on neuronal viability. J Biol Chem 2003;278(37):34783–34793
16. Spencer JP, Schroeter H, Crossthwaithe AJ, Kuhnle G, Williams RJ, Rice-Evans C. Contrasting influences of glucuronidation and O-methylation of epicatechin on hydrogen peroxide-induced cell death in neurons and fibroblasts. Free Radic Biol Med 2001;31(9):1139–1146
17. Hou Z, Lambert JD, Chin KV, Yang CS. Effects of tea polyphenols on signal transduction pathways related to cancer chemoprevention. Mutat Res 2004;555(1–2):3–19

18. Lambert JD, Yang CS. Mechanisms of cancer prevention by tea constituents. J Nutr 2003;133(10):3262S–3267S
19. Kong AN, Owuor E, Yu R, et al. Induction of xenobiotic enzymes by the MAP kinase pathway and the antioxidant or electrophile response element (ARE/EpRE). Drug Metab Rev 2001;33(3–4):255–271
20. Walle UK, Walle T. Induction of human UDP-glucuronosyltransferase UGT1A1 by flavonoids-structural requirements. Drug Metab Dispos 2002;30(5):564–569
21. Chen JJ, Ye ZQ, Koo MW. Growth inhibition and cell cycle arrest effects of epigallocatechin gallate in the NBT-II bladder tumour cell line. BJU Int 2004;93(7):1082–1086
22. Wang W, VanAlstyne PC, Irons KA, Chen S, Stewart JW, Birt DF. Individual and interactive effects of apigenin analogs on G2/M cell-cycle arrest in human colon carcinoma cell lines. Nutr Cancer 2004;48(1):106–114
23. Stewart ZA, Westfall MD, Pietenpol JA. Cell-cycle dysregulation and anticancer therapy. Trends Pharmacol Sci 2003;24(3):139–145
24. Sah JF, Balasubramanian S, Eckert RL, Rorke EA. Epigallocatechin-3-gallate inhibits epidermal growth factor receptor signaling pathway. Evidence for direct inhibition of ERK1/2 and AKT kinases. J Biol Chem 2004;279(13):12755–12762
25. Kavanagh KT, Hafer LJ, Kim DW, et al. Green tea extracts decrease carcinogen-induced mammary tumor burden in rats and rate of breast cancer cell proliferation in culture. J Cell Biochem 2001;82(3):387–398
26. Ramos S. Effects of dietary flavonoids on apoptotic pathways related to cancer chemoprevention. J Nutr Biochem 2007;18(7):427–442
27. Bagli E, Stefaniotou M, Morbidelli L, et al. Luteolin inhibits vascular endothelial growth factor-induced angiogenesis; inhibition of endothelial cell survival and proliferation by targeting phosphatidylinositol 3'-kinase activity. Cancer Res 2004;64(21):7936–7946
28. Kim MH. Flavonoids inhibit VEGF/bFGF-induced angiogenesis in vitro by inhibiting the matrix-degrading proteases. J Cell Biochem 2003;89(3):529–538
29. O'Leary KA, de Pascual-Tereasa S, Needs PW, Bao YP, O'Brien NM, Williamson G. Effect of flavonoids and vitamin E on cyclooxygenase-2 (COX-2) transcription. Mutat Res 2004;551(1–2):245–254
30. Sakata K, Hirose Y, Qiao Z, Tanaka T, Mori H. Inhibition of inducible isoforms of cyclooxygenase and nitric oxide synthase by flavonoid hesperidin in mouse macrophage cell line. Cancer Lett 2003;199(2):139–145
31. Cho SY, Park SJ, Kwon MJ, et al. Quercetin suppresses proinflammatory cytokines production through MAP kinases and NF-kappaB pathway in lipopolysaccharide-stimulated macrophage. Mol Cell Biochem 2003;243(1–2):153–160
32. Steele VE, Hawk ET, Viner JL, Lubet RA. Mechanisms and applications of non-steroidal anti-inflammatory drugs in the chemoprevention of cancer. Mutat Res 2003;523–524:137–144
33. Blake GJ, Ridker PM. C-reactive protein and other inflammatory risk markers in acute coronary syndromes. J Am Coll Cardiol 2003; 41(4, Suppl S):37S–42S
34. Choi JS, Choi YJ, Park SH, Kang JS, Kang YH. Flavones mitigate tumor necrosis factor-alpha-induced adhesion molecule upregulation in cultured human endothelial cells: role of nuclear factor-kappa B. J Nutr 2004;134(5):1013–1019
35. Ludwig A, Lorenz M, Grimbo N, et al. The tea flavonoid epigallocatechin-3-gallate reduces cytokine-induced VCAM-1 expression and monocyte adhesion to endothelial cells. Biochem Biophys Res Commun 2004;316(3):659–665
36. Stocker R, Keaney JF Jr. Role of oxidative modifications in atherosclerosis. Physiol Rev 2004;84(4):1381–1478
37. Anter E, Thomas SR, Schulz E, Shapira OM, Vita JA, Keaney JF Jr. Activation of endothelial nitric-oxide synthase by the p38 MAPK in response to black tea polyphenols. J Biol Chem 2004;279(45):46637–46643
38. Duffy SJ, Vita JA. Effects of phenolics on vascular endothelial function. Curr Opin Lipidol 2003;14(1):21–27
39. Deana R, Turetta L, Donella-Deana A, et al. Green tea epigallocatechin-3-gallate inhibits platelet signalling pathways triggered by both proteolytic and non-proteolytic agonists. Thromb Haemost 2003;89(5):866–874
40. Bucki R, Pastore JJ, Giraud F, Sulpice JC, Janmey PA. Flavonoid inhibition of platelet procoagulant activity and phosphoinositide synthesis. J Thromb Haemost 2003;1(8):1820–1828
41. Hubbard GP, Wolffram S, Lovegrove JA, Gibbins JM. The role of polyphenolic compounds in the diet as inhibitors of platelet function. Proc Nutr Soc 2003; 62(2):469–478
42. Geleijnse JM, Launer LJ, Van der Kuip DA, Hofman A, Witteman JC. Inverse association of tea and flavonoid intakes with incident myocardial infarction: the Rotterdam Study. Am J Clin Nutr 2002;75(5):880–886
43. Hertog MG, Feskens EJ, Kromhout D. Antioxidant flavonols and coronary heart disease risk. Lancet 1997;349(9053):699
44. Hirvonen T, Pietinen P, Virtanen M, et al. Intake of flavonols and flavones and risk of coronary heart disease in male smokers. Epidemiology 2001;12(1):62–67
45. Knekt P, Kumpulainen J, Järvinen R, et al. Flavonoid intake and risk of chronic diseases. Am J Clin Nutr 2002;76(3):560–568
46. Yochum L, Kushi LH, Meyer K, Folsom AR. Dietary flavonoid intake and risk of cardiovascular disease in postmenopausal women. Am J Epidemiol 1999; 149(10):943–949
47. Hertog MG, Sweetnam PM, Fehily AM, Elwood PC, Kromhout D. Antioxidant flavonols and ischemic heart disease in a Welsh population of men: the Caerphilly Study. Am J Clin Nutr 1997;65(5):1489–1494
48. Rimm EB, Katan MB, Ascherio A, Stampfer MJ, Willett WC. Relation between intake of flavonoids and risk for coronary heart disease in male health professionals. Ann Intern Med 1996;125(5):384–389
49. Sesso HD, Gaziano JM, Liu S, Buring JE. Flavonoid intake and the risk of cardiovascular disease in women. Am J Clin Nutr 2003;77(6):1400–1408
50. Mink PJ, Scrafford CG, Barraj LM, et al. Flavonoid intake and cardiovascular disease mortality: a prospective study in postmenopausal women. Am J Clin Nutr 2007;85(3):895–909
51. Lin J, Rexrode KM, Hu F, et al. Dietary intakes of flavonols and flavones and coronary heart disease in US women. Am J Epidemiol 2007;165(11):1305–1313
52. Keli SO, Hertog MG, Feskens EJ, Kromhout D. Dietary flavonoids, antioxidant vitamins, and incidence of

stroke: the Zutphen study. Arch Intern Med 1996;156(6):637–642

53. Hirvonen T, Virtamo J, Korhonen P, Albanes D, Pietinen P. Intake of flavonoids, carotenoids, vitamins C and E, and risk of stroke in male smokers. Stroke 2000;31(10):2301–2306

54. Knekt P, Isotupa S, Rissanen H, et al. Quercetin intake and the incidence of cerebrovascular disease. Eur J Clin Nutr 2000;54(5):415–417

55. Liu RH. Health benefits of fruit and vegetables are from additive and synergistic combinations of phytochemicals. Am J Clin Nutr 2003; 78(3, Suppl):517S–520S

56. Vita JA. Tea consumption and cardiovascular disease: effects on endothelial function. J Nutr 2003; 133(10):3293S–3297S

57. Duffy SJ, Keaney JF Jr, Holbrook M, et al. Short- and long-term black tea consumption reverses endothelial dysfunction in patients with coronary artery disease. Circulation 2001;104(2):151–156

58. Hodgson JM, Puddey IB, Burke V, Watts GF, Beilin LJ. Regular ingestion of black tea improves brachial artery vasodilator function. Clin Sci (Lond) 2002; 102(2):195–201

59. Stein JH, Keevil JG, Wiebe DA, Aeschlimann S, Folts JD. Purple grape juice improves endothelial function and reduces the susceptibility of LDL cholesterol to oxidation in patients with coronary artery disease. Circulation 1999;100(10):1050–1055

60. Engler MB, Engler MM, Chen CY, et al. Flavonoid-rich dark chocolate improves endothelial function and increases plasma epicatechin concentrations in healthy adults. J Am Coll Nutr 2004;23(3):197–204

61. Wang-Polagruto JF, Villablanca AC, Polagruto JA, et al. Chronic consumption of flavanol-rich cocoa improves endothelial function and decreases vascular cell adhesion molecule in hypercholesterolemic postmenopausal women. J Cardiovasc Pharmacol 2006;47 (Suppl 2):S177–S186; discussion S206–S209

62. Balzer J, Rassaf T, Heiss C, et al. Sustained benefits in vascular function through flavanol-containing cocoa in medicated diabetic patients a double-masked, randomized, controlled trial. J Am Coll Cardiol 2008; 51(22):2141–2149

63. Schroeter H, Heiss C, Balzer J, et al. (-)-Epicatechin mediates beneficial effects of flavanol-rich cocoa on vascular function in humans. Proc Natl Acad Sci U S A 2006;103(4):1024–1029

64. Taubert D, Roesen R, Lehmann C, Jung N, Schömig E. Effects of low habitual cocoa intake on blood pressure and bioactive nitric oxide: a randomized controlled trial. JAMA 2007;298(1):49–60

65. Freese R, Vaarala O, Turpeinen AM, Mutanen M. No difference in platelet activation or inflammation markers after diets rich or poor in vegetables, berries and apple in healthy subjects. Eur J Nutr 2004; 43(3):175–182

66. Janssen K, Mensink RP, Cox FJ, et al. Effects of the flavonoids quercetin and apigenin on hemostasis in healthy volunteers: results from an in vitro and a dietary supplement study. Am J Clin Nutr 1998; 67(2):255–262

67. Duffy SJ, Vita JA, Holbrook M, Swerdloff PL, Keaney JF Jr. Effect of acute and chronic tea consumption on platelet aggregation in patients with coronary artery disease. Arterioscler Thromb Vasc Biol 2001;21(6): 1084–1089

68. Hodgson JM, Puddey IB, Burke V, Beilin LJ, Mori TA, Chan SY. Acute effects of ingestion of black tea on postprandial platelet aggregation in human subjects. Br J Nutr 2002;87(2):141–145

69. Freedman JE, Parker C III, Li L, et al. Select flavonoids and whole juice from purple grapes inhibit platelet function and enhance nitric oxide release. Circulation 2001;103(23):2792–2798

70. Keevil JG, Osman HE, Reed JD, Folts JD. Grape juice, but not orange juice or grapefruit juice, inhibits human platelet aggregation. J Nutr 2000;130(1):53–56

71. Polagruto JA, Schramm DD, Wang-Polagruto JF, Lee L, Keen CL. Effects of flavonoid-rich beverages on prostacyclin synthesis in humans and human aortic endothelial cells: association with ex vivo platelet function. J Med Food 2003;6(4):301–308

72. Innes AJ, Kennedy G, McLaren M, Bancroft AJ, Belch JJ. Dark chocolate inhibits platelet aggregation in healthy volunteers. Platelets 2003;14(5):325–327

73. Rein D, Paglieroni TG, Pearson DA, et al. Cocoa and wine polyphenols modulate platelet activation and function. J Nutr 2000;130(8S Suppl):2120S–2126S

74. Rein D, Paglieroni TG, Wun T, et al. Cocoa inhibits platelet activation and function. Am J Clin Nutr 2000;72(1):30–35

75. Murphy KJ, Chronopoulos AK, Singh I, et al. Dietary flavanols and procyanidin oligomers from cocoa (Theobroma cacao) inhibit platelet function. Am J Clin Nutr 2003;77(6):1466–1473

76. Yang CS, Yang GY, Landau JM, Kim S, Liao J. Tea and tea polyphenols inhibit cell hyperproliferation, lung tumorigenesis, and tumor progression. Exp Lung Res 1998;24(4):629–639

77. Balasubramanian S, Govindasamy S. Inhibitory effect of dietary flavonol quercetin on 7,12-dimethylbenz[a] anthracene-induced hamster buccal pouch carcinogenesis. Carcinogenesis 1996;17(4):877–879

78. Li ZG, Shimada Y, Sato F, et al. Inhibitory effects of epigallocatechin-3-gallate on N-nitrosomethylbenzylamine-induced esophageal tumorigenesis in F344 rats. Int J Oncol 2002;21(6):1275–1283

79. Yamane T, Nakatani H, Kikuoka N, et al. Inhibitory effects and toxicity of green tea polyphenols for gastrointestinal carcinogenesis. Cancer 1996; 77(8, Suppl):1662–1667

80. Guo JY, Li X, Browning JD Jr, et al. Dietary soy isoflavones and estrone protect ovariectomized ERalphaKO and wild-type mice from carcinogen-induced colon cancer. J Nutr 2004;134(1):179–182

81. Huang MT, Xie JG, Wang ZY, et al. Effects of tea, decaffeinated tea, and caffeine on UVB light-induced complete carcinogenesis in SKH-1 mice: demonstration of caffeine as a biologically important constituent of tea. Cancer Res 1997;57(13):2623–2629

82. Gupta S, Hastak K, Ahmad N, Lewin JS, Mukhtar H. Inhibition of prostate carcinogenesis in TRAMP mice by oral infusion of green tea polyphenols. Proc Natl Acad Sci U S A 2001;98(18):10350–10355

83. Haddad AQ, Venkateswaran V, Viswanathan L, Teahan SJ, Fleshner NE, Klotz LH. Novel antiproliferative flavonoids induce cell cycle arrest in human prostate cancer cell lines. Prostate Cancer Prostatic Dis 2006;9(1):68–76

84. Yamagishi M, Natsume M, Osakabe N, et al. Effects of cacao liquor proanthocyanidins on PhIP-induced mutagenesis in vitro, and in vivo mammary and pancreatic tumorigenesis in female Sprague-Dawley rats. Cancer Lett 2002;185(2):123–130

85. Ross JA, Kasum CM. Dietary flavonoids: bioavailability, metabolic effects, and safety. Annu Rev Nutr 2002;22:19–34

86. Hertog MG, Feskens EJ, Hollman PC, Katan MB, Kromhout D. Dietary flavonoids and cancer risk in the Zutphen Elderly Study. Nutr Cancer 1994;22(2):175–184

87. Arts IC, Hollman PC, Bueno De Mesquita HB, Feskens EJ, Kromhout D. Dietary catechins and epithelial cancer incidence: the Zutphen elderly study. Int J Cancer 2001;92(2):298–302

88. Goldbohm RA, Hertog MG, Brants HA, van Poppel G, van den Brandt PA. Consumption of black tea and cancer risk: a prospective cohort study. J Natl Cancer Inst 1996;88(2):93–100

89. Arts IC, Jacobs DR Jr, Gross M, Harnack LJ, Folsom AR. Dietary catechins and cancer incidence among postmenopausal women: the Iowa Women's Health Study (United States). Cancer Causes Control 2002; 13(4):373–382

90. Higdon JV, Frei B. Tea catechins and polyphenols: health effects, metabolism, and antioxidant functions. Crit Rev Food Sci Nutr 2003;43(1):89–143

91. De Stefani E, Ronco A, Mendilaharsu M, Deneo-Pellegrini H. Diet and risk of cancer of the upper aerodigestive tract–II. Nutrients. Oral Oncol 1999; 35(1):22–26

92. Garcia-Closas R, Gonzalez CA, Agudo A, Riboli E. Intake of specific carotenoids and flavonoids and the risk of gastric cancer in Spain. Cancer Causes Control 1999;10(1):71–75

93. Lagiou P, Samoli E, Lagiou A, et al. Flavonoids, vitamin C and adenocarcinoma of the stomach. Cancer Causes Control 2004;15(1):67–72

94. Peterson J, Lagiou P, Samoli E, et al. Flavonoid intake and breast cancer risk: a case–control study in Greece. Br J Cancer 2003;89(7):1255–1259

95. Garcia R, Gonzalez CA, Agudo A, Riboli E. High intake of specific carotenoids and flavonoids does not reduce the risk of bladder cancer. Nutr Cancer 1999;35(2):212–214

96. Garcia-Closas R, Agudo A, Gonzalez CA, Riboli E. Intake of specific carotenoids and flavonoids and the risk of lung cancer in women in Barcelona, Spain. Nutr Cancer 1998;32(3):154–158

97. Ramassamy C. Emerging role of polyphenolic compounds in the treatment of neurodegenerative diseases: a review of their intracellular targets. Eur J Pharmacol 2006;545(1):51–64

98. Youdim KA, Qaiser MZ, Begley DJ, Rice-Evans CA, Abbott NJ. Flavonoid permeability across an in situ model of the blood-brain barrier. Free Radic Biol Med 2004;36(5):592–604

99. Schmitt-Schillig S, Schaffer S, Weber CC, Eckert GP, Müller WE. Flavonoids and the aging brain. J Physiol Pharmacol 2005;56(Suppl 1):23–36

100. Goyarzu P, Malin DH, Lau FC, et al. Blueberry supplemented diet: effects on object recognition memory and nuclear factor-kappa B levels in aged rats. Nutr Neurosci 2004;7(2):75–83

101. Joseph JA, Denisova NA, Arendash G, et al. Blueberry supplementation enhances signaling and prevents behavioral deficits in an Alzheimer disease model. Nutr Neurosci 2003;6(3):153–162

102. Joseph JA, Shukitt-Hale B, Denisova NA, et al. Reversals of age-related declines in neuronal signal transduction, cognitive, and motor behavioral deficits with blueberry, spinach, or strawberry dietary supplementation. J Neurosci 1999;19(18):8114–8121

103. Patil CS, Singh VP, Satyanarayan PS, Jain NK, Singh A, Kulkarni SK. Protective effect of flavonoids against aging- and lipopolysaccharide-induced cognitive impairment in mice. Pharmacology 2003;69(2):59–67

104. Laurin D, Masaki KH, Foley DJ, White LR, Launer LJ. Midlife dietary intake of antioxidants and risk of late-life incident dementia: the Honolulu-Asia Aging Study. Am J Epidemiol 2004;159(10):959–967

105. White LR, Petrovitch H, Ross GW, et al. Brain aging and midlife tofu consumption. J Am Coll Nutr 2000;19(2):242–255

106. de Rijk MC, Breteler MM, den Breeijen JH, et al. Dietary antioxidants and Parkinson disease. The Rotterdam Study. Arch Neurol 1997;54(6):762–765

107. Engelhart MJ, Geerlings MI, Ruitenberg A, et al. Dietary intake of antioxidants and risk of Alzheimer disease. JAMA 2002;287(24):3223–3229

108. Commenges D, Scotet V, Renaud S, Jacqmin-Gadda H, Barberger-Gateau P, Dartigues JF. Intake of flavonoids and risk of dementia. Eur J Epidemiol 2000; 16(4):357–363

109. Letenneur L, Proust-Lima C, Le Gouge A, Dartigues JF, Barberger-Gateau P. Flavonoid intake and cognitive decline over a 10-year period. Am J Epidemiol 2007;165(12):1364–1371

110. Kreijkamp-Kaspers S, Kok L, Grobbee DE, et al. Effect of soy protein containing isoflavones on cognitive function, bone mineral density, and plasma lipids in postmenopausal women: a randomized controlled trial. JAMA 2004;292(1):65–74

111. Casini ML, Marelli G, Papaleo E, Ferrari A, D'Ambrosio F, Unfer V. Psychological assessment of the effects of treatment with phytoestrogens on postmenopausal women: a randomized, double-blind, crossover, placebo-controlled study. Fertil Steril 2006;85(4):972–978

112. Gu L, Kelm MA, Hammerstone JF, et al. Concentrations of proanthocyanidins in common foods and estimations of normal consumption. J Nutr 2004; 134(3):613–617

113. US Department of Agriculture. USDA Database for the Flavonoid Content of Selected Foods. March 2003. Available at: http://www.nal.usda.gov/fnic/foodcomp/Data/Flav/flav.html. Accessed May 3, 2012

114. US Department of Agriculture. USDA Database for the Proanthocyanidin Content of Selected Foods. August, 2004. Available at: http://www.nal.usda.gov/fnic/foodcomp/Data/PA/PA.html. Accessed May 3, 2010

115. Vrhovsek U, Rigo A, Tonon D, Mattivi F. Quantitation of polyphenols in different apple varieties. J Agric Food Chem 2004;52(21):6532–6538

116. Moyer RA, Hummer KE, Finn CE, Frei B, Wrolstad RE. Anthocyanins, phenolics, and antioxidant capacity in diverse small fruits: vaccinium, rubus, and ribes. J Agric Food Chem 2002;50(3):519–525

117. Lee HS. Characterization of major anthocyanins and the color of red-fleshed Budd Blood orange (Citrus sinensis). J Agric Food Chem 2002;50(5):1243–1246

118. Ryan JM, Revilla E. Anthocyanin composition of Cabernet Sauvignon and Tempranillo grapes at different stages of ripening. J Agric Food Chem 2003; 51(11):3372–3378

119. Henning SM, Fajardo-Lira C, Lee HW, Youssefian AA, Go VL, Heber D. Catechin content of 18 teas and a green tea extract supplement correlates with the antioxidant capacity. Nutr Cancer 2003;45(2):226–235

120. Hendler SS, Rorvik DR, eds. PDR for Nutritional Supplements. Montvale, NJ: Medical Economics Company, Inc; 2001
121. Shoskes DA, Zeitlin SI, Shahed A, Rajfer J. Quercetin in men with category III chronic prostatitis: a preliminary prospective, double-blind, placebo-controlled trial. Urology 1999;54(6):960–963
122. Ferry DR, Smith A, Malkhandi J, et al. Phase I clinical trial of the flavonoid quercetin: pharmacokinetics and evidence for in vivo tyrosine kinase inhibition. Clin Cancer Res 1996;2(4):659–668
123. Bonkovsky HL. Hepatotoxicity associated with supplements containing Chinese green tea (Camellia sinensis). Ann Intern Med 2006;144(1):68–71
124. Javaid A, Bonkovsky HL. Hepatotoxicity due to extracts of Chinese green tea (Camellia sinensis): a growing concern. J Hepatol 2006;45(2):334–335, author reply 335–336
125. Jatoi A, Ellison N, Burch PA, et al. A phase II trial of green tea in the treatment of patients with androgen independent metastatic prostate carcinoma. Cancer 2003;97(6):1442–1446
126. Pisters KM, Newman RA, Coldman B, et al. Phase I trial of oral green tea extract in adult patients with solid tumors. J Clin Oncol 2001;19(6):1830–1838
127. Chow HH, Cai Y, Hakim IA, et al. Pharmacokinetics and safety of green tea polyphenols after multiple-dose administration of epigallocatechin gallate and polyphenon E in healthy individuals. Clin Cancer Res 2003;9(9):3312–3319
128. Bailey DG, Dresser GK. Interactions between grapefruit juice and cardiovascular drugs. Am J Cardiovasc Drugs 2004;4(5):281–297
129. Dahan A, Altman H. Food-drug interaction: grapefruit juice augments drug bioavailability—mechanism, extent and relevance. Eur J Clin Nutr 2004; 58(1):1–9
130. Zhou S, Lim LY, Chowbay B. Herbal modulation of P-glycoprotein. Drug Metab Rev 2004;36(1):57–104
131. Marzolini C, Paus E, Buclin T, Kim RB. Polymorphisms in human MDR1 (P-glycoprotein): recent advances and clinical relevance. Clin Pharmacol Ther 2004;75(1):13–33
132. Hurrell RF, Reddy M, Cook JD. Inhibition of nonhaem iron absorption in man by polyphenolic-containing beverages. Br J Nutr 1999;81(4):289–295
133. Zijp IM, Korver O, Tijburg LB. Effect of tea and other dietary factors on iron absorption. Crit Rev Food Sci Nutr 2000;40(5):371–398
134. Song J, Kwon O, Chen S, et al. Flavonoid inhibition of sodium-dependent vitamin C transporter 1 (SVCT1) and glucose transporter isoform 2 (GLUT2), intestinal transporters for vitamin C and glucose. J Biol Chem 2002;277(18):15252–15260

12 Soy Isoflavones

Isoflavones are polyphenolic compounds that are capable of exerting estrogen-like effects. For this reason, they are classified as phytoestrogens—plant-derived compounds with estrogenic activity.[1] Legumes, particularly soybeans, are the richest sources of isoflavones in the human diet. In soybeans, isoflavones are present as glycosides (bound to a sugar molecule). Fermentation or digestion of soybeans or soy products results in release of the sugar molecule from the isoflavone glycoside, leaving an isoflavone aglycone. Soy isoflavone glycosides are called *daidzin, genistin,* and *glycitin*; the aglycones are called *genistein, daidzein,* and *glycitein,* respectively (**Fig. 12.1**). Unless otherwise indicated, quantities of isoflavones specified in this article refer to aglycones—not glycosides.

Bioavailability and Metabolism

The biological effects of soy isoflavones are strongly influenced by their metabolism, which is dependent on the activity of bacteria that colonize the human intestine.[2] For example, the soy isoflavone daidzein may be metabolized in the intestine to equol (**Fig. 12.2**), a metabolite that has greater estrogenic activity than daidzein, and to other metabolites that are less estrogenic. Studies that measure urinary equol excretion after soy consumption indicate that only approximately 33% of individuals from Western populations metabolize daidzein to equol.[3] Thus, individual differences in the metabolism of isoflavones could have important implications for the biological activities of these phytoestrogens.

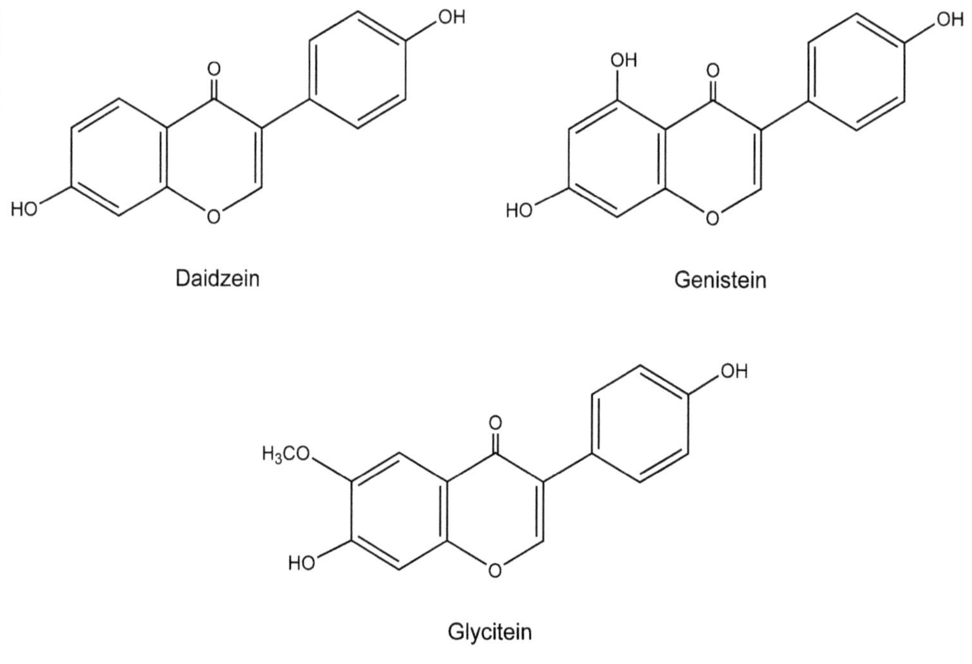

Daidzein

Genistein

Glycitein

Fig. 12.1 Chemical structures of the soy isoflavones, daidzein, genistein, and glycitein, in their aglycone forms.

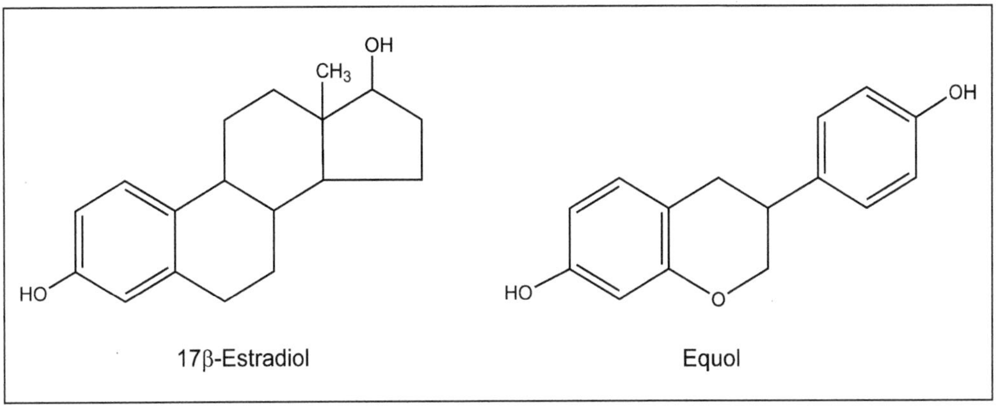

Fig. 12.2 Chemical structures of 17 β-estradiol, an endogenous estrogen, and equol, a bacterial metabolite of daidzein that has estrogenic activity.

Biological Activities

Estrogenic and Antiestrogenic Activities

Soy isoflavones are known to have weak estrogenic or hormone-like activity. Estrogens are signaling molecules that exert their effects by binding to estrogen receptors within cells. The estrogen–receptor complex interacts with DNA to change the expression of estrogen-responsive genes. Estrogen receptors are present in numerous tissues other than those associated with reproduction, including bone, liver, heart, and brain.[4] Soy isoflavones and other phytoestrogens can bind to estrogen receptors, mimicking the effects of estrogen in some tissues and antagonizing (blocking) the effects of estrogen in others.[5] Scientists are interested in the tissue-selective activities of phytoestrogens because antiestrogenic effects in reproductive tissue could help reduce the risk of hormone-associated cancers (breast, uterine, and prostate), while estrogenic effects in other tissues could help maintain bone density and improve blood lipid profiles (cholesterol levels). The extent to which soy isoflavones exert estrogenic and antiestrogenic effects in humans is currently the focus of considerable scientific research.

Estrogen-Receptor-Independent Activities

Soy isoflavones and their metabolites also have biological activities that are unrelated to their interactions with estrogen receptors.[6] By inhibiting the synthesis and activity of certain enzymes involved in estrogen metabolism, soy isoflavones may alter the biological activity of endogenous estrogens and androgens.[7–9] Soy isoflavones have also been found to inhibit tyrosine kinases,[10] enzymes that play critical roles in the signaling pathways that stimulate cell proliferation. Additionally, isoflavones can act as antioxidants in vitro,[11] but the extent to which they contribute to the antioxidant status of humans is not yet clear. Plasma F_2-isoprostanes, biomarkers of lipid peroxidation in vivo, were significantly lower after 2 weeks of daily consumption of soy protein containing 56 mg of isoflavones than after consumption of soy protein providing only 2 mg of isoflavones.[12] However, daily supplementation with 50–100 mg of isolated soy isoflavones did not significantly alter plasma or urinary F_2-isoprostane levels.[13,14]

Disease Prevention

Cardiovascular Disease

Serum Cholesterol

Although controlled clinical trials conducted prior to 1995 suggested that substituting 25–50 g/day of soy protein for animal protein lowered serum low-density lipoprotein (LDL) cholesterol by approximately 13%,[15] more recent and better controlled trials indicate that the LDL-cholesterol-lowering effect of soy protein is much more modest. A review in 2000 of 22 randomized controlled trials concluded that substituting 50 g/day of soy protein for animal protein lowered LDL cholesterol by only approximately 3%.[16] There is limited evidence that soy protein containing isoflavones is more effective than soy protein without isoflavones in lowering LDL cholesterol,[17,18] but the consumption of soy isoflavones alone (as supplements or extracts) does not appear to have favorable effects on serum lipid profiles.[16,19–21] For more information on soy protein and cholesterol, see Chapter 3.

Arterial Function

The preservation of normal arterial function plays an important role in cardiovascular disease prevention. The ability of arteries to dilate in response to nitric oxide produced by the endothelial cells that line their inner surface (endothelium-mediated vasodilation) is compromised in people at high risk for cardiovascular disease.[22] To date, results of randomized controlled trials on the effect of soy isoflavones on arterial function have been mixed. However, most placebo-controlled trials found no significant improvement in endothelium-mediated vasodilation when postmenopausal women were supplemented with up to 80 mg/day of soy isoflavones[23–25] or up to 60 g/day of soy protein containing isoflavones.[26–30] Arterial stiffness is another measure of arterial function. Measurements of arterial stiffness assess the distensibility of arteries, and a strong association between arterial stiffness and atherosclerosis has been observed.[31] In placebo-controlled clinical trials, supplementing the diet of postmenopausal women with 80 mg/day of a soy isoflavone extract for 5 weeks significantly decreased arterial stiffness,[32] as did supplementation of men and postmenopausal women at 40 g/day of soy protein, providing 118 mg/day of soy isoflavones for 3 months.[29] Although most studies have not found supplementation with soy protein or isoflavones to improve endothelium-mediated vasodilation, preliminary research suggests that soy isoflavone supplementation may decrease arterial stiffness. However, a recent randomized, controlled, crossover trial in hypertensive individuals found that supplementation with soy protein containing 118 mg/day of isoflavones for 6 months did not improve measures of arterial function, including arterial stiffness.[33] More research is needed to determine whether supplementation with soy isoflavones improves arterial function.

Hormone-Associated Cancers

Breast Cancer

The incidence of breast cancer in Asia, where average isoflavone intakes from soy foods range from 25 mg/day to 50 mg/day,[34] is lower than breast cancer rates in the Western countries where average isoflavone intakes in non-Asian women are less than 2 mg/day.[35,36] However, many other hereditary and lifestyle factors could contribute to this difference. Epidemiological studies of dietary soy and breast cancer have reported conflicting results. A few studies suggest that a higher soy intake during adolescence may lower risk of developing breast cancer later in life.[37,38] See Chapter 3 for more information about soy consumption and breast cancer risk. At present, there is little evidence that taking soy isoflavone supplements decreases the risk of breast cancer.

Endometrial Cancer

Because the development of endometrial (uterine) cancer is related to prolonged exposure to unopposed estrogens (estrogen not counterbalanced with the hormone progesterone), it has been suggested that high intakes of phytoestrogens with antiestrogenic activity could be protective against endometrial cancer.[39] In support of this idea, three retrospective case–control studies found that women with endometrial cancer had lower intakes of soy isoflavones from foods compared with cancer-free control groups.[39–41] However, giving soy protein supplements to postmenopausal women, providing 120 mg/day of isoflavones for 6 months did not prevent endometrial hyperplasia induced by the administration of exogenous estradiol.[42] Although limited evidence from case–control studies suggests an inverse relationship between consumption of soy foods and endometrial cancer, there is no evidence from intervention trials that taking soy isoflavone supplements decreases the risk of endometrial cancer.

Prostate Cancer

Mortality from prostate cancer is much higher in the United States than in Asian countries, such as Japan and China.[43] However, epidemiological studies do not provide consistent evidence that high intakes of soy foods are associated with reduced prostate cancer risk. See Chapter 3 for more information about soy foods and prostate cancer risk. The results of cell culture and animal studies suggest a potential role for soy isoflavones in limiting the progression of prostate cancer.[44] Although soy isoflavone supplementation for up to 1 year did not significantly decrease serum concentration of prostate-specific antigen (PSA) in men without confirmed prostate cancer,[45–47] soy isoflavone supplementation appeared to slow the rising serum PSA concentration associated with prostate tumor growth in two small studies of patients with prostate cancer.[48,49] One small, short-term (<1 month) study in patients with prostate cancer found that men randomized to receive a high-phytoestrogen diet experienced a statistically significant improvement in PSA concentrations compared with men randomized to receive a low-phytoestrogen diet.[50] A trial of soy milk supplementation (141 mg/day isoflavones) in men with PSA-specific recurrent prostate cancer found that PSA levels increased by an average of 20% over a 12-month period compared with a 56% yearly increase prior to the study.[51] A review published in 2006 found that isoflavone supplementation in prostate cancer patients favorably affected PSA concentrations in four out of eight trials.[52] Additionally, a recent meta-analysis of eight studies found that consumption of isoflavones was associated with a reduction in risk of prostate cancer, but the association was not statistically significant.[53] Although such preliminary findings are encouraging, the results of larger randomized controlled trials, which are currently ongoing, are needed to determine whether soy isoflavone supplementation can play a role in the prevention or treatment of prostate cancer.[54]

Osteoporosis

Although hip fracture rates are generally lower among Asian populations consuming soy foods than among Western populations, it is not yet clear whether increasing soy isoflavone consumption in Western populations helps to prevent osteoporosis.[55] The results of short-term clinical trials (≤6 months) assessing the effects of increased soy intake on biochemical markers of bone formation and bone resorption are inconsistent. Some controlled trials in postmenopausal women have found that increasing intakes of soy foods, soy protein, or soy isoflavones improves markers of bone resorption and formation[56–59] or attenuates bone loss,[59,60] but other trials have found no significant benefit of increasing soy intake.[61–64] Randomized controlled trials of longer duration are required to determine whether increased soy intake can actually prevent losses in bone mineral density (BMD) or osteoporotic fracture. Two controlled clinical trials found that BMD losses over 6 months were significantly lower in postmenopausal women given supplements of soy protein containing isoflavones than in those given supplements with equal amounts of milk protein,[62,65] but two longer trials found that BMD loss did not significantly differ between postmenopausal women given supplements with soy protein containing isoflavones and those supplemented with milk protein.[66,67] A 2-year clinical trial found that daily consumption of soy milk containing isoflavones significantly decreased BMD loss in the lumbar spine compared with daily consumption of soy milk without isoflavones,[68] but three other studies found that BMD loss did not significantly differ between postmenopausal women taking soy protein supplements containing isoflavones and those taking soy protein supplements without or with negligible amounts of isoflavones.[68–70] Loss of bone mineral content at the hip over 1 year was lower in Taiwanese women who took 80 mg/day of isolated soy isoflavones compared with placebo, but the difference was significant only in those women who were at least 4 years past menopause, had lower body weights, or had lower calcium intakes.[71] Another study in Taiwanese women found that those taking 100 mg/day of isolated soy isoflavones for 1 year experienced less bone loss compared with the control group, but women taking 200 mg/day of supplemental isoflavones did not experience any benefit.[72] Yet, a randomized controlled trial in European postmenopausal women found that supplementation with isoflavone-enriched foods (110 mg/day of isoflavones) for 1 year had no significant effect on BMD.[73] A recent placebo-controlled trial in postmenopausal women, aged >60 years, found that neither supplemental soy protein (18 g/day) nor isoflavones (105 mg/day), alone or in combination, significantly affected BMD over a 1-year period.[74] To date, results of studies are conflicting, but a recent meta-analysis of nine randomized controlled trials (trial duration: 1–12 months) concluded that soy isoflavones at doses up to 90 mg/day inhibit bone resorption and stimulate bone formation.[75] Some authors have proposed that the effect of soy isoflavones on bone health may be dependent on whether or not the individual produces the isoflavone metabolite, equol (see the Bioavailability and Metabolism section above).[76–79] This could possibly explain disparate results among clinical trials. Thus, while there is some evidence that isoflavone-rich diets have bone-sparing effects, it is not known whether increasing soy isoflavone intake appreciably decreases the risk of osteoporosis or osteoporotic fracture.

Cognitive Decline

Scientific research on the effect of soy isoflavones on cognitive function is limited. An observational study that examined the relationship between soy intake and cognitive function found that Hawaiian men who reported consuming tofu at least twice weekly during midlife were more likely to have poor cognitive test scores 20–25 years later than those who reported consuming tofu less than twice a week.[80] In an Indonesian study of elderly men and women, consumption of tofu was associated with worse memory, while consumption of tempeh was associated with improved memory.[81] In contrast, the results of several small clinical trials in postmenopausal women suggest that increasing soy isoflavone intake may result in modest improvements in performance on some cognitive tests for up to 6 months. Postmenopausal women given soy extracts, providing 60 mg/day of soy isoflavones for 6–12 weeks, performed better on cognitive tests of picture recall (short-term memory), learning rule reversals (mental flexibility), and a planning task, compared with women given a placebo.[82,83] In a longer trial, postmenopausal women given supplements that provided 110 mg/day of soy isoflavones for 6 months performed better on a test of verbal fluency than women given placebos.[84] In a crossover trial lasting 6 months, women receiving 60 mg/day of soy isoflavones experi-

enced significant improvements in cognitive performance and overall mood compared with when the women were given a placebo.[85] However, in larger placebo-controlled trials of postmenopausal women, giving 80 mg/day of isoflavones for 6 months or 99 mg/day of isoflavones for 1 year did not affect performance on a battery of cognitive function tests, including tests for memory, attention, verbal fluency, motor control, and dementia.[67,86] A recent review of eight trials, seven of which were conducted in postmenopausal women, found half reported that soy isoflavone treatment was associated with improvements in cognitive function.[87]

Disease Treatment

Menopausal Symptoms

Hot flushes (flashes) are the primary reason that women seek medical attention for menopausal symptoms.[88] Concern over potential adverse effects of hormone replacement therapy[89,90] has led to increased interest in the use of phytoestrogen supplements by women experiencing menopausal symptoms.[91] The effects of increasing soy isoflavone intake on the frequency of hot flushes have been examined in several randomized controlled trials.[92–94] To date, at least four reviews of such trials have been published. A review published in 2002 found that only one out of eight randomized controlled trials of soy foods reported a significant reduction in the frequency of hot flushes, while three out of five controlled trials of soy isoflavone extracts reported a significant reduction in hot flush frequency.[95] In general, any reductions observed were modest (10%–20%) compared with placebo. A 2004 systematic review that examined 10 randomized controlled trials found that only four trials reported beneficial effects of soy preparations in the treatment of menopausal symptoms like hot flushes.[94] More recently, another systematic review and meta-analysis of 12 randomized controlled trials found that soy isoflavone supplementation was associated with a small reduction in the number of hot flushes; this analysis found that women with a higher number of daily flushes experienced the greatest benefit from isoflavone therapy.[93] One review that analyzed various trials according to the specific isoflavones contained in the supplements found that use of supplements containing

Table 12.1 Total isoflavone aglycone, daidzein, and genistein content of selected foods[107]

Food	Serving	Total Isoflavones (mg)	Daidzein (mg)	Genistein (mg)
Soy protein concentrate, aqueous washed	3.5 oz (100 g)	102	43	56
Miso	½ cup	59	22	34
Soybeans, boiled	½ cup	47	23	24
Tempeh	3 oz	37	15	21
Soybeans, dry roasted	1 oz (28 g)	37	15	19
Soy milk	1 cup	23	11	15
Tofu yogurt	½ cup	21	7	12
Tofu	3 oz	20	8	12
Soy protein concentrate, alcohol washed	3.5 oz (100 g)	12	7	5
Meatless (soy) hot dog	1 hot dog	11	2	6
Meatless (soy) sausage	3 links (75 g)	3	0.6	2
Soy cheese, mozzarella	1 oz	2	0.3	1

primarily genistein reduced symptoms of hot flushes.[96] Interestingly, a recent study found that only women who produced the isoflavone metabolite, equol (see the Bioavailability and Metabolism section above), which was detected in the urine, experienced improvements in menopausal symptoms like hot flushes following soy isoflavone supplementation.[97] Breast cancer survivors in particular may experience more frequent and severe hot flushes related to therapies aimed at preventing recurrence of breast cancer.[98] However, none of the randomized controlled trials in breast cancer survivors found that soy isoflavone supplementation was significantly more effective than a placebo in decreasing the frequency or severity of hot flushes.[99–102] To date, studies on the effect of soy isoflavone consumption on menopausal symptoms have reported mixed results.

Sources

Food Sources

Isoflavones are found in small amounts in several legumes, grains, and vegetables, but soybeans are by far the most concentrated source of isoflavones in the human diet.[103,104] Recent surveys suggest that average dietary isoflavone intakes in Japan, China, and other Asian countries range from 25 mg/day to 50 mg/day.[34] Dietary isofla-

vone intakes are considerably lower in Western countries, where studies have found average isoflavone intakes to be as low as 2 mg/day.[35,36] Traditional Asian foods made from soybeans include tofu, tempeh, miso, and natto. Edamame refers to varieties of soybeans that are harvested and eaten in their green phase. Soy products that are gaining popularity in Western countries include soy-based meat substitutes, soy milk, soy cheese, and soy yogurt.

The isoflavone content of a soy protein isolate depends on the method used to isolate it. Soy protein isolates prepared by an ethanol wash process generally lose most of their associated isoflavones, while those prepared by aqueous wash processes tend to retain them.[105] Some foods that are rich in soy isoflavones are listed in Table 12.1, along with their isoflavone content.[106] Because the isoflavone content of soy foods can vary considerably between brands and between different lots of the same brand,[105] these values should be viewed only as a guide. Given the potential health implications of diets rich in soy isoflavones, accurate and consistent labeling of the soy isoflavone content of soy foods is needed.

Supplements

Soy isoflavone extracts and supplements are available as dietary supplements without a prescription in the United States. These products are not standardized, and the amounts of soy isoflavones they provide may vary considerably. Moreover, quality control may be an issue with some of these products.[107] When isoflavone supplements available in the United States were tested for their isoflavone content by an independent laboratory, the isoflavone content in the product differed by more than 10% from the amount claimed on the label in approximately 50% of the products tested.[108]

Infant Formulas

Soy-based infant formulas are made from soy protein isolate and contain significant amounts of soy isoflavones. In 1997, the total isoflavone content of soy-based infant formulas that were commercially available in the United States ranged from 32 mg/L to 47 mg/L (approx. 34 fl oz).[109]

Safety

For many years, soy isoflavones have been consumed by humans as part of soy-based diets, without any evidence of adverse effects.[104] The 75th percentile of dietary isoflavone intake has been reported to be as high as 65 mg/day in some Asian populations.[110] Although diets rich in soy or soy-containing products appear safe and potentially beneficial, the long-term safety of very high supplemental doses of soy isoflavones is not yet known. One study in older men and women found that 100 mg/day of soy isoflavones for 6 months was well tolerated.[111] Yet, long-term studies are needed to evaluate the safety of isoflavones.

Adverse Effects

Safety for Breast Cancer Survivors

The safety of high intakes of soy isoflavones and other phytoestrogens for breast cancer survivors is an area of considerable debate among scientists and clinicians.[98,112] The effects of high intakes of soy isoflavones on breast cancer recurrence and survival of breast cancer patients have not been well studied. The results of cell culture and animal studies are conflicting, but some have found that soy isoflavones can stimulate the growth of estrogen-receptor-positive (ER+)

breast cancer cells.[113,114] High intakes of the soy isoflavone, genistein, interfered with the ability of tamoxifen to inhibit the growth of ER+ breast cancer cells implanted in mice,[115] but it is not known if a similar effect would be seen in humans. A recent prospective study in 5042 female breast cancer survivors in China, who were followed for a median of 3.9 years, found that consumption of isoflavone-rich soy foods was significantly associated with a 29% lower risk of death and a 32% lower risk of cancer recurrence.[116] In this study, soy isoflavone consumption was associated with a nonsignificant, 21% reduction in risk of death and a significant, 23% reduction in risk of cancer recurrence.[116] Very limited data from clinical trials suggest that increased consumption of soy isoflavones (38–45 mg/day) can have estrogenic effects in human breast tissue.[117,118] However, a study in women with biopsy-confirmed breast cancer found that supplementation with 200 mg/day of soy isoflavones did not increase tumor growth over the next 2–6 weeks before surgery when compared with a control group that did not take soy isoflavones.[119] Given the available data, some experts think that women with a history of breast cancer, particularly ER+ breast cancer, should not increase their consumption of phytoestrogens, including soy isoflavones.[98] However, other experts argue that there is not enough evidence to discourage breast cancer survivors from consuming soy foods in moderation,[112] and the recent study mentioned above[116] indicates that moderate consumption of soy foods (11 g/day of soy protein) may even be beneficial to breast cancer survivors. Due to conflicting results, more research is needed to determine the safety of high soy isoflavone intake in breast cancer survivors.

Soy-Based Infant Formulas

Infant formula made from soy protein isolate has been commercially available since the mid-1960s.[120] As much as 25% of the infant formula sold in the United States is soy-based formula.[121] Since infants fed soy-based formulas are exposed to relatively high levels of isoflavones, which they can absorb and metabolize, concern has been raised regarding potential long-term effects on growth and development, as well as reproductive and immune function.[109,122] The results of at least six clinical trials comparing infants who were fed soy-based formula with infants fed cow's-milk-based formula indicate that soy-based formula supports normal growth and development in the first year of life.[123] A prospective study evaluating growth and development in children fed breast milk, cow's-milk-based formula, or soy-based formula is currently under way at the Arkansas Children's Nutrition Center. Five years into the study, adverse effects of soy formula have not been observed, and no differences in growth and development among the various groups have been noted.[124] In addition, one retrospective study of 811 men and women aged 20–34 years found no differences in height, weight, time of puberty, general health, or pregnancy outcomes between those fed soy-based formula as infants and those fed cow's-milk-based formula, although women fed soy-based formula reported significantly greater use of asthma or allergy drugs than women fed cow's milk formula.[125] The American Academy of Pediatrics recently published a report that reviews the indications and contraindications for the use of soy-based formulas.[121] At present, there is no convincing evidence that infants fed soy-based formula are at greater risk for adverse effects than infants fed cow's milk-based formula. However, long-term studies on the growth and development of infants fed soy-based formula are currently ongoing.[126,127]

Thyroid Function

In cell culture and animal studies, soy isoflavones have been found to inhibit the activity of thyroid peroxidase, an enzyme required for thyroid hormone synthesis.[128,129] However, high intakes of soy isoflavones do not appear to increase the risk of hypothyroidism, as long as dietary iodine consumption is adequate.[130] Since the addition of iodine to soy-based formulas in the 1960s, there have been no further reports of hypothyroidism in infants fed on soy formula.[131] Several clinical trials, mostly in premenopausal and postmenopausal women with sufficient iodine intakes, have not found that increased consumption of soy isoflavones results in clinically significant changes in circulating thyroid hormone levels.[132–136]

Pregnancy

To date, studies have not examined the effect of an isoflavone-rich diet on fetal development or pregnancy outcomes in humans, and the safety of isoflavone supplements during pregnancy has not been established.

Drug Interactions

Because colonic bacteria play an important role in the metabolism of soy isoflavones, antibiotic therapy could decrease their biological activity.[137] Some evidence from animal studies suggests that high intakes of soy isoflavones, particularly genistein, can interfere with the antitumor effects of tamoxifen (Nolvadex).[115] Until more is known about potential interactions in humans, those taking tamoxifen or other selective estrogen receptor modulators to treat or prevent breast cancer should avoid soy protein supplements or isoflavone extracts (see the Safety for Breast Cancer Survivors section above). High intakes of soy protein may interfere with the efficacy of the anticoagulant medication warfarin. There is one case report of an individual on warfarin who developed subtherapeutic international normalized ratio (INR; prothrombin time) values upon consuming approximately 16 oz of soy milk daily for 4 weeks.[138] INR values returned to therapeutic levels 2 weeks after discontinuing soy milk. The amount of levothyroxine required for adequate thyroid hormone replacement has been found to increase in infants with congenital hypothyroidism fed soy formula.[131,139] Taking levothyroxine at the same time as a soy protein supplement also increased the levothyroxine dose required for adequate thyroid hormone replacement in an adult with hypothyroidism.[140]

Summary

- Isoflavones are a class of phytoestrogens—plant-derived compounds with estrogenic activity. Soybeans and soy products are the richest sources of isoflavones in the human diet.
- The results of randomized controlled trials suggest that substituting 50 g/day of soy protein for animal protein results in only a modest 3% reduction of low-density lipoprotein cholesterol. Isolated soy isoflavone supplements do not appear to have favorable effects on serum lipid profiles.
- Consumption of soy isoflavones, at doses of <90 mg/day, may inhibit bone resorption and stimulate bone formation.

- Overall, the results of numerous observational studies do not support the idea that high soy isoflavone intakes in adults are protective against breast cancer. Limited research suggests that higher intakes of soy foods early in life may decrease the risk of breast cancer in adulthood.
- Although scientists are interested in the potential for soy isoflavones to prevent or inhibit the progression of prostate cancer, evidence from observational studies that soy isoflavones are protective against prostate cancer is limited and inconsistent.
- To date, studies on the effect of soy isoflavone consumption on menopausal symptoms have reported mixed results.
- Some health effects of soy isoflavones may be dependent on whether or not the isoflavone metabolite equol is produced.
- Although diets rich in soy or soy-containing products appear safe and potentially beneficial, the long-term safety of high doses of soy isoflavone supplements is not yet known.
- At present, there is no convincing evidence that infants fed soy-based formula are at greater risk for adverse effects than infants fed cow's-milk-based formula.

References

1. Lampe JW. Isoflavonoid and lignan phytoestrogens as dietary biomarkers. J Nutr 2003;133(Suppl 3):956S–964S
2. Rowland I, Faughnan M, Hoey L, Wähälä K, Williamson G, Cassidy A. Bioavailability of phyto-oestrogens. Br J Nutr 2003;89(Suppl 1):S45–S58
3. Setchell KD, Brown NM, Lydeking-Olsen E. The clinical importance of the metabolite equol-a clue to the effectiveness of soy and its isoflavones. J Nutr 2002;132(12):3577–3584
4. National Cancer Institute. Understanding Cancer Series: Estrogen Receptors/SERMs. National Cancer Institute. Available at: http://www.cancer.gov/cancertopics/understandingcancer/estrogenreceptors. Accessed May 3, 2012
5. Wang LQ. Mammalian phytoestrogens: enterodiol and enterolactone. J Chromatogr B Analyt Technol Biomed Life Sci 2002;777(1–2):289–309
6. Barnes S, Boersma B, Patel R, et al. Isoflavonoids and chronic disease: mechanisms of action. Biofactors 2000;12(1–4):209–215
7. Kao YC, Zhou C, Sherman M, Laughton CA, Chen S. Molecular basis of the inhibition of human aromatase (estrogen synthetase) by flavone and isoflavone phytoestrogens: A site-directed mutagenesis study. Environ Health Perspect 1998;106(2):85–92
8. Whitehead SA, Cross JE, Burden C, Lacey M. Acute and chronic effects of genistein, tyrphostin and lavendus-

tin A on steroid synthesis in luteinized human granulosa cells. Hum Reprod 2002;17(3):589–594
9. Holzbeierlein JM, McIntosh J, Thrasher JB. The role of soy phytoestrogens in prostate cancer. Curr Opin Urol 2005;15(1):17–22
10. Akiyama T, Ishida J, Nakagawa S, et al. Genistein, a specific inhibitor of tyrosine-specific protein kinases. J Biol Chem 1987;262(12):5592–5595
11. Ruiz-Larrea MB, Mohan AR, Paganga G, Miller NJ, Bolwell GP, Rice-Evans CA. Antioxidant activity of phytoestrogenic isoflavones. Free Radic Res 1997; 26(1):63–70
12. Wiseman H, O'Reilly JD, Adlercreutz H, et al. Isoflavone phytoestrogens consumed in soy decrease F(2)-isoprostane concentrations and increase resistance of low-density lipoprotein to oxidation in humans. Am J Clin Nutr 2000;72(2):395–400
13. Hodgson JM, Puddey IB, Croft KD, Mori TA, Rivera J, Beilin LJ. Isoflavonoids do not inhibit in vivo lipid peroxidation in subjects with high-normal blood pressure. Atherosclerosis 1999;145(1):167–172
14. Djuric Z, Chen G, Doerge DR, Heilbrun LK, Kucuk O. Effect of soy isoflavone supplementation on markers of oxidative stress in men and women. Cancer Lett 2001;172(1):1–6
15. Anderson JW, Johnstone BM, Cook-Newell ME. Meta-analysis of the effects of soy protein intake on serum lipids. N Engl J Med 1995;333(5):276–282
16. Sacks FM, Lichtenstein A, Van Horn L, Harris W, Kris-Etherton P, Winston M; American Heart Association Nutrition Committee. Soy protein, isoflavones, and cardiovascular health: an American Heart Association Science Advisory for professionals from the Nutrition Committee. Circulation 2006;113(7):1034–1044
17. Zhan S, Ho SC. Meta-analysis of the effects of soy protein containing isoflavones on the lipid profile. Am J Clin Nutr 2005;81(2):397–408
18. Zhuo XG, Melby MK, Watanabe S. Soy isoflavone intake lowers serum LDL cholesterol: a meta-analysis of 8 randomized controlled trials in humans. J Nutr 2004;134(9):2395–2400
19. Lichtenstein AH, Jalbert SM, Adlercreutz H, et al. Lipoprotein response to diets high in soy or animal protein with and without isoflavones in moderately hypercholesterolemic subjects. Arterioscler Thromb Vasc Biol 2002;22(11):1852–1858
20. Weggemans RM, Trautwein EA. Relation between soy-associated isoflavones and LDL and HDL cholesterol concentrations in humans: a meta-analysis. Eur J Clin Nutr 2003;57(8):940–946
21. Dewell A, Hollenbeck PL, Hollenbeck CB. Clinical review: a critical evaluation of the role of soy protein and isoflavone supplementation in the control of plasma cholesterol concentrations. J Clin Endocrinol Metab 2006;91(3):772–780
22. Landmesser U, Hornig B, Drexler H. Endothelial function: a critical determinant in atherosclerosis? Circulation 2004; 109(21, Suppl 1): II27–II33
23. Squadrito F, Altavilla D, Crisafulli A, et al. Effect of genistein on endothelial function in postmenopausal women: a randomized, double-blind, controlled study. Am J Med 2003;114(6):470–476
24. Simons LA, von Konigsmark M, Simons J, Celermajer DS. Phytoestrogens do not influence lipoprotein levels or endothelial function in healthy, postmenopausal women. Am J Cardiol 2000;85(11):1297–1301
25. Katz DL, Evans MA, Njike VY, et al. Raloxifene, soy phytoestrogens and endothelial function in post-

menopausal women. Climacteric 2007;10(6):500–507

26. Kreijkamp-Kaspers S, Kok L, Bots ML, Grobbee DE, Lampe JW, van der Schouw YT. Randomized controlled trial of the effects of soy protein containing isoflavones on vascular function in postmenopausal women. Am J Clin Nutr 2005;81(1):189–195

27. Steinberg FM, Guthrie NL, Villablanca AC, Kumar K, Murray MJ. Soy protein with isoflavones has favorable effects on endothelial function that are independent of lipid and antioxidant effects in healthy postmenopausal women. Am J Clin Nutr 2003;78(1):123–130

28. Blum A, Lang N, Vigder F, et al. Effects of soy products on endothelium-dependent vasodilatation and lipid profile in postmenopausal women with mild hypercholesterolemia. Clin Invest Med 2003;26(1):20–26

29. Teede HJ, Dalais FS, Kotsopoulos D, Liang YL, Davis S, McGrath BP. Dietary soy has both beneficial and potentially adverse cardiovascular effects: a placebo-controlled study in men and postmenopausal women. J Clin Endocrinol Metab 2001;86(7):3053–3060

30. Evans M, Njike VY, Hoxley M, Pearson M, Katz DL. Effect of soy isoflavone protein and soy lecithin on endothelial function in healthy postmenopausal women. Menopause 2007;14(1):141–149

31. van Popele NM, Grobbee DE, Bots ML, et al. Association between arterial stiffness and atherosclerosis: the Rotterdam Study. Stroke 2001;32(2):454–460

32. Nestel PJ, Yamashita T, Sasahara T, et al. Soy isoflavones improve systemic arterial compliance but not plasma lipids in menopausal and perimenopausal women. Arterioscler Thromb Vasc Biol 1997; 17(12):3392–3398

33. Teede HJ, Giannopoulos D, Dalais FS, Hodgson J, McGrath BP. Randomised, controlled, cross-over trial of soy protein with isoflavones on blood pressure and arterial function in hypertensive subjects. J Am Coll Nutr 2006;25(6):533–540

34. Messina M, Nagata C, Wu AH. Estimated Asian adult soy protein and isoflavone intakes. Nutr Cancer 2006;55(1):1–12

35. van Erp-Baart MA, Brants HA, Kiely M, et al. Isoflavone intake in four different European countries: the VENUS approach. Br J Nutr 2003;89(Suppl 1):S25–S30

36. de Kleijn MJ, van der Schouw YT, Wilson PW, et al. Intake of dietary phytoestrogens is low in postmenopausal women in the United States: the Framingham study(1–4). J Nutr 2001;131(6):1826–1832

37. Shu XO, Jin F, Dai Q, et al. Soyfood intake during adolescence and subsequent risk of breast cancer among Chinese women. Cancer Epidemiol Biomarkers Prev 2001;10(5):483–488

38. Wu AH, Wan P, Hankin J, Tseng CC, Yu MC, Pike MC. Adolescent and adult soy intake and risk of breast cancer in Asian-Americans. Carcinogenesis 2002; 23(9):1491–1496

39. Horn-Ross PL, John EM, Canchola AJ, Stewart SL, Lee MM. Phytoestrogen intake and endometrial cancer risk. J Natl Cancer Inst 2003;95(15):1158–1164

40. Goodman MT, Wilkens LR, Hankin JH, Lyu LC, Wu AH, Kolonel LN. Association of soy and fiber consumption with the risk of endometrial cancer. Am J Epidemiol 1997;146(4):294–306

41. Xu WH, Zheng W, Xiang YB, et al. Soya food intake and risk of endometrial cancer among Chinese women in Shanghai: population based case-control study. BMJ 2004;328(7451):1285

42. Murray MJ, Meyer WR, Lessey BA, Oi RH, DeWire RE, Fritz MA. Soy protein isolate with isoflavones does not prevent estradiol-induced endometrial hyperplasia in postmenopausal women: a pilot trial. Menopause 2003;10(5):456–464

43. Messina MJ. Emerging evidence on the role of soy in reducing prostate cancer risk. Nutr Rev 2003;61(4): 117–131

44. Steiner C, Arnould S, Scalbert A, Manach C. Isoflavones and the prevention of breast and prostate cancer: new perspectives opened by nutrigenomicc. Br J Nutr 2008;99 (E Suppl 1):ES78–ES108

45. Adams KF, Chen C, Newton KM, Potter JD, Lampe JW. Soy isoflavones do not modulate prostate-specific antigen concentrations in older men in a randomized controlled trial. Cancer Epidemiol Biomarkers Prev 2004;13(4):644–648

46. Jenkins DJ, Kendall CW, D'Costa MA, et al. Soy consumption and phytoestrogens: effect on serum prostate specific antigen when blood lipids and oxidized low-density lipoprotein are reduced in hyperlipidemic men. J Urol 2003;169(2):507–511

47. Urban D, Irwin W, Kirk M, et al. The effect of isolated soy protein on plasma biomarkers in elderly men with elevated serum prostate specific antigen. J Urol 2001;165(1):294–300

48. Fischer L, Mahoney C, Jeffcoat AR, et al. Clinical characteristics and pharmacokinetics of purified soy isoflavones: multiple-dose administration to men with prostate neoplasia. Nutr Cancer 2004;48(2):160–170

49. Hussain M, Banerjee M, Sarkar FH, et al. Soy isoflavones in the treatment of prostate cancer. Nutr Cancer 2003;47(2):111–117

50. Dalais FS, Meliala A, Wattanapenpaiboon N, et al. Effects of a diet rich in phytoestrogens on prostate-specific antigen and sex hormones in men diagnosed with prostate cancer. Urology 2004;64(3):510–515

51. Pendleton JM, Tan WW, Anai S, et al. Phase II trial of isoflavone in prostate-specific antigen recurrent prostate cancer after previous local therapy. BMC Cancer 2008;8:132

52. Messina M, Kucuk O, Lampe JW. An overview of the health effects of isoflavones with an emphasis on prostate cancer risk and prostate-specific antigen levels. J AOAC Int 2006;89(4):1121–1134

53. Yan L, Spitznagel EL. Soy consumption and prostate cancer risk in men: a revisit of a meta-analysis. Am J Clin Nutr 2009;89(4):1155–1163

54. Goetzl MA, Van Veldhuizen PJ, Thrasher JB. Effects of soy phytoestrogens on the prostate. Prostate Cancer Prostatic Dis 2007;10(3):216–223

55. Setchell KD, Lydeking-Olsen E. Dietary phytoestrogens and their effect on bone: evidence from in vitro and in vivo, human observational, and dietary intervention studies. Am J Clin Nutr 2003; 78(3, Suppl):593S–609S

56. Chiechi LM, Secreto G, D'Amore M, et al. Efficacy of a soy rich diet in preventing postmenopausal osteoporosis: the Menfis randomized trial. Maturitas 2002;42(4):295–300

57. Scheiber MD, Liu JH, Subbiah MT, Rebar RW, Setchell KD. Dietary inclusion of whole soy foods results in significant reductions in clinical risk factors for osteoporosis and cardiovascular disease in normal postmenopausal women. Menopause 2001;8(5):384–392

58. Arjmandi BH, Khalil DA, Smith BJ, et al. Soy protein has a greater effect on bone in postmenopausal women not on hormone replacement therapy, as evidenced by reducing bone resorption and urinary cal-

cium excretion. J Clin Endocrinol Metab 2003;88(3): 1048–1054

59. Harkness LS, Fiedler K, Sehgal AR, Oravec D, Lerner E. Decreased bone resorption with soy isoflavone supplementation in postmenopausal women. J Womens Health (Larchmt) 2004;13(9):1000–1007

60. Ye YB, Tang XY, Verbruggen MA, Su YX. Soy isoflavones attenuate bone loss in early postmenopausal Chinese women: a single-blind randomized, placebo-controlled trial. Eur J Nutr 2006;45(6):327–334

61. Wangen KE, Duncan AM, Merz-Demlow BE, et al. Effects of soy isoflavones on markers of bone turnover in premenopausal and postmenopausal women. J Clin Endocrinol Metab 2000;85(9):3043–3048

62. Alekel DL, Germain AS, Peterson CT, Hanson KB, Stewart JW, Toda T. Isoflavone-rich soy protein isolate attenuates bone loss in the lumbar spine of perimenopausal women. Am J Clin Nutr 2000;72(3):844–852

63. Dalais FS, Ebeling PR, Kotsopoulos D, McGrath BP, Teede HJ. The effects of soy protein containing isoflavones on lipids and indices of bone resorption in postmenopausal women. Clin Endocrinol (Oxf) 2003;58(6):704–709

64. Cheong JM, Martin BR, Jackson GS, et al. Soy isoflavones do not affect bone resorption in postmenopausal women: a dose-response study using a novel approach with 41Ca. J Clin Endocrinol Metab 2007;92(2):577–582

65. Potter SM, Baum JA, Teng H, Stillman RJ, Shay NF, Erdman JW Jr. Soy protein and isoflavones: their effects on blood lipids and bone density in postmenopausal women. Am J Clin Nutr 1998; 68(6, Suppl):1375S–1379S

66. Arjmandi BH, Lucas EA, Khalil DA, et al. One year soy protein supplementation has positive effects on bone formation markers but not bone density in postmenopausal women. Nutr J 2005;4(1):8

67. Kreijkamp-Kaspers S, Kok L, Grobbee DE, et al. Effect of soy protein containing isoflavones on cognitive function, bone mineral density, and plasma lipids in postmenopausal women: a randomized controlled trial. JAMA 2004;292(1):65–74

68. Lydeking-Olsen E, Beck-Jensen JE, Setchell KD, Holm-Jensen T. Soymilk or progesterone for prevention of bone loss—a 2 year randomized, placebo-controlled trial. Eur J Nutr 2004;43(4):246–257

69. Gallagher JC, Satpathy R, Rafferty K, Haynatzka V. The effect of soy protein isolate on bone metabolism. Menopause 2004;11(3):290–298

70. Newton KM, LaCroix AZ, Levy L, et al. Soy protein and bone mineral density in older men and women: a randomized trial. Maturitas 2006;55(3):270–277

71. Chen YM, Ho SC, Lam SS, Ho SS, Woo JL. Beneficial effect of soy isoflavones on bone mineral content was modified by years since menopause, body weight, and calcium intake: a double-blind, randomized, controlled trial. Menopause 2004;11(3):246–254

72. Huang HY, Yang HP, Yang HT, Yang TC, Shieh MJ, Huang SY. One-year soy isoflavone supplementation prevents early postmenopausal bone loss but without a dose-dependent effect. J Nutr Biochem 2006;17(8):509–517

73. Brink E, Coxam V, Robins S, Wahala K, Cassidy A, Branca F; PHYTOS Investigators. Long-term consumption of isoflavone-enriched foods does not affect bone mineral density, bone metabolism, or hormonal status in early postmenopausal women: a randomized, double-blind, placebo controlled study. Am J Clin Nutr 2008;87(3):761–770

74. Kenny AM, Mangano KM, Abourizk RH, et al. Soy proteins and isoflavones affect bone mineral density in older women: a randomized controlled trial. Am J Clin Nutr 2009;90(1):234–242

75. Ma DF, Qin LQ, Wang PY, Katoh R. Soy isoflavone intake inhibits bone resorption and stimulates bone formation in menopausal women: meta-analysis of randomized controlled trials. Eur J Clin Nutr 2008; 62(2):155–161

76. Wu J, Oka J, Ezaki J, et al. Possible role of equol status in the effects of isoflavone on bone and fat mass in postmenopausal Japanese women: a double-blind, randomized, controlled trial. Menopause 2007; 14(5):866–874

77. Vatanparast H, Chilibeck PD. Does the effect of soy phytoestrogens on bone in postmenopausal women depend on the equol-producing phenotype? Nutr Rev 2007;65(6 Pt 1):294–299

78. Ishimi Y. Soybean isoflavones in bone health. Forum Nutr 2009;61:104–116

79. Frankenfeld CL, McTiernan A, Thomas WK, et al. Postmenopausal bone mineral density in relation to soy isoflavone-metabolizing phenotypes. Maturitas 2006;53(3):315–324

80. White LR, Petrovitch H, Ross GW, et al. Brain aging and midlife tofu consumption. J Am Coll Nutr 2000;19(2):242–255

81. Hogervorst E, Sadjimim T, Yesufu A, Kreager P, Rahardjo TB. High tofu intake is associated with worse memory in elderly Indonesian men and women. Dement Geriatr Cogn Disord 2008;26(1):50–57

82. Duffy R, Wiseman H, File SE. Improved cognitive function in postmenopausal women after 12 weeks of consumption of a soya extract containing isoflavones. Pharmacol Biochem Behav 2003;75(3):721–729

83. File SE, Hartley DE, Elsabagh S, Duffy R, Wiseman H. Cognitive improvement after 6 weeks of soy supplements in postmenopausal women is limited to frontal lobe function. Menopause 2005;12(2):193–201

84. Kritz-Silverstein D, Von Mühlen D, Barrett-Connor E, Bressel MA. Isoflavones and cognitive function in older women: the SOy and Postmenopausal Health In Aging (SOPHIA) Study. Menopause 2003;10(3):196–202

85. Casini ML, Marelli G, Papaleo E, Ferrari A, D'Ambrosio F, Unfer V. Psychological assessment of the effects of treatment with phytoestrogens on postmenopausal women: a randomized, double-blind, crossover, placebo-controlled study. Fertil Steril 2006;85(4):972–978

86. Ho SC, Chan AS, Ho YP, et al. Effects of soy isoflavone supplementation on cognitive function in Chinese postmenopausal women: a double-blind, randomized, controlled trial. Menopause 2007;14(3 Pt 1):489–499

87. Zhao L, Brinton RD. WHI and WHIMS follow-up and human studies of soy isoflavones on cognition. Expert Rev Neurother 2007;7(11):1549–1564

88. Tice JA, Ettinger B, Ensrud K, Wallace R, Blackwell T, Cummings SR. Phytoestrogen supplements for the treatment of hot flashes: the Isoflavone Clover Extract (ICE) Study: a randomized controlled trial. JAMA 2003;290(2):207–214

89. Nelson HD, Humphrey LL, Nygren P, Teutsch SM, Allan JD. Postmenopausal hormone replacement therapy: scientific review. JAMA 2002;288(7):872–881

90. Farquhar C, Marjoribanks J, Lethaby A, Suckling JA, Lamberts Q. Long term hormone therapy for perimenopausal and postmenopausal women. Cochrane Database Syst Rev 2009; (2):CD004143

91. Nelson HD, Vesco KK, Haney E, et al. Nonhormonal therapies for menopausal hot flashes: systematic review and meta-analysis. JAMA 2006;295(17):2057–2071

92. Kronenberg F, Fugh-Berman A. Complementary and alternative medicine for menopausal symptoms: a review of randomized, controlled trials. Ann Intern Med 2002;137(10):805–813

93. Howes LG, Howes JB, Knight DC. Isoflavone therapy for menopausal flushes: a systematic review and meta-analysis. Maturitas 2006;55(3):203–211

94. Huntley AL, Ernst E. Soy for the treatment of perimenopausal symptoms—a systematic review. Maturitas 2004;47(1):1–9

95. Krebs EE, Ensrud KE, MacDonald R, Wilt TJ. Phytoestrogens for treatment of menopausal symptoms: a systematic review. Obstet Gynecol 2004;104(4):824–836

96. Williamson-Hughes PS, Flickinger BD, Messina MJ, Empie MW. Isoflavone supplements containing predominantly genistein reduce hot flash symptoms: a critical review of published studies. Menopause 2006;13(5):831–839

97. Jou HJ, Wu SC, Chang FW, Ling PY, Chu KS, Wu WH. Effect of intestinal production of equol on menopausal symptoms in women treated with soy isoflavones. Int J Gynaecol Obstet 2008;102(1):44–49

98. Duffy C, Cyr M. Phytoestrogens: potential benefits and implications for breast cancer survivors. J Womens Health (Larchmt) 2003;12(7):617–631

99. MacGregor CA, Canney PA, Patterson G, McDonald R, Paul J. A randomised double-blind controlled trial of oral soy supplements versus placebo for treatment of menopausal symptoms in patients with early breast cancer. Eur J Cancer 2005;41(5):708–714

100. Nikander E, Kilkkinen A, Metsä-Heikkilä M, et al. A randomized placebo-controlled crossover trial with phytoestrogens in treatment of menopause in breast cancer patients. Obstet Gynecol 2003;101(6):1213–1220

101. Van Patten CL, Olivotto IA, Chambers GK, et al. Effect of soy phytoestrogens on hot flashes in postmenopausal women with breast cancer: a randomized, controlled clinical trial. J Clin Oncol 2002;20(6):1449–1455

102. Quella SK, Loprinzi CL, Barton DL, et al. Evaluation of soy phytoestrogens for the treatment of hot flashes in breast cancer survivors: A North Central Cancer Treatment Group Trial. J Clin Oncol 2000;18(5):1068–1074

103. Fletcher RJ. Food sources of phyto-oestrogens and their precursors in Europe. Br J Nutr 2003;89(Suppl 1):S39–S43

104. Munro IC, Harwood M, Hlywka JJ, et al. Soy isoflavones: a safety review. Nutr Rev 2003;61(1):1–33

105. Setchell KD, Cole SJ. Variations in isoflavone levels in soy foods and soy protein isolates and issues related to isoflavone databases and food labeling. J Agric Food Chem 2003;51(14):4146–4155

106. United States Department of Agriculture Nutrient Data Laboratory. USDA-Iowa State University Isoflavones Database, 6/2002. Available at: http://www.nal.usda.gov/fnic/foodcomp/Data/isoflav/isoflav.html. Accessed May 3, 2012

107. Chua R, Anderson K, Chen J, Hu M. Quality, labeling accuracy, and cost comparison of purified soy isoflavonoid products. J Altern Complement Med 2004;10(6):1053–1060

108. Setchell KD, Brown NM, Desai P, et al. Bioavailability of pure isoflavones in healthy humans and analysis of commercial soy isoflavone supplements. J Nutr 2001; 131(4, Suppl):1362S–1375S

109. Setchell KD, Zimmer-Nechemias L, Cai J, Heubi JE. Isoflavone content of infant formulas and the metabolic fate of these phytoestrogens in early life. Am J Clin Nutr 1998; 68(6, Suppl):1453S–1461S

110. Chen Z, Zheng W, Custer LJ, et al. Usual dietary consumption of soy foods and its correlation with the excretion rate of isoflavonoids in overnight urine samples among Chinese women in Shanghai. Nutr Cancer 1999;33(1):82–87

111. Gleason CE, Carlsson CM, Barnet JH, et al. A preliminary study of the safety, feasibility and cognitive efficacy of soy isoflavone supplements in older men and women. Age Ageing 2009;38(1):86–93

112. Messina MJ, Loprinzi CL. Soy for breast cancer survivors: a critical review of the literature. J Nutr 2001; 131(11, Suppl):3095S–3108S

113. Allred CD, Allred KF, Ju YH, Virant SM, Helferich WG. Soy diets containing varying amounts of genistein stimulate growth of estrogen-dependent (MCF-7) tumors in a dose-dependent manner. Cancer Res 2001;61(13):5045–5050

114. Ju YH, Allred CD, Allred KF, Karko KL, Doerge DR, Helferich WG. Physiological concentrations of dietary genistein dose-dependently stimulate growth of estrogen-dependent human breast cancer (MCF-7) tumors implanted in athymic nude mice. J Nutr 2001;131(11):2957–2962

115. Ju YH, Doerge DR, Allred KF, Allred CD, Helferich WG. Dietary genistein negates the inhibitory effect of tamoxifen on growth of estrogen-dependent human breast cancer (MCF-7) cells implanted in athymic mice. Cancer Res 2002;62(9):2474–2477

116. Shu XO, Zheng Y, Cai H, et al. Soy food intake and breast cancer survival. JAMA 2009;302(22):2437–2443

117. Petrakis NL, Barnes S, King EB, et al. Stimulatory influence of soy protein isolate on breast secretion in pre- and postmenopausal women. Cancer Epidemiol Biomarkers Prev 1996;5(10):785–794

118. Hargreaves DF, Potten CS, Harding C, et al. Two-week dietary soy supplementation has an estrogenic effect on normal premenopausal breast. J Clin Endocrinol Metab 1999;84(11):4017–4024

119. Sartippour MR, Rao JY, Apple S, et al. A pilot clinical study of short-term isoflavone supplements in breast cancer patients. Nutr Cancer 2004;49(1):59–65

120. American Academy of Pediatrics. Committee on Nutrition. Soy protein-based formulas: recommendations for use in infant feeding. Pediatrics 1998;101(1 Pt 1):148–153

121. Bhatia J, Greer F; American Academy of Pediatrics Committee on Nutrition. Use of soy protein-based formulas in infant feeding. Pediatrics 2008;121(5):1062–1068

122. Setchell KD, Zimmer-Nechemias L, Cai J, Heubi JE. Isoflavone content of infant formulas and the metabolic fate of these phytoestrogens in early life. Am J Clin Nutr 1998; 68(6, Suppl):1453S–1461S

123. Mendez MA, Anthony MS, Arab L. Soy-based formulae and infant growth and development: a review. J Nutr 2002;132(8):2127–2130

124. Badger TM, Gilchrist JM, Pivik RT, et al. The health implications of soy infant formula. Am J Clin Nutr 2009;89(5):1668S–1672S

125. Strom BL, Schinnar R, Ziegler EE, et al. Exposure to soy-based formula in infancy and endocrinological and reproductive outcomes in young adulthood. JAMA 2001;286(7):807–814

126. US Department of Agriculture, Agricultural Research Service. Study Examines Long-Term Health Effects of Soy Infant Formula. 2004. Available at: http://www.ars.usda.gov/is/AR/archive/jan04/soy0104.htm. Accessed May 3, 2012

127. Turck D. Soy protein for infant feeding: what do we know? Curr Opin Clin Nutr Metab Care 2007; 10(3):360–365

128. Divi RL, Chang HC, Doerge DR. Anti-thyroid isoflavones from soybean: isolation, characterization, and mechanisms of action. Biochem Pharmacol 1997; 54(10):1087–1096

129. Doerge DR, Sheehan DM. Goitrogenic and estrogenic activity of soy isoflavones. Environ Health Perspect 2002;110(Suppl 3):349–353

130. Messina M, Redmond G. Effects of soy protein and soybean isoflavones on thyroid function in healthy adults and hypothyroid patients: a review of the relevant literature. Thyroid 2006;16(3):249–258

131. Chorazy PA, Himelhoch S, Hopwood NJ, Greger NG, Postellon DC. Persistent hypothyroidism in an infant receiving a soy formula: case report and review of the literature. Pediatrics 1995;96(1 Pt 1):148–150

132. Bruce B, Messina M, Spiller GA. Isoflavone supplements do not affect thyroid function in iodine-replete postmenopausal women. J Med Food 2003; 6(4):309–316

133. Persky VW, Turyk ME, Wang L, et al. Effect of soy protein on endogenous hormones in postmenopausal women. Am J Clin Nutr 2002;75(1):145–153

134. Duncan AM, Merz BE, Xu X, Nagel TC, Phipps WR, Kurzer MS. Soy isoflavones exert modest hormonal effects in premenopausal women. J Clin Endocrinol Metab 1999;84(1):192–197

135. Duncan AM, Underhill KE, Xu X, Lavalleur J, Phipps WR, Kurzer MS. Modest hormonal effects of soy isoflavones in postmenopausal women. J Clin Endocrinol Metab 1999;84(10):3479–3484

136. Dillingham BL, McVeigh BL, Lampe JW, Duncan AM. Soy protein isolates of varied isoflavone content do not influence serum thyroid hormones in healthy young men. Thyroid 2007;17(2):131–137

137. Natural Medicines Comprehensive Database. Soy. 2004. Available at: http://www.naturaldatabase.com/monograph.asp?mono_id=975&brand_id=. Accessed May 3, 2012

138. Cambria-Kiely JA. Effect of soy milk on warfarin efficacy. Ann Pharmacother 2002;36(12):1893–1896

139. Jabbar MA, Larrea J, Shaw RA. Abnormal thyroid function tests in infants with congenital hypothyroidism: the influence of soy-based formula. J Am Coll Nutr 1997;16(3):280–282

140. Bell DS, Ovalle F. Use of soy protein supplement and resultant need for increased dose of levothyroxine. Endocr Pract 2001;7(3):193–194

13 Isothiocyanates

Cruciferous vegetables, such as broccoli, cabbage, and kale, are rich sources of sulfur-containing compounds called *glucosinolates*. Isothiocyanates are biologically active hydrolysis (breakdown) products of glucosinolates. Cruciferous vegetables contain a variety of glucosinolates, each of which forms a different isothiocyanate when hydrolyzed (**Fig. 13.1**).[1] For example, broccoli is a good source of glucoraphanin, the glucosinolate precursor of sulforaphane (SFN), and sinigrin, the glucosinolate precursor of allyl isothiocyanate (AITC).[2] Watercress is a rich source of gluconasturtiin, the precursor of phenethyl isothiocyanate (PEITC), while garden cress is rich in glucotropaeolin, the precursor of benzyl isothiocyanate (BITC). At present, scientists are interested in the cancer-preventive activities of vegetables that are rich in glucosinolates (see Chapter 2), as well as individual isothiocyanates.[3]

Bioavailability and Metabolism

Myrosinase, a class of enzymes that catalyzes the hydrolysis of glucosinolates, is physically separated from glucosinolates in intact plant cells.[4] When cruciferous vegetables are chopped or chewed, myrosinase can interact with glucosinolates and release isothiocyanates from their precursors (**Fig. 13.1**). Thorough chewing of raw cruciferous vegetables increases glucosinolate contact with plant myrosinase and increases the amount of isothiocyanates absorbed.[5] Even when plant myrosinase is completely inactivated by heat, the myrosinase activity of human intestinal bacteria allows for some formation and absorption of isothiocyanates.[6] However, the absorption and excretion of isothiocyanates is substantially lower from cooked than from raw cruciferous vegetables[5,7,8] (see the Food Sources section below). During metabolism, isothiocyanates are conjugated (bound) to glutathione, an activity that is promoted by a family of enzymes called *glutathione S-transferases* (GSTs), and further

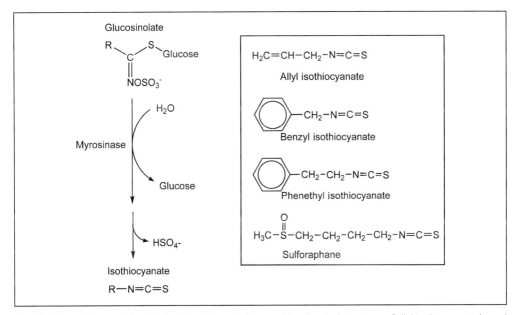

Fig. 13.1 Myrosinase-catalyzed hydrolysis of glucosinolates and the chemical structures of allyl isothiocyanate, benzyl isothiocyanate, phenethyl isothiocyanate, and sulforaphane.

metabolized to mercapturic acids. These isothiocyanate metabolites can be measured in the urine and are highly correlated with dietary intake of cruciferous vegetables.[9] There is also some evidence that isothiocyanate metabolites contribute to the biological activity of isothiocyanates.[3,10]

Biological Activities

Effects on Biotransformation Enzymes Involved in Carcinogen Metabolism

Biotransformation enzymes play important roles in the metabolism and elimination of a variety of chemicals, including drugs, toxins, and carcinogens. In general, phase I biotransformation enzymes catalyze reactions that increase the reactivity of hydrophobic (fat-soluble) compounds, preparing them for reactions catalyzed by phase II biotransformation enzymes. Reactions catalyzed by phase II enzymes generally increase water solubility and promote the elimination of the compound from the body.[11]

Inhibition of Phase I Biotransformation Enzymes

Some procarcinogens (carcinogen precursors) require biotransformation by phase I enzymes, such as those of the cytochrome P450 (CYP) family, to become active carcinogens that are capable of binding DNA and inducing mutations. Inhibition of specific CYP enzymes involved in carcinogen activation inhibits the development of cancer in animal models.[3] Isothiocyanates, including PEITC and BITC, have been found in animal studies to inhibit carcinogen activation by CYP enzymes.[12,13] Cell culture studies have also shown that SFN inhibits certain CYP enzymes.[14] A small clinical trial in smokers found evidence that consumption of 170 g/day (6 oz/day) of watercress, which is rich in the glucosinolate precursor of PEITC, decreased the activation of a procarcinogen found in tobacco.[15]

Induction of Phase II Biotransformation Enzymes

Many isothiocyanates, particularly SFN, are potent inducers of phase II enzymes in cultured human cells.[2,14] Phase II enzymes, including GSTs, uridine diphosphate (UDP)-glucuronosyl trans-

ferases (UGTs), quinone reductase, and γ-glutamatyl cysteine ligase, play important roles in protecting cells from DNA damage by carcinogens and reactive oxygen species.[16] The genes for these and other phase II enzymes contain a specific sequence of DNA called an *antioxidant response element* (ARE). Isothiocyanates have been shown to increase phase II enzyme activity by increasing the transcription of genes that contain an ARE.[17] Limited data from clinical trials suggest that glucosinolate-rich foods can increase phase II enzyme activity in humans. When smokers consumed 170 g/day (6 oz/day) of watercress, urinary excretion of glucuronidated nicotine metabolites increased significantly, suggesting UGT activity increased.[18] Brussels sprouts are rich in several glucosinolates, including precursors of AITC and SFN. Consumption of 300 g/day (11 oz/day) of Brussels sprouts for a week significantly increased plasma and intestinal GST levels in nonsmoking men.[19,20]

Preservation of Normal Cell-Cycle Regulation

After a cell divides, it passes through a sequence of stages known as the *cell cycle*, before dividing again. Following DNA damage, the cell cycle can be transiently arrested to allow for DNA repair or, if the damage cannot be repaired, activation of pathways leading to cell death (apoptosis).[21] Defective cell-cycle regulation may result in the propagation of mutations that contribute to the development of cancer. Several isothiocyanates, including AITC, BITC, PEITC, and SFN, have been found to induce cell-cycle arrest in cultured cells.[2]

Inhibition of Proliferation and Induction of Apoptosis

Unlike normal cells, cancer cells proliferate rapidly and lose the ability to respond to cell death signals that initiate apoptosis. Isothiocyanates have been found to inhibit proliferation and induce apoptosis in several cancer cell lines.[3,22,23]

Inhibition of Histone Deacetylation

In the nucleus of a cell, DNA is coiled around basic proteins called *histones*. In general, acetylation of histones by histone acetyl transferases makes DNA more accessible to transcription factors, which bind DNA and activate gene transcription. Deacetylation of histones by histone deacetylases restricts the access of transcription factors to DNA. Acetylation and deacetylation of nuclear histones is an important cellular mechanism for regulating gene transcription.[24] However, the balance between histone acetyl transferase and histone deacetylase activities that exists in normal cells may be disrupted in cancer cells. Compounds that inhibit histone deacetylases can potentially suppress the development of cancer by inducing the transcription of tumor suppressor proteins that promote differentiation and apoptosis in transformed (precancerous) cells.[25] SFN and AITC metabolites have been found to inhibit histone deacetylase activity in cultured cancer cells.[10,26–28] Moreover, in vivo evidence for SFN inhibiting histone deacetylase came from a mouse model using prostate cancer xenografts.[29] In humans, histone deacetylase activity was inhibited in blood cells following ingestion of 68 g (1 cup) of SFN-rich broccoli sprouts.[29]

Anti-inflammatory Activity

Inflammation promotes cellular proliferation and inhibits apoptosis, increasing the risk of developing cancer.[30] SFN and PEITC have been found to decrease the secretion of inflammatory signaling molecules by white blood cells; these compounds have also been shown to decrease DNA binding of nuclear factor kappa B (NF-κB), a pro-inflammatory transcription factor.[31,32]

Antibacterial Activity

Helicobacter pylori

Bacterial infection with *Helicobacter pylori* (*H. pylori*) is associated with a marked increase in the risk of gastric cancer.[33] In the test tube and in tissue culture, purified SFN inhibited the growth and killed multiple strains of *H. pylori*, including antibiotic-resistant strains.[34] In an animal model of *H. pylori* infection, SFN administration for 5 days eradicated *H. pylori* from eight out of 11 xenografts of human gastric tissue implanted in immune-compromised mice.[35] However, in a small clinical trial, consumption of up to 56 g/day (2 oz/day) of glucoraphanin-rich broccoli sprouts for 1 week was associated with *H. pylori* eradication in only three out of nine patients with gastritis.[36] Further research is needed to determine whether SFN or foods rich in its precursor, glucobrassicin, will be helpful in the treatment of *H. pylori* infection in humans.

Disease Prevention

Cancer

Naturally occurring isothiocyanates and their metabolites have been found to inhibit the development of chemically induced cancers of the lung, liver, esophagus, stomach, small intestine, colon, and mammary gland (breast) in a variety of animal models.[3,12] Although epidemiological studies provide some evidence that higher intakes of cruciferous vegetables are associated with decreased cancer risk in humans,[37] it is difficult to determine whether such protective effects are related to isothiocyanates or other factors associated with consumption of cruciferous vegetables (see Chapter 2). Investigators have attempted to calculate human isothiocyanate exposure based on assessments of cruciferous vegetable intake and measurements of the maximal amounts of isothiocyanates that can be liberated from various cruciferous vegetables in the laboratory.[38] Case–control studies using this technique found that dietary isothiocyanate intakes were significantly lower in Chinese women[39] and US men[40] diagnosed with lung cancer than in cancer-free control groups.

Assessing dietary intake of cruciferous vegetables may not accurately measure an individual exposure to isothiocyanates, since other factors may alter the amount of isothiocyanates formed and absorbed (see the Bioavailability and Metabolism section above). Measuring urinary excretion of isothiocyanates and their metabolites may provide a better assessment of isothiocyanate exposure,[9,41,42] but few studies have examined the relationships between urinary isothiocyanate excretion and cancer risk. In a prospective study, Chinese men with detectable levels of urinary isothiocyanates at baseline were at significantly lower risk of developing lung cancer over the next 10 years than men with undetectable levels.[43] A case–control study found that urinary isothiocyanate excretion was significantly lower in Chinese women diagnosed with breast cancer than in a cancer-free control group.[44] In contrast, cruciferous vegetable intake estimated from a food frequency questionnaire was not associated with breast cancer risk in the same study.

Genetic Variation in Isothiocyanate Metabolism and Cancer Risk

GSTs are a family of phase II biotransformation enzymes that promote the metabolism and elimination of isothiocyanates and other compounds from the body. Genetic variations (polymorphisms) that affect the activity of GST enzymes have been identified in humans. Null variants of the *GSTM1* gene and *GSTT1* gene contain large deletions, and individuals who inherit two copies of the *GSTM1*-null or *GSTT1*-null gene cannot produce the corresponding GST enzyme.[45] Lower GST activity in such individuals could result in slower elimination and thus longer exposure to isothiocyanates after cruciferous vegetable consumption.[9] In support of this idea, several epidemiological studies found that inverse associations between isothiocyanate intake from cruciferous vegetables and the risk of lung cancer[39,40,43,46,47] or colon cancer[48–50] were more

Table 13.1 Total glucosinolate content of selected cruciferous vegetables[52]

Vegetable (Raw)	Serving	Total Glucosinolates (mg)
Brussels sprouts	½ cup	104
Garden cress	½ cup	98
Mustard greens	½ cup	79
Turnip	½ cup	60
Cabbage, Savoy	½ cup	35
Kale	½ cup	34
Cabbage, red	½ cup	29
Broccoli	½ cup	27
Bok choy (pak choi)	½ cup	19
Watercress	½ cup	16

pronounced in *GSTM1*-null or *GSTT1*-null individuals. These findings suggest a protective role for isothiocyanates that may be enhanced in individuals who eliminate them more slowly from the body.

Sources

Food Sources

Cruciferous Vegetables

Cruciferous vegetables, such as bok choy, broccoli, Brussels sprouts, cabbage, cauliflower, horseradish, kale, kohlrabi, mustard, radish, rutabaga, turnip, and watercress, are rich sources of glucosinolate precursors of isothiocyanates.[51] Unlike some other phytochemicals, glucosinolates are present in relatively high concentrations in commonly consumed portions of cruciferous vegetables. For example ½ cup of raw broccoli might provide more than 25 mg of total glucosinolates. Total glucosinolate contents of selected cruciferous vegetables are presented in Table 13.1.[52] Some cruciferous vegetables are better sources of specific glucosinolates (and isothiocyanates) than others. Vegetables that are relatively good sources of some of the isothiocyanates that are currently under study for their cancer-preventive properties are listed in Table 13.2. Amounts of isothiocyanates formed from glucosinolates in foods are variable and depend partly on food processing and preparation (see the Effects of Cooking section below). Consumption of five or more weekly servings of cruciferous vegetables has been associated with significant reductions in cancer risk in some prospective cohort studies.[53–55]

Broccoli Sprouts

The amount of glucoraphanin, the precursor of SFN, in broccoli seeds remains more or less constant as those seeds germinate and grow into

Table 13.2 Some food sources of selected isothiocyanates and their glucosinolate precursors[12]

Isothiocyanate	Glucosinolate (Precursor)	Food Sources
Allyl isothiocyanate (AITC)	Sinigrin	Broccoli, Brussels sprouts, cabbage, horseradish, mustard, radish
Benzyl isothiocyanate (BITC)	Glucotropaeolin	Cabbage, garden cress, Indian cress
Phenethyl isothiocyanate (PEITC)	Gluconasturtiin	Watercress
Sulforaphane (SFN)	Glucoraphanin	Broccoli, Brussels sprouts, cabbage

mature plants. Thus, 3-day-old broccoli sprouts are concentrated sources of glucoraphanin, which contain 10 to 100 times more glucoraphanin by weight than mature broccoli plants.[56] Broccoli sprouts that are certified to contain at least 73 mg of glucoraphanin (also called *sulforaphane glucosinolate*) per 1-oz serving are available in some health food and grocery stores.

Effects of Cooking

Glucosinolates are water-soluble compounds that may be leached into cooking water. Boiling cruciferous vegetables for 9–15 minutes resulted in 18%–59% decreases in the total glucosinolate content of cruciferous vegetables.[52] Cooking methods that use less water, such as steaming or microwaving, may reduce glucosinolate losses.[57] However, some cooking practices, including boiling,[5] steaming,[7,58] and microwaving at high power (750–900 W),[8,58,59] may inactivate myrosinase, the enzyme that catalyzes glucosinolate hydrolysis. Even in the absence of plant myrosinase activity, the myrosinase activity of human intestinal bacteria results in some glucosinolate hydrolysis.[6] However, several studies in humans have found that inactivation of myrosinase in cruciferous vegetables substantially decreases the bioavailability of isothiocyanates.[5,7,8]

Supplements

Dietary supplements containing extracts of broccoli sprouts, broccoli, and other cruciferous vegetables are available without a prescription. Some products are standardized to contain a minimum amount of glucosinolates and/or sulforaphane. However, the bioavailability of isothiocyanates derived from these supplements is not known.

Safety

Adverse Effects

No serious adverse effects of isothiocyanates in humans have been reported. The majority of animal studies have found that isothiocyanates inhibited the development of cancer when given prior to the chemical carcinogen (pre-initiation) However, very high intakes of PEITC or BITC (25–250 times higher than average human dietary isothiocyanate intakes) have been found to promote bladder cancer in rats when given after a

chemical carcinogen (post-initiation).[60] The relevance of these findings to human urinary bladder cancer is not clear, since at least one prospective cohort study found cruciferous vegetable consumption to be inversely associated with the risk of bladder cancer in men.[55]

Pregnancy and Lactation

Although high dietary intakes of glucosinolates from cruciferous vegetables are not known to have adverse effects during pregnancy or lactation, there is no information on the safety of purified isothiocyanates or supplements containing high doses of glucosinolates and/or isothiocyanates during pregnancy or lactation in humans.

Drug Interactions

Isothiocyanates are not known to interact with any drugs or medications. However, the potential for isothiocyanates to inhibit various isoforms of the CYP family of enzymes raises the potential for interactions with drugs that are CYP substrates.[61]

Summary

- Isothiocyanates are derived from the hydrolysis (breakdown) of glucosinolates—sulfur-containing compounds found in cruciferous vegetables.
- Cruciferous vegetables contain a variety of glucosinolates, each of which forms a different isothiocyanate when hydrolyzed.
- Isothiocyanates, such as sulforaphane, may help prevent cancer by promoting the elimination of potential carcinogens from the body and by enhancing the transcription of tumor suppressor proteins.
- Epidemiological studies provide some evidence that human exposure to isothiocyanates through cruciferous vegetable consumption may decrease cancer risk, but the protective effects may be influenced by individual genetic variation in the metabolism and elimination of isothiocyanates from the body.
- Glucosinolates are present in relatively high concentrations in cruciferous vegetables, but cooking, particularly boiling and microwaving at high power, may decrease the bioavailability of isothiocyanates.

References

1. Fahey JW, Zalcmann AT, Talalay P. The chemical diversity and distribution of glucosinolates and isothiocyanates among plants. Phytochemistry 2001;56(1):5–51

2. Zhang Y. Cancer-preventive isothiocyanates: measurement of human exposure and mechanism of action. Mutat Res 2004;555(1–2):173–190

3. Hecht SS. Chemoprevention by isothiocyanates. In: Kelloff GJ, Hawk ET, Sigman CC, eds. Promising Cancer Chemopreventive Agents, Vol 1: Cancer Chemopreventive Agents. Totowa, NJ: Humana Press; 2004:21–35

4. Holst B, Williamson G. A critical review of the bioavailability of glucosinolates and related compounds. Nat Prod Rep 2004;21(3):425–447

5. Shapiro TA, Fahey JW, Wade KL, Stephenson KK, Talalay P. Chemoprotective glucosinolates and isothiocyanates of broccoli sprouts: metabolism and excretion in humans. Cancer Epidemiol Biomarkers Prev 2001;10(5):501–508

6. Shapiro TA, Fahey JW, Wade KL, Stephenson KK, Talalay P. Human metabolism and excretion of cancer chemoprotective glucosinolates and isothiocyanates of cruciferous vegetables. Cancer Epidemiol Biomarkers Prev 1998;7(12):1091–1100

7. Conaway CC, Getahun SM, Liebes LL, et al. Disposition of glucosinolates and sulforaphane in humans after ingestion of steamed and fresh broccoli. Nutr Cancer 2000;38(2):168–178

8. Rouzaud G, Young SA, Duncan AJ. Hydrolysis of glucosinolates to isothiocyanates after ingestion of raw or microwaved cabbage by human volunteers. Cancer Epidemiol Biomarkers Prev 2004;13(1):125–131

9. Seow A, Shi CY, Chung FL, et al. Urinary total isothiocyanate (ITC) in a population-based sample of middle-aged and older Chinese in Singapore: relationship with dietary total ITC and glutathione S-transferase M1/T1/P1 genotypes. Cancer Epidemiol Biomarkers Prev 1998;7(9):775–781

10. Myzak MC, Karplus PA, Chung FL, Dashwood RH. A novel mechanism of chemoprotection by sulforaphane: inhibition of histone deacetylase. Cancer Res 2004;64(16):5767–5774

11. Lampe JW, Peterson S. Brassica, biotransformation and cancer risk: genetic polymorphisms alter the preventive effects of cruciferous vegetables. J Nutr 2002;132(10):2991–2994

12. Conaway CC, Yang YM, Chung FL. Isothiocyanates as cancer chemopreventive agents: their biological activities and metabolism in rodents and humans. Curr Drug Metab 2002;3(3):233–255

13. Hecht SS. Inhibition of carcinogenesis by isothiocyanates. Drug Metab Rev 2000;32(3–4):395–411

14. Fimognari C, Hrelia P. Sulforaphane as a promising molecule for fighting cancer. Mutat Res 2007;635(2–3):90–104

15. Hecht SS, Chung FL, Richie JP Jr, et al. Effects of watercress consumption on metabolism of a tobacco-specific lung carcinogen in smokers. Cancer Epidemiol Biomarkers Prev 1995;4(8):877–884

16. Kensler TW, Talalay P. Inducers of enzymes that protect against carcinogens and oxidants: drug- and food-based approaches with dithiolethiones and sulforaphane. In: Kelloff GJ, Hawk ET, Sigman CC, eds. Promising Cancer Chemopreventive Agents, Vol 1: Cancer Chemopreventive Agents. Totowa, NJ: Humana Press; 2004:3–20

17. Dinkova-Kostova AT, Holtzclaw WD, Cole RN, et al. Direct evidence that sulfhydryl groups of Keap1 are the sensors regulating induction of phase 2 enzymes that protect against carcinogens and oxidants. Proc Natl Acad Sci U S A 2002;99(18):11908–11913

18. Hecht SS, Carmella SG, Murphy SE. Effects of watercress consumption on urinary metabolites of nicotine in smokers. Cancer Epidemiol Biomarkers Prev 1999;8(10):907–913

19. Nijhoff WA, Grubben MJ, Nagengast FM, et al. Effects of consumption of Brussels sprouts on intestinal and lymphocytic glutathione S-transferases in humans. Carcinogenesis 1995;16(9):2125–2128

20. Nijhoff WA, Mulder TP, Verhagen H, van Poppel G, Peters WH. Effects of consumption of brussels sprouts on plasma and urinary glutathione S-transferase class-alpha and -pi in humans. Carcinogenesis 1995;16(4):955–957

21. Stewart ZA, Westfall MD, Pietenpol JA. Cell-cycle dysregulation and anticancer therapy. Trends Pharmacol Sci 2003;24(3):139–145

22. Nakamura Y, Miyoshi N. Cell death induction by isothiocyanates and their underlying molecular mechanisms. Biofactors 2006;26(2):123–134

23. Zhang Y, Yao S, Li J. Vegetable-derived isothiocyanates: anti-proliferative activity and mechanism of action. Proc Nutr Soc 2006;65(1):68–75

24. Mei S, Ho AD, Mahlknecht U. Role of histone deacetylase inhibitors in the treatment of cancer (Review). Int J Oncol 2004;25(6):1509–1519

25. Marks PA, Richon VM, Miller T, Kelly WK. Histone deacetylase inhibitors. Adv Cancer Res 2004;91:137–168

26. Lea MA, Rasheed M, Randolph VM, Khan F, Shareef A, desBordes C. Induction of histone acetylation and inhibition of growth of mouse erythroleukemia cells by S-allylmercaptocysteine. Nutr Cancer 2002;43(1):90–102

27. Myzak MC, Hardin K, Wang R, Dashwood RH, Ho E. Sulforaphane inhibits histone deacetylase activity in BPH-1, LnCaP and PC-3 prostate epithelial cells. Carcinogenesis 2006;27(4):811–819

28. Pledgie-Tracy A, Sobolewski MD, Davidson NE. Sulforaphane induces cell type-specific apoptosis in human breast cancer cell lines. Mol Cancer Ther 2007;6(3):1013–1021

29. Myzak MC, Tong P, Dashwood WM, Dashwood RH, Ho E. Sulforaphane retards the growth of human PC-3 xenografts and inhibits HDAC activity in human subjects. Exp Biol Med (Maywood) 2007;232(2):227–234

30. Steele VE, Hawk ET, Viner JL, Lubet RA. Mechanisms and applications of non-steroidal anti-inflammatory drugs in the chemoprevention of cancer. Mutat Res 2003;523–524:137–144

31. Gerhäuser C, Klimo K, Heiss E, et al. Mechanism-based in vitro screening of potential cancer chemopreventive agents. Mutat Res 2003;523–524:163–172

32. Heiss E, Herhaus C, Klimo K, Bartsch H, Gerhäuser C. Nuclear factor kappa B is a molecular target for sulforaphane-mediated anti-inflammatory mechanisms. J Biol Chem 2001;276(34):32008–32015

33. Normark S, Nilsson C, Normark BH, Hornef MW. Persistent infection with Helicobacter pylori and the development of gastric cancer. Adv Cancer Res 2003;90:63–89

34. Fahey JW, Haristoy X, Dolan PM, et al. Sulforaphane inhibits extracellular, intracellular, and antibiotic-resistant strains of Helicobacter pylori and prevents benzo[a]pyrene-induced stomach tumors. Proc Natl Acad Sci U S A 2002;99(11):7610–7615

35. Haristoy X, Angioi-Duprez K, Duprez A, Lozniewski A. Efficacy of sulforaphane in eradicating Helicobacter pylori in human gastric xenografts implanted in nude mice. Antimicrob Agents Chemother 2003;47(12):3982–3984

36. Galan MV, Kishan AA, Silverman AL. Oral broccoli sprouts for the treatment of Helicobacter pylori infection: a preliminary report. Dig Dis Sci 2004;49(7–8):1088–1090

37. Verhoeven DT, Goldbohm RA, van Poppel G, Verhagen H, van den Brandt PA. Epidemiological studies on brassica vegetables and cancer risk. Cancer Epidemiol Biomarkers Prev 1996;5(9):733–748

38. Jiao D, Yu MC, Hankin JH, Low SH, Chung FL. Total isothiocyanate contents in cooked vegetables frequently consumed in Singapore. J Agric Food Chem 1998;46(3):1055–1058

39. Zhao B, Seow A, Lee EJ, et al. Dietary isothiocyanates, glutathione S-transferase -M1, -T1 polymorphisms and lung cancer risk among Chinese women in Singapore. Cancer Epidemiol Biomarkers Prev 2001;10(10):1063–1067

40. Spitz MR, Duphorne CM, Detry MA, et al. Dietary intake of isothiocyanates: evidence of a joint effect with glutathione S-transferase polymorphisms in lung cancer risk. Cancer Epidemiol Biomarkers Prev 2000;9(10):1017–1020

41. Fowke JH, Hebert JR, Fahey JW. Urinary excretion of dithiocarbamates and self-reported Cruciferous vegetable intake: application of the 'method of triads' to a food-specific biomarker. Public Health Nutr 2002;5(6):791–799

42. Kristensen M, Krogholm KS, Frederiksen H, Bügel SH, Rasmussen SE. Urinary excretion of total isothiocyanates from cruciferous vegetables shows high dose-response relationship and may be a useful biomarker for isothiocyanate exposure. Eur J Nutr 2007;46(7):377–382

43. London SJ, Yuan JM, Chung FL, et al. Isothiocyanates, glutathione S-transferase M1 and T1 polymorphisms, and lung-cancer risk: a prospective study of men in Shanghai, China. Lancet 2000;356(9231):724–729

44. Fowke JH, Shu XO, Dai Q, et al. Urinary isothiocyanate excretion, brassica consumption, and gene polymorphisms among women living in Shanghai, China. Cancer Epidemiol Biomarkers Prev 2003;12(12):1536–1539

45. Coles BF, Kadlubar FF. Detoxification of electrophilic compounds by glutathione S-transferase catalysis: determinants of individual response to chemical carcinogens and chemotherapeutic drugs? Biofactors 2003;17(1–4):115–130

46. Lewis S, Brennan P, Nyberg F, et al. Re: Spitz, M. R., Duphorne, C. M., Detry, M. A., et al. Dietary intake of isothiocyanates: evidence of a joint effect with glutathione S-transferase polymorphisms in lung cancer risk. Cancer Epidemiol. Biomark. Prev., 9: 1017–1020, 2000. Cancer Epidemiol Biomarkers Prev 2001;10(10):1105–1106

47. Brennan P, Hsu CC, Moullan N, et al. Effect of cruciferous vegetables on lung cancer in patients stratified by genetic status: a mendelian randomisation approach. Lancet 2005;366(9496):1558–1560

48. Seow A, Yuan JM, Sun CL, Van Den Berg D, Lee HP, Yu MC. Dietary isothiocyanates, glutathione S-transferase polymorphisms and colorectal cancer risk in the Singapore Chinese Health Study. Carcinogenesis 2002;23(12):2055–2061

49. Slattery ML, Kampman E, Samowitz W, Caan BJ, Potter JD. Interplay between dietary inducers of GST and the GSTM-1 genotype in colon cancer. Int J Cancer 2000;87(5):728–733

50. Turner F, Smith G, Sachse C, et al. Vegetable, fruit and meat consumption and potential risk modifying genes in relation to colorectal cancer. Int J Cancer 2004;112(2):259–264

51. Fenwick GR, Heaney RK, Mullin WJ. Glucosinolates and their breakdown products in food and food plants. Crit Rev Food Sci Nutr 1983;18(2):123–201

52. McNaughton SA, Marks GC. Development of a food composition database for the estimation of dietary intakes of glucosinolates, the biologically active constituents of cruciferous vegetables. Br J Nutr 2003;90(3):687–697

53. Feskanich D, Ziegler RG, Michaud DS, et al. Prospective study of fruit and vegetable consumption and risk of lung cancer among men and women. J Natl Cancer Inst 2000;92(22):1812–1823

54. Giovannucci E, Rimm EB, Liu Y, Stampfer MJ, Willett WC. A prospective study of cruciferous vegetables and prostate cancer. Cancer Epidemiol Biomarkers Prev 2003;12(12):1403–1409

55. Michaud DS, Spiegelman D, Clinton SK, Rimm EB, Willett WC, Giovannucci EL. Fruit and vegetable intake and incidence of bladder cancer in a male prospective cohort. J Natl Cancer Inst 1999;91(7):605–613

56. Fahey JW, Zhang Y, Talalay P. Broccoli sprouts: an exceptionally rich source of inducers of enzymes that protect against chemical carcinogens. Proc Natl Acad Sci U S A 1997;94(19):10367–10372

57. Song L, Thornalley PJ. Effect of storage, processing and cooking on glucosinolate content of Brassica vegetables. Food Chem Toxicol 2007;45(2):216–224

58. Rungapamestry V, Duncan AJ, Fuller Z, Ratcliffe B. Changes in glucosinolate concentrations, myrosinase activity, and production of metabolites of glucosinolates in cabbage (Brassica oleracea Var. capitata) cooked for different durations. J Agric Food Chem 2006;54(20):7628–7634

59. Verkerk R, Dekker M. Glucosinolates and myrosinase activity in red cabbage (Brassica oleracea L. var. Capitata f. rubra DC.) after various microwave treatments. J Agric Food Chem 2004;52(24):7318–7323

60. Okazaki K, Umemura T, Imazawa T, Nishikawa A, Masegi T, Hirose M. Enhancement of urinary bladder carcinogenesis by combined treatment with benzyl isothiocyanate and N-butyl-N-(4-hydroxybutyl)nitrosamine in rats after initiation. Cancer Sci 2003;94(11):948–952

61. Natural Medicines Comprehensive Database. Sulforaphane. Available at: http://naturaldatabase.com. Accessed May 4, 2012

14 Indole-3-Carbinol

Cruciferous vegetables differ from other classes of vegetables in that they are rich sources of sulfur-containing compounds known as *glucosinolates* (see Chapter 2 and Chapter 13). Because epidemiological studies provide some evidence that diets rich in cruciferous vegetables are associated with lower risk of several types of cancer, scientists are interested in the potential cancer-preventive activities of compounds derived from glucosinolates.[1] Among these compounds is indole-3-carbinol (I3C), a compound derived from the enzymatic hydrolysis (breakdown) of an indole glucosinolate, commonly known as *glucobrassicin*.[2]

Bioavailability and Metabolism

Several commonly consumed cruciferous vegetables, including broccoli, Brussels sprouts, and cabbage, are good sources of glucobrassicin—the glucosinolate precursor of I3C. Myrosinase, an enzyme that catalyzes the hydrolysis of glucosinolates, is physically separated from glucosinolates in intact plant cells.[3] When plant cells are damaged, as when cruciferous vegetables are chopped or chewed, the interaction of myrosinase and glucobrassicin results in the formation of I3C (**Fig. 14.1**). In the acidic environment of the stomach, I3C molecules can combine with each other to form a complex mixture of biologically active compounds, known collectively as *acid condensation products*.[4] Although numerous acid condensation products of I3C have been identi-

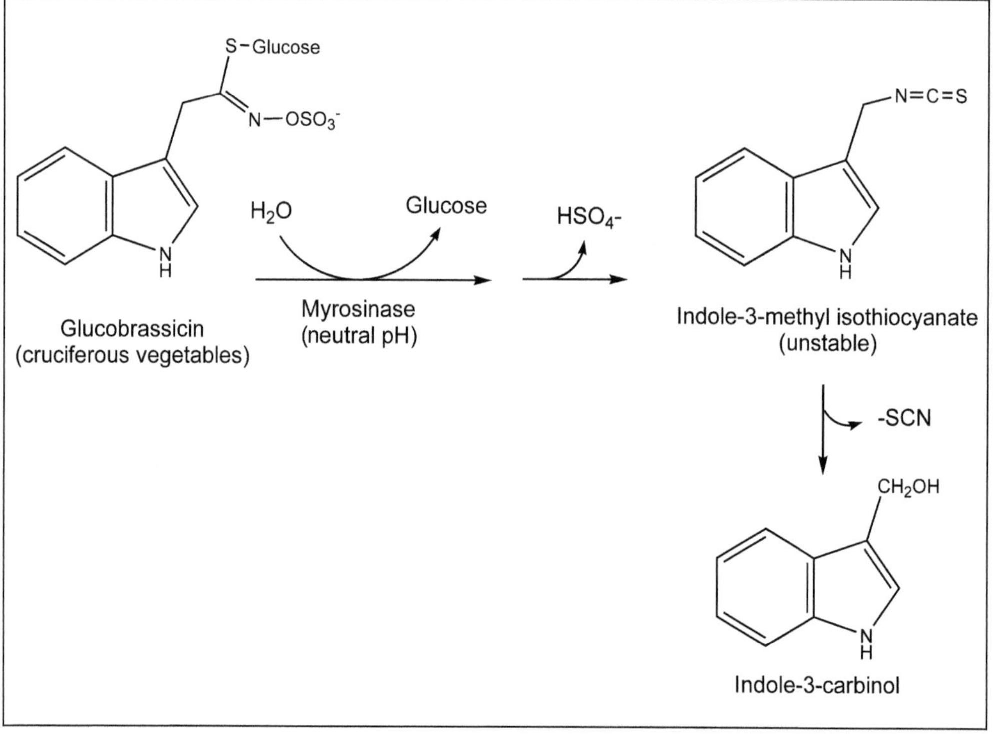

Fig. 14.1 The hydrolysis of glucobrassicin by myrosinase at neutral pH results in an unstable indole isothiocyanate that degrades to form indole-3-carbinol and a thiocyanate ion.

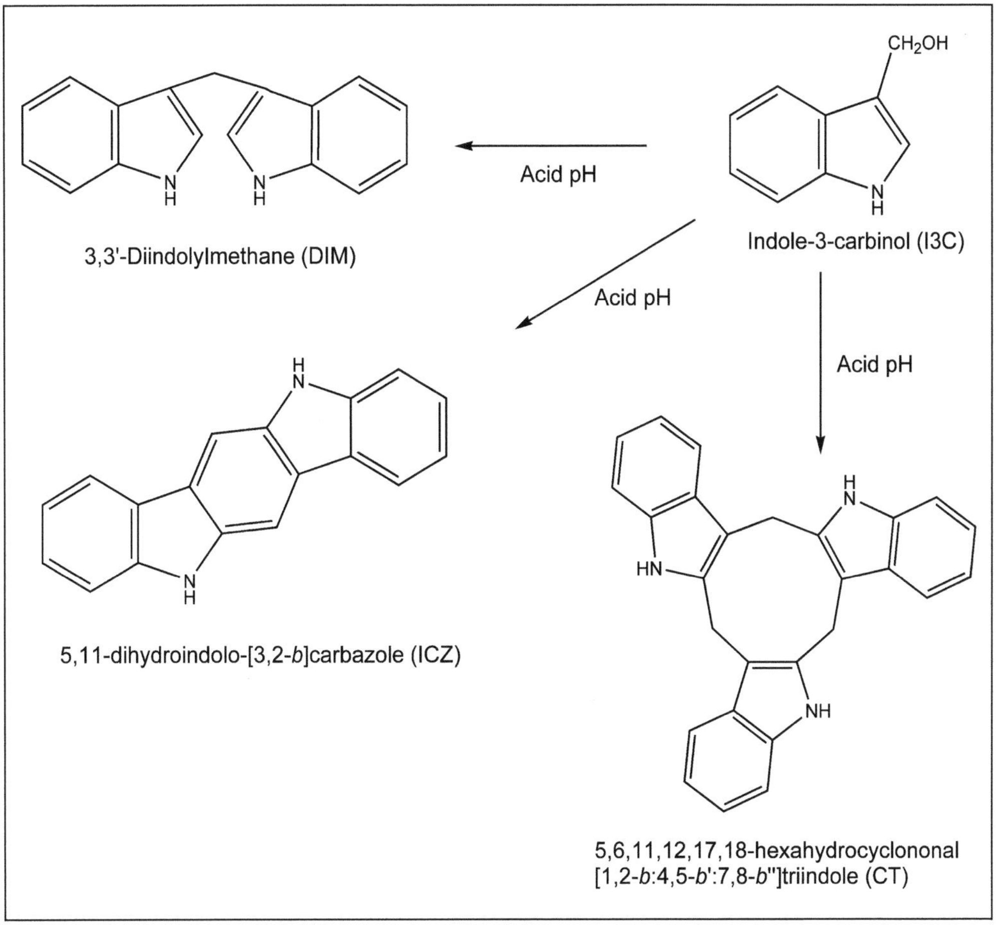

Fig. 14.2 Some acid condensation products of indole-3-carbinol.

fied, some of the most prominent include the dimer 3,3′-diindolylmethane (DIM) and a cyclic trimer (CT) (**Fig. 14.2**). The biological activities of individual acid condensation products differ from those of I3C and are responsible for the biological effects attributed to I3C.[5] When plant myrosinase is inactivated (e.g., by boiling), glucosinolate hydrolysis still occurs to a lesser degree, due to the myrosinase activity of human intestinal bacteria.[6] Thus, when cruciferous vegetables are cooked in a manner that inactivates myrosinase, glucobrassicin hydrolysis by intestinal bacteria still results in some I3C formation (see the Food Sources section below). However, acid condensation products are less likely to form in the more alkaline environment of the intestine.

Biological Activities

Effects on Biotransformation Enzymes Involved in Carcinogen Metabolism

Biotransformation enzymes play major roles in the metabolism and elimination of many biologically active compounds, including steroid hormones, carcinogens, toxins, and drugs. In general, phase I biotransformation enzymes, including the cytochrome P450 (CYP) family, catalyze reactions that increase the reactivity of hydrophobic (fat-soluble) compounds, which prepares them for reactions catalyzed by phase II biotransformation enzymes. Reactions catalyzed by phase II enzymes generally increase water solubility and promote the elimination of these compounds.[7]

Acid condensation products of I3C, particularly DIM and indolo[3,2-*b*]carbazole (ICZ), can bind to a protein in the cytoplasm of cells called the *aryl hydrocarbon receptor* (AhR).[5,8] Binding allows the AhR to enter the nucleus where it forms a complex with the AhR nuclear translocator (Arnt) protein. This AhR–Arnt complex binds to specific DNA sequences in genes, known as *xenobiotic response elements* (XREs) and enhances their transcription.[9] Genes for several CYP enzymes and several phase II enzymes are known to contain XREs. Thus, oral consumption of I3C results in the formation of acid condensation products that can increase the activity of certain phase I and phase II enzymes.[8,10,11] Increasing the activity of biotransformation enzymes is generally considered a beneficial effect because the elimination of potential carcinogens or toxins is enhanced. However, there is a potential for adverse effects because some procarcinogens require biotransformation by phase I enzymes to become active carcinogens.[12]

Alterations in Estrogen Activity and Metabolism

Endogenous estrogens, including 17β-estradiol, exert their estrogenic effects by binding to estrogen receptors (ERs). Within the nucleus, the estrogen–ER complex can bind to DNA sequences in genes known as *estrogen response elements*, recruit coactivator molecules, and thus enhance the transcription of estrogen-responsive genes.[13] Some ER-mediated effects, such as those that promote cellular proliferation in the breast and uterus, can increase the risk of developing estrogen-sensitive cancers.[14]

Effects on Estrogen Receptor Activity

When added to breast cancer cells in culture, I3C has been found to inhibit the transcription of estrogen-responsive genes stimulated by 17β-estradiol.[15,16] Acid condensation products of I3C that bind and activate AhR may also inhibit the transcription of estrogen-responsive genes by competing for coactivators or increasing ER degradation.[9,17] In contrast, some studies in cell culture[18,19] and animal models[20] have found that acid condensation products of I3C actually enhance the transcription of estrogen-responsive genes. Further research is needed to determine the nature of the stimulatory and inhibitory effects of I3C and its acid condensation products on estrogen-responsive gene transcription under conditions that are relevant to human cancer risk (see the Cancer section below).

Effects on Estrogen Metabolism

The endogenous estrogen 17β-estradiol can be irreversibly metabolized to 16α-hydroxyestrone (16αOHE1) or 2-hydroxyestrone (2OHE1). In contrast to 2OHE1, 16αOHE1 is highly estrogenic and has been found to stimulate the proliferation of several estrogen-sensitive cancer cell lines.[21,22] It has been hypothesized that shifting the metabolism of 17β-estradiol toward 2OHE1, and away from 16αOHE1, could decrease the risk of estrogen-sensitive cancers, such as breast cancer.[23] In controlled clinical trials, oral supplementation with 300–400 mg/day of I3C has consistently increased urinary 2OHE1 levels or urinary 2OHE1:16αOHE1 ratios in women.[24–29] Supplementation with 108 mg/day of DIM also increased urinary 2OHE1 levels in postmenopausal women.[30] However, the relationship between urinary 2OHE1:16αOHE1 ratios and breast cancer risk is not clear. Although women with breast cancer had lower urinary ratios of 2OHE1:16αOHE1 in several small case–control studies,[31–33] larger case–control and prospective cohort studies have not found significant associations between urinary 2OHE1:16αOHE1 ratios and breast cancer risk.[34–36]

Induction of Cell-Cycle Arrest

Once a cell divides, it passes through a sequence of stages—collectively known as the *cell cycle*—before it divides again. Following DNA damage, the cell cycle can be transiently arrested at damage checkpoints, which allows for DNA repair or activation of pathways leading to cell death (apoptosis) if the damage is irreparable.[37] Defective cell-cycle regulation may result in the propagation of mutations that contribute to the development of cancer. The addition of I3C to prostate and breast cancer cells in culture has been found to induce cell-cycle arrest.[38,39] However, the physiological relevance of these cell culture studies is unclear, since little or no I3C is available to tissues after oral administration (see the Bioavailability and Metabolism section above).[40]

Induction of Apoptosis

Unlike normal cells, cancerous cells lose their ability to respond to death signals that initiate apoptosis. I3C and DIM have been found to induce apoptosis when added to cultured prostate,[38] breast,[41–43] pancreatic,[44] and cervical cancer cells.[45]

Inhibition of Tumor Invasion and Angiogenesis

Limited evidence in cell culture experiments suggests that I3C and DIM can inhibit the invasion of normal tissue by cancer cells[46] and also inhibit the development of new blood vessels (angiogenesis) required by rapidly growing tumors.[47,48]

Disease Prevention

Cancer

Epidemiological Studies

Epidemiological studies provide some support for the hypothesis that higher intakes of cruciferous vegetables are associated with lower risk for some types of cancer.[49] However, cruciferous vegetables are relatively good sources of other nutrients and phytochemicals that may have protective effects against cancer, including vitamin C, folate, selenium, carotenoids, and fiber (see Chapter 2). Moreover, cruciferous vegetables provide a variety of glucosinolates that may be hydrolyzed to a variety of potentially protective isothiocyanates, in addition to indole-3-carbinol (see Chapter 13).[50] Consequently, evidence for an inverse association between cruciferous vegetable intake and cancer risk provides relatively little information about the specific effects of I3C on cancer risk.

Animal Studies

In most animal models, exposure to a chemical carcinogen is required to cause cancer. When administered before or at the same time as the carcinogen, oral I3C has been found to inhibit the development of cancer in a variety of animal models and tissues, including cancers of the mammary gland (breast),[51,52] uterus,[53] stomach,[54] colon,[55,56] lung,[57] and liver.[58,59] However, several studies have found that I3C actually pro-

moted or enhanced the development of cancer when administered chronically after the carcinogen (post-initiation). The cancer-promoting effects of I3C were first reported in a trout model of liver cancer.[60,61] However, I3C has also been found to promote cancer of the liver,[62–64] thyroid,[64] colon,[65,66] and uterus[67] in rats. More recently, inclusion of I3C in the maternal diet was found to protect the offspring from lymphoma and lung tumors induced by dibenzo[a,l]pyrene, a polycyclic aromatic hydrocarbon.[68] Polycyclic aromatic hydrocarbons are chemical pollutants formed during incomplete combustion of organic substances, such as coal, oil, wood, and tobacco.[69] Although the long-term effects of I3C supplementation on cancer risk in humans are not known, the contradictory results of animal studies have led several experts to caution against the widespread use of I3C and DIM supplements in humans until their potential risks and benefits are better understood.[62,70,71]

Disease Treatment

Diseases Related to Human Papilloma Virus Infection

Cervical Intraepithelial Neoplasia

Infection with certain strains of human papilloma virus (HPV) is an important risk factor for cervical cancer.[72] Transgenic mice that express cancer-promoting HPV genes develop cervical cancer with chronic 17β-estradiol administration. In this model, feeding I3C markedly reduced the number of mice that developed cervical cancer.[73] A small placebo-controlled trial in women examined the effect of oral I3C supplementation on the progression of precancerous cervical lesions classified as cervical intraepithelial neoplasia (CIN) 2 or CIN 3.[74] After 12 weeks, four out of the eight women who took 200 mg/day I3C had complete regression of CIN and four out of the nine who took 400 mg/day had complete regression, while none of the ten who took a placebo had complete regression. HPV was present in seven out of the ten women in the placebo group, seven out of eight women in the 200 mg I3C group, and eight out of nine women in the 400 mg I3C group.[74] Although these preliminary results are encouraging, larger controlled clinical trials are needed to determine the efficacy of I3C supplementation for preventing the progression of pre-cancerous lesions of the cervix.[75]

Vulvar Intraepithelial Neoplasia

HPV infection can also lead to vulvar intraepithelial neoplasia (VIN).[76] A small randomized trial in 12 women with VIN found that supplementation with 200 mg/day or 400 mg/day of I3C for 6 months improved overall symptoms and decreased lesion size and degree of aggressive histopathology.[77] While the results of this preliminary trial are promising, more clinical trials are needed to determine whether I3C might be an effective treatment for VIN.

Recurrent Respiratory Papillomatosis

Recurrent respiratory papillomatosis (RRP) is a rare disease of children and adults, which is characterized by generally benign growths (papillomas) in the respiratory tract caused by HPV infection.[78] These papillomas occur most commonly on or around the vocal cords in the larynx (voice box), but they may also affect the trachea, bronchi, and lungs. The most common treatment for RRP is surgical removal of the papillomas. Since papillomas often recur, adjunct treatments may be used to help prevent or reduce recurrences.[79] In immune-compromised mice transplanted with HPV-infected laryngeal tissue, only 25% of the mice fed I3C developed laryngeal papillomas compared with 100% of the control mice.[80] In a small observational study of RRP patients, increased urinary 2OHE1:16αOHE1 ratios resulting from increased cruciferous vegetable consumption were associated with less severe RRP.[81] Most recently, an uncontrolled pilot study examined the effect of I3C supplementation (400 mg/day for adults and 10 mg/kg daily for children) on papilloma recurrence in RRP patients.[82] Over a 5-year follow-up period, 11 of the original 49 patients experienced no recurrence, 10 experienced a reduction in the rate of recurrence, 12 experienced no improvement, and 12 were lost to follow-up.[83] Although the low toxicity of I3C makes it an attractive adjunct therapy for RRP, controlled clinical trials are needed to determine whether I3C is effective in preventing or reducing the recurrence of respiratory papillomas.

Systemic Lupus Erythematosus

Systemic lupus erythematosus (SLE) is an autoimmune disorder characterized by chronic inflammation that may result in damage to the joints, skin, kidneys, heart, lungs, blood vessels, or brain.[84] Estrogen is thought to play a role in the pathology of SLE because the disorder is much more common in women than men, and its onset is most common during the reproductive years when endogenous estrogen levels are highest.[85] The potential for I3C supplementation to shift endogenous estrogen metabolism toward the less estrogenic metabolite 2OHE1, and away from the highly estrogenic metabolite 16αOHE1 (see the Estrogen Metabolism section above), led to interest in its use in SLE.[24] In an animal model of SLE, I3C feeding decreased the severity of renal (kidney) disease and prolonged survival.[86] A small uncontrolled trial of I3C supplementation (375 mg/day) in female SLE patients found that I3C increased urinary 2OHE1:16αOHE1 ratios, but the trial found no significant change in SLE symptoms after 3 months.[86] Controlled clinical trials are needed to determine whether I3C supplementation might benefit SLE patients.

Sources

Food Sources

Glucobrassicin, the glucosinolate precursor of I3C, is found in several cruciferous vegetables, including broccoli, Brussels sprouts, cabbage, cauliflower, collard greens, kale, kohlrabi, mustard greens, radish, rutabaga, and turnip.[87,88] Although glucosinolates are present in relatively high concentrations in cruciferous vegetables, glucobrassicin makes up only approximately 8%–12% of the total glucosinolates.[89] See Chapter 13, **Table 13.1**, for the total glucosinolate contents of selected cruciferous vegetables. The amount of I3C formed from glucobrassicin in foods is variable and depends, in part, on the processing and preparation of foods.

Effects of Cooking

Glucosinolates are water-soluble compounds that may be leached into cooking water. Boiling cruciferous vegetables for 9–15 minutes resulted in 18%–59% decreases in the total glucosinolate content of cruciferous vegetables.[90] Cooking methods that use less water, such as steaming or microwaving, may reduce glucosinolate losses. Some cooking practices, including boiling,[91] steaming,[92] and microwaving at high power (850–900 W),[93,94] may inactivate myrosinase, the enzyme that catalyzes glucosinolate hydrolysis. Even in the absence of plant myrosinase activity, the myrosinase activity of human intestinal bacteria results in some glucosinolate hydrolysis.[6] However, studies in humans have found that inactivation of myrosinase in cruciferous vegetables substantially decreases the bioavailability of glucosinolate hydrolysis products known as *isothiocyanates*.[91–93] Since the formation of I3C also depends on glucosinolate hydrolysis, it is very likely that the bioavailability of I3C and its acid condensation products would also be decreased by myrosinase inactivation.

Supplements

Indole-3-Carbinol (I3C)

I3C is available without a prescription as a dietary supplement. I3C supplementation increased urinary 2OHE1 levels in adults at doses of 300–400 mg/day.[28] I3C doses of 200 mg/day or 400 mg/day improved the regression of CIN in a preliminary clinical trial.[74] I3C in doses up to 400 mg/day has been used to treat RRP.[82,83] These supplemental levels are well above dietary levels, which commonly range from 20 mg to 120 mg daily.[95]

3,3'-Diindolylmethane (DIM)

DIM is available without a prescription as a dietary supplement. In a small clinical trial, DIM supplementation at a dose of 108 mg/day for 30 days increased urinary 2OHE1 excretion in postmenopausal women with a history of breast cancer.[30]

Safety

Adverse Effects

Slight increases in the serum concentrations of a liver enzyme (alanine aminotransferase; ALT) were observed in two women who took unspecified doses of I3C supplements for 4 weeks.[28] One person reported a skin rash while taking 375 mg/day of I3C.[24] High doses of I3C (800 mg/day) were associated with symptoms of disequilibrium and

tremor, which resolved when the dose was decreased.[82] I3C supplementation enhanced the development of cancer in some animal models when given after the carcinogen[62,64,65,67] (see the Cancer section above). The effects of I3C or DIM supplementation on cancer risk in humans are not known.

Pregnancy and Lactation

The safety of I3C or DIM supplements during pregnancy or lactation has not been established.

Drug Interactions

No drug interactions in humans have been reported. However, preliminary evidence that I3C and DIM can increase the activity of CYP1A2[96,97] suggests the potential for I3C or DIM supplementation to decrease serum concentrations of medications metabolized by CYP1A2. Both I3C and DIM modestly increase the activity of CYP3A4 in rats when administered chronically.[98] This observation raises the potential for adverse drug interactions in humans, since CYP3A4 is involved in the metabolism of approximately 50% of therapeutic drugs.

Summary

- Indole-3-carbinol (I3C) is derived from the hydrolysis (breakdown) of glucobrassicin, a compound found in cruciferous vegetables.
- In the acidic environment of the stomach, I3C molecules can combine with each other to form several biologically active acid condensation products, such as 3,3'-diindolylmethane (DIM).
- I3C has been found to inhibit the development of cancer in animals when given before or at the same time as a carcinogen. However, in some cases, I3C enhanced the development of cancer in animals when administered after a carcinogen.
- The contradictory results of animal studies have led some experts to caution against the widespread use of I3C and DIM supplements for cancer prevention in humans until their potential risks and benefits are better understood.
- Although I3C and DIM supplementation have been found to alter urinary estrogen metabo-

lite profiles in women, the effects of I3C and DIM on breast cancer risk are not known.

- Results of small preliminary trials in humans suggest that I3C supplementation may help treat conditions related to human papilloma virus infection, such as cervical intraepithelial neoplasia and recurrent respiratory papillomatosis. However, randomized controlled trials are needed to determine whether I3C supplementation is beneficial.

References

1. Verhoeven DT, Verhagen H, Goldbohm RA, van den Brandt PA, van Poppel G. A review of mechanisms underlying anticarcinogenicity by brassica vegetables. Chem Biol Interact 1997;103(2):79–129
2. Kim YS, Milner JA. Targets for indole-3-carbinol in cancer prevention. J Nutr Biochem 2005;16(2):65–73
3. Holst B, Williamson G. A critical review of the bioavailability of glucosinolates and related compounds. Nat Prod Rep 2004;21(3):425–447
4. Shertzer HG, Senft AP. The micronutrient indole-3-carbinol: implications for disease and chemoprevention. Drug Metabol Drug Interact 2000;17(1–4): 159–188
5. Bjeldanes LF, Kim JY, Grose KR, Bartholomew JC, Bradfield CA. Aromatic hydrocarbon responsiveness-receptor agonists generated from indole-3-carbinol in vitro and in vivo: comparisons with 2,3,7,8-tetrachlorodibenzo-p-dioxin. Proc Natl Acad Sci U S A 1991; 88(21):9543–9547
6. Shapiro TA, Fahey JW, Wade KL, Stephenson KK, Talalay P. Human metabolism and excretion of cancer chemoprotective glucosinolates and isothiocyanates of cruciferous vegetables. Cancer Epidemiol Biomarkers Prev 1998;7(12):1091–1100
7. Lampe JW, Peterson S. Brassica, biotransformation and cancer risk: genetic polymorphisms alter the preventive effects of cruciferous vegetables. J Nutr 2002;132(10):2991–2994
8. Bonnesen C, Eggleston IM, Hayes JD. Dietary indoles and isothiocyanates that are generated from cruciferous vegetables can both stimulate apoptosis and confer protection against DNA damage in human colon cell lines. Cancer Res 2001;61(16):6120–6130
9. Safe S. Molecular biology of the Ah receptor and its role in carcinogenesis. Toxicol Lett 2001;120(1–3):1–7
10. Nho CW, Jeffery E. The synergistic upregulation of phase II detoxification enzymes by glucosinolate breakdown products in cruciferous vegetables. Toxicol Appl Pharmacol 2001;174(2):146–152
11. Wallig MA, Kingston S, Staack R, Jefferey EH. Induction of rat pancreatic glutathione S-transferase and quinone reductase activities by a mixture of glucosinolate breakdown derivatives found in Brussels sprouts. Food Chem Toxicol 1998;36(5):365–373
12. Baird WM, Hooven LA, Mahadevan B. Carcinogenic polycyclic aromatic hydrocarbon-DNA adducts and mechanism of action. Environ Mol Mutagen 2005;45(2–3):106–114
13. Jordan VC, Gapstur S, Morrow M. Selective estrogen receptor modulation and reduction in risk of breast cancer, osteoporosis, and coronary heart disease. J Natl Cancer Inst 2001;93(19):1449–1457
14. Liehr JG. Is estradiol a genotoxic mutagenic carcinogen? Endocr Rev 2000;21(1):40–54
15. Ashok BT, Chen Y, Liu X, Bradlow HL, Mittelman A, Tiwari RK. Abrogation of estrogen-mediated cellular and biochemical effects by indole-3-carbinol. Nutr Cancer 2001;41(1–2):180–187
16. Meng Q, Yuan F, Goldberg ID, Rosen EM, Auborn K, Fan S. Indole-3-carbinol is a negative regulator of estrogen receptor-alpha signaling in human tumor cells. J Nutr 2000;130(12):2927–2931
17. Chen I, McDougal A, Wang F, Safe S. Aryl hydrocarbon receptor-mediated antiestrogenic and antitumorigenic activity of diindolylmethane. Carcinogenesis 1998;19(9):1631–1639
18. Leong H, Riby JE, Firestone GL, Bjeldanes LF. Potent ligand-independent estrogen receptor activation by 3,3′-diindolylmethane is mediated by cross talk between the protein kinase A and mitogen-activated protein kinase signaling pathways. Mol Endocrinol 2004;18(2):291–302
19. Riby JE, Feng C, Chang YC, Schaldach CM, Firestone GL, Bjeldanes LF. The major cyclic trimeric product of indole-3-carbinol is a strong agonist of the estrogen receptor signaling pathway. Biochemistry 2000; 39(5):910–918
20. Shilling AD, Carlson DB, Katchamart S, Williams DE. 3,3′-diindolylmethane, a major condensation product of indole-3-carbinol, is a potent estrogen in the rainbow trout. Toxicol Appl Pharmacol 2001;170(3):191–200
21. Telang NT, Suto A, Wong GY, Osborne MP, Bradlow HL. Induction by estrogen metabolite 16 alpha-hydroxyestrone of genotoxic damage and aberrant proliferation in mouse mammary epithelial cells. J Natl Cancer Inst 1992;84(8):634–638
22. Yuan F, Chen DZ, Liu K, Sepkovic DW, Bradlow HL, Auborn K. Anti-estrogenic activities of indole-3-carbinol in cervical cells: implication for prevention of cervical cancer. Anticancer Res 1999;19(3A):1673–1680
23. Bradlow HL, Telang NT, Sepkovic DW, Osborne MP. 2-hydroxyestrone: the 'good' estrogen. J Endocrinol 1996;150(Suppl):S259–S265
24. McAlindon TE, Gulin J, Chen T, Klug T, Lahita R, Nuite M. Indole-3-carbinol in women with SLE: effect on estrogen metabolism and disease activity. Lupus 2001;10(11):779–783
25. Bradlow HL, Michnovicz JJ, Halper M, Miller DG, Wong GY, Osborne MP. Long-term responses of women to indole-3-carbinol or a high fiber diet. Cancer Epidemiol Biomarkers Prev 1994;3(7):591–595
26. Michnovicz JJ. Increased estrogen 2-hydroxylation in obese women using oral indole-3-carbinol. Int J Obes Relat Metab Disord 1998;22(3):227–229
27. Michnovicz JJ, Adlercreutz H, Bradlow HL. Changes in levels of urinary estrogen metabolites after oral indole-3-carbinol treatment in humans. J Natl Cancer Inst 1997;89(10):718–723
28. Wong GY, Bradlow L, Sepkovic D, Mehl S, Mailman J, Osborne MP. Dose-ranging study of indole-3-carbinol for breast cancer prevention. J Cell Biochem Suppl 1997;28–29:111–116
29. Reed GA, Peterson KS, Smith HJ, et al. A phase I study of indole-3-carbinol in women: tolerability and effects. Cancer Epidemiol Biomarkers Prev 2005; 14(8):1953–1960

30. Dalessandri KM, Firestone GL, Fitch MD, Bradlow HL, Bjeldanes LF. Pilot study: effect of 3,3′-diindolylmethane supplements on urinary hormone metabolites in postmenopausal women with a history of early-stage breast cancer. Nutr Cancer 2004;50(2):161–167

31. Ho GH, Luo XW, Ji CY, Foo SC, Ng EH. Urinary 2/16 alpha-hydroxyestrone ratio: correlation with serum insulin-like growth factor binding protein-3 and a potential biomarker of breast cancer risk. Ann Acad Med Singapore 1998;27(2):294–299

32. Kabat GC, Chang CJ, Sparano JA, et al. Urinary estrogen metabolites and breast cancer: a case-control study. Cancer Epidemiol Biomarkers Prev 1997; 6(7):505–509

33. Schneider J, Kinne D, Fracchia A, et al. Abnormal oxidative metabolism of estradiol in women with breast cancer. Proc Natl Acad Sci U S A 1982;79(9):3047–3051

34. Cauley JA, Zmuda JM, Danielson ME, et al. Estrogen metabolites and the risk of breast cancer in older women. Epidemiology 2003;14(6):740–744

35. Meilahn EN, De Stavola B, Allen DS, et al. Do urinary oestrogen metabolites predict breast cancer? Guernsey III cohort follow-up. Br J Cancer 1998;78(9):1250–1255

36. Ursin G, London S, Stanczyk FZ, et al. Urinary 2-hydroxyestrone/16alpha-hydroxyestrone ratio and risk of breast cancer in postmenopausal women. J Natl Cancer Inst 1999;91(12):1067–1072

37. Stewart ZA, Westfall MD, Pietenpol JA. Cell-cycle dysregulation and anticancer therapy. Trends Pharmacol Sci 2003;24(3):139–145

38. Chinni SR, Li Y, Upadhyay S, Koppolu PK, Sarkar FH. Indole-3-carbinol (I3C) induced cell growth inhibition, G1 cell cycle arrest and apoptosis in prostate cancer cells. Oncogene 2001;20(23):2927–2936

39. Cover CM, Hsieh SJ, Tran SH, et al. Indole-3-carbinol inhibits the expression of cyclin-dependent kinase-6 and induces a G1 cell cycle arrest of human breast cancer cells independent of estrogen receptor signaling. J Biol Chem 1998;273(7):3838–3847

40. Stresser DM, Williams DE, Griffin DA, Bailey GS. Mechanisms of tumor modulation by indole-3-carbinol. Disposition and excretion in male Fischer 344 rats. Drug Metab Dispos 1995;23(9):965–975

41. Hong C, Firestone GL, Bjeldanes LF. Bcl-2 family-mediated apoptotic effects of 3,3′-diindolylmethane (DIM) in human breast cancer cells. Biochem Pharmacol 2002;63(6):1085–1097

42. Howells LM, Gallacher-Horley B, Houghton CE, Manson MM, Hudson EA. Indole-3-carbinol inhibits protein kinase B/Akt and induces apoptosis in the human breast tumor cell line MDA MB468 but not in the non-tumorigenic HBL100 line. Mol Cancer Ther 2002; 1(13):1161–1172

43. Rahman KW, Sarkar FH. Inhibition of nuclear translocation of nuclear factor-kappaB contributes to 3,3′-diindolylmethane-induced apoptosis in breast cancer cells. Cancer Res 2005;65(1):364–371

44. Abdelrahim M, Newman K, Vanderlaag K, Samudio I, Safe S. 3,3′-diindolylmethane (DIM) and its derivatives induce apoptosis in pancreatic cancer cells through endoplasmic reticulum stress-dependent upregulation of DR5. Carcinogenesis 2006;27(4):717–728

45. Chen D, Carter TH, Auborn KJ. Apoptosis in cervical cancer cells: implications for adjunct anti-estrogen therapy for cervical cancer. Anticancer Res 2004; 24(5A):2649–2656

46. Meng Q, Goldberg ID, Rosen EM, Fan S. Inhibitory effects of Indole-3-carbinol on invasion and migration in human breast cancer cells. Breast Cancer Res Treat 2000;63(2):147–152

47. Chang X, Tou JC, Hong C, et al. 3,3′-Diindolylmethane inhibits angiogenesis and the growth of transplantable human breast carcinoma in athymic mice. Carcinogenesis 2005;26(4):771–778

48. Wu HT, Lin SH, Chen YH. Inhibition of cell proliferation and in vitro markers of angiogenesis by indole-3-carbinol, a major indole metabolite present in cruciferous vegetables. J Agric Food Chem 2005; 53(13):5164–5169

49. Verhoeven DT, Goldbohm RA, van Poppel G, Verhagen H, van den Brandt PA. Epidemiological studies on brassica vegetables and cancer risk. Cancer Epidemiol Biomarkers Prev 1996;5(9):733–748

50. Fahey JW, Zalcmann AT, Talalay P. The chemical diversity and distribution of glucosinolates and isothiocyanates among plants. Phytochemistry 2001;56(1):5–51

51. Grubbs CJ, Steele VE, Casebolt T, et al. Chemoprevention of chemically-induced mammary carcinogenesis by indole-3-carbinol. Anticancer Res 1995;15(3):709–716

52. Bradlow HL, Michnovicz J, Telang NT, Osborne MP. Effects of dietary indole-3-carbinol on estradiol metabolism and spontaneous mammary tumors in mice. Carcinogenesis 1991;12(9):1571–1574

53. Kojima T, Tanaka T, Mori H. Chemoprevention of spontaneous endometrial cancer in female Donryu rats by dietary indole-3-carbinol. Cancer Res 1994;54(6):1446–1449

54. Wattenberg LW, Loub WD. Inhibition of polycyclic aromatic hydrocarbon-induced neoplasia by naturally occurring indoles. Cancer Res 1978;38(5):1410–1413

55. Wargovich MJ, Chen CD, Jimenez A, et al. Aberrant crypts as a biomarker for colon cancer: evaluation of potential chemopreventive agents in the rat. Cancer Epidemiol Biomarkers Prev 1996;5(5):355–360

56. Guo D, Schut HA, Davis CD, Snyderwine EG, Bailey GS, Dashwood RH. Protection by chlorophyllin and indole-3-carbinol against 2-amino-1-methyl-6-phenylimidazo[4,5-b]pyridine (PhIP)-induced DNA adducts and colonic aberrant crypts in the F344 rat. Carcinogenesis 1995;16(12):2931–2937

57. Morse MA, LaGreca SD, Amin SG, Chung FL. Effects of indole-3-carbinol on lung tumorigenesis and DNA methylation induced by 4-(methylnitrosamino)-1-(3-pyridyl)-1-butanone (NNK) and on the metabolism and disposition of NNK in A/J mice. Cancer Res 1990;50(9):2613–2617

58. Dashwood RH, Arbogast DN, Fong AT, Hendricks JD, Bailey GS. Mechanisms of anti-carcinogenesis by indole-3-carbinol: detailed in vivo DNA binding dose-response studies after dietary administration with aflatoxin B1. Carcinogenesis 1988;9(3):427–432

59. Oganesian A, Hendricks JD, Williams DE. Long term dietary indole-3-carbinol inhibits diethylnitrosamine-initiated hepatocarcinogenesis in the infant mouse model. Cancer Lett 1997;118(1):87–94

60. Dashwood RH, Fong AT, Williams DE, Hendricks JD, Bailey GS. Promotion of aflatoxin B1 carcinogenesis by the natural tumor modulator indole-3-carbinol: influence of dose, duration, and intermittent exposure on indole-3-carbinol promotional potency. Cancer Res 1991;51(9):2362–2365

61. Oganesian A, Hendricks JD, Pereira CB, Orner GA, Bailey GS, Williams DE. Potency of dietary indole-3-carbinol as a promoter of aflatoxin B1-initiated hepatocarcinogenesis: results from a 9000 animal tumor study. Carcinogenesis 1999;20(3):453–458

62. Stoner G, Casto B, Ralston S, Roebuck B, Pereira C, Bailey G. Development of a multi-organ rat model for evaluating chemopreventive agents: efficacy of indole-3-carbinol. Carcinogenesis 2002;23(2):265–272

63. Kim DJ, Lee KK, Han BS, Ahn B, Bae JH, Jang JJ. Biphasic modifying effect of indole-3-carbinol on diethylnitrosamine-induced preneoplastic glutathione S-transferase placental form-positive liver cell foci in Sprague-Dawley rats. Jpn J Cancer Res 1994; 85(6):578–583

64. Kim DJ, Han BS, Ahn B, et al. Enhancement by indole-3-carbinol of liver and thyroid gland neoplastic development in a rat medium-term multiorgan carcinogenesis model. Carcinogenesis 1997;18(2):377–381

65. Pence BC, Buddingh F, Yang SP. Multiple dietary factors in the enhancement of dimethylhydrazine carcinogenesis: main effect of indole-3-carbinol. J Natl Cancer Inst 1986;77(1):269–276

66. Suzui M, Inamine M, Kaneshiro T, et al. Indole-3-carbinol inhibits the growth of human colon carcinoma cells but enhances the tumor multiplicity and volume of azoxymethane-induced rat colon carcinogenesis. Int J Oncol 2005;27(5):1391–1399

67. Yoshida M, Katashima S, Ando J, et al. Dietary indole-3-carbinol promotes endometrial adenocarcinoma development in rats initiated with N-ethyl-N'-nitro-N-nitrosoguanidine, with induction of cytochrome P450s in the liver and consequent modulation of estrogen metabolism. Carcinogenesis 2004;25(11): 2257–2264

68. Yu Z, Mahadevan B, Löhr CV, et al. Indole-3-carbinol in the maternal diet provides chemoprotection for the fetus against transplacental carcinogenesis by the polycyclic aromatic hydrocarbon dibenzo[a,l]pyrene. Carcinogenesis 2006;27(10):2116–2123

69. Agency for Toxic Substances and Disease Registry Toxicological Profile for Polycyclic Aromatic Hydrocarbons (PAHs). Atlanta, GA: US Department of Health and Human Services; 1995. Available at: http://www.atsdr.cdc.gov/toxprofiles/tp69.pdf. Accessed May 3, 2012

70. Dashwood RH. Indole-3-carbinol: anticarcinogen or tumor promoter in brassica vegetables? Chem Biol Interact 1998;110(1–2):1–5

71. Lee BM, Park KK. Beneficial and adverse effects of chemopreventive agents. Mutat Res 2003;523–524: 265–278

72. Bosch FX, de Sanjosé S. Chapter 1: Human papillomavirus and cervical cancer—burden and assessment of causality. J Natl Cancer Inst Monogr 2003; (31):3–13

73. Jin L, Qi M, Chen DZ, et al. Indole-3-carbinol prevents cervical cancer in human papilloma virus type 16 (HPV16) transgenic mice. Cancer Res 1999; 59(16):3991–3997

74. Bell MC, Crowley-Nowick P, Bradlow HL, et al. Placebo-controlled trial of indole-3-carbinol in the treatment of CIN. Gynecol Oncol 2000;78(2):123–129

75. Stanley M. Chapter 17: Genital human papillomavirus infections—current and prospective therapies. J Natl Cancer Inst Monogr 2003; (31):117–124

76. Hørding U, Junge J, Poulsen H, Lundvall F. Vulvar intraepithelial neoplasia III: a viral disease of undetermined progressive potential. Gynecol Oncol 1995; 56(2):276–279

77. Naik R, Nixon S, Lopes A, Godfrey K, Hatem MH, Monaghan JM. A randomized phase II trial of indole-3-carbinol in the treatment of vulvar intraepithelial neoplasia. Int J Gynecol Cancer 2006;16(2):786–790

78. What is recurrent respiratory papillomatosis? Recurrent Respiratory Papillomatosis Foundation. Available at: http://rrpf.org/whatisRRP.html. Accessed May 3, 2012

79. Auborn KJ. Therapy for recurrent respiratory papillomatosis. Antivir Ther 2002;7(1):1–9

80. Newfield L, Goldsmith A, Bradlow HL, Auborn K. Estrogen metabolism and human papillomavirus-induced tumors of the larynx: chemo-prophylaxis with indole-3-carbinol. Anticancer Res 1993;13(2):337–341

81. Auborn K, Abramson A, Bradlow HL, Sepkovic D, Mullooly V. Estrogen metabolism and laryngeal papillomatosis: a pilot study on dietary prevention. Anticancer Res 1998;18(6B):4569–4573

82. Rosen CA, Woodson GE, Thompson JW, Hengesteg AP, Bradlow HL. Preliminary results of the use of indole-3-carbinol for recurrent respiratory papillomatosis. Otolaryngol Head Neck Surg 1998;118(6):810–815

83. Rosen CA, Bryson PC. Indole-3-carbinol for recurrent respiratory papillomatosis: long-term results. J Voice 2004;18(2):248–253

84. Nass T. Lupus: A Patient Care Guide for Nurses and Other Health Professionals 3rd ed. Bethesda, MD: National Institute of Arthritis and Musculoskeletal and Skin Diseases; 2001. Available at: http://www.niams.nih.gov/hi/topics/lupus/lupusguide/outline.htm. Accessed May 3, 2012

85. McMurray RW, May W. Sex hormones and systemic lupus erythematosus: review and meta-analysis. Arthritis Rheum 2003;48(8):2100–2110

86. Auborn KJ, Qi M, Yan XJ, et al. Lifespan is prolonged in autoimmune-prone (NZB/NZW) F1 mice fed a diet supplemented with indole-3-carbinol. J Nutr 2003;133(11):3610–3613

87. Carlson DG, Daxenbichler ME, Etten CH, Kwolek WF, Williams PH. Glucosinolates in crucifer vegetables: broccoli, Brussels sprouts, cauliflower, collards, kale, mustard greens, and kohlrabi. J Am Soc Hortic Sci 1987;112(1):173–178

88. Fenwick GR, Heaney RK, Mullin WJ. Glucosinolates and their breakdown products in food and food plants. Crit Rev Food Sci Nutr 1983;18(2):123–201

89. Kushad MM, Brown AF, Kurilich AC, et al. Variation of glucosinolates in vegetable crops of Brassica oleracea. J Agric Food Chem 1999;47(4):1541–1548

90. McNaughton SA, Marks GC. Development of a food composition database for the estimation of dietary intakes of glucosinolates, the biologically active constituents of cruciferous vegetables. Br J Nutr 2003;90(3):687–697

91. Shapiro TA, Fahey JW, Wade KL, Stephenson KK, Talalay P. Chemoprotective glucosinolates and isothiocyanates of broccoli sprouts: metabolism and excretion in humans. Cancer Epidemiol Biomarkers Prev 2001;10(5):501–508

92. Conaway CC, Getahun SM, Liebes LL, et al. Disposition of glucosinolates and sulforaphane in humans after ingestion of steamed and fresh broccoli. Nutr Cancer 2000;38(2):168–178

93. Rouzaud G, Young SA, Duncan AJ. Hydrolysis of glucosinolates to isothiocyanates after ingestion of raw or microwaved cabbage by human volunteers. Cancer Epidemiol Biomarkers Prev 2004;13(1):125–131

94. Verkerk R, Dekker M. Glucosinolates and myrosinase activity in red cabbage (Brassica oleracea L. var. Capitata f. rubra DC.) after various microwave treatments. J Agric Food Chem 2004;52(24):7318–7323

95. Natural Medicines Online Database. Indole-3-Carbinol. 2008. Available at: http://naturaldatabase.therapeuticresearch.com/nd/Search.aspx?cs=&s=ND&pt=100&id=1027&ds=&lang=0. Accessed May 3, 2012

96. He YH, Friesen MD, Ruch RJ, Schut HA. Indole-3-carbinol as a chemopreventive agent in 2-amino-1-methyl-6-phenylimidazo[4,5-b]pyridine (PhIP) carcinogenesis: inhibition of PhIP-DNA adduct formation, acceleration of PhIP metabolism, and induction of cytochrome P450 in female F344 rats. Food Chem Toxicol 2000;38(1):15–23

97. Lake BG, Tredger JM, Renwick AB, Barton PT, Price RJ. 3,3′-Diindolylmethane induces CYP1A2 in cultured precision-cut human liver slices. Xenobiotica 1998; 28(8):803–811

98. Leibelt DA, Hedstrom OR, Fischer KA, Pereira CB, Williams DE. Evaluation of chronic dietary exposure to indole-3-carbinol and absorption-enhanced 3,3′-diindolylmethane in Sprague-Dawley rats. Toxicol Sci 2003;74(1):10–21

15 Lignans

The enterolignans, enterodiol and enterolactone (**Fig. 15.1**), are formed by the action of intestinal bacteria on lignan precursors found in plants.[1] Because enterodiol and enterolactone can mimic some of the effects of estrogens, their plant-derived precursors are classified as phytoestrogens. Lignan precursors that have been identified in the human diet include pinoresinol, lariciresinol, secoisolariciresinol, matairesinol (**Fig. 15.2**), and others. Secoisolariciresinol and matairesinol were among the first lignan precursors identified in the human diet and are therefore the most extensively studied. Lignan precursors are found in a wide variety of foods, including flaxseeds, sesame seeds, legumes, whole grains, fruits, and vegetables. While most research on phytoestrogen-rich diets has focused on soy isoflavones, lignans are the principal source of dietary phytoestrogens in typical Western diets.[2,3]

Bioavailability and Metabolism

When plant lignans are ingested, they can be metabolized by intestinal bacteria to the enterolignans, enterodiol and enterolactone in the intestinal lumen.[4] Enterodiol can also be converted to enterolactone by intestinal bacteria. Not surprisingly, antibiotic use has been associated with lower serum enterolactone levels.[5] Thus, enterolactone levels measured in serum and urine reflect the activity of intestinal bacteria in addition to dietary intake of plant lignans. Because data on the lignan content of foods are limited, serum and urinary enterolactone levels are sometimes used as markers of dietary lignan intake. A pharmacokinetic study that measured plasma and urinary levels of enterodiol and enterolactone after a single dose (0.9 mg/kg of body weight) of secoisolariciresinol, the principal lignan in flaxseed, found that at least 40% was available to the body as enterodiol and enterolactone.[6] Plasma enterodiol concentrations peaked at 73 nmol/L an average of 15 hours after ingestion of secoisolariciresinol, and plasma enterolactone concentrations peaked at 56 nmol/L an average of 20 hours after ingestion. Thus, substantial amounts of ingested plant lignans are available to humans in the form of enterodiol and enterolactone. Considerable variation among individuals in urinary and serum enterodiol:enterolactone ratios has been observed in flaxseed feeding studies, suggesting that some individuals convert most enterodiol to enterolactone, while others convert relatively little.[1] It is likely that individual differences in the metabolism of lignans, possibly due to gut microbes, influence the biological activities and health effects of these compounds.

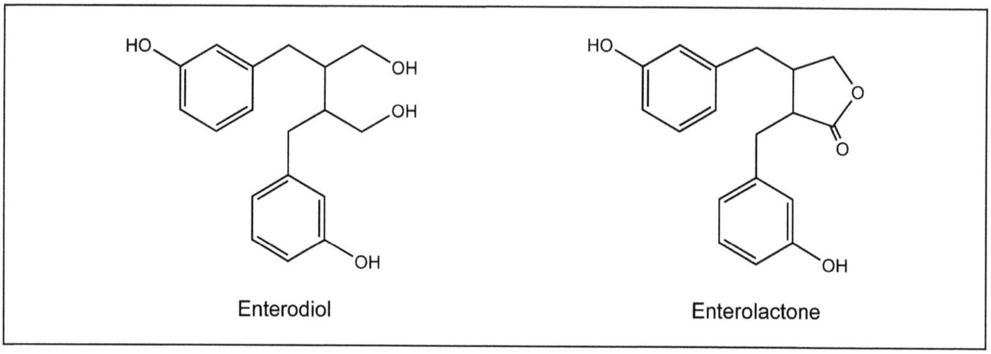

Fig. 15.1 Chemical structures of the lignans, enterodiol and enterolactone.

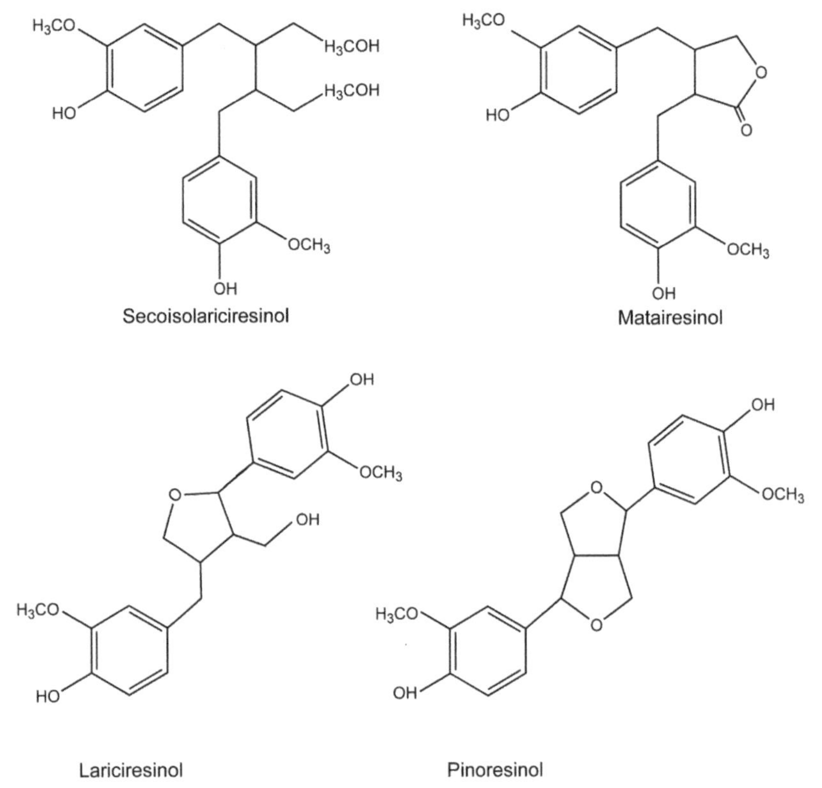

Fig. 15.2 Chemical structures of secoisolariciresinol, matairesinol, lariciresinol, and pinoresinol, plant lignans that are precursors for lignans.

Biological Activities

Estrogenic and Antiestrogenic Activities

Estrogens are signaling molecules (hormones) that exert their effects by binding to estrogen receptors within cells. The estrogen–receptor complex interacts with DNA to change the expression of estrogen-responsive genes. Estrogen receptors are present in numerous tissues other than those associated with reproduction, including bone, liver, heart and brain.[7] Although phytoestrogens can also bind to estrogen receptors, their estrogenic activity is much weaker than that of endogenous estrogens, and they may actually block or antagonize the effects of estrogen in some tissues.[8] Scientists are interested in the tissue-selective activities of phytoestrogens because antiestrogenic effects in reproductive tissue could

help reduce the risk of hormone-associated cancers (breast, uterine, ovarian, and prostate), while estrogenic effects in bone could help maintain bone density. The enterolignans, enterodiol and enterolactone, are known to have weak estrogenic activity. At present, the extent to which enterolignans exert weak estrogenic and/or antiestrogenic effects in humans is not well understood.

Estrogen-Receptor-Independent Activities

Enterolignans also have biological activities that are unrelated to their interactions with estrogen receptors. By altering the activity of enzymes involved in estrogen metabolism, lignans may change the biological activity of endogenous estrogens.[9] Lignans can act as antioxidants in the test tube, but the significance of such antioxidant activity in humans is not clear because lignans are rapidly and extensively metabolized.[4] Although one cross-sectional study found that a biomarker of oxidative damage was inversely associated with serum enterolactone levels in men,[10] it is not clear whether this effect was related to enterolactone or other antioxidants present in lignan-rich foods.

Disease Prevention

Cardiovascular Disease

Diets rich in foods containing plant lignans (whole grains, nuts and seeds, legumes, fruits, and vegetables) have been consistently associated with reductions in the risk of cardiovascular disease. However, it is likely that numerous nutrients and phytochemicals found in these foods contribute to their cardioprotective effects. In a prospective cohort study of 1889 Finnish men followed for an average of 12 years, those with the highest serum enterolactone levels (a marker of plant lignan intake) were significantly less likely to die from coronary heart disease (CHD) or cardiovascular disease than those with the lowest levels.[11] However, a recent study in male smokers did not find strong support for an association between serum enterolactone levels and CHD.[12] Flaxseeds are among the richest sources of plant lignans in the human diet, but they are also good sources of other nutrients and phytochemicals with cardioprotective effects, such as omega-3 fatty acids and fiber. Four small clinical trials found that adding 30–50 g/day of flaxseed to the usual diet for 4–12 weeks resulted in modest 8%–14% decreases in low-density lipoprotein (LDL) cholesterol levels,[13–16] while four other trials did not observe significant reductions in LDL cholesterol after adding 30–40 g/day of flaxseed to the diet.[17–20] More recently, a double-blind, randomized controlled trial in adults aged 44 to 75 found that supplementation with 40 g/day of flaxseed led to significant reductions in LDL cholesterol after 5 weeks, but cholesterol reductions were not statistically significant following 10 weeks of supplementation.[21] Additionally, a 1-year clinical trial in menopausal women reported that supplementation with 40 g/day of flaxseed did not lower LDL cholesterol compared with a placebo containing wheat germ.[22] Most of

these trials used ground or crushed flaxseed, which is much more bioavailable than whole flaxseed.[23] Although the results of prospective cohort studies consistently indicate that diets rich in whole grains, nuts, fruits, and vegetables are associated with significant reductions in cardiovascular disease risk, it is not yet clear whether lignans themselves are cardioprotective.

Hormone-Associated Cancers

Breast cancer

Overall, there is little evidence that dietary intake of plant lignans is significantly associated with breast cancer risk; studies to date have reported conflicting results. Two prospective cohort studies examining plant lignan intake and breast cancer found no association.[24,25] A more recent prospective study reported no association between total lignan intake and breast cancer in premenopausal women.[26] In another prospective analysis, the same group of authors found postmenopausal women in the highest quartile of dietary lignan intake had a 17% lower risk of breast cancer compared with women in the lowest quartile, but this protective association was only observed in women with estrogen-positive and progesterone-positive tumors.[27] A recent meta-analysis did not find an overall association between dietary lignan intake and breast cancer, but when the analysis was limited to postmenopausal women, the authors reported a 15% reduction in risk of breast cancer with high lignan intake.[28] Several studies, mainly case–control studies, have examined the relationship between blood or urine levels of enterolactone and breast cancer; results of these studies are conflicting.[29–31] Moreover, a recent meta-analysis did not find an association between blood levels of enterolactone and breast cancer.[28] At present, it is not clear whether high intakes of plant lignans or high circulating levels of enterolignans offer significant protective effects against breast cancer.

Endometrial and Ovarian Cancer

In a case–control study of lignans and endometrial cancer, US women with the highest intakes of plant lignans had the lowest risk of endometrial cancer, but the reduction in risk was statistically significant in postmenopausal women only.[32] Yet, a recent prospective case–control study in three different countries (US, Sweden, and Italy) did not find an association between circulating enterolactone, a marker of lignan intake, and endometrial cancer in premenopausal or postmenopausal women.[33] In the only case–control study of lignans and ovarian cancer, US women with the highest intakes of plant lignans had the lowest risk of ovarian cancer.[34] However, high intakes of other phytochemicals associated with plant-based diets like fiber, carotenoids, and phytosterols were also associated with decreased ovarian cancer risk. Although these studies support the hypothesis that diets rich in plant foods may be helpful in decreasing the risk of hormone-associated cancers, they do not provide strong evidence that lignans are protective against endometrial or ovarian cancer.

Prostate Cancer

Although dietary lignans are the principal source of phytoestrogens in the typical Western diet, relationships between dietary lignan intake and prostate cancer risk have not been well studied. Three prospective case–control studies examined the relationship between circulating enterolactone concentrations, a marker of lignan intake, and the subsequent development of prostate cancer in Scandinavian men.[35–37] In all three studies, initial serum enterolactone concentrations in men who were diagnosed with prostate cancer 5–14 years later were not significantly different from serum enterolactone levels in matched control groups of men who did not develop prostate cancer. In a retrospective case–control study, recalled dietary lignan intake did not differ between US men diagnosed with prostate cancer and a matched control group.[38] More recently, serum enterolactone levels were not significantly associated with risk of prostate cancer in a case–control study in Swedish men.[39] Additionally, two prospective, European case–control studies did not find an association between serum enterolactone and prostate cancer.[40,41] However, a case–control study conducted in Scotland found that higher serum enterolactone concentrations were associated with a lower risk of prostate cancer.[42] At present, limited data from epidemiological studies do not support a relationship between dietary lignan intake and prostate cancer risk.

Osteoporosis

Research on the effects of dietary lignan intake on osteoporosis risk is very limited. In two small observational studies, urinary enterolactone excretion was used as a marker of dietary lignan intake. One study of 75 postmenopausal Korean women, who were classified as osteoporotic, osteopenic, or normal on the basis of bone mineral density (BMD) measurements, found that urinary enterolactone excretion was positively associated with BMD of the lumbar spine and hip.[43] However, a study of 50 postmenopausal Dutch women found that higher levels of urinary enterolactone excretion were associated with higher rates of bone loss.[44] In two separate placebo-controlled trials, supplementation of postmenopausal women with 25–40 g/day of ground flaxseed for 3–4 months did not significantly alter biochemical markers of bone formation or bone resorption (loss).[19,45] More research is necessary to determine whether high dietary intakes of plant lignans can decrease the risk or severity of osteoporosis.

Sources

Food Sources

Lignans are present in a wide variety of plant foods, including seeds (flax, pumpkin, sunflower, poppy, sesame), whole grains (rye, oats, barley), bran (wheat, oat, rye), beans, fruits (particularly berries), and vegetables.[30,46] Secoisolariciresinol and matairesinol were the first plant lignans identified in foods.[47] Pinoresinol and lariciresinol, two recently identified plant lignans, contribute substantially to total dietary lignan intakes. A survey of 4660 Dutch men and women during 1997 and 1998 found that the median total lignan intake was 0.98 mg/day.[48] Lariciresinol and pinoresinol contributed approximately 75% to the total lignan intake, while secoisolariciresinol and matairesinol contributed only approximately 25%. Plant lignans are the principal source of phytoestrogens in the diets of people who do not typically consume soy foods. The daily phytoestrogen intake of postmenopausal women in the United States was estimated to be less than 1 mg/day, with 80% from lignans and 20% from isoflavones.[49]

Flaxseed is by far the richest dietary source of plant lignans,[50] and lignan bioavailability can be

Table 15.1   Total lignan content[a] of selected foods[51]

Food	Serving	Total Lignans (mg)
Flaxseeds	1 oz	85.5
Sesame seeds	1 oz	11.2
Curly kale	½ cup, chopped	0.8
Broccoli	½ cup, chopped	0.6
Apricots	½ cup, sliced	0.4
Cabbage	½ cup, chopped	0.3
Brussels sprouts	½ cup, chopped	0.3
Strawberries	½ cup	0.2
Tofu	¼ block (4 oz)	0.2
Dark rye bread	1 slice	0.1

[a] Secoisolariciresinol, matairesinol, pinoresinol, and lariciresinol.

improved by crushing or milling flaxseed.[23] Lignans are not associated with the oil fraction of foods, so flaxseed oils do not typically provide lignans unless ground flaxseed has been added to the oil. A variety of factors may affect the lignan contents of plants, including geographic location, climate, maturity, and storage conditions. Table 15.1 provides the total lignan (secoisolariciresinol, matairesinol, pinoresinol, and lariciresinol) content of selected lignan-rich foods.[51]

Supplements

Dietary supplements containing lignans derived from flaxseed are available in the United States without a prescription. One such supplement provides 50 mg of secoisolariciresinol diglycoside per capsule.

Safety

Adverse Effects

Lignan precursors in foods are not known to have any adverse effects. Flaxseeds, which are rich in lignan precursors as well as fiber, may increase stool frequency or cause diarrhea in doses of 45–50 g/day in adults.[13,52] The safety of lignan supplements in pregnant or lactating women has not been established. Therefore, lignan supplements should be avoided by women who are pregnant, breast-feeding, or trying to conceive.

Summary

- Lignans are polyphenols found in plants.
- Lignan precursors are found in a wide variety of plant-based foods, including seeds, whole grains, legumes, fruits, and vegetables.
- Flaxseeds are the richest dietary source of lignan precursors.
- When consumed, lignan precursors are converted to the enterolignans, enterodiol and enterolactone, by bacteria that normally colonize the human intestine.
- Enterodiol and enterolactone have weak estrogenic activity but may also exert biological effects through nonestrogenic mechanisms.
- Lignan-rich foods are part of a healthful dietary pattern, but the role of lignans in the prevention of hormone-associated cancers, osteoporosis, and cardiovascular diseases is not yet clear.

References

1. Lampe JW. Isoflavonoid and lignan phytoestrogens as dietary biomarkers. J Nutr 2003;133(Suppl 3):956S–964S
2. de Kleijn MJ, van der Schouw YT, Wilson PW, Grobbee DE, Jacques PF. Dietary intake of phytoestrogens is associated with a favorable metabolic cardiovascular risk profile in postmenopausal US women: the Framingham study. J Nutr 2002;132(2):276–282
3. Valsta LM, Kilkkinen A, Mazur W, et al. Phyto-oestrogen database of foods and average intake in Finland. Br J Nutr 2003;89(Suppl 1):S31–S38
4. Rowland I, Faughnan M, Hoey L, Wähälä K, Williamson G, Cassidy A. Bioavailability of phyto-oestrogens. Br J Nutr 2003;89(Suppl 1):S45–S58
5. Kilkkinen A, Pietinen P, Klaukka T, Virtamo J, Korhonen P, Adlercreutz H. Use of oral antimicrobials decreases serum enterolactone concentration. Am J Epidemiol 2002;155(5):472–477
6. Kuijsten A, Arts IC, Vree TB, Hollman PC. Pharmacokinetics of enterolignans in healthy men and women consuming a single dose of secoisolariciresinol diglucoside. J Nutr 2005;135(4):795–801
7. National Cancer Institute. Understanding Cancer Series: Estrogen Receptors/SERMs. National Cancer Institute. Available at: http://www.cancer.gov/cancer topics/understandingcancer/estrogenreceptors. Accessed May 3, 2012
8. Wang LQ. Mammalian phytoestrogens: enterodiol and enterolactone. J Chromatogr B Analyt Technol Biomed Life Sci 2002;777(1–2):289–309
9. Brooks JD, Thompson LU. Mammalian lignans and genistein decrease the activities of aromatase and 17beta-hydroxysteroid dehydrogenase in MCF-7 cells. J Steroid Biochem Mol Biol 2005;94(5):461–467
10. Vanharanta M, Voutilainen S, Nurmi T, et al. Association between low serum enterolactone and increased

plasma F2-isoprostanes, a measure of lipid peroxidation. Atherosclerosis 2002;160(2):465–469

11. Vanharanta M, Voutilainen S, Rissanen TH, Adlercreutz H, Salonen JT. Risk of cardiovascular disease-related and all-cause death according to serum concentrations of enterolactone: Kuopio Ischaemic Heart Disease Risk Factor Study. Arch Intern Med 2003;163(9):1099–1104

12. Kilkkinen A, Erlund I, Virtanen MJ, Alfthan G, Ariniemi K, Virtamo J. Serum enterolactone concentration and the risk of coronary heart disease in a case-cohort study of Finnish male smokers. Am J Epidemiol 2006;163(8):687–693

13. Cunnane SC, Hamadeh MJ, Liede AC, Thompson LU, Wolever TM, Jenkins DJ. Nutritional attributes of traditional flaxseed in healthy young adults. Am J Clin Nutr 1995;61(1):62–68

14. Arjmandi BH, Khan DA. Juma S et al. Whole flaxseed consumption lowers serum LDL-cholesterol and lipoprotein(a) concentrations in postmenopausal women. Nutr Res 1998;18:1203–1214

15. Jenkins DJ, Kendall CW, Vidgen E, et al. Health aspects of partially defatted flaxseed, including effects on serum lipids, oxidative measures, and ex vivo androgen and progestin activity: a controlled crossover trial. Am J Clin Nutr 1999;69(3):395–402

16. Patade A, Devareddy L, Lucas EA, Korlagunta K, Daggy BP, Arjmandi BH. Flaxseed reduces total and LDL cholesterol concentrations in Native American postmenopausal women. J Womens Health (Larchmt) 2008;17(3):355–366

17. Clark WF, Kortas C, Heidenheim AP, Garland J, Spanner E, Parbtani A. Flaxseed in lupus nephritis: a two-year nonplacebo-controlled crossover study. J Am Coll Nutr 2001; 20(2, Suppl):143–148

18. Lemay A, Dodin S, Kadri N, Jacques H, Forest JC. Flaxseed dietary supplement versus hormone replacement therapy in hypercholesterolemic menopausal women. Obstet Gynecol 2002;100(3):495–504

19. Lucas EA, Wild RD, Hammond LJ, et al. Flaxseed improves lipid profile without altering biomarkers of bone metabolism in postmenopausal women. J Clin Endocrinol Metab 2002;87(4):1527–1532

20. Stuglin C, Prasad K. Effect of flaxseed consumption on blood pressure, serum lipids, hemopoietic system and liver and kidney enzymes in healthy humans. J Cardiovasc Pharmacol Ther 2005;10(1):23–27

21. Bloedon LT, Balikai S, Chittams J, et al. Flaxseed and cardiovascular risk factors: results from a double blind, randomized, controlled clinical trial. J Am Coll Nutr 2008;27(1):65–74

22. Dodin S, Lemay A, Jacques H, Légaré F, Forest JC, Mâsse B. The effects of flaxseed dietary supplement on lipid profile, bone mineral density, and symptoms in menopausal women: a randomized, double-blind, wheat germ placebo-controlled clinical trial. J Clin Endocrinol Metab 2005;90(3):1390–1397

23. Kuijsten A, Arts IC, van't Veer P, Hollman PC. The relative bioavailability of enterolignans in humans is enhanced by milling and crushing of flaxseed. J Nutr 2005;135(12):2812–2816

24. Horn-Ross PL, Hoggatt KJ, West DW, et al. Recent diet and breast cancer risk: the California Teachers Study (USA). Cancer Causes Control 2002;13(5):407–415

25. Keinan-Boker L, van Der Schouw YT, Grobbee DE, Peeters PH. Dietary phytoestrogens and breast cancer risk. Am J Clin Nutr 2004;79(2):282–288

26. Touillaud MS, Thiébaut AC, Niravong M, Boutron-Ruault MC, Clavel-Chapelon F. No association between

dietary phytoestrogens and risk of premenopausal breast cancer in a French cohort study. Cancer Epidemiol Biomarkers Prev 2006;15(12):2574–2576

27. Touillaud MS, Thiébaut AC, Fournier A, Niravong M, Boutron-Ruault MC, Clavel-Chapelon F. Dietary lignan intake and postmenopausal breast cancer risk by estrogen and progesterone receptor status. J Natl Cancer Inst 2007;99(6):475–486

28. Velentzis LS, Cantwell MM, Cardwell C, Keshtgar MR, Leathem AJ, Woodside JV. Lignans and breast cancer risk in pre- and post-menopausal women: meta-analyses of observational studies. Br J Cancer 2009;100(9):1492–1498

29. Velentzis LS, Woodside JV, Cantwell MM, Leathem AJ, Keshtgar MR. Do phytoestrogens reduce the risk of breast cancer and breast cancer recurrence? What clinicians need to know. Eur J Cancer 2008;44(13):1799–1806

30. Adlercreutz H. Lignans and human health. Crit Rev Clin Lab Sci 2007;44(5–6):483–525

31. Boccardo F, Puntoni M, Guglielmini P, Rubagotti A. Enterolactone as a risk factor for breast cancer: a review of the published evidence. Clin Chim Acta 2006; 365(1–2):58–67

32. Horn-Ross PL, John EM, Canchola AJ, Stewart SL, Lee MM. Phytoestrogen intake and endometrial cancer risk. J Natl Cancer Inst 2003;95(15):1158–1164

33. Zeleniuch-Jacquotte A, Lundin E, Micheli A, et al. Circulating enterolactone and risk of endometrial cancer. Int J Cancer 2006;119(10):2376–2381

34. McCann SE, Freudenheim JL, Marshall JR, Graham S. Risk of human ovarian cancer is related to dietary intake of selected nutrients, phytochemicals and food groups. J Nutr 2003;133(6):1937–1942

35. Kilkkinen A, Virtamo J, Virtanen MJ, Adlercreutz H, Albanes D, Pietinen P. Serum enterolactone concentration is not associated with prostate cancer risk in a nested case-control study. Cancer Epidemiol Biomarkers Prev 2003;12(11 Pt 1):1209–1212

36. Stattin P, Adlercreutz H, Tenkanen L, et al. Circulating enterolactone and prostate cancer risk: a Nordic nested case-control study. Int J Cancer 2002;99(1):124–129

37. Stattin P, Bylund A, Biessy C, Kaaks R, Hallmans G, Adlercreutz H. Prospective study of plasma enterolactone and prostate cancer risk (Sweden). Cancer Causes Control 2004;15(10):1095–1102

38. Strom SS, Yamamura Y, Duphorne CM, et al. Phytoestrogen intake and prostate cancer: a case-control study using a new database. Nutr Cancer 1999; 33(1):20–25

39. Hedelin M, Klint A, Chang ET, et al. Dietary phytoestrogen, serum enterolactone and risk of prostate cancer: the cancer prostate Sweden study (Sweden). Cancer Causes Control 2006;17(2):169–180

40. Travis RC, Spencer EA, Allen NE, et al. Plasma phytoestrogens and prostate cancer in the European Prospective Investigation into Cancer and Nutrition. Br J Cancer 2009;100(11):1817–1823

41. Ward H, Chapelais G, Kuhnle GG, Luben R, Khaw KT, Bingham S. Lack of prospective associations between plasma and urinary phytoestrogens and risk of prostate or colorectal cancer in the European Prospective into Cancer-Norfolk study. Cancer Epidemiol Biomarkers Prev 2008;17(10):2891–2894

42. Heald CL, Ritchie MR, Bolton-Smith C, Morton MS, Alexander FE. Phyto-oestrogens and risk of prostate cancer in Scottish men. Br J Nutr 2007;98(2):388–396

43. Kim MK, Chung BC, Yu VY, et al. Relationships of urinary phyto-oestrogen excretion to BMD in postmenopausal women. Clin Endocrinol (Oxf) 2002;56(3):321–328

44. Kardinaal AF, Morton MS, Brüggemann-Rotgans IE, van Beresteijn EC. Phyto-oestrogen excretion and rate of bone loss in postmenopausal women. Eur J Clin Nutr 1998;52(11):850–855

45. Brooks JD, Ward WE, Lewis JE, et al. Supplementation with flaxseed alters estrogen metabolism in postmenopausal women to a greater extent than does supplementation with an equal amount of soy. Am J Clin Nutr 2004;79(2):318–325

46. Meagher LP, Beecher GR. Assessment of data on the lignan content of foods. J Food Compost Anal 2000;13(6):935–947

47. Ososki AL, Kennelly EJ. Phytoestrogens: a review of the present state of research. Phytother Res 2003;17(8):845–869

48. Milder IE, Feskens EJ, Arts IC, Bueno de Mesquita HB, Hollman PC, Kromhout D. Intake of the plant lignans secoisolariciresinol, matairesinol, lariciresinol, and pinoresinol in Dutch men and women. J Nutr 2005;135(5):1202–1207

49. de Kleijn MJ, van der Schouw YT, Wilson PW, et al. Intake of dietary phytoestrogens is low in postmenopausal women in the United States: the Framingham study(1–4). J Nutr 2001;131(6):1826–1832

50. Thompson LU. Experimental studies on lignans and cancer. Baillieres Clin Endocrinol Metab 1998; 12(4):691–705

51. Milder IE, Arts IC, van de Putte B, Venema DP, Hollman PC. Lignan contents of Dutch plant foods: a database including lariciresinol, pinoresinol, secoisolariciresinol and matairesinol. Br J Nutr 2005;93(3):393–402

52. Clark WF, Parbtani A, Huff MW, et al. Flaxseed: a potential treatment for lupus nephritis. Kidney Int 1995;48(2):475–480

16 Fiber

All dietary fibers are resistant to digestion in the small intestine, meaning they arrive at the colon intact.[1] Although most fibers are carbohydrates, one important factor that determines their susceptibility to digestion by human enzymes is the conformation of the chemical bonds between sugar molecules (glycosidic bonds). Humans lack digestive enzymes capable of hydrolyzing most β-glycosidic bonds, which explains why amylose, a glucose polymer with α-1,4 glycosidic bonds, is digestible by human enzymes, while cellulose, a glucose polymer with β-1,4 glycosidic bonds, is indigestible (**Fig. 16.1**).

Definitions of Fiber

Although nutritional scientists and clinicians generally agree that a healthy diet should include plenty of fiber-rich foods, agreement on the actual definition of fiber has been more difficult to achieve.[2–4] In the 1970s, dietary fiber was defined as remnants of plant cells that are resistant to digestion by human enzymes.[5] This definition includes a component of some plant cell walls called lignin, as well as indigestible carbohydrates found in plants. However, this definition omits indigestible carbohydrates derived from animal sources (e.g., chitin) and synthetic (e.g., fructooligosaccharides) and digestible carbohydrates that are inaccessible to human digestive enzymes (e.g., resistant starch).[6] These com-

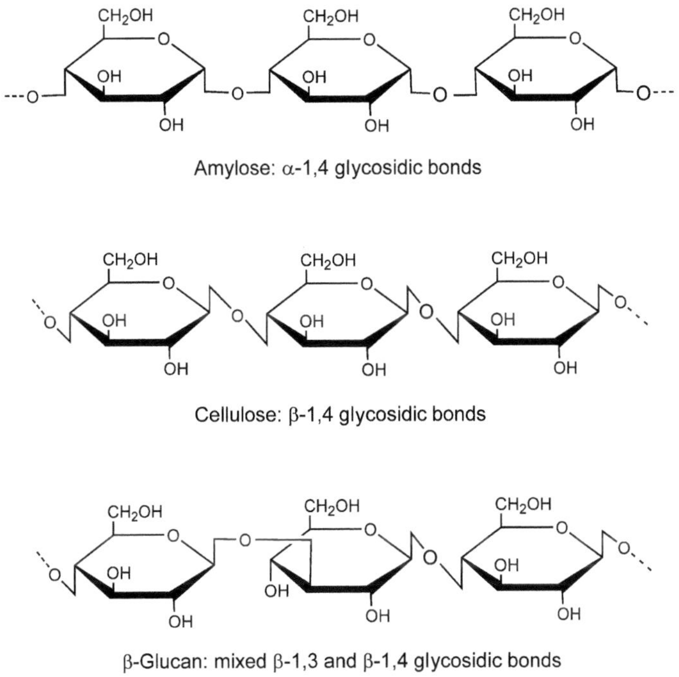

Fig. 16.1 Chemical structures of amylase (a digestible carbohydrate), cellulose (a fiber that is not digestible by human enzymes), and β-glucan (a fiber).[7]

pounds share many of the characteristics of fiber present in plant foods.

US Institute of Medicine Classification System

Before establishing intake recommendations for fiber in 2001, a panel of experts convened by the Institute of Medicine developed definitions of fiber that made a distinction between fiber that occurs naturally in plant foods (dietary fiber) and isolated or synthetic fibers that may be added to foods or used as dietary supplements (functional fiber).[4] However, these distinctions are controversial, and there are other classification systems for dietary fiber (see the section on Other Classification Systems below).

Dietary Fiber

- **Lignin:** lignin is not a carbohydrate; rather, it is a polyphenolic compound with a complex three-dimensional structure that is found in the cell walls of woody plants and seeds.[7]
- **Cellulose:** cellulose is a glucose polymer with β-1,4 glycosidic bonds, found in all plant cell walls (**Fig. 16.1**).[6]
- **β-Glucans:** β-glucans are glucose polymers with a mixture of β-1,4 glycosidic bonds and β-1,3 glycosidic bonds (**Fig. 16.1**). Oats and barley are particularly rich in β-glucans.[7]
- **Hemicelluloses:** hemicelluloses are a diverse group of polysaccharides (sugar polymers) containing six-carbon sugars (hexoses) and five-carbon sugars (pentoses).[6] Like cellulose, hemicelluloses are found in plant cell walls.
- **Pectins:** pectins are viscous polysaccharides that are particularly abundant in fruits and berries.[4]
- **Gums:** gums are viscous polysaccharides often found in seeds.[4]
- **Inulin and oligofructose:** inulin is a mixture of fructose chains that vary in length and often terminate with a glucose molecule.[8] Oligofructose is a mixture of shorter fructose chains that may terminate in glucose or fructose. Inulin and oligofructose occur naturally in plants, such as onions and Jerusalem artichokes.
- **Resistant starch:** naturally occurring resistant starch is sequestered in plant cell walls and is therefore inaccessible to human digestive enzymes.[4] Bananas and legumes are sources of naturally occurring resistant starch. Resistant starch may also be formed by food processing or by cooling and reheating.

Functional Fiber

According to the Institute of Medicine's definition, functional fiber "consists of isolated, nondigestible carbohydrates that have beneficial physiological effects in humans."[4] Functional fibers may be nondigestible carbohydrates that have been isolated or extracted from a natural plant or animal source, or they may be manufactured or synthesized. However, designation as a functional fiber by the Institute of Medicine requires the presentation of sufficient evidence of physiological benefit in humans. Fibers identified as potential functional fibers by the Institute of Medicine include:

- Isolated or extracted forms of the dietary fibers listed above.
- **Psyllium:** psyllium refers to viscous mucilage, which is isolated from the husks of psyllium seeds. The husks are usually isolated from the seeds of *Plantago ovata* or blond psyllium. Psyllium is also known as *ispaghula husk*.[4]
- **Chitin and chitosan:** chitin is a nondigestible carbohydrate extracted from the exoskeletons of crustaceans, such as crabs and lobsters. It is a long polymer of acetylated glucosamine units linked by β-1,4 glycosidic bonds. Deacetylation of chitin is used to produce chitosan, a nondigestible glucosamine polymer.[9]
- **Fructooligosaccharides:** fructooligosaccharides are short, synthetic fructose chains terminating with a glucose unit. They are used as food additives.[8]
- **Polydextrose and polyols:** polydextrose and polyols are synthetic polysaccharides used as bulking agents and sugar substitutes in foods.[4]
- **Resistant dextrins:** resistant dextrins, also called *resistant maltodextrins*, are indigestible polysaccharides formed when starch is heated and treated with enzymes. They are used as food additives.[4]

Total Fiber

Total fiber is defined by the Institute of Medicine as "the sum of dietary fiber and functional fiber."[4]

Other Classification Systems

Viscous and Nonviscous Fiber

Some fibers form very viscous solutions or gels in water. This property is linked to the ability of some fibers to slow the emptying of the stomach, delay the absorption of some nutrients in the small intestine, and lower serum cholesterol. Viscous fibers include pectins, β-glucans, some gums (e.g., guar gum), and mucilages (e.g., psyllium). Cellulose, lignin, and some hemicelluloses are nonviscous fibers.[6,7]

Fermentable and Nonfermentable Fiber

Some fibers are readily fermented by bacteria that normally colonize the colon. In addition to increasing the amount of bacteria in the colon, fermentation results in the formation of short-chain fatty acids (acetate, propionate, and butyrate) and gases.[1] Short-chain fatty acids can be absorbed and metabolized to produce energy. Interestingly, the preferred energy source for colonocytes (epithelial cells that line the colon) is butyrate. Pectins, β-glucans, guar gum, inulin, and oligofructose are readily fermented, while cellulose and lignin are resistant to fermentation in the colon.[6,7] Foods that are rich in fermentable fibers include oats and barley, as well as fruits and vegetables. Cereal fibers that are rich in cellulose, such as wheat bran, are relatively resistant to bacterial fermentation.[1]

Soluble and Insoluble Fiber

"Soluble fiber" originated as an analytical term.[10] Soluble fibers are dispersible in water, while insoluble fibers are not. Originally, the solubility of fiber was thought to predict its physiological effects. For example, it was thought that soluble fibers were more likely to form viscous gels and were more easily fermented by colonic bacteria. Further research has revealed that solubility does not reliably predict the physiological effects of fiber. However, the terms "soluble" and "insoluble" fiber are still used by many nutrition and health-care professionals, as well as the US Food and Drug Administration (FDA) for nutrition labeling. β-glucans, gums, mucilages (e.g., psyllium), pectins, and some hemicelluloses are soluble fibers, while cellulose, lignin, some pectins, and some hemicelluloses are insoluble fibers.[10] Oat products and legumes (dry beans, peas, and lentils) are rich sources of soluble fiber.

Biological Activities

Lowering Serum Cholesterol

Numerous controlled clinical trials have found that increasing the intake of viscous dietary fibers, particularly from legumes (beans, peas, and lentils)[11–13] and oat products,[14–19] decreases serum total and low-density lipoprotein (LDL) cholesterol. These findings led the FDA to approve health claims like the following on labels of foods containing at least 0.75 g/serving of soluble fiber from whole oats: "Soluble fiber from foods such as oat bran, as part of a diet low in saturated fat and cholesterol, may reduce the risk of heart disease."[20] Supplementation with viscous fibers, such as pectin, guar gum, and psyllium, has also been found to decrease total and LDL cholesterol levels when compared with low-fiber placebos.[17,21–26] Although many of these studies examined relatively high fiber intakes, a meta-analysis that combined the results of 67 controlled trials found that even a modest, 10-g per day increase in viscous fiber intake resulted in reductions in LDL cholesterol averaging 22 mg/dL (0.57 mmol/L) and reductions in total cholesterol averaging 17 mg/dL (0.45 mmol/L).[17]

Decreasing Postprandial Glycemia

The addition of viscous dietary fiber[27,28] and isolated viscous fibers[29–32] to a carbohydrate-containing meal has been found to result in significant improvements in blood glucose and insulin responses in numerous controlled clinical trials.[33] Large, rapid increases in blood glucose levels are potent signals to the β-cells of the pancreas to increase insulin secretion. Over time, recurrent elevations in blood glucose and excessive insulin secretion are thought to increase the risk of developing type 2 diabetes mellitus (DM), as well as cardiovascular disease (see the Disease Prevention section below). When the carbohydrate content of two meals is equal, the presence of fiber, particularly viscous fiber, generally results in smaller but more sustained increases in blood glucose and thus significantly lower insulin levels.[33]

Softening Stool

Increasing intakes of dietary fibers and fiber supplements can prevent or ameliorate constipation by softening and adding bulk to stool and by speeding its passage through the colon.[34] Wheat bran and fruits and vegetables are the fiber sources that have been most consistently found to increase stool bulk and shorten transit time.[35] Fiber supplements that have been found to be effective in treating constipation include cellulose and psyllium.[4] Sufficient fluid intake is also required to maximize the stool-softening effect of increased fiber intake.[36] In addition to increasing fiber intake, drinking at least 64 oz (approx. 2 L) of fluid daily is usually recommended to help prevent and treat constipation.[37]

Disease Prevention

Observational studies that have identified associations between high fiber intakes and reductions in chronic disease risk have generally assessed only fiber-rich foods, rather than fiber itself, making it difficult to determine whether observed benefits are related to fiber or other nutrients and phytochemicals commonly found in fiber-rich foods. In contrast, intervention trials often use isolated fibers to determine whether a specific fiber component has beneficial health effects.

Cardiovascular Disease

Prospective cohort studies have consistently found that high intakes of fiber-rich foods are associated with significant reductions in coronary heart disease (CHD) risk[38–48] and cardiovascular-related mortality.[48–51] A pooled analysis of 10 prospective cohort studies of dietary fiber intake in the United States and Europe found that each 10 g/day increase in total dietary fiber intake was associated with a 14% decrease in the risk of coronary events, such as myocardial infarction (MI), and a 24% decrease in deaths from CHD.[51] This inverse association between fiber intake and CHD death was particularly high for cereal fiber and fruit fiber. Three large prospective cohort studies[42,43,45] found that dietary fiber intakes of approximately 14 g per 1000 kcal of energy were associated with substantial (16%–33%) decreases

in the risk of CHD; these results are the basis for the Institute of Medicine's adequate intake (AI) recommendation for fiber (see the Intake Recommendations section below).[4]

Although the cholesterol-lowering effect of viscous dietary fibers and fiber supplements probably contributes to the cardioprotective effects of dietary fiber, other mechanisms are likely to play a role. Beneficial effects of fiber consumption on blood glucose and insulin responses may also contribute to observed reductions in CHD risk.[52] Low-fiber, high-glycemic-load diets are associated with higher serum triglyceride levels and lower high-density lipoprotein (HDL) cholesterol levels, two risk factors for cardiovascular disease.[53,54] Fiber-rich diets that are rich in certain micronutrients like magnesium and potassium may also help lower blood pressure, another important risk factor for cardiovascular disease; some observational studies have found inverse associations between dietary fiber intake and blood pressure[55] or hypertension.[56] A meta-analysis of 24 randomized, placebo-controlled trials found that dietary fiber supplementation (average of 11.5 g/day) lowered systolic blood pressure (SBP) by 1.13 mmHg and diastolic blood pressure (DBP) by 1.26 mmHg.[57] Similarly, another meta-analysis of 25 randomized controlled trials found that an increase in dietary fiber (median increase of 10.7 g/day compared with the control group) was associated with a 1.15 mmHg reduction in SBP and a 1.65 mmHg reduction in DBP.[58] Both analyses reported that the reductions in DBP, but not SBP, were statistically significant. Additionally, recent studies have indicated that higher consumption of dietary fiber may lower levels of C-reactive protein,[59,60] a biomarker of inflammation that is strongly associated with the risk of cardiovascular events, such as MI and stroke.[61] Thus, several mechanisms might contribute to the cardioprotective effect of high-fiber foods. Although viscous dietary fibers and fiber supplements appear to be most effective in lowering LDL cholesterol levels, large epidemiological studies provide strong and consistent evidence that diets rich in all fiber from whole grains, legumes, fruits, and nonstarchy vegetables can significantly reduce CHD risk.[62]

Type 2 Diabetes Mellitus

Increasing intakes of refined carbohydrates and decreasing intakes of fiber in the United States have paralleled the increasing prevalence of type 2 DM to near epidemic proportions.[63] Numerous prospective cohort studies have found that that diets rich in fiber, particularly cereal fiber from whole grains, are associated with significant reductions in the risk of developing type 2 DM.[64–74] Although no intervention trials have evaluated the effect of increasing dietary fiber intake alone on type 2 DM prevention, two important intervention trials found that a combination of lifestyle modifications that included increasing fiber intake decreased the risk of developing type 2 DM in adults with impaired glucose tolerance.[75,76] Although multiple factors, including obesity, inactivity, and genetics, increase the risk of developing type 2 DM, the results of observational studies and intervention trials indicate that fiber-rich diets improve glucose tolerance and decrease the risk of type 2 DM, particularly in high-risk individuals.

Cancer

Colorectal Cancer

The majority of case–control studies conducted prior to 1990 found the incidence of colorectal cancer was lower in people with higher fiber intakes.[77,78] A recent nested case–control study found an inverse association between dietary fiber intake and risk of colorectal cancer when fiber intake was assessed by food diaries but not when assessed by food-frequency questionnaires.[79] To date, most prospective cohort studies have not found significant associations between measures of dietary fiber intake and colorectal cancer risk.[80–89] A pooled analysis of 13 prospective cohort studies, which analyzed data from 725 628 adults, did not find high dietary fiber intake to be protective against colorectal cancer when other dietary factors were taken into account.[90] However, the largest prospective study on diet and cancer to date, which included 519 978 men and women participating in the European Prospective Investigation into Cancer and Nutrition (EPIC) study, found that dietary fiber from foods was protective against development of colon cancer.[91] This EPIC study was not included in the earlier pooled analysis mentioned

above that reported no association between dietary fiber intake and colorectal cancer.[90]

In addition, four controlled clinical trials have failed to demonstrate a protective effect of fiber consumption on the recurrence of colorectal adenomas (precancerous polyps). The rate of recurrence of colorectal adenomas over a 4-year period was not significantly different between those who consumed approximately 33 g/day of fiber from a fruit- and vegetable-rich, low-fat diet and those in a control group who consumed approximately 19 g/day of fiber.[92] In another trial, there was no significant difference in the rate of colorectal adenoma recurrence over a 3-year period between those supplemented with 13.5 g/day of wheat-bran fiber and those supplemented with 2 g/day of wheat-bran fiber.[93] More recently, a 4-year intervention trial found that supplementation with 7.5 g/day of wheat bran had no effect on colorectal adenoma recurrence.[94] Surprisingly, in another intervention trial, supplementation with 3.5 g/day of psyllium for 3 years resulted in a significant increase in adenoma recurrence compared with placebo.[95]

The reasons for the discrepancies between the findings of case–control studies with those of most prospective cohort studies and recent intervention trials have generated considerable debate among scientists. Potential reasons for the lack of a protective effect of dietary fiber observed in these studies include the possibility that the type or the amount of fiber consumed by most people in these studies was inadequate to prevent colorectal cancer,[4] or that other dietary factors like fat may interact with fiber, influencing its effects on colorectal cancer.[1,96] The methods used to assess fiber intake in observational studies may also contribute to the disparate results.[79] Clearly, more research is needed to sort out the complex effects of dietary fiber and fiber supplements on colorectal cancer risk and progression.

Breast Cancer

Several early case–control studies found significant inverse associations between dietary fiber intake and breast cancer incidence,[97–100] but many prospective cohort studies have not found dietary fiber intake to be associated with significant reductions in breast cancer risk.[101–108] Three studies have reported a protective effect of dietary fiber on breast cancer risk. A prospective cohort study in the United Kingdom found that dietary fiber intake was inversely associated with risk of breast cancer in premenopausal women but not in postmenopausal women.[109] Additionally, a prospective cohort study in Sweden found that postmenopausal women with the highest fiber intakes (averaging approximately 26 g/day) had a risk of breast cancer that was 40% lower than that of women with the lowest fiber intakes (averaging approximately 13 g/day).[110] Women with the highest fiber and lowest fat intakes had the very lowest risk of breast cancer. More recently, a prospective study in a cohort of more than 185000 postmenopausal women in the United States found that those with the highest intakes of dietary fiber (median, 26 g/day) had a 13% lower risk of all forms of breast cancer and a 44% lower risk of hormone receptor-negative tumors (ER-/PR-) compared with those with the lowest intakes of dietary fiber (median 11 g/day).[111] A 2011 meta-analysis of 10 prospective cohort studies found a modest, 11% lower risk of breast cancer in women with the highest intakes of dietary fiber.[112] The results of small, short-term intervention trials in premenopausal and postmenopausal women suggested that low-fat (10%–25% of energy), high-fiber (25–40 g/day) diets could decrease circulating estrogen levels by increasing the excretion of estrogens and by promoting the metabolism of estrogens to less estrogenic forms.[113,114] However, it is not known whether fiber-associated effects on endogenous estrogen levels have a clinically significant impact on breast cancer risk.[4] Overall, observational studies examining dietary fiber intake and breast cancer incidence have reported mixed results. In such studies, it is possible that the association may be confounded by consumption of fiber-rich foods, such as fruits and vegetables.

Diverticular Disease

Some observational studies have associated high fiber intakes with a decreased risk of diverticulosis, a relatively common condition that is characterized by the formation of small pouches (diverticula) in the colon.[115,116] However, a recent cross-sectional study of 2104 adults found that those with the highest fiber intakes, measured by food frequency questionnaires, had a higher prevalence of diverticula (assessed by colonoscopy) compared with those with the lowest fiber intakes.[117] Although most people with diverticulosis experience no symptoms, approximately 15%–20% may develop pain or inflammation, known as *diverticulitis*.[118] In a large prospective cohort study, men with the highest insoluble fiber intakes (median 22.7 g/day) had a 37% lower risk of developing symptomatic diverticular disease compared with men with the lowest insoluble fiber intakes (median 10.1 g/day). The protective effect of dietary fiber against diverticular disease was strongest for cellulose and lignin.[119] More research is needed to clarify the association between dietary fiber and diverticular disease.

Weight Control

In addition to providing less energy, there is some evidence that higher fiber intakes can help to prevent weight gain or promote weight loss by extending the feeling of fullness after a meal (satiety).[120] Observational studies have found that adults with higher intakes of dietary fiber are leaner[121,122] and less likely to be obese than adults with low fiber intakes.[123,124] One large prospective cohort study found that women whose intake of high-fiber foods increased by an average of 9 g/day over a 12-year period were half as likely to experience a major weight gain of at least 55 lb (25 kg) than those whose intake of high-fiber foods decreased by an average of 3 g/day.[125] The results of short-term clinical trials examining the effect of increased fiber intake on weight loss have been mixed. Overall, a systematic review of clinical trials conducted prior to 2001 found that increasing fiber intake from foods or supplements by 14 g/day resulted in a 10% decrease in energy intake and weight losses averaging approximately 4 lb (1.9 kg) over 4 months.[120] However, some more recent clinical trials did not find fiber-rich cereal[126] or fiber supplements[127] enhanced weight loss. A 2011 systematic review of 61 randomized controlled trials examined the effect of different fiber types on body weight.[128] This analysis found that dextrins and marine polysaccharides reduced body weight in all of the studies, while chitosan, arabinoxylans, and fructans reduced body weight in at least two-thirds of the studies. Average weight reductions were greatest for the fructans and marine polysaccharides groups (approximately 1.3 kg or 2.8 lb/4 weeks for a 79 kg person in both groups). For all fiber types combined, the average weight reduction was only 0.3 g (0.7 lb) per 4 weeks for a 79-kg person.[128] Although people with higher intakes of fiber-rich foods, particularly whole grains, appear more likely to maintain a healthy body weight, the role of fiber alone in long-term weight control is not yet clear. Effects on body weight might depend on the specific type of dietary fiber.

All-Cause Mortality

Several prospective cohort studies have found higher intakes of dietary fiber to be associated with a lower risk of mortality from all causes. A recent report from the National Institutes of Health American Association of Retired Persons (NIH-AARP) Diet and Health Study, which followed 388 122 older adults for an average of 9 years, found that men and women in the highest quintiles of dietary fiber intake had a 22% lower risk of mortality when compared with the lowest quintiles of dietary fiber intake.[50] Smaller prospective studies have also reported an inverse association between total fiber intake and all-cause mortality,[44,48,129] and an inverse association between cereal fiber intake and all-cause mortality was found in the Nurses' Health Study, which included more than 50 000 participants.[130] However, no association was found between total fiber intake or soluble fiber intake and mortality from all causes in the National Health and Nutrition Examination Survey (NHANES) I Epidemiologic Follow-Up Study—a prospective study that assessed fiber intake by a single, 24-hour dietary recall method.[46]

Disease Treatment

Diabetes Mellitus

Numerous controlled clinical trials in people who have type 1 or type 2 DM have found that increasing fiber intake from foods[131,132] or viscous fiber supplements[133-135] improves markers of glycemic control, particularly postprandial glucose levels and serum lipid profiles. A meta-analysis that combined the results of 23 clinical trials comparing the effects of high-fiber diets (>20 g/1000 kcal) with those of low-fiber diets (<10 g/1000 kcal) in patients with diabetes found that high-fiber diets lowered postprandial blood glucose concentrations by 13%–21%, serum LDL

cholesterol concentrations by 8%–16%, and serum triglyceride concentrations by 8%–13%.[136] Based on the evidence from this meta-analysis, the authors recommended a dietary fiber intake of 25–50 g/day (15–25 g/1000 kcal) for individuals with diabetes, which is consistent with the recommendations of many international diabetes organizations of at least 25–35 g/day.[137-139] In general, the results of controlled clinical trials support recommendations that people with diabetes aim for high fiber intakes by increasing their consumption of whole grains, legumes, nuts, fruits, and nonstarchy vegetables. Since there is little evidence from clinical trials that increasing nonviscous fiber alone is beneficial,[140] individuals with diabetes should avoid increasing fiber intake exclusively from nonviscous sources, such as wheat bran.[136]

Irritable Bowel Syndrome

Irritable bowel syndrome (IBS) is a functional disorder of the intestines, characterized by episodes of abdominal pain or discomfort associated with a change in bowel movements, such as constipation or diarrhea.[141] Although people diagnosed with IBS are often encouraged by healthcare providers to increase dietary fiber intake, the results of controlled clinical trials of psyllium, methylcellulose, and wheat bran have been mixed.[142-144] A systematic review and meta-analysis of 12 randomized controlled trials found a beneficial effect of fiber that was limited to ispaghula husk (psyllium).[143] More recently, a 3-month randomized, placebo-controlled trial in 275 patients with IBS found that supplementation with psyllium (10 g/day) improved symptoms of abdominal pain or discomfort in the first 2 months of supplementation and also improved symptom severity after 3 months' supplementation.[145] Compared with placebo, supplementation with insoluble bran fiber (10 g/day) improved abdominal pain or discomfort only after 3 months' supplementation and had no effect on symptom severity.[145] Additionally, a systematic review of 17 randomized controlled trials of fiber supplements in IBS patients found that supplementation with soluble fiber, mainly from psyllium, significantly improved a global measure of IBS symptoms, while supplementation with insoluble fiber, such as corn bran or wheat bran, did not improve IBS symptoms.[146] In general, fi-

Table 16.1 Total fiber content of selected fiber-rich foods[150]

Food	Serving	Total Dietary Fiber (g)
100% (wheat) bran cereal	½ cup	12.5
Navy beans, cooked from dried	½ cup	9.6
Split peas, cooked from dried	½ cup	8.1
Lentils, cooked from dried	½ cup	7.8
Kidney beans, canned	½ cup	6.8
Asian pear	1 small	4.4
Apple with skin	1 medium	4.4
English muffin, whole-wheat	1	4.4
Bulgur, cooked	½ cup	4.1
Raspberries, raw	½ cup	4.0
Sweet potato, baked with peel	1 medium	3.8
Spinach, frozen, cooked	½ cup	3.5
Almonds	1 oz	3.5

ber supplements improved constipation in IBS patients but did not improve IBS-associated abdominal pain. Thus, the results of randomized controlled trials suggest that increasing soluble or viscous fiber intake gradually to 12–30 g/day may be beneficial for patients in whom constipation is the predominant symptom of IBS.[147] However, fiber supplements could actually exacerbate symptoms in those in whom diarrhea predominates.[148] A few clinical trials have found that partially hydrolyzed guar gum (5 g/day), a water-soluble, non-gelling fiber, may improve IBS symptoms in patients with diarrhea and in those with constipation-predominant IBS.[149] IBS patients should be advised to increase fiber intake gradually, since increasing their intake of viscous, readily fermented fibers could increase gas production and bloating.

Sources

Food Sources

Dietary fiber intakes in the United States average 16–18 g/day for men and 12–14 g/day for women—well below recommended intake levels (see the Intake Recommendations section below).[4] Good sources of dietary fiber include legumes, nuts, whole grains, bran products, fruits, and nonstarchy vegetables. Legumes, whole grains, and nuts are generally more concentrated sources of fiber than fruits and vegetables. All plant-based foods contain mixtures of soluble and insoluble fiber.[10] Oat products and legumes are rich sources of soluble and viscous fiber. Wheat bran and whole grains are rich sources of insoluble and nonviscous fiber. The total fiber content of some fiber-rich foods is presented in Table 16.1.[150] Some strategies for increasing dietary fiber intake include increasing fruit and nonstarchy vegetable intake, increasing intake of legumes, eating whole-grain cereal or oatmeal for breakfast, substituting whole grains for refined grains, and substituting nuts or popcorn for less healthy snacks.

Isolated Fibers and Supplements

β-Glucans

β-Glucans are viscous, easily fermented, soluble fibers found naturally in oats, barley, mushrooms, yeast, bacteria, and algae.[151] β-Glucans extracted from oats, mushrooms, and yeast are available in a variety of nutritional supplements without a prescription.

Pectin

Pectins are viscous fibers, most often extracted from citrus peels and apple pulp. Pectins are widely used as gelling agents in foods but are also available as dietary supplements without a prescription.[9]

Inulins and Oligofructose

Inulins and oligofructose, extracted from chicory root or synthesized from sucrose, are used as food additives.[8] Isolated inulin is added to replace fat in products like salad dressing, while sweet-tasting oligofructose is added to products like fruit yogurts and desserts. Inulins and oligofructose are highly fermentable fibers that are also classified as prebiotics because of their ability to stimulate the growth of potentially beneficial *Bifidobacteria* species in the human colon.[152] Encouraging the growth of *Bifidobacteria* could promote intestinal health by suppressing the growth of pathogenic bacteria known to cause diarrhea, or by enhancing the immune response.[153] Although several dietary supplements containing inulins and oligofructose are marketed as prebiotics, the health benefits of prebiotics have not yet been convincingly demonstrated in humans.[154,155]

Guar Gum

Guar gum is a viscous, fermentable fiber derived from the Indian cluster bean.[4] It is used as a thickener or emulsifier in many food products. Dietary supplements containing guar gum have been marketed as weight-loss aids, but a meta-analysis that combined the results of 11 randomized controlled trials found that guar gum supplements were not effective in reducing body weight.[156]

Psyllium

Psyllium, a viscous, soluble fiber isolated from psyllium seed husks, is available without a prescription in laxatives, ready-to-eat cereals, and dietary supplements.[9] The FDA has approved health claims like the following on the labels of foods containing at least 1.7 g/serving of soluble fiber from psyllium: "Diets low in saturated fat and cholesterol that include 7 g/day of soluble fiber from psyllium may reduce the risk of heart disease."[20]

Chitosan

Chitosan is an indigestible glucosamine polymer derived from chitin. When administered with food in animal studies, chitosan decreased fat absorption.[157] Consequently, chitosan has been marketed as a dietary supplement to promote weight loss and lower cholesterol. Controlled clinical trials in humans have not generally found chitosan supplementation to be more effective than placebo in promoting weight loss.[158] While some clinical trials in humans have found chitosan supplementation to result in modest reductions in total and LDL cholesterol levels compared with placebo,[159,160] others found no improvement.[161,162] Chitosan is available as a dietary supplement without a prescription in the United States.

Note:

All fiber supplements should be taken with sufficient fluids. Most clinicians recommend taking fiber supplements with at least 8 oz (240 mL) of water and consuming a total of at least 64 oz (approx. 2 L) of fluid daily.[163,164]

Safety

Adverse Effects

Dietary Fiber

Some people experience abdominal cramping, bloating, or gas when they abruptly increase their dietary fiber intakes.[163,164] These symptoms can be minimized or avoided by increasing the intake of fiber-rich foods gradually and increasing fluid intake to at least 64 oz/day (approx. 2 L). There have been rare reports of intestinal obstruction related to large intakes of oat bran or wheat bran, usually in people with impaired intestinal motility or difficulty chewing.[165–168] The Institute of Medicine has not established a tolerable upper intake level for dietary or functional fiber.[4]

Isolated Fibers and Fiber Supplements

Gastrointestinal symptoms. The following fibers have been found to cause gastrointestinal distress, including abdominal cramping, bloating, gas, and diarrhea: guar gum, inulin and oligofructose, fructooligosaccharides, polydextrose, resistant starch, and psyllium.[4] Use of a guar-gum-containing supplement for weight loss has been associated with esophageal and small bowel obstruction.[169] Additionally, several cases of intestinal obstruction by psyllium have been reported when taken with insufficient fluids or by people with impaired swallowing or gastrointestinal motility.[170,171]

Colorectal adenomas. One randomized controlled trial in patients with a history of colorectal adenomas (precancerous polyps) found that supplementation with 3.5 g/day of psyllium for 3 years resulted in a significant increase in colorectal adenoma recurrence compared with placebo (see the section on Colorectal Cancer above).[95]

Table 16.2   US Institute of Medicine adequate intake recommendations for total fiber[4]

Life Stage	Age	Males (g/day)	Females (g/day)
Infants	0–6 months	ND[a]	ND
Infants	7–12 months	ND	ND
Children	1–3 years	19	19
Children	4–8 years	25	25
Children	9–13 years	31	26
Adolescents	14–18 years	38	26
Adults	19–50 years	38	25
Adults	51 years and older	30	21
Pregnancy	All ages	–	28
Breast-feeding	All ages	–	29

[a] Not determined.

Allergy and anaphylaxis. Since chitin and chitosan may be isolated from the exoskeletons of crustaceans, such as crabs and lobsters, people with shellfish allergies should avoid taking chitin or chitosan supplements.[9] Anaphylaxis has been reported after intravenous administration of inulin,[172] as well as ingestion of margarine containing inulin extracted from chicory.[173] Anaphylaxis has also been reported after the ingestion of cereals containing psyllium, and asthma has occasionally been reported in people with occupational exposure to psyllium powder.[174]

Drug Interactions

Psyllium may reduce the absorption of lithium, carbamazepine (Tegretol), digoxin (Lanoxin), and warfarin (Coumadin) when taken at the same time.[9] Guar gum may slow the absorption of digoxin, acetaminophen (paracetamol, Tylenol), and bumetanide (Bumex) and decrease the absorption of metformin (Glucophage), penicillin, and some formulations of glibenclamide (Glynase) when taken at the same time.[175] Pectin may decrease the absorption of lovastatin (Mevacor) when taken at the same time.[176] Concomitant administration of kaolin-pectin has been reported to decrease the absorption of clindamycin, tetracyclines, and digoxin, but it is not known whether kaolin or pectin is responsible for the interaction.[9] In general, medications should be taken at least 1 hour before or 2 hours after fiber supplements.

Nutrient Interactions

The addition of cereal fiber to meals has generally been found to decrease the absorption of iron, zinc, calcium, and magnesium in the same meal, but this effect appears to be related to the phytate present in the cereal fiber rather than the fiber itself.[177] In general, dietary fiber as part of a balanced diet has not been found to adversely affect the calcium, magnesium, iron, or zinc status of healthy people at recommended intake levels.[4] Evidence from animal studies and limited research in humans suggests that inulin and oligofructose may enhance calcium absorption.[178,179] The addition of pectin and guar gum to a meal significantly reduced the absorption of the carotenoids β-carotene, lycopene, and lutein from that meal.[180,181]

Intake Recommendations

Adequate Intake

In light of consistent evidence from prospective cohort studies that fiber-rich diets are associated with significant reductions in cardiovascular disease risk, the Food and Nutrition Board of the US Institute of Medicine established its first recommended intake levels for fiber in 2001.[4] The adequate intake (AI) recommendations for total fiber intake are based on the findings of several large prospective cohort studies that dietary fiber intakes of approximately 14 g for every 1000 calories (kcal) consumed were associated with significant reductions in the risk of CHD,[42,43,45] as well as type 2 DM.[66,67] For adults aged 50 years and younger, the AI recommendation for total fiber intake is 38 g/day for men and 25 g/day for women. For adults aged over 50 years, the recommendation is 30 g/day for men and 21 g/day for women. The AI recommendations for males and females of all ages are presented in Table 16.2.[4]

Summary

- Dietary fiber is a diverse group of compounds, including lignin and complex carbohydrates, that cannot be digested by human enzymes in the small intestine.
- Although each class of fiber is chemically unique, scientists have tried to classify fibers on the basis of their solubility, viscosity, and fermentability, to better understand their physiological effects.
- Viscous fibers, such as those found in oat products and legumes, can lower serum low-density lipoprotein cholesterol levels and normalize blood glucose and insulin responses.
- High fiber intakes promote bowel health by preventing constipation and diverticular disease.
- Large prospective cohort studies provide strong and consistent evidence that diets rich in fiber from whole grains, legumes, fruits, and nonstarchy vegetables can reduce the risk of cardiovascular disease and type 2 diabetes.
- Although the results of case–control studies suggested that colorectal cancer was more prevalent in people with low-fiber intakes, more recent findings from large prospective cohort studies and four clinical intervention trials do not support an association between fiber intake and the risk of colorectal cancer.
- Observational studies on dietary fiber intake and breast cancer incidence have reported inconsistent findings.
- Numerous controlled clinical trials in people with type 1 and type 2 diabetes have found that increasing fiber intake improves glycemic control and serum lipid profiles.
- In 2001, the Food and Nutrition Board of the Institute of Medicine established an adequate intake (AI) recommendation for total daily fiber intake. For adults who are aged 50 years and younger, the AI recommendation for total fiber intake is 38 g/day for men and 25 g/day for women. For adults aged over 50 years, the recommendation is 30 g/day for men and 21 g/day for women.

References

1. Lupton JR. Microbial degradation products influence colon cancer risk: the butyrate controversy. J Nutr 2004;134(2):479–482
2. Ha MA, Jarvis MC, Mann JI. A definition for dietary fibre. Eur J Clin Nutr 2000;54(12):861–864
3. DeVries JW. On defining dietary fibre. Proc Nutr Soc 2003;62(1):37–43
4. Institute of Medicine. Dietary, Functional, and Total Fiber. Dietary Reference Intakes for Energy, Carbohydrate, Fiber, Fat, Fatty Acids, Cholesterol, Protein, and Amino Acids. Washington, DC: National Academies Press; 2002:265–334
5. Trowell H. Dietary fibre, ischaemic heart disease and diabetes mellitus. Proc Nutr Soc 1973;32(3):151–157
6. Lupton JR, Turner ND. Dietary fiber. In: Stipanuk MH, ed. Biochemical and Physiological Aspects of Human Nutrition. Philadelphia: WB Saunders; 2000:143–154
7. Gallaher CM, Schneeman BO. Dietary fiber. In: Bowman BA, Russell RM, eds. Present Knowledge in Nutrition. 8th ed. Washington, DC: ILSI Press; 2001:83–91
8. Niness KR. Inulin and oligofructose: what are they? J Nutr 1999; 129(7, Suppl):1402S–1406S
9. Hendler SS, Rorvik DR, eds. PDR for Nutritional Supplements. 2nd ed. Montvale, NJ: Physicians' Desk Reference Inc.; 2008
10. Marlett JA. Content and composition of dietary fiber in 117 frequently consumed foods. J Am Diet Assoc 1992;92(2):175–186
11. Bazzano LA, Thompson AM, Tees MT, Nguyen CH, Winham DM. Non-soy legume consumption lowers cholesterol levels: a meta-analysis of randomized controlled trials. Nutr Metab Cardiovasc Dis 2011; 21(2):94–103
12. Zhang Z, Lanza E, Kris-Etherton PM, et al. A high legume low glycemic index diet improves serum lipid profiles in men. Lipids 2010;45(9):765–775
13. Anderson JW, Major AW. Pulses and lipaemia, short- and long-term effect: potential in the prevention of cardiovascular disease. Br J Nutr 2002;88(Suppl 3): S263–S271
14. Wolever TM, Tosh SM, Gibbs AL, et al. Physicochemical properties of oat β-glucan influence its ability to reduce serum LDL cholesterol in humans: a randomized clinical trial. Am J Clin Nutr 2010;92(4):723–732
15. Naumann E, van Rees AB, Onning G, Oste R, Wydra M, Mensink RP. Beta-glucan incorporated into a fruit drink effectively lowers serum LDL-cholesterol concentrations. Am J Clin Nutr 2006;83(3):601–605
16. Ripsin CM, Keenan JM, Jacobs DR Jr, et al. Oat products and lipid lowering. A meta-analysis. JAMA 1992; 267(24):3317–3325
17. Brown L, Rosner B, Willett WW, Sacks FM. Cholesterol-lowering effects of dietary fiber: a meta-analysis. Am J Clin Nutr 1999;69(1):30–42
18. Queenan KM, Stewart ML, Smith KN, Thomas W, Fulcher RG, Slavin JL. Concentrated oat beta-glucan, a fermentable fiber, lowers serum cholesterol in hyper-

cholesterolemic adults in a randomized controlled trial. Nutr J 2007;6:6

19. Reyna-Villasmil N, Bermúdez-Pirela V, Mengual-Moreno E, et al. Oat-derived beta-glucan significantly improves HDLC and diminishes LDLC and non-HDL cholesterol in overweight individuals with mild hypercholesterolemia. Am J Ther 2007;14(2):203–212

20. Food and Drug Administration, HHS. Food labeling: health claims; soluble dietary fiber from certain foods and coronary heart disease. Final rule. Fed Regist 2003;68(144):44207–44209

21. Wei ZH, Wang H, Chen XY, et al. Time- and dose-dependent effect of psyllium on serum lipids in mild-to-moderate hypercholesterolemia: a meta-analysis of controlled clinical trials. Eur J Clin Nutr 2009; 63(7):821–827

22. Pal S, Khossousi A, Binns C, Dhaliwal S, Ellis V. The effect of a fibre supplement compared to a healthy diet on body composition, lipids, glucose, insulin and other metabolic syndrome risk factors in overweight and obese individuals. Br J Nutr 2011;105(1):90–100

23. Anderson JW, Allgood LD, Lawrence A, et al. Cholesterol-lowering effects of psyllium intake adjunctive to diet therapy in men and women with hypercholesterolemia: meta-analysis of 8 controlled trials. Am J Clin Nutr 2000;71(2):472–479

24. Butt MS, Shahzadi N, Sharif MK, Nasir M. Guar gum: a miracle therapy for hypercholesterolemia, hyperglycemia and obesity. Crit Rev Food Sci Nutr 2007; 47(4):389–396

25. Theuwissen E, Mensink RP. Water-soluble dietary fibers and cardiovascular disease. Physiol Behav 2008;94(2):285–292

26. Bazzano LA. Effects of soluble dietary fiber on low-density lipoprotein cholesterol and coronary heart disease risk. Curr Atheroscler Rep 2008;10(6):473–477

27. Schäfer G, Schenk U, Ritzel U, Ramadori G, Leonhardt U. Comparison of the effects of dried peas with those of potatoes in mixed meals on postprandial glucose and insulin concentrations in patients with type 2 diabetes. Am J Clin Nutr 2003;78(1):99–103

28. Kabir M, Oppert JM, Vidal H, et al. Four-week low-glycemic index breakfast with a modest amount of soluble fibers in type 2 diabetic men. Metabolism 2002;51(7):819–826

29. Brand-Miller JC, Atkinson FS, Gahler RJ, Kacinik V, Lyon MR, Wood S. Effects of PGX, a novel functional fibre, on acute and delayed postprandial glycaemia. Eur J Clin Nutr 2010;64(12):1488–1493

30. Jenkins AL, Kacinik V, Lyon MR, Wolever TM. Reduction of postprandial glycemia by the novel viscous polysaccharide PGX, in a dose-dependent manner, independent of food form. J Am Coll Nutr 2010; 29(2):92–98

31. Williams JA, Lai CS, Corwin H, et al. Inclusion of guar gum and alginate into a crispy bar improves postprandial glycemia in humans. J Nutr 2004;134(4):886–889

32. Sierra M, Garcia JJ, Fernández N, Diez MJ, Calle AP, Sahagún AM. Effects of ispaghula husk and guar gum on postprandial glucose and insulin concentrations in healthy subjects. Eur J Clin Nutr 2001;55(4):235–243

33. Wolever TM, Jenkins DA. Effect of dietary fiber and foods on carbohydrate metabolism. In: Spiller GA, ed. CRC Handbook of Dietary Fiber in Human Nutrition. 3rd ed. Boca Raton, FL: CRC Press; 2001:321–360

34. Marlett JA, McBurney MI, Slavin JL; American Dietetic Association. Position of the American Dietetic Asso-

ciation: health implications of dietary fiber. J Am Diet Assoc 2002;102(7):993–1000

35. Cummings JH. The effect of dietary fiber on fecal weight and composition. In: Spiller GA, ed. Fiber in Human Nutrition. 3rd ed. Boca Raton, FL: CRC Press; 2001:183–252

36. Anti M, Pignataro G, Armuzzi A, et al. Water supplementation enhances the effect of high-fiber diet on stool frequency and laxative consumption in adult patients with functional constipation. Hepatogastroenterology 1998;45(21):727–732

37. American Academy of Family Physicians. Constipation. Available at: http://familydoctor.org/037.xml. Accessed May 3, 2012

38. Fraser GE, Sabaté J, Beeson WL, Strahan TM. A possible protective effect of nut consumption on risk of coronary heart disease. The Adventist Health Study. Arch Intern Med 1992;152(7):1416–1424

39. Humble CG, Malarcher AM, Tyroler HA. Dietary fiber and coronary heart disease in middle-aged hypercholesterolemic men. Am J Prev Med 1993;9(4):197–202

40. Jacobs DR Jr, Meyer KA, Kushi LH, Folsom AR. Whole-grain intake may reduce the risk of ischemic heart disease death in postmenopausal women: the Iowa Women's Health Study. Am J Clin Nutr 1998; 68(2):248–257

41. Khaw KT, Barrett-Connor E. Dietary fiber and reduced ischemic heart disease mortality rates in men and women: a 12-year prospective study. Am J Epidemiol 1987;126(6):1093–1102

42. Pietinen P, Rimm EB, Korhonen P, et al. Intake of dietary fiber and risk of coronary heart disease in a cohort of Finnish men. The Alpha-Tocopherol, Beta-Carotene Cancer Prevention Study. Circulation 1996;94(11):2720–2727

43. Rimm EB, Ascherio A, Giovannucci E, Spiegelman D, Stampfer MJ, Willett WC. Vegetable, fruit, and cereal fiber intake and risk of coronary heart disease among men. JAMA 1996;275(6):447–451

44. Todd S, Woodward M, Tunstall-Pedoe H, Bolton-Smith C. Dietary antioxidant vitamins and fiber in the etiology of cardiovascular disease and all-causes mortality: results from the Scottish Heart Health Study. Am J Epidemiol 1999;150(10):1073–1080

45. Wolk A, Manson JE, Stampfer MJ, et al. Long-term intake of dietary fiber and decreased risk of coronary heart disease among women. JAMA 1999;281(21): 1998–2004

46. Bazzano LA, He J, Ogden LG, Loria CM, Whelton PK; National Health and Nutrition Examination Survey I Epidemiologic Follow-up Study. Dietary fiber intake and reduced risk of coronary heart disease in US men and women: the National Health and Nutrition Examination Survey I Epidemiologic Follow-up Study. Arch Intern Med 2003;163(16):1897–1904

47. Mozaffarian D, Kumanyika SK, Lemaitre RN, Olson JL, Burke GL, Siscovick DS. Cereal, fruit, and vegetable fiber intake and the risk of cardiovascular disease in elderly individuals. JAMA 2003;289(13):1659–1666

48. Streppel MT, Ocké MC, Boshuizen HC, Kok FJ, Kromhout D. Dietary fiber intake in relation to coronary heart disease and all-cause mortality over 40 y: the Zutphen Study. Am J Clin Nutr 2008;88(4):1119–1125

49. Eshak ES, Iso H, Date C, et al; JACC Study Group. Dietary fiber intake is associated with reduced risk of mortality from cardiovascular disease among Japanese men and women. J Nutr 2010;140(8):1445–1453

50. Park Y, Subar AF, Hollenbeck A, Schatzkin A. Dietary fiber intake and mortality in the NIH-AARP diet and health study. Arch Intern Med 2011;171(12):1061–1068

51. Pereira MA, O'Reilly E, Augustsson K, et al. Dietary fiber and risk of coronary heart disease: a pooled analysis of cohort studies. Arch Intern Med 2004; 164(4):370–376

52. Liu S, Willett WC. Dietary glycemic load and atherothrombotic risk. Curr Atheroscler Rep 2002;4(6):454–461

53. Ford ES, Liu S. Glycemic index and serum high-density lipoprotein cholesterol concentration among US adults. Arch Intern Med 2001;161(4):572–576

54. Liu S, Manson JE, Stampfer MJ, et al. Dietary glycemic load assessed by food-frequency questionnaire in relation to plasma high-density-lipoprotein cholesterol and fasting plasma triacylglycerols in postmenopausal women. Am J Clin Nutr 2001;73(3):560–566

55. Ascherio A, Hennekens C, Willett WC, et al. Prospective study of nutritional factors, blood pressure, and hypertension among US women. Hypertension 1996;27(5):1065–1072

56. Ascherio A, Rimm EB, Giovannucci EL, et al. A prospective study of nutritional factors and hypertension among US men. Circulation 1992;86(5):1475–1484

57. Streppel MT, Arends LR, van 't Veer P, Grobbee DE, Geleijnse JM. Dietary fiber and blood pressure: a meta-analysis of randomized placebo-controlled trials. Arch Intern Med 2005;165(2):150–156

58. Whelton SP, Hyre AD, Pedersen B, Yi Y, Whelton PK, He J. Effect of dietary fiber intake on blood pressure: a meta-analysis of randomized, controlled clinical trials. J Hypertens 2005;23(3):475–481

59. King DE, Egan BM, Woolson RF, Mainous AG III, Al-Solaiman Y, Jesri A. Effect of a high-fiber diet vs a fiber-supplemented diet on C-reactive protein level. Arch Intern Med 2007;167(5):502–506

60. Ma Y, Griffith JA, Chasan-Taber L, et al. Association between dietary fiber and serum C-reactive protein. Am J Clin Nutr 2006;83(4):760–766

61. Patel VB, Robbins MA, Topol EJ. C-reactive protein: a 'golden marker' for inflammation and coronary artery disease. Cleve Clin J Med 2001;68(6):521–524, 527–534

62. Lupton JR, Turner ND. Dietary fiber and coronary disease: does the evidence support an association? Curr Atheroscler Rep 2003;5(6):500–505

63. Gross LS, Li L, Ford ES, Liu S. Increased consumption of refined carbohydrates and the epidemic of type 2 diabetes in the United States: an ecologic assessment. Am J Clin Nutr 2004;79(5):774–779

64. Wannamethee SG, Whincup PH, Thomas MC, Sattar N. Associations between dietary fiber and inflammation, hepatic function, and risk of type 2 diabetes in older men: potential mechanisms for the benefits of fiber on diabetes risk. Diabetes Care 2009; 32(10):1823–1825

65. Hopping BN, Erber E, Grandinetti A, Verheus M, Kolonel LN, Maskarinec G. Dietary fiber, magnesium, and glycemic load alter risk of type 2 diabetes in a multiethnic cohort in Hawaii. J Nutr 2010;140(1):68–74

66. Salmerón J, Ascherio A, Rimm EB, et al. Dietary fiber, glycemic load, and risk of NIDDM in men. Diabetes Care 1997;20(4):545–550

67. Salmerón J, Manson JE, Stampfer MJ, Colditz GA, Wing AL, Willett WC. Dietary fiber, glycemic load, and risk of non-insulin-dependent diabetes mellitus in women. JAMA 1997;277(6):472–477

68. Meyer KA, Kushi LH, Jacobs DR Jr, Slavin J, Sellers TA, Folsom AR. Carbohydrates, dietary fiber, and incident type 2 diabetes in older women. Am J Clin Nutr 2000;71(4):921–930

69. Stevens J, Ahn K, Juhaeri, Houston D, Steffan L, Couper D. Dietary fiber intake and glycemic index and incidence of diabetes in African-American and white adults: the ARIC study. Diabetes Care 2002; 25(10):1715–1721

70. Montonen J, Knekt P, Järvinen R, Aromaa A, Reunanen A. Whole-grain and fiber intake and the incidence of type 2 diabetes. Am J Clin Nutr 2003;77(3):622–629

71. Schulze MB, Liu S, Rimm EB, Manson JE, Willett WC, Hu FB. Glycemic index, glycemic load, and dietary fiber intake and incidence of type 2 diabetes in younger and middle-aged women. Am J Clin Nutr 2004;80(2):348–356

72. Ventura E, Davis J, Byrd-Williams C, et al. Reduction in risk factors for type 2 diabetes mellitus in response to a low-sugar, high-fiber dietary intervention in overweight Latino adolescents. Arch Pediatr Adolesc Med 2009;163(4):320–327

73. Krishnan S, Rosenberg L, Singer M, et al. Glycemic index, glycemic load, and cereal fiber intake and risk of type 2 diabetes in US black women. Arch Intern Med 2007;167(21):2304–2309

74. Schulze MB, Schulz M, Heidemann C, Schienkiewitz A, Hoffmann K, Boeing H. Fiber and magnesium intake and incidence of type 2 diabetes: a prospective study and meta-analysis. Arch Intern Med 2007; 167(9):956–965

75. Knowler WC, Barrett-Connor E, Fowler SE, et al; Diabetes Prevention Program Research Group. Reduction in the incidence of type 2 diabetes with lifestyle intervention or metformin. N Engl J Med 2002; 346(6):393–403

76. Tuomilehto J, Lindström J, Eriksson JG, et al; Finnish Diabetes Prevention Study Group. Prevention of type 2 diabetes mellitus by changes in lifestyle among subjects with impaired glucose tolerance. N Engl J Med 2001;344(18):1343–1350

77. Trock B, Lanza E, Greenwald P. Dietary fiber, vegetables, and colon cancer: critical review and meta-analyses of the epidemiologic evidence. J Natl Cancer Inst 1990;82(8):650–661

78. Howe GR, Benito E, Castelleto R, et al. Dietary intake of fiber and decreased risk of cancers of the colon and rectum: evidence from the combined analysis of 13 case-control studies. J Natl Cancer Inst 1992; 84(24):1887–1896

79. Dahm CC, Keogh RH, Spencer EA, et al. Dietary fiber and colorectal cancer risk: a nested case-control study using food diaries. J Natl Cancer Inst 2010;102(9):614–626

80. Steinmetz KA, Kushi LH, Bostick RM, Folsom AR, Potter JD. Vegetables, fruit, and colon cancer in the Iowa Women's Health Study. Am J Epidemiol 1994; 139(1):1–15

81. Kato I, Akhmedkhanov A, Koenig K, Toniolo PG, Shore RE, Riboli E. Prospective study of diet and female colorectal cancer: the New York University Women's Health Study. Nutr Cancer 1997;28(3):276–281

82. Pietinen P, Malila N, Virtanen M, et al. Diet and risk of colorectal cancer in a cohort of Finnish men. Cancer Causes Control 1999;10(5):387–396

83. Terry P, Giovannucci E, Michels KB, et al. Fruit, vegetables, dietary fiber, and risk of colorectal cancer. J Natl Cancer Inst 2001;93(7):525–533

84. Mai V, Flood A, Peters U, Lacey JV Jr, Schairer C, Schatzkin A. Dietary fibre and risk of colorectal cancer in the Breast Cancer Detection Demonstration Project (BCDDP) follow-up cohort. Int J Epidemiol 2003;32(2):234–239

85. Lin J, Zhang SM, Cook NR, et al. Dietary intakes of fruit, vegetables, and fiber, and risk of colorectal cancer in a prospective cohort of women (United States). Cancer Causes Control 2005;16(3):225–233

86. Michels KB, Fuchs CS, Giovannucci E, et al. Fiber intake and incidence of colorectal cancer among 76,947 women and 47,279 men. Cancer Epidemiol Biomarkers Prev 2005;14(4):842–849

87. Shin A, Li H, Shu XO, Yang G, Gao YT, Zheng W. Dietary intake of calcium, fiber and other micronutrients in relation to colorectal cancer risk: Results from the Shanghai Women's Health Study. Int J Cancer 2006;119(12):2938–2942

88. Otani T, Iwasaki M, Ishihara J, Sasazuki S, Inoue M, Tsugane S; Japan Public Health Center-Based Prospective Study Group. Dietary fiber intake and subsequent risk of colorectal cancer: the Japan Public Health Center-based prospective study. Int J Cancer 2006;119(6):1475–1480

89. Schatzkin A, Mouw T, Park Y, et al. Dietary fiber and whole-grain consumption in relation to colorectal cancer in the NIH-AARP Diet and Health Study. Am J Clin Nutr 2007;85(5):1353–1360

90. Park Y, Hunter DJ, Spiegelman D, et al. Dietary fiber intake and risk of colorectal cancer: a pooled analysis of prospective cohort studies. JAMA 2005;294(22):2849–2857

91. Bingham SA, Day NE, Luben R, et al; European Prospective Investigation into Cancer and Nutrition. Dietary fibre in food and protection against colorectal cancer in the European Prospective Investigation into Cancer and Nutrition (EPIC): an observational study. Lancet 2003;361(9368):1496–1501

92. Schatzkin A, Lanza E, Corle D, et al; Polyp Prevention Trial Study Group. Lack of effect of a low-fat, high-fiber diet on the recurrence of colorectal adenomas. N Engl J Med 2000;342(16):1149–1155

93. Alberts DS, Martínez ME, Roe DJ, et al. Lack of effect of a high-fiber cereal supplement on the recurrence of colorectal adenomas. Phoenix Colon Cancer Prevention Physicians' Network. N Engl J Med 2000;342(16):1156–1162

94. Ishikawa H, Akedo I, Otani T, et al. Randomized trial of dietary fiber and Lactobacillus casei administration for prevention of colorectal tumors. Int J Cancer 2005;116(5):762–767

95. Bonithon-Kopp C, Kronborg O, Giacosa A, Räth U, Faivre J; European Cancer Prevention Organisation Study Group. Calcium and fibre supplementation in prevention of colorectal adenoma recurrence: a randomised intervention trial. Lancet 2000;356(9238):1300–1306

96. Giovannucci E, Stampfer MJ, Colditz G, Rimm EB, Willett WC. Relationship of diet to risk of colorectal adenoma in men. J Natl Cancer Inst 1992;84(2):91–98

97. Van 't Veer P, Kolb CM, Verhoef P, et al. Dietary fiber, beta-carotene and breast cancer: results from a case-control study. Int J Cancer 1990;45(5):825–828

98. Baghurst PA, Rohan TE. High-fiber diets and reduced risk of breast cancer. Int J Cancer 1994;56(2):173–176

99. Yuan JM, Wang QS, Ross RK, Henderson BE, Yu MC. Diet and breast cancer in Shanghai and Tianjin, China. Br J Cancer 1995;71(6):1353–1358

100. Ronco A, De Stefani E, Boffetta P, Deneo-Pellegrini H, Mendilaharsu M, Leborgne F. Vegetables, fruits, and related nutrients and risk of breast cancer: a case-control study in Uruguay. Nutr Cancer 1999;35(2):111–119

101. Belle FN, Kampman E, McTiernan A, et al. Dietary fiber, carbohydrates, glycemic index, and glycemic load in relation to breast cancer prognosis in the HEAL cohort. Cancer Epidemiol Biomarkers Prev 2011;20(5):890–899

102. Graham S, Zielezny M, Marshall J, et al. Diet in the epidemiology of postmenopausal breast cancer in the New York State Cohort. Am J Epidemiol 1992;136(11):1327–1337

103. Terry P, Jain M, Miller AB, Howe GR, Rohan TE. No association among total dietary fiber, fiber fractions, and risk of breast cancer. Cancer Epidemiol Biomarkers Prev 2002;11(11):1507–1508

104. Cho E, Spiegelman D, Hunter DJ, Chen WY, Colditz GA, Willett WC. Premenopausal dietary carbohydrate, glycemic index, glycemic load, and fiber in relation to risk of breast cancer. Cancer Epidemiol Biomarkers Prev 2003;12(11 Pt 1):1153–1158

105. Holmes MD, Liu S, Hankinson SE, Colditz GA, Hunter DJ, Willett WC. Dietary carbohydrates, fiber, and breast cancer risk. Am J Epidemiol 2004;159(8):732–739

106. Lajous M, Boutron-Ruault MC, Fabre A, Clavel-Chapelon F, Romieu I. Carbohydrate intake, glycemic index, glycemic load, and risk of postmenopausal breast cancer in a prospective study of French women. Am J Clin Nutr 2008;87(5):1384–1391

107. Wen W, Shu XO, Li H, et al. Dietary carbohydrates, fiber, and breast cancer risk in Chinese women. Am J Clin Nutr 2009;89(1):283–289

108. Maruti SS, Lampe JW, Potter JD, Ready A, White E. A prospective study of bowel motility and related factors on breast cancer risk. Cancer Epidemiol Biomarkers Prev 2008;17(7):1746–1750

109. Cade JE, Burley VJ, Greenwood DC; UK Women's Cohort Study Steering Group. Dietary fibre and risk of breast cancer in the UK Women's Cohort Study. Int J Epidemiol 2007;36(2):431–438

110. Mattisson I, Wirfält E, Johansson U, Gullberg B, Olsson H, Berglund G. Intakes of plant foods, fibre and fat and risk of breast cancer—a prospective study in the Malmö Diet and Cancer cohort. Br J Cancer 2004;90(1):122–127

111. Park Y, Brinton LA, Subar AF, Hollenbeck A, Schatzkin A. Dietary fiber intake and risk of breast cancer in postmenopausal women: the National Institutes of Health-AARP Diet and Health Study. Am J Clin Nutr 2009;90(3):664–671

112. Dong JY, He K, Wang P, Qin LQ. Dietary fiber intake and risk of breast cancer: a meta-analysis of prospective cohort studies. Am J Clin Nutr 2011;94(3):900–905

113. Rock CL, Flatt SW, Thomson CA, et al. Effects of a high-fiber, low-fat diet intervention on serum concentrations of reproductive steroid hormones in women with a history of breast cancer. J Clin Oncol 2004;22(12):2379–2387

114. Kasim-Karakas SE, Almario RU, Gregory L, Todd H, Wong R, Lasley BL. Effects of prune consumption on the ratio of 2-hydroxyestrone to 16alpha-hydroxyestrone. Am J Clin Nutr 2002;76(6):1422–1427

115. Korzenik JR. Case closed? Diverticulitis: epidemiology and fiber. J Clin Gastroenterol 2006;40(Suppl 3):S112–S116

116. Bogardus ST Jr. What do we know about diverticular disease? A brief overview. J Clin Gastroenterol 2006;40(Suppl 3):S108–S111

117. Peery AF, Barrett PR, Park D, et al. A high-fiber diet does not protect against asymptomatic diverticulosis. Gastroenterology 2012;142(2):266–272.e1

118. Farrell RJ, Farrell JJ, Morrin MM. Diverticular disease in the elderly. Gastroenterol Clin North Am 2001;30(2):475–496

119. Aldoori WH, Giovannucci EL, Rockett HR, Sampson L, Rimm EB, Willett WC. A prospective study of dietary fiber types and symptomatic diverticular disease in men. J Nutr 1998;128(4):714–719

120. Howarth NC, Saltzman E, Roberts SB. Dietary fiber and weight regulation. Nutr Rev 2001;59(5):129–139

121. Du H, van der A DL, Boshuizen HC, et al. Dietary fiber and subsequent changes in body weight and waist circumference in European men and women. Am J Clin Nutr 2010;91(2):329–336

122. Appleby PN, Thorogood M, Mann JI, Key TJ. Low body mass index in non-meat eaters: the possible roles of animal fat, dietary fibre and alcohol. Int J Obes Relat Metab Disord 1998;22(5):454–460

123. Miller WC, Niederpruem MG, Wallace JP, Lindeman AK. Dietary fat, sugar, and fiber predict body fat content. J Am Diet Assoc 1994;94(6):612–615

124. Davis JN, Hodges VA, Gillham MB. Normal-weight adults consume more fiber and fruit than their age- and height-matched overweight/obese counterparts. J Am Diet Assoc 2006;106(6):833–840

125. Liu S, Willett WC, Manson JE, Hu FB, Rosner B, Colditz G. Relation between changes in intakes of dietary fiber and grain products and changes in weight and development of obesity among middle-aged women. Am J Clin Nutr 2003;78(5):920–927

126. Saltzman E, Moriguti JC, Das SK, et al. Effects of a cereal rich in soluble fiber on body composition and dietary compliance during consumption of a hypocaloric diet. J Am Coll Nutr 2001;20(1):50–57

127. Howarth NC, Saltzman E, McCrory MA, et al. Fermentable and nonfermentable fiber supplements did not alter hunger, satiety or body weight in a pilot study of men and women consuming self-selected diets. J Nutr 2003;133(10):3141–3144

128. Wanders AJ, van den Borne JJ, de Graaf C, et al. Effects of dietary fibre on subjective appetite, energy intake and body weight: a systematic review of randomized controlled trials. Obes Rev 2011;12(9):724–739

129. Lubin F, Lusky A, Chetrit A, Dankner R. Lifestyle and ethnicity play a role in all-cause mortality. J Nutr 2003;133(4):1180–1185

130. Baer HJ, Glynn RJ, Hu FB, et al. Risk factors for mortality in the nurses' health study: a competing risks analysis. Am J Epidemiol 2011;173(3):319–329

131. Giacco R, Parillo M, Rivellese AA, et al. Long-term dietary treatment with increased amounts of fiber-rich low-glycemic index natural foods improves blood glucose control and reduces the number of hypoglycemic events in type 1 diabetic patients. Diabetes Care 2000;23(10):1461–1466

132. Chandalia M, Garg A, Lutjohann D, von Bergmann K, Grundy SM, Brinkley LJ. Beneficial effects of high dietary fiber intake in patients with type 2 diabetes mellitus. N Engl J Med 2000;342(19):1392–1398

133. Groop PH, Aro A, Stenman S, Groop L. Long-term effects of guar gum in subjects with non-insulin-dependent diabetes mellitus. Am J Clin Nutr 1993; 58(4):513–518

134. Sierra M, García JJ, Fernández N, Diez MJ, Calle AP. Therapeutic effects of psyllium in type 2 diabetic patients. Eur J Clin Nutr 2002;56(9):830–842

135. Anderson JW, Allgood LD, Turner J, Oeltgen PR, Daggy BP. Effects of psyllium on glucose and serum lipid responses in men with type 2 diabetes and hypercholesterolemia. Am J Clin Nutr 1999;70(4):466–473

136. Anderson JW, Randles KM, Kendall CW, Jenkins DJ. Carbohydrate and fiber recommendations for individuals with diabetes: a quantitative assessment and meta-analysis of the evidence. J Am Coll Nutr 2004;23(1):5–17

137. American Diabetes Association Task Force for Writing Nutrition Principles and Recommendations for the Management of Diabetes and Related Complications. American Diabetes Association position statement: evidence-based nutrition principles and recommendations for the treatment and prevention of diabetes and related complications. J Am Diet Assoc 2002;102(1):109–118

138. Nutrition Subcommittee of the British Diabetic Association's Professional Advisory Committee. Dietary recommendations for people with diabetes: an update for the 1990s. Diabet Med 1992;9(2):189–202

139. National Nutrition Committee. Canadian Diabetes Association. Guidelines for the Nutritional Management of Diabetes Mellitus in the New Millennium: A Position Statement by the Canadian Diabetes Association. Can J Diabetes Care 1999;23(3):56–69

140. Jenkins DJ, Kendall CW, Augustin LS, et al. Effect of wheat bran on glycemic control and risk factors for cardiovascular disease in type 2 diabetes. Diabetes Care 2002;25(9):1522–1528

141. Horwitz BJ, Fisher RS. The irritable bowel syndrome. N Engl J Med 2001;344(24):1846–1850

142. Jailwala J, Imperiale TF, Kroenke K. Pharmacologic treatment of the irritable bowel syndrome: a systematic review of randomized, controlled trials. Ann Intern Med 2000;133(2):136–147

143. Ford AC, Talley NJ, Spiegel BM, et al. Effect of fibre, antispasmodics, and peppermint oil in the treatment of irritable bowel syndrome: systematic review and meta-analysis. BMJ 2008;337:a2313

144. Quartero AO, Meineche-Schmidt V, Muris J, Rubin G, de Wit N. Bulking agents, antispasmodic and antidepressant medication for the treatment of irritable bowel syndrome. Cochrane Database Syst Rev 2005; (2):CD003460

145. Bijkerk CJ, de Wit NJ, Muris JW, Whorwell PJ, Knottnerus JA, Hoes AW. Soluble or insoluble fibre in irritable bowel syndrome in primary care? Randomised placebo controlled trial. BMJ 2009;339: b3154

146. Bijkerk CJ, Muris JW, Knottnerus JA, Hoes AW, de Wit NJ. Systematic review: the role of different types of fibre in the treatment of irritable bowel syndrome. Aliment Pharmacol Ther 2004;19(3):245–251

147. Viera AJ, Hoag S, Shaughnessy J. Management of irritable bowel syndrome. Am Fam Physician 2002; 66(10):1867–1874

148. Mertz HR. Irritable bowel syndrome. N Engl J Med 2003;349(22):2136–2146

149. Giannini EG, Mansi C, Dulbecco P, Savarino V. Role of partially hydrolyzed guar gum in the treatment of irritable bowel syndrome. Nutrition 2006;22(3):334–342

150. US Department of Agriculture, Agricultural Research Service. National Nutrient Database for Standard Reference. Release 24. Available at: http://ndb.nal.usda.gov/ndb/foods/list. Accessed May 3, 2012

151. Hendler SS, Rorvik DR, eds. PDR for Nutritional Supplements. Montvale, NJ: Medical Economics Company, Inc; 2001

152. Gibson GR, Beatty ER, Wang X, Cummings JH. Selective stimulation of bifidobacteria in the human colon by oligofructose and inulin. Gastroenterology 1995;108(4):975–982

153. Kolida S, Tuohy K, Gibson GR. Prebiotic effects of inulin and oligofructose. Br J Nutr 2002;87(Suppl 2): S193–S197

154. Cummings JH, Macfarlane GT. Gastrointestinal effects of prebiotics. Br J Nutr 2002;87(Suppl 2):S145–S151

155. Duggan C, Penny ME, Hibberd P, et al. Oligofructose-supplemented infant cereal: 2 randomized, blinded, community-based trials in Peruvian infants. Am J Clin Nutr 2003;77(4):937–942

156. Pittler MH, Ernst E. Guar gum for body weight reduction: meta-analysis of randomized trials. Am J Med 2001;110(9):724–730

157. Gallaher CM, Munion J, Hesslink R Jr, Wise J, Gallaher DD. Cholesterol reduction by glucomannan and chitosan is mediated by changes in cholesterol absorption and bile acid and fat excretion in rats. J Nutr 2000;130(11):2753–2759

158. Pittler MH, Ernst E. Dietary supplements for body-weight reduction: a systematic review. Am J Clin Nutr 2004;79(4):529–536

159. Bokura H, Kobayashi S. Chitosan decreases total cholesterol in women: a randomized, double-blind, placebo-controlled trial. Eur J Clin Nutr 2003;57(5):721–725

160. Wuolijoki E, Hirvelä T, Ylitalo P. Decrease in serum LDL cholesterol with microcrystalline chitosan. Methods Find Exp Clin Pharmacol 1999;21(5):357–361

161. Metso S, Ylitalo R, Nikkilä M, Wuolijoki E, Ylitalo P, Lehtimäki T. The effect of long-term microcrystalline chitosan therapy on plasma lipids and glucose concentrations in subjects with increased plasma total cholesterol: a randomised placebo-controlled double-blind crossover trial in healthy men and women. Eur J Clin Pharmacol 2003;59(10):741–746

162. Ho SC, Tai ES, Eng PH, Tan CE, Fok AC. In the absence of dietary surveillance, chitosan does not reduce plasma lipids or obesity in hypercholesterolaemic obese Asian subjects. Singapore Med J 2001;42(1):6–10

163. American Academy of Family Physicians. Fiber: How to Increase the Amount in Your Diet. Available at: http://familydoctor.org/familydoctor/en/prevention-wellness/food-nutrition/nutrients/fiber-how-to-increase-the-amount-in-your-diet.html. Accessed May 3, 2012

164. Papazian R. Bulking Up Fiber's Healthful Reputation. Food and Drug Administration. Available at: http://www.fda.gov/fdac/features/1997/597_fiber.html. Accessed Sep 14, 2004

165. Rosario PG, Gerst PH, Prakash K, Albu E. Dentureless distention: oat bran bezoars cause obstruction. J Am Geriatr Soc 1990;38(5):608

166. Miller DL, Miller PF, Dekker JJ. Small-bowel obstruction from bran cereal. JAMA 1990;263(6):813–814

167. Cooper SG, Tracey EJ. Small-bowel obstruction caused by oat-bran bezoar. N Engl J Med 1989; 320(17):1148–1149

168. McClurken JB, Carp NZ. Bran-induced small-intestinal obstruction in a patient with no history of abdominal operation. Arch Surg 1988;123(1):98–100

169. Lewis JH. Esophageal and small bowel obstruction from guar gum-containing "diet pills": analysis of 26 cases reported to the Food and Drug Administration. Am J Gastroenterol 1992;87(10):1424–1428

170. Agha FP, Nostrant TT, Fiddian-Green RG. "Giant colonic bezoar:" a medication bezoar due to psyllium seed husks. Am J Gastroenterol 1984;79(4):319–321

171. Schneider RP. Perdiem causes esophageal impaction and bezoars. South Med J 1989;82(11):1449–1450

172. Chandra R, Barron JL. Anaphylactic reaction to intravenous sinistrin (Inutest). Ann Clin Biochem 2002; 39(Pt 1):76

173. Gay-Crosier F, Schreiber G, Hauser C. Anaphylaxis from inulin in vegetables and processed food. N Engl J Med 2000;342(18):1372

174. Khalili B, Bardana EJ Jr, Yunginger JW. Psyllium-associated anaphylaxis and death: a case report and review of the literature. Ann Allergy Asthma Immunol 2003;91(6):579–584

175. Fugh-Berman A. Herb-drug interactions. Lancet 2000;355(9198):134–138

176. Richter WO, Jacob BG, Schwandt P. Interaction between fibre and lovastatin. Lancet 1991;338(8768):706

177. Greger JL. Nondigestible carbohydrates and mineral bioavailability. J Nutr 1999; 129(7, Suppl):1434S–1435S

178. Bosscher D, Van Caillie-Bertrand M, Van Cauwenbergh R, Deelstra H. Availabilities of calcium, iron, and zinc from dairy infant formulas is affected by soluble dietary fibers and modified starch fractions. Nutrition 2003;19(7–8):641–645

179. Scholz-Ahrens KE, Schrezenmeir J. Inulin, oligofructose and mineral metabolism - experimental data and mechanism. Br J Nutr 2002;87(Suppl 2):S179–S186

180. Rock CL, Swendseid ME. Plasma beta-carotene response in humans after meals supplemented with dietary pectin. Am J Clin Nutr 1992;55(1):96–99

181. Riedl J, Linseisen J, Hoffmann J, Wolfram G. Some dietary fibers reduce the absorption of carotenoids in women. J Nutr 1999;129(12):2170–2176

17 Organosulfur Compounds from Garlic

Garlic (*Allium sativum* L.) has been used for culinary and medicinal purposes by many cultures for centuries.[1] Garlic is a particularly rich source of organosulfur compounds, which are thought to be responsible for its flavor and aroma, as well as its potential health benefits.[2] Consumer interest in the health benefits of garlic is strong enough to place it among the best-selling herbal supplements in the United States.[3] Scientists are interested in the potential for organosulfur compounds derived from garlic to prevent and treat chronic diseases, such as cancer and cardiovascular disease.[4]

Two classes of organosulfur compounds are found in whole garlic cloves: (1) γ-glutamylcysteines, and (2) cysteine sulfoxides. Allylcysteine sulfoxide (alliin) accounts for approximately 80% of the cysteine sulfoxides in garlic.[1] When raw garlic cloves are crushed, chopped, or chewed, an enzyme known as *alliinase* is released. Alliinase catalyzes the formation of sulfenic acids from cysteine sulfoxides (**Fig. 17.1**). Sulfenic acids spontaneously react with each other to form unstable compounds called *thiosulfinates*. In the case of alliin, the resulting sulfenic acids react with each other to form a thiosulfinate known as *allicin* (half-life in crushed garlic at 23°C is 2.5 days). The formation of thiosulfinates is very rapid and has been found to be complete within 10–60 seconds of crushing garlic. Allicin breaks down in vitro to form a variety of fat-soluble organosulfur compounds (**Fig. 17.1**), including diallyl trisulfide (DATS), diallyl disulfide (DADS), and diallyl sulfide (DAS), or in the presence of oil or organic solvents, ajoene and vinyldithiins.[2] Crushing garlic does not change its γ-glutamylcysteine content. Water-soluble organosulfur compounds, such as *S*-allylcysteine, are formed from γ-glutamylcysteines during long-term incubation of crushed garlic in aqueous solutions, as in the manufacture of aged garlic extracts (see the Sources section below).

Bioavailability and Metabolism

Allicin-Derived Compounds

The absorption and metabolism of allicin and allicin-derived compounds are only partially understood.[5] Although several biological activities have been attributed to various allicin-derived compounds, it is not yet clear which of these compounds or metabolites actually reach target tissues.[1] Animal studies using radiolabeled compounds indicate that allicin or its breakdown products are absorbed intestinally.[6,7] However, allicin and allicin-derived compounds, including diallylsufides, ajoene, and vinyldithiins, have never been detected in human blood, urine, or stool, even after the consumption of up to 25 g of fresh garlic or 60 mg of pure allicin.[1] These findings suggest that allicin and allicin-derived compounds are rapidly metabolized. The concentration of allyl methyl sulfide in the breath has been proposed as an indicator of the bioavailability of allicin and allicin-derived compounds.[5] Human consumption of crushed garlic and equivalent amounts of allicin, DATS, DADS, and allyl methyl sulfide resulted in similar increases in breath concentrations of allyl methyl sulfide,[5] suggesting that allicin and allicin-derived compounds are metabolized to allyl methyl sulfide, a volatile compound that can be measured in exhaled air.

γ-Glutamylcysteines and S-Allylcysteine

γ-Glutamylcysteines are thought to be absorbed intact and hydrolyzed to *S*-allylcysteine and *S*-1-propenylcysteine, since metabolites of these compounds have been measured in human urine after garlic consumption.[8,9] The consumption of aged garlic extract, a commercial garlic preparation that contains *S*-allylcysteine, has been found to increase plasma *S*-allylcysteine concentrations in humans.[10,11]

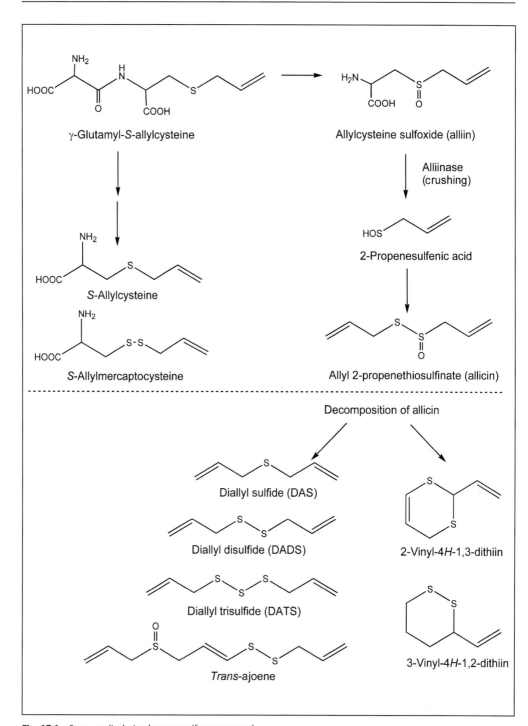

Fig. 17.1 Some garlic-derived organosulfur compounds.

Biological Activities

Related to Cardiovascular Disease Prevention

Inhibition of Cholesterol Synthesis

Garlic and garlic-derived organosulfur compounds have been found to decrease the synthesis of cholesterol by hepatocytes (liver cells).[12] Several garlic-derived organosulfur compounds, including S-allylcysteine and ajoene, have been found to inhibit 3-hydroxy-3-methyl-glutaryl-coenzyme A reductase (HMG-CoA reductase), a critical enzyme in the cholesterol biosynthesis pathway.[13,14] Garlic-derived compounds may also inhibit other enzymes in this pathway, including sterol 4-α-methyl oxidase.[15]

Inhibition of Platelet Aggregation

A variety of garlic-derived organosulfur compounds have been found to inhibit platelet aggregation in the test tube.[16,17]

Anti-inflammatory Activity

Inflammation appears to play an important role in the pathology of cardiovascular disease.[18] Garlic-derived organosulfur compounds have been found to inhibit the activity of the inflammatory enzymes, cyclooxygenase and lipoxygenase, in vitro (reviewed in [19]) and to decrease the expression of inducible nitric oxide synthase (iNOS) in inflammatory white blood cells (macrophages).[20,21] More recently, organosulfur compounds have been found to decrease the production of inflammatory signaling molecules in cultured macrophages[22] and human whole blood.[23]

Inhibition of Arterial Smooth Muscle Proliferation

The proliferation and migration of normally quiescent arterial smooth muscle cells are central features of vascular diseases, including atherosclerosis and coronary restenosis.[24] Although the significance of these findings for human cardiovascular disease is not yet clear, limited cell culture research suggests that organosulfur compounds from garlic may inhibit the proliferation and migration of vascular smooth muscle cells.[13,25,26]

Antioxidant Activity

Several organosulfur compounds have been found to have antioxidant activity in the test tube, and there is some evidence that organosulfur compounds can stimulate the synthesis of glutathione, an important intracellular antioxidant.[27] Although garlic oil supplementation in hypertensive adults was reported to decrease a biomarker of in vivo lipid (fat) oxidation in a small uncontrolled trial,[28] it is not yet clear whether garlic-derived organosulfur compounds have clinically important antioxidant effects in vivo.

Hydrogen Sulfide-Mediated Vasodilatory Activity

The preservation of normal arterial function plays an important role in prevention of cardiovascular disease. Hydrogen sulfide, a gaseous signaling molecule produced by some cells within the body, acts as a vasodilator (relaxes blood vessels) and thus may have cardioprotective properties.[29,30] A recent study found that garlic-derived compounds are converted to hydrogen sulfide by red blood cells in vitro.[31] However, human consumption of a high dose of raw garlic does not increase breath hydrogen sulfide levels, suggesting that significant metabolism of garlic compounds to hydrogen sulfide does not occur in vivo.[32]

Biological Activities Related to Cancer

Effects on Carcinogen Metabolism

Inhibition of phase I biotransformation enzymes. Some chemical carcinogens do not become active carcinogens until they have been metabolized by phase I biotransformation enzymes, such as those belonging to the cytochrome P450 (CYP) family. Inhibition of specific CYP enzymes involved in carcinogen activation inhibits the development of cancer in some animal models.[33] In particular, DAS and its metabolites have been found to inhibit CYP2E1 activity in vitro[34] and when administered orally at high doses to animals.[35,36] Oral administration of garlic oil and DAS to humans has also resulted in evidence of decreased CYP2E1 activity.[37,38]

Induction of phase II biotransformation enzymes. Reactions catalyzed by phase II biotransformation enzymes generally promote the elimination of drugs, toxins, and carcinogens from the body. Consequently, increasing the activity of phase II enzymes, such as glutathione *S*-transferase and quinone reductase, may help prevent cancer by enhancing the elimination of potential carcinogens.[39] In animal studies, oral administration of garlic preparations and organosulfur compounds increases the activity of phase II enzymes in a variety of tissues.[40–42] The genes for several phase II enzymes contain a specific sequence of DNA called an *antioxidant response element* (ARE). Research suggests that allyl sulfides, particularly DATS, promote the translocation of a transcription factor known as Nrf2 to the nucleus, where it binds ARE and increases the transcription of ARE-containing genes.[43,44] Although very high doses of organosulfur compounds were administered in most animal studies, at least one study found that quinone reductase activity increased in the gastrointestinal tracts of mice given a dose of DADS that might be achieved by human intake.[45]

Enhanced cellular glutathione synthesis. Glutathione is an important intracellular antioxidant and is also required for some phase II biotransformation reactions. There is some evidence from cell culture and animal studies that garlic-derived organosulfur compounds increase intracellular glutathione concentrations.[43,46] Like the genes for many phase II enzymes, the gene for a critical enzyme in glutathione synthesis also contains an ARE. Thus, organosulfur compounds may increase cellular glutathione synthesis by promoting the nuclear translocation and binding of the Nrf2 transcription factor to genes containing AREs (see the Induction of phase II biotransformation enzymes section above).

Induction of Cell-Cycle Arrest

Unregulated cell division is a hallmark of human cancers.[47] In normal cells, the cell cycle is tightly regulated to ensure faithful DNA replication and chromosomal segregation prior to cell division. Following DNA damage, the cell cycle can be transiently arrested to allow for DNA repair or activation of pathways leading to cell death (apoptosis). Organosulfur compounds, including DATS, DADS, ajoene, and *S*-allylmercaptocysteine

(SAMC), have been found to induce cell-cycle arrest when added to cancer cells in cell culture experiments.[48–50]

Induction of Apoptosis

Apoptosis is a normal physiological process for the self-destruction of cells that are genetically damaged or no longer necessary. Precancerous and cancerous cells are resistant to signals that induce apoptosis.[51] Garlic-derived organosulfur compounds, including allicin, ajoene, DAS, DADS, DATS, and SAMC, have been found to induce apoptosis when added to various cancer cell lines grown in culture (reviewed in [48,51]). Oral administration of aqueous garlic extract and *S*-allylcysteine has been reported to enhance apoptosis in an animal model of oral cancer.[52,53]

Antimicrobial Activity

Garlic extracts have been found to have antibacterial and antifungal properties.[54,55] Thiosulfinates, particularly allicin, are thought to play an important role in the antimicrobial activity of garlic.[55–57] Allicin-derived compounds, including DATS and ajoene, also have some antimicrobial activity in vitro, although generally less than allicin.[1] To date, randomized controlled trials have not provided strong evidence that oral garlic preparations have significant antibacterial activity in humans[58–60]; however, clinical trials using allicin-rich garlic preparations (raw or cooked garlic) have not been conducted. A small randomized controlled trial found that application of 1% ajoene cream to the skin twice daily was as effective in treating tinea pedis (athlete's foot) as 1% terbinafine (Lamisil) cream.[61]

Disease Prevention

Cardiovascular Disease

Interest in garlic and its potential to prevent cardiovascular disease began with observations that people living near the Mediterranean had lower mortality from cardiovascular disease.[62] Garlic is a common ingredient in Mediterranean cuisine, but several characteristics of the "Mediterranean diet" have been proposed to explain its cardioprotective effects. Although few epidemiological studies have examined associations between garlic consumption and cardiovascular disease risk, numerous intervention trials have explored the effects of garlic supplementation on risk factors for cardiovascular disease.

Serum Lipid Profiles

More than 40 randomized controlled trials have examined the effects of supplementation with various garlic preparations on serum lipid profiles in individuals with elevated and normal serum cholesterol levels.[63] Although many of these trials had methodological limitations, the results of several meta-analyses indicate that garlic supplementation results in modest (6%–11%) reductions in serum total cholesterol, low-density lipoprotein (LDL) cholesterol, and triglyceride levels, compared with placebo.[63–65] The most comprehensive meta-analysis to date found that the modest reductions in serum cholesterol levels, which were evident up to 3 months after starting supplementation, were no longer statistically significant after 6 months of supplementation.[63] Several recent clinical trials have not found that the use of garlic supplements results in statistically or clinically significant improvements in serum lipid profiles when compared with a placebo.[66–74] The most recent and largest trial included high doses of raw garlic and a garlic supplement with high allicin bioavailability. However, neither supplement had a significant effect on serum lipids after 6 months in individuals with moderate hypercholesterolemia.[74] Hence, garlic consumption strongly appears to have no effect on serum lipids, except possibly in individuals with very high levels of LDL cholesterol.

Platelet Aggregation

Platelet aggregation is one of the first steps in the formation of blood clots that can occlude coronary or cerebral arteries, leading to myocardial infarction (heart attack) or ischemic stroke, respectively. Most randomized controlled trials have found that garlic supplementation results in significant reductions in measures of ex-vivo platelet aggregation. Four out of five trials found that supplementation with dehydrated garlic or garlic oil macerates significantly decreased spontaneous platelet aggregation compared with placebo.[63] More recently, supplementation with aged garlic extract inhibited ex-vivo platelet aggregation induced by physiological activators in two separate trials.[11,75]

Blood Pressure

The majority of controlled clinical trials have not found that garlic supplementation significantly reduces systolic or diastolic blood pressure in people with normal or high blood pressure.[63,76] Only three out of 23 randomized controlled trials identified in a systematic review[63] reported statistically significant reductions in diastolic blood pressure,[77–79] and only one reported a statistically significant reduction in systolic blood pressure.[77] At present, there is little evidence to support the use of garlic supplementation to prevent or treat hypertension.

Garlic and Atherosclerosis

Two studies have attempted to assess the effect of garlic supplementation on the progression of atherosclerosis in humans. One study in Germany used ultrasound imaging to assess the effect of 900 mg/day of dehydrated garlic on the progression of atherosclerotic plaque in the carotid and femoral arteries.[80] After 4 years, the increase in plaque volume was significantly greater in women taking the placebo than in women taking the garlic supplement, but there was no significant difference between men taking garlic or placebo.[81] In a smaller pilot study, investigators measured coronary artery calcium using electron beam tomography to assess the effect of supplementation with aged garlic extract on the progression of atherosclerosis in 19 adults already taking HMG-CoA reductase inhibitors (statins).[82] After 1 year, increases in coronary calcium were significantly lower in those taking aged garlic extract (4 mL/day) than in those taking a placebo. Although coronary calcium scores are correlated with the severity of coronary atherosclerosis, the predictive value of this technique is still under investigation.[83] Both studies were funded by companies that market garlic supplements.

Summary: Cardiovascular Disease

In summary, the results of randomized controlled trials suggest that garlic supplementation inhibits platelet aggregation and modestly improves serum lipid profiles when taken for 3 months. It is not yet known whether garlic supplementation can reduce atherosclerosis or prevent cardiovascular events, such as myocardial infarction or stroke.

Cancer

Gastric Cancer

In an area of China associated with low mortality from gastric (stomach) cancer, 82% of men and 74% of women reportedly consumed garlic at least three times weekly. In contrast, in an area of China known for its high mortality from gastric cancer, only 1% of men and women consumed garlic at least three times weekly.[84] Three out of four case–control studies in Europe and Asia found that past garlic consumption was significantly lower in people diagnosed with gastric cancer than in cancer-free control groups.[85–87] A meta-analysis that combined the results of case–control studies found that those with the highest garlic intakes had a risk of gastric cancer that was approximately 50% lower than in those with low garlic intakes.[88] In contrast, a prospective cohort study in the Netherlands found no association between the use of garlic supplements and risk of gastric cancer.[89] However, it is important to note that one study reported that the composition of sulfur compounds in various commercially available garlic supplements sold in Europe varied by more than 12-fold.[90] More recently, a randomized, double-blind, placebo-controlled intervention study in China found that supplementation with aged garlic extract and steam-distilled garlic oil for 7.3 years did not reduce the prevalence of precancerous gastric lesions or the incidence of gastric cancer.[60] The amount of garlic compounds consumed as supplements is probably considerably lower than the amount consumed in garlic food. Thus, regular consumption of garlic food may be needed to observe any anti-cancer effects.

Helicobacter pylori **infection and gastric cancer.** Infection with some strains of *Helicobacter pylori* bacteria markedly increases the risk of gastric cancer. Although garlic preparations and organosulfur compounds have been found to inhibit the growth of *H. pylori* in the laboratory, there is little evidence that high garlic intakes or garlic supplementation can prevent or eradicate *H. pylori* infection in humans.[91,92] Higher intakes of garlic were not associated with a significantly lower prevalence of *H. pylori* infection in China or Turkey.[93,94] Moreover, clinical trials using garlic cloves,[95] aged garlic extract,[59] steam-distilled garlic oil,[59,96] garlic oil macerate,[97] or garlic pow-

der[98] have not found garlic supplementation to be effective in eradicating *H. pylori* infection in humans.

Colorectal Cancer

Three out of four case–control studies found that garlic intake was significantly lower in people diagnosed with colorectal cancer than in cancer-free control groups.[99–101] In contrast, three prospective cohort studies found no association between garlic consumption and colorectal cancer risk.[102–104] However, garlic consumption was generally low in these cohorts, and one study assessed only the garlic supplement use.[102] A meta-analysis that combined the results of case–control and prospective studies found that the risk of colorectal cancer was approximately 30% lower in those with the highest garlic intakes compared with those with the lowest intakes.[88] An analysis of data from case–control studies conducted in Italy and Switzerland found a similar 26% reduction in risk for those with the highest garlic intake compared with the lowest.[105] Colorectal adenomas (polyps) are precancerous lesions. One case–control study of adults undergoing sigmoidoscopy found that those with colorectal adenomas consumed significantly less garlic than those in whom no colorectal adenomas were found.[106] A small preliminary intervention trial in 37 patients with colorectal adenomas examined whether supplementation with aged garlic extract for 12 months affected adenoma size and recurrence. Both the number and size of adenomas were significantly reduced in patients given a high dose of aged garlic extract (2.4 mL/day) compared with those given a much lower dose (0.16 mL/day).[107,108] Larger randomized controlled trials are needed to determine whether garlic or garlic extracts can substantially reduce adenoma recurrence.

Summary: Cancer

The results of epidemiological studies in human populations suggest that high intakes of garlic and other *Allium* vegetables may help protect against gastric and colorectal cancer, but evidence that high intakes of garlic can reduce the risk of other types of cancer in humans is limited and inconsistent.[88,109] Although garlic and organosulfur compounds have been found to inhibit the development of chemically induced cancers in animal models of oral, esophageal, gastric, colon, uterine, breast, prostate,[110] and skin cancer,[51] it is not known whether garlic-derived organosulfur compounds can prevent or slow the development of cancer in humans.

Sources

Food Sources

Allium vegetables, including garlic and onions, are the richest sources of organosulfur compounds in the human diet.[109] To date, the majority of scientific research relating to the health effects of organosulfur compounds has focused on those derived from garlic. Fresh garlic cloves contain approximately 2–6 mg/g of γ-glutamyl-*S*-allylcysteine (0.2%–0.6% fresh weight) and 6–14 mg/g of alliin (0.6%–1.4% fresh weight). Garlic cloves yield approximately 2500–4500 µg of allicin per gram of fresh weight when crushed. One fresh garlic clove weighs 2–4 g.[1]

Effects of Cooking

The enzyme alliinase can be inactivated by heat. In one study, microwave cooking of unpeeled, uncrushed garlic completely destroyed alliinase enzyme activity.[111] An in vitro study found that prolonged oven heating or boiling (i.e., 6 minutes or longer) suppressed the inhibitory effect of uncrushed and crushed garlic on platelet aggregation, but crushed garlic retained more antiaggre-gatory activity compared with uncrushed garlic.[112] Administering raw garlic to rats significantly decreased the amount of DNA damage caused by a chemical carcinogen, but heating uncrushed garlic cloves for 60 seconds in a microwave oven or 45 minutes in a convection oven prior to administration blocked the protective effect of garlic.[113] The protective effect of garlic against DNA damage can be partially conserved by crushing garlic and allowing it to stand for 10 minutes prior to microwave heating for 60 seconds or by cutting the tops off garlic cloves and allowing them to stand for 10 minutes before heating in a convection oven. Because organosulfur compounds derived from alliinase-catalyzed reactions appear to play a role in some of the biological effects of garlic, some scientists recommend that crushed or chopped garlic be allowed to "stand" for at least 10 minutes prior to cooking.[111]

Supplements

Several different types of garlic preparations are available commercially, and each type provides a different profile of organosulfur compounds depending on how it was processed (**Table 17.1**). Not all garlic preparations are standardized, and even standardized brands may vary with respect to the amount and the bioavailability of the organosulfur compounds they provide.[1]

Table 17.1 Principal organosulfur compounds in commercial garlic preparations[1]

Product	Principal Organosulfur Compounds	Delivers Allicin-Derived Compounds?
Fresh garlic cloves	Cysteine sulfoxides (alliin)	Yes, when chopped, crushed, or chewed raw
	γ-Glutamylcysteines	Minimally, when garlic cloves are cooked before crushing or chopping
Powdered garlic (tablets)	Cysteine sulfoxides (alliin)	Varies greatly among commercial products. Enteric-coated tablets that pass the USP[a] allicin-release test are likely to provide the most
	γ-Glutamylcysteines	
Steam-distilled garlic oil (capsules)	Diallyl disulfide Diallyl trisulfide Allyl methyl trisulfide	Yes
Garlic oil macerate (capsules)	Vinyldithiins Ajoene Diallyl trisulfide	Yes
Aged garlic extract (tablets or capsules)	S-Allylcysteine S-Allylmercaptocysteine S-1-Propenylcysteine	Minimally

[a] United States Pharmacopeia Convention.

Powdered (Dehydrated) Garlic

Powdered or dehydrated garlic is made from garlic cloves that are usually sliced and dried at a low temperature to prevent alliinase inactivation.[114] The dried garlic is pulverized and often made into tablets. To meet United States Pharmacopeia Convention (USP) standards, powdered garlic supplements must contain no less than 0.1% γ-glutamyl-S-allylcysteine and no less than 0.3% alliin (dry weight).[115] Although powdered garlic supplements do not actually contain allicin, the manufacturer may provide a value for the "allicin potential" or "allicin yield" of a supplement on the label. These values represent the maximum achievable allicin yield of a supplement.[116] It is determined by dissolving powdered garlic in water at room temperature and measuring the allicin content after 30 minutes.[115] Because alliinase is inactivated at the acidic pH of the stomach, most powdered garlic tablets are enteric coated to keep them from dissolving before they reach the neutral pH of the intestine. It has been argued that it is more appropriate to measure "allicin release" using a USP method for assessing drug release from enteric-coated tablets under conditions that mimic those of the stomach and intestine.[115] Allicin release by this method has been shown to parallel true bioavailability.[116] Most tablet brands have been found to produce little allicin under these conditions, due mainly to low alliinase activity and prolonged disintegration times.[116,117] Many manufacturers provide information on the "allicin potential" of their powdered garlic supplements, but few provide information on the "allicin release." Several controlled clinical trials have examined the effect of powdered or dehydrated garlic supplements on cardiovascular risk factors (see the Cardiovascular Disease section above). The most commonly used doses ranged from 600 mg/day to 900 mg/day and provided 3600–5400 µg/day of potential allicin.[63]

Garlic Fluid Extracts (Aged Garlic Extract)

When garlic cloves are incubated in a solution of ethanol and water for up to 20 months, allicin is mainly converted to allyl sulfides, which are lost by evaporation or converted to other compounds.[114] The resulting extract contains primarily water-soluble organosulfur compounds, such as S-allylcysteine and SAMC.[118] Garlic fluid extracts, including aged garlic extracts, are standardized to their S-allylcysteine content. In controlled clinical trials, aged garlic extract at doses of 2.4–7.2 g/day resulted in short-term reductions in ex-vivo platelet aggregation[11] and reductions in serum cholesterol levels up to 12 weeks.[119]

Steam-Distilled Garlic Oil

Steam distillation of crushed garlic cloves results in a product that contains mainly allyl sulfides, including DATS, DADS, and DAS.[114] These fat-soluble steam-distillation products are usually dissolved in vegetable oil.

Garlic Oil Macerates

Incubation of crushed garlic cloves in oil at room temperature results in the formation of vinyldithiins and ajoene from allicin, in addition to allyl sulfides, such as DADS and DATS.[1] Ether extracts are similar in composition to garlic oil macerates, but more concentrated.[76]

Safety

Adverse Effects

The most commonly reported adverse effects of oral ingestion of garlic and garlic supplements are breath and body odor.[63,120] Gastrointestinal symptoms have also been reported, including heartburn, abdominal pain, nausea, vomiting, flatulence, and diarrhea.[121] The most serious adverse effects associated with oral garlic supplementation are related to uncontrolled bleeding. Several cases of serious postoperative or spontaneous bleeding associated with garlic supplementation have been reported in the medical literature.[122–125] Garlic may trigger allergic responses in some individuals, including asthma in people with occupational exposure to garlic powder or dust.[126] Exposure of the skin to garlic has been reported to cause contact dermatitis in some individuals.[120,127] More serious skin lesions, including blisters and burns, have also been reported with topical exposure to garlic for 6 hours or more.

Pregnancy and Lactation

No adverse effects on pregnancy outcomes have been reported when garlic is consumed in the diet. Although no adverse pregnancy outcomes were reported in a study of Iranian women who took dehydrated garlic tablets (800 mg/day) for 2 months during the third trimester of pregnancy,[128] the safety of garlic supplements in pregnancy has not been established. There is some evidence that garlic consumption alters the odor and possibly the flavor of breast milk. In a controlled crossover trial, oral consumption of 1.5 g of garlic extract by lactating women increased the perceived intensity of breast-milk odor.[129] Infants spent more time breast-feeding after their mothers consumed the garlic extract compared with a placebo, but the amount of milk consumed and number of feedings was not significantly different. Additionally, it is not known if topical use of garlic is safe during pregnancy or lactation.

Drug Interactions

Anticoagulant Medications

Garlic may enhance the anticoagulant effects of warfarin (Coumadin). There have been two case reports in which prothrombin time (international normalized ratio—INR) increased in patients who started taking garlic tablets or garlic oil without changing their warfarin dose or other habits.[130] However, a study in closely monitored patients on warfarin therapy found that garlic fluid extracts (aged garlic extract) did not increase hemorrhagic risk.[131] Since garlic supplements have been found to inhibit platelet aggregation,[63] there is a potential for additive effects when garlic supplements are taken together with other medications or supplements that inhibit platelet aggregation, such as high-dose fish oil or vitamin E.[132] More research is needed to determine whether garlic supplements are safe for people on anticoagulant therapy.

HIV Protease Inhibitors

Giving supplements of garlic caplets twice daily (allicin yield, 7200 μg/day) for 3 weeks to healthy volunteers of resulted in a 50% decrease in the bioavailability of the protease inhibitor, saquinavir (Fortovase).[133] Although saquinavir undergoes significant metabolism by CYP3A4, supplementation with garlic extract for 2 weeks did not significantly alter a measure of CYP3A4 activity in healthy volunteers.[134] Garlic extract supplementation (10 mg/day) for 4 days did not significantly alter single-dose pharmacokinetics of the protease inhibitor, ritonavir (Norvir), but further research is needed to determine steady-state interactions between well-characterized garlic supplements and ritonavir.[135]

Summary

- Garlic (*Allium sativum* L.) is a particularly rich source of organosulfur compounds, which are currently under investigation for their potential to prevent and treat disease.
- Crushing or chopping garlic releases an enzyme called *alliinase* that catalyzes the formation of allicin. Allicin rapidly breaks down to form a variety of organosulfur compounds.
- Since cooking can inactivate alliinase, some scientists recommend letting garlic stand for 10 minutes after chopping or crushing before cooking it.
- Several different types of garlic supplements are available commercially, and each type provides a different profile of organosulfur compounds depending on how it was processed.
- The results of randomized controlled trials suggest that garlic supplementation inhibits platelet aggregation, but it is not known whether garlic supplementation can prevent cardiovascular disease.
- The results of a few epidemiological studies suggest that high intakes of garlic and other *Allium* vegetables (e.g., onions and leeks) may help protect against gastric and colorectal cancer, but it is not known whether garlic-derived organosulfur compounds are effective in preventing or treating human cancers.

References

1. Lawson LD. Garlic: a review of its medicinal effects and indicated active compounds. In: Lawson LD, Bauer R, eds. Phytomedicines of Europe: Chemistry and Biological Activity. Washington, DC: American Chemical Society; 1998:177–209
2. Block E. The chemistry of garlic and onions. Sci Am 1985;252(3):114–119
3. Blumenthal M. Herb sales down 7.4 percent in mainstream market. HerbalGram 2005;6663
4. Tapiero H, Townsend DM, Tew KD. Organosulfur compounds from alliaceae in the prevention of human pathologies. Biomed Pharmacother 2004;58(3):183–193
5. Lawson LD, Wang ZJ. Allicin and allicin-derived garlic compounds increase breath acetone through allyl methyl sulfide: use in measuring allicin bioavailability. J Agric Food Chem 2005;53(6):1974–1983

6. Germain E, Auger J, Ginies C, Siess MH, Teyssier C. In vivo metabolism of diallyl disulphide in the rat: identification of two new metabolites. Xenobiotica 2002;32(12):1127–1138

7. Lachmann G, Lorenz D, Radeck W, Steiper M. The pharmacokinetics of the S35 labeled labeled garlic constituents alliin, allicin and vinyldithiine [in German]. Arzneimittelforschung 1994;44(6):734–743

8. de Rooij BM, Boogaard PJ, Rijksen DA, Commandeur JN, Vermeulen NP. Urinary excretion of N-acetyl-S-allyl-L-cysteine upon garlic consumption by human volunteers. Arch Toxicol 1996;70(10):635–639

9. Jandke J, Spiteller G. Unusual conjugates in biological profiles originating from consumption of onions and garlic. J Chromatogr A 1987;421(1):1–8

10. Kodera Y, Suzuki A, Imada O, et al. Physical, chemical, and biological properties of s-allylcysteine, an amino acid derived from garlic. J Agric Food Chem 2002;50(3):622–632

11. Steiner M, Li W. Aged garlic extract, a modulator of cardiovascular risk factors: a dose-finding study on the effects of AGE on platelet functions. J Nutr 2001;131(3s):980S–984S

12. Gebhardt R, Beck H. Differential inhibitory effects of garlic-derived organosulfur compounds on cholesterol biosynthesis in primary rat hepatocyte cultures. Lipids 1996;31(12):1269–1276

13. Ferri N, Yokoyama K, Sadilek M, et al. Ajoene, a garlic compound, inhibits protein prenylation and arterial smooth muscle cell proliferation. Br J Pharmacol 2003;138(5):811–818

14. Liu L, Yeh YY. S-alk(en)yl cysteines of garlic inhibit cholesterol synthesis by deactivating HMG-CoA reductase in cultured rat hepatocytes. J Nutr 2002;132(6):1129–1134

15. Singh DK, Porter TD. Inhibition of sterol 4alpha-methyl oxidase is the principal mechanism by which garlic decreases cholesterol synthesis. J Nutr 2006; 136(3, Suppl):759S–764S

16. Chan KC, Hsu CC, Yin MC. Protective effect of three diallyl sulphides against glucose-induced erythrocyte and platelet oxidation, and ADP-induced platelet aggregation. Thromb Res 2002;108(5–6):317–322

17. Lawson LD, Ransom DK, Hughes BG. Inhibition of whole blood platelet-aggregation by compounds in garlic clove extracts and commercial garlic products. Thromb Res 1992;65(2):141–156

18. Blake GJ, Ridker PM. C-reactive protein and other inflammatory risk markers in acute coronary syndromes. J Am Coll Cardiol 2003; 41(4, Suppl S)37S–42S

19. Ali M, Thomson M, Afzal M. Garlic and onions: their effect on eicosanoid metabolism and its clinical relevance. Prostaglandins Leukot Essent Fatty Acids 2000;62(2):55–73

20. Dirsch VM, Kiemer AK, Wagner H, Vollmar AM. Effect of allicin and ajoene, two compounds of garlic, on inducible nitric oxide synthase. Atherosclerosis 1998; 139(2):333–339

21. Kim KM, Chun SB, Koo MS, et al. Differential regulation of NO availability from macrophages and endothelial cells by the garlic component S-allyl cysteine. Free Radic Biol Med 2001;30(7):747–756

22. Chang HP, Huang SY, Chen YH. Modulation of cytokine secretion by garlic oil derivatives is associated with suppressed nitric oxide production in stimulated macrophages. J Agric Food Chem 2005;53(7):2530–2534

23. Keiss HP, Dirsch VM, Hartung T, et al. Garlic (Allium sativum L.) modulates cytokine expression in lipopolysaccharide-activated human blood thereby inhibiting NF-kappaB activity. J Nutr 2003;133(7):2171–2175

24. Hedin U, Roy J, Tran PK. Control of smooth muscle cell proliferation in vascular disease. Curr Opin Lipidol 2004;15(5):559–565

25. Campbell JH, Efendy JL, Smith NJ, Campbell GR. Molecular basis by which garlic suppresses atherosclerosis. J Nutr 2001;131(3s):1006S–1009S

26. Golovchenko I, Yang CH, Goalstone ML, Draznin B. Garlic extract methylallyl thiosulfinate blocks insulin potentiation of platelet-derived growth factor-stimulated migration of vascular smooth muscle cells. Metabolism 2003;52(2):254–259

27. Banerjee SK, Mukherjee PK, Maulik SK. Garlic as an antioxidant: the good, the bad and the ugly. Phytother Res 2003;17(2):97–106

28. Dhawan V, Jain S. Effect of garlic supplementation on oxidized low density lipoproteins and lipid peroxidation in patients of essential hypertension. Mol Cell Biochem 2004;266(1–2):109–115

29. Pryor WA, Houk KN, Foote CS, et al. Free radical biology and medicine: it's a gas, man! Am J Physiol Regul Integr Comp Physiol 2006;291(3):R491–R511

30. Lefer DJ. A new gaseous signaling molecule emerges: cardioprotective role of hydrogen sulfide. Proc Natl Acad Sci U S A 2007;104(46):17907–17908

31. Benavides GA, Squadrito GL, Mills RW, et al. Hydrogen sulfide mediates the vasoactivity of garlic. Proc Natl Acad Sci U S A 2007;104(46):17977–17982

32. Suarez F, Springfield J, Furne J, Levitt M. Differentiation of mouth versus gut as site of origin of odoriferous breath gases after garlic ingestion. Am J Physiol 1999;276(2 Pt 1):G425–G430

33. Yang CS, Chhabra SK, Hong JY, Smith TJ. Mechanisms of inhibition of chemical toxicity and carcinogenesis by diallyl sulfide (DAS) and related compounds from garlic. J Nutr 2001;131(3s):1041S–1045S

34. Brady JF, Ishizaki H, Fukuto JM, et al. Inhibition of cytochrome P-450 2E1 by diallyl sulfide and its metabolites. Chem Res Toxicol 1991;4(6):642–647

35. Jeong HG, Lee YW. Protective effects of diallyl sulfide on N-nitrosodimethylamine-induced immunosuppression in mice. Cancer Lett 1998;134(1):73–79

36. Park KA, Kweon S, Choi H. Anticarcinogenic effect and modification of cytochrome P450 2E1 by dietary garlic powder in diethylnitrosamine-initiated rat hepatocarcinogenesis. J Biochem Mol Biol 2002;35(6):615–622

37. Gurley BJ, Gardner SF, Hubbard MA, et al. Cytochrome P450 phenotypic ratios for predicting herb-drug interactions in humans. Clin Pharmacol Ther 2002; 72(3):276–287

38. Loizou GD, Cocker J. The effects of alcohol and diallyl sulphide on CYP2E1 activity in humans: a phenotyping study using chlorzoxazone. Hum Exp Toxicol 2001;20(7):321–327

39. Munday R, Munday CM. Induction of phase II enzymes by aliphatic sulfides derived from garlic and onions: an overview. Methods Enzymol 2004; 382:449–456

40. Andorfer JH, Tchaikovskaya T, Listowsky I. Selective expression of glutathione S-transferase genes in the murine gastrointestinal tract in response to dietary organosulfur compounds. Carcinogenesis 2004 ;25 (3):359–367

41. Hatono S, Jimenez A, Wargovich MJ. Chemopreventive effect of S-allylcysteine and its relationship to the detoxification enzyme glutathione S-transferase. Carcinogenesis 1996;17(5):1041–1044

42. Munday R, Munday CM. Relative activities of organosulfur compounds derived from onions and garlic in increasing tissue activities of quinone reductase and glutathione transferase in rat tissues. Nutr Cancer 2001;40(2):205–210

43. Chen C, Pung D, Leong V, et al. Induction of detoxifying enzymes by garlic organosulfur compounds through transcription factor Nrf2: effect of chemical structure and stress signals. Free Radic Biol Med 2004;37(10):1578–1590

44. Fisher CD, Augustine LM, Maher JM, et al. Induction of drug-metabolizing enzymes by garlic and allyl sulfide compounds via activation of constitutive androstane receptor and nuclear factor E2-related factor 2. Drug Metab Dispos 2007;35(6):995–1000

45. Munday R, Munday CM. Low doses of diallyl disulfide, a compound derived from garlic, increase tissue activities of quinone reductase and glutathione transferase in the gastrointestinal tract of the rat. Nutr Cancer 1999;34(1):42–48

46. Kweon S, Park KA, Choi H. Chemopreventive effect of garlic powder diet in diethylnitrosamine-induced rat hepatocarcinogenesis. Life Sci 2003;73(19):2515–2526

47. Stewart ZA, Westfall MD, Pietenpol JA. Cell-cycle dysregulation and anticancer therapy. Trends Pharmacol Sci 2003;24(3):139–145

48. Herman-Antosiewicz A, Singh SV. Signal transduction pathways leading to cell cycle arrest and apoptosis induction in cancer cells by Allium vegetable-derived organosulfur compounds: a review. Mutat Res 2004;555(1–2):121–131

49. Knowles LM, Milner JA. Possible mechanism by which allyl sulfides suppress neoplastic cell proliferation. J Nutr 2001;131(3s):1061S–1066S

50. Arunkumar A, Vijayababu MR, Srinivasan N, Aruldhas MM, Arunakaran J. Garlic compound, diallyl disulfide induces cell cycle arrest in prostate cancer cell line PC-3. Mol Cell Biochem 2006;288(1–2):107–113

51. Wu X, Kassie F, Mersch-Sundermann V. Induction of apoptosis in tumor cells by naturally occurring sulfur-containing compounds. Mutat Res 2005;589(2):81–102

52. Balasenthil S, Rao KS, Nagini S. Apoptosis induction by S-allylcysteine, a garlic constituent, during 7,12-dimethylbenz[a]anthracene-induced hamster buccal pouch carcinogenesis. Cell Biochem Funct 2002;20(3):263–268

53. Balasenthil S, Rao KS, Nagini S. Garlic induces apoptosis during 7,12-dimethylbenz[a]anthracene-induced hamster buccal pouch carcinogenesis. Oral Oncol 2002;38(5):431–436

54. Fenwick GR, Hanley AB. The genus Allium–Part 3. Crit Rev Food Sci Nutr 1985;23(1):1–73

55. Harris JC, Cottrell SL, Plummer S, Lloyd D. Antimicrobial properties of Allium sativum (garlic). Appl Microbiol Biotechnol 2001;57(3):282–286

56. Ankri S, Mirelman D. Antimicrobial properties of allicin from garlic. Microbes Infect 1999;1(2):125–129

57. Cavallito CJ, Bailey JH. Allicin, the antibacterial principle of Allium sativum. I. Isolation, physical properties and antibacterial action. J Am Chem Soc 1944;66(11):1950–1951

58. Martin KW, Ernst E. Herbal medicines for treatment of bacterial infections: a review of controlled clinical trials. J Antimicrob Chemother 2003;51(2):241–246

59. Gail MH, Pfeiffer RM, Brown LM, et al. Garlic, vitamin, and antibiotic treatment for Helicobacter pylori: a randomized factorial controlled trial. Helicobacter 2007;12(5):575–578

60. You WC, Brown LM, Zhang L, et al. Randomized double-blind factorial trial of three treatments to reduce the prevalence of precancerous gastric lesions. J Natl Cancer Inst 2006;98(14):974–983

61. Ledezma E, Marcano K, Jorquera A, Padilla M, Pulgar M, Apitz-Castro R; De Sousa L. Efficacy of ajoene in the treatment of tinea pedis: a double-blind and comparative study with terbinafine. J Am Acad Dermatol 2000;43(5 Pt 1):829–832

62. Keys A. Wine, garlic, and CHD in seven countries. Lancet 1980;1(8160):145–146

63. Ackermann RT, Mulrow CD, Ramirez G, Gardner CD, Morbidoni L, Lawrence VA. Garlic shows promise for improving some cardiovascular risk factors. Arch Intern Med 2001;161(6):813–824

64. Alder R, Lookinland S, Berry JA, Williams M. A systematic review of the effectiveness of garlic as an anti-hyperlipidemic agent. J Am Acad Nurse Pract 2003;15(3):120–129

65. Stevinson C, Pittler MH, Ernst E. Garlic for treating hypercholesterolemia. A meta-analysis of randomized clinical trials. Ann Intern Med 2000;133(6):420–429

66. Berthold HK, Sudhop T, von Bergmann K. Effect of a garlic oil preparation on serum lipoproteins and cholesterol metabolism: a randomized controlled trial. JAMA 1998;279(23):1900–1902

67. Gardner CD, Chatterjee LM, Carlson JJ. The effect of a garlic preparation on plasma lipid levels in moderately hypercholesterolemic adults. Atherosclerosis 2001;154(1):213–220

68. Kannar D, Wattanapenpaiboon N, Savige GS, Wahlqvist ML. Hypocholesterolemic effect of an enteric-coated garlic supplement. J Am Coll Nutr 2001;20(3):225–231

69. McCrindle BW, Helden E, Conner WT. Garlic extract therapy in children with hypercholesterolemia. Arch Pediatr Adolesc Med 1998;152(11):1089–1094

70. Neil HA, Silagy CA, Lancaster T, et al. Garlic powder in the treatment of moderate hyperlipidaemia: a controlled trial and meta-analysis. J R Coll Physicians Lond 1996;30(4):329–334

71. Turner B, Mølgaard C, Marckmann P. Effect of garlic (Allium sativum) powder tablets on serum lipids, blood pressure and arterial stiffness in normo-lipidaemic volunteers: a randomised, double-blind, placebo-controlled trial. Br J Nutr 2004;92(4):701–706

72. Zhang L, Gail MH, Wang YQ, et al. A randomized factorial study of the effects of long-term garlic and micronutrient supplementation and of 2-wk antibiotic treatment for Helicobacter pylori infection on serum cholesterol and lipoproteins. Am J Clin Nutr 2006;84(4):912–919

73. van Doorn MB, Espirito Santo SM, Meijer P, et al. Effect of garlic powder on C-reactive protein and plasma lipids in overweight and smoking subjects. Am J Clin Nutr 2006;84(6):1324–1329

74. Gardner CD, Lawson LD, Block E, et al. Effect of raw garlic vs commercial garlic supplements on plasma lipid concentrations in adults with moderate hypercholesterolemia: a randomized clinical trial. Arch Intern Med 2007;167(4):346–353

75. Rahman K, Billington D. Dietary supplementation with aged garlic extract inhibits ADP-induced platelet aggregation in humans. J Nutr 2000; 130(11): 2662–2665

76. Brace LD. Cardiovascular benefits of garlic (Allium sativum L). J Cardiovasc Nurs 2002;16(4):33–49

77. Adler AJ, Holub BJ. Effect of garlic and fish-oil supplementation on serum lipid and lipoprotein concentrations in hypercholesterolemic men. Am J Clin Nutr 1997;65(2):445–450

78. Auer W, Eiber A, Hertkorn E, et al. Hypertension and hyperlipidaemia: garlic helps in mild cases. Br J Clin Pract Suppl 1990;69:3–6

79. Vorberg G, Schneider B. Therapy with garlic: results of a placebo-controlled, double-blind study. Br J Clin Pract Suppl 1990;69:7–11

80. Koscielny J, Klüssendorf D, Latza R, et al. The antiatherosclerotic effect of Allium sativum. Atherosclerosis 1999;144(1):237–249

81. Siegel G, Klüssendorf D. The anti-atheroslerotic effect of Allium sativum: statistics re-evaluated. Atherosclerosis 2000;150(2):437–438

82. Budoff MJ, Takasu J, Flores FR, et al. Inhibiting progression of coronary calcification using Aged Garlic Extract in patients receiving statin therapy: a preliminary study. Prev Med 2004;39(5):985–991

83. Vliegenthart R. Non-invasive assessment of coronary calcification. Eur J Epidemiol 2004;19(12):1063–1072

84. Takezaki T, Gao CM, Ding JH, Liu TK, Li MS, Tajima K. Comparative study of lifestyles of residents in high and low risk areas for gastric cancer in Jiangsu Province, China; with special reference to allium vegetables. J Epidemiol 1999;9(5):297–305

85. Buiatti E, Palli D, Decarli A, et al. A case-control study of gastric cancer and diet in Italy. Int J Cancer 1989;44(4):611–616

86. Kim HJ, Chang WK, Kim MK, Lee SS, Choi BY. Dietary factors and gastric cancer in Korea: a case-control study. Int J Cancer 2002;97(4):531–535

87. You WC, Blot WJ, Chang YS, et al. Allium vegetables and reduced risk of stomach cancer. J Natl Cancer Inst 1989;81(2):162–164

88. Fleischauer AT, Poole C, Arab L. Garlic consumption and cancer prevention: meta-analyses of colorectal and stomach cancers. Am J Clin Nutr 2000;72(4): 1047–1052

89. Dorant E, van den Brandt PA, Goldbohm RA, Sturmans F. Consumption of onions and a reduced risk of stomach carcinoma. Gastroenterology 1996;110(1): 12–20

90. Lawson LD, Wang ZJ, Hughes BG. Identification and HPLC quantitation of the sulfides and dialk(en)yl thiosulfinates in commercial garlic products. Planta Med 1991;57(4):363–370

91. Cañizares P, Gracia I, Gómez LA, et al. Allyl-thiosulfinates, the bacteriostatic compounds of garlic against Helicobacter pylori. Biotechnol Prog 2004; 20(1):397–401

92. O'Gara EA, Hill DJ, Maslin DJ. Activities of garlic oil, garlic powder, and their diallyl constituents against Helicobacter pylori. Appl Environ Microbiol 2000; 66(5):2269–2273

93. Salih BA, Abasiyanik FM. Does regular garlic intake affect the prevalence of Helicobacter pylori in asymptomatic subjects? Saudi Med J 2003;24(8):842–845

94. You WC, Zhang L, Gail MH, et al. Helicobacter pylori infection, garlic intake and precancerous lesions in a Chinese population at low risk of gastric cancer. Int J Epidemiol 1998;27(6):941–944

95. Graham DY, Anderson SY, Lang T. Garlic or jalapeño peppers for treatment of Helicobacter pylori infection. Am J Gastroenterol 1999;94(5):1200–1202

96. McNulty CA, Wilson MP, Havinga W, Johnston B, O'Gara EA, Maslin DJ. A pilot study to determine the effectiveness of garlic oil capsules in the treatment of dyspeptic patients with Helicobacter pylori. Helicobacter 2001;6(3):249–253

97. Aydin A, Ersöz G, Tekesin O, Akçiçek E, Tuncyürek M. Garlic oil and Helicobacter pylori infection. Am J Gastroenterol 2000;95(2):563–564

98. Ernst E. Is garlic an effective treatment for Helicobacter pylori infection? Arch Intern Med 1999; 159(20):2484–2485

99. Hu JF, Liu YY, Yu YK, Zhao TZ, Liu SD, Wang QQ. Diet and cancer of the colon and rectum: a case-control study in China. Int J Epidemiol 1991;20(2):362–367

100. Iscovich JM, L'Abbé KA, Castelleto R, et al. Colon cancer in Argentina. I: Risk from intake of dietary items. Int J Cancer 1992;51(6):851–857

101. Levi F, Pasche C, La Vecchia C, Lucchini F, Franceschi S. Food groups and colorectal cancer risk. Br J Cancer 1999;79(7–8):1283–1287

102. Dorant E, van den Brandt PA, Goldbohm RA. A prospective cohort study on the relationship between onion and leek consumption, garlic supplement use and the risk of colorectal carcinoma in The Netherlands. Carcinogenesis 1996;17(3):477–484

103. Giovannucci E, Rimm EB, Stampfer MJ, Colditz GA, Ascherio A, Willett WC. Intake of fat, meat, and fiber in relation to risk of colon cancer in men. Cancer Res 1994;54(9):2390–2397

104. Steinmetz KA, Kushi LH, Bostick RM, Folsom AR, Potter JD. Vegetables, fruit, and colon cancer in the Iowa Women's Health Study. Am J Epidemiol 1994; 139(1):1–15

105. Galeone C, Pelucchi C, Levi F, et al. Onion and garlic use and human cancer. Am J Clin Nutr 2006; 84(5):1027–1032

106. Witte JS, Longnecker MP, Bird CL, Lee ER, Frankl HD, Haile RW. Relation of vegetable, fruit, and grain consumption to colorectal adenomatous polyps. Am J Epidemiol 1996;144(11):1015–1025

107. Tanaka S, Haruma K, Kunihiro M, et al. Effects of aged garlic extract (AGE) on colorectal adenomas: a double-blinded study. Hiroshima J Med Sci 2004;53(3–4):39–45

108. Tanaka S, Haruma K, Yoshihara M, et al. Aged garlic extract has potential suppressive effect on colorectal adenomas in humans. J Nutr 2006; 136(3, Suppl): 821S–826S

109. Bianchini F, Vainio H. Allium vegetables and organosulfur compounds: do they help prevent cancer? Environ Health Perspect 2001;109(9):893–902

110. Arunkumar A, Vijayababu MR, Venkataraman P, Senthilkumar K, Arunakaran J. Chemoprevention of rat prostate carcinogenesis by diallyl disulfide, an organosulfur compound of garlic. Biol Pharm Bull 2006;29(2):375–379

111. Song K, Milner JA. The influence of heating on the anticancer properties of garlic. J Nutr 2001; 131(3s):1054S–1057S

112. Cavagnaro PF, Camargo A, Galmarini CR, Simon PW. Effect of cooking on garlic (Allium sativum L.) antiplatelet activity and thiosulfinates content. J Agric Food Chem 2007;55(4):1280–1288

113. Song K, Milner JA. Heating garlic inhibits its ability to suppress 7, 12-dimethylbenz(a)anthracene-induced DNA adduct formation in rat mammary tissue. J Nutr 1999;129(3):657–661

114. Staba EJ, Lash L, Staba JE. A commentary on the effects of garlic extraction and formulation on product composition. J Nutr 2001;131(3s):1118S–1119S

115. Dietary Supplements. Garlic. The United States Pharmacopeia. Vol 28. Rockville, MD: United States Pharmacopeial Convention, Inc; 2005:2087–2092

116. Lawson LD, Wang ZJ. Low allicin release from garlic supplements: a major problem due to the sensitivities of alliinase activity. J Agric Food Chem 2001;49(5):2592–2599

117. Lawson LD, Wang ZJ, Papadimitriou D. Allicin release under simulated gastrointestinal conditions from garlic powder tablets employed in clinical trials on serum cholesterol. Planta Med 2001;67(1):13–18

118. Amagase H, Petesch BL, Matsuura H, Kasuga S, Itakura Y. Intake of garlic and its bioactive components. J Nutr 2001;131(3s):955S–962S

119. Steiner M, Khan AH, Holbert D, Lin RI. A double-blind crossover study in moderately hypercholesterolemic men that compared the effect of aged garlic extract and placebo administration on blood lipids. Am J Clin Nutr 1996;64(6):866–870

120. Borrelli F, Capasso R, Izzo AA. Garlic (Allium sativum L.): adverse effects and drug interactions in humans. Mol Nutr Food Res 2007;51(11):1386–1397

121. Mulrow C, Lawrence V, Ackermann R, et al. Garlic: Effects on Cardiovascular Risks and Disease, Protective Effects against Cancer, and Clinical Adverse Effects. Rockville, MD: Agency for Healthcare Research and Quality; 2000 [Evidence Report/Technology Assessment No. 20]. Available at: http://www.ncbi. nlm.nih.gov/books/NBK11910/. Accessed May 7, 2012

122. Burnham BE. Garlic as a possible risk for postoperative bleeding. Plast Reconstr Surg 1995;95(1):213

123. Carden SM, Good WV, Carden PA, Good RM. Garlic and the strabismus surgeon. Clin Experiment Ophthalmol 2002;30(4):303–304

124. German K, Kumar U, Blackford HN. Garlic and the risk of TURP bleeding. Br J Urol 1995;76(4):518

125. Rose KD, Croissant PD, Parliament CF, Levin MB. Spontaneous spinal epidural hematoma with associated platelet dysfunction from excessive garlic ingestion: a case report. Neurosurgery 1990;26(5):880–882

126. Añibarro B, Fontela JL, De La Hoz F. Occupational asthma induced by garlic dust. J Allergy Clin Immunol 1997;100(6 Pt 1):734–738

127. Jappe U, Bonnekoh B, Hausen BM, Gollnick H. Garlic-related dermatoses: case report and review of the literature. Am J Contact Dermat 1999;10(1):37–39

128. Ziaei S, Hantoshzadeh S, Rezasoltani P, Lamyian M. The effect of garlic tablet on plasma lipids and platelet aggregation in nulliparous pregnants at high risk of preeclampsia. Eur J Obstet Gynecol Reprod Biol 2001;99(2):201–206

129. Mennella JA, Beauchamp GK. Maternal diet alters the sensory qualities of human milk and the nursling's behavior. Pediatrics 1991;88(4):737–744

130. Sunter WH. Warfarin and garlic. [Letter] Pharm J 1991;246:722

131. Macan H, Uykimpang R, Alconcel M, et al. Aged garlic extract may be safe for patients on warfarin therapy. J Nutr 2006; 136(3, Suppl):793S–795S

132. Izzo AA, Ernst E. Interactions between herbal medicines and prescribed drugs: a systematic review. Drugs 2001;61(15):2163–2175

133. Piscitelli SC, Burstein AH, Welden N, Gallicano KD, Falloon J. The effect of garlic supplements on the pharmacokinetics of saquinavir. Clin Infect Dis 2002;34(2):234–238

134. Markowitz JS, Devane CL, Chavin KD, Taylor RM, Ruan Y, Donovan JL. Effects of garlic (Allium sativum L.) supplementation on cytochrome P450 2D6 and 3A4 activity in healthy volunteers. Clin Pharmacol Ther 2003;74(2):170–177

135. Gallicano K, Foster B, Choudhri S. Effect of short-term administration of garlic supplements on single-dose ritonavir pharmacokinetics in healthy volunteers. Br J Clin Pharmacol 2003;55(2):199–202

18 Phytosterols

Throughout much of human evolution, it is likely that large amounts of plant foods were consumed.[1] In addition to being rich in fiber and plant protein, the diets of our ancestors were also rich in phytosterols—plant-derived sterols that are similar in structure and function to cholesterol. There is increasing evidence that the reintroduction of plant foods providing phytosterols into the modern diet can improve serum lipid (cholesterol) profiles and reduce the risk of cardiovascular disease.[2]

Although cholesterol is the predominant sterol in animals, including humans, a variety of sterols are found in plants.[3] Nutritionists recognize two classes of phytosterols: (1) sterols, which have a double bond in the sterol ring; and (2) stanols, which lack a double bond in the sterol ring (Fig. 18.1). The most abundant sterols in plants and the human diet are sitosterol and campesterol. Stanols are also present in plants, but they comprise only approximately 10% of total dietary phytosterols. Cholesterol in human blood and tis-

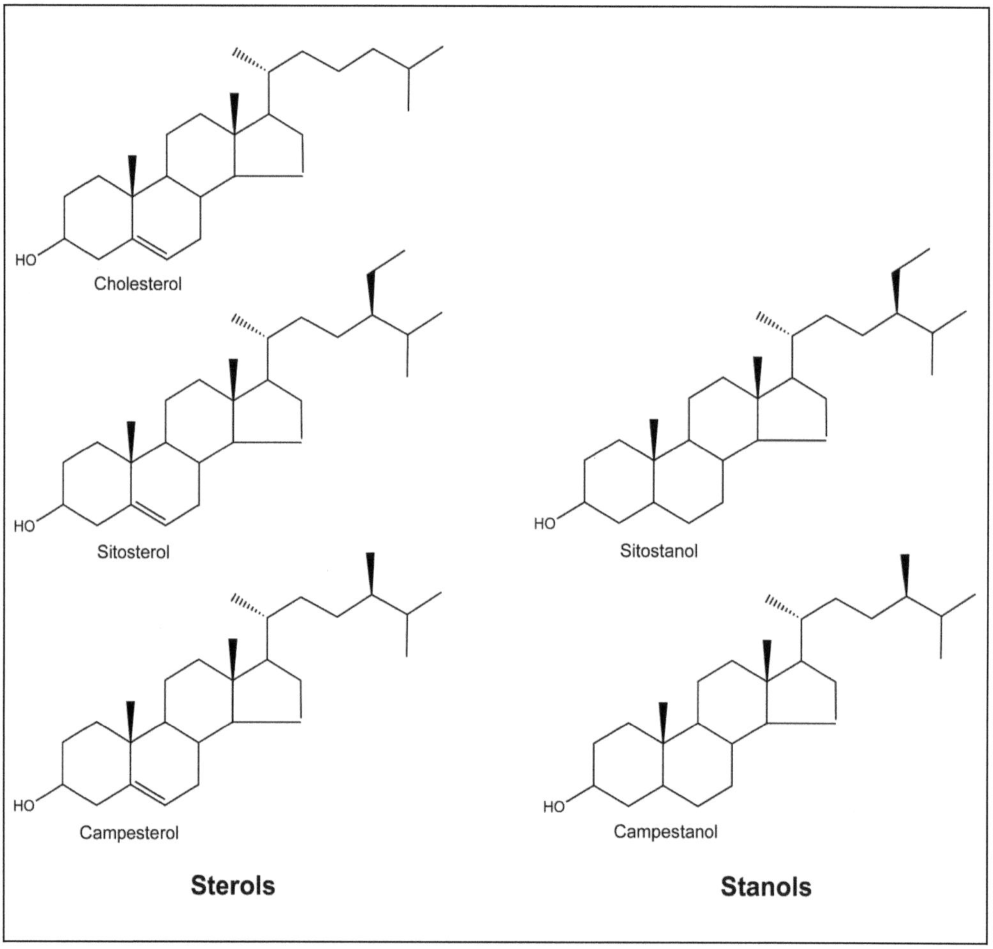

Fig. 18.1 Chemical structure of cholesterol compared with plant sterols (sitosterol and campesterol) and plant stanols (sitostanol and campestanol).

sues is derived from the diet as well as endogenous cholesterol synthesis. In contrast, all phytosterols in human blood and tissues are derived from the diet because humans cannot synthesize phytosterols.[4]

Definitions

Phytosterols. A collective term for plant-derived sterols and stanols.
Plant sterols or stanols. Terms generally applied to plant-derived sterols or stanols; these phytochemicals are added to foods or supplements.
Plant sterol or stanol esters. Plant sterols or stanols that have been esterified by creating an ester bond between a fatty acid and the sterol or stanol. Esterification occurs in intestinal cells and is also an industrial process. Esterification makes plant sterols and stanols more fat soluble so they are easily incorporated into fat-containing foods, including margarines and salad dressings. In this chapter, the weights of plant sterol and stanol esters are expressed as the equivalent weights of free (unesterified) sterols and stanols.

Bioavailability and Metabolism

Absorption and Metabolism of Dietary Cholesterol

Dietary cholesterol must be incorporated into mixed micelles to be absorbed by the cells that line the intestine (enterocytes).[5] Mixed micelles are mixtures of bile salts, lipids (fats), and sterols formed in the small intestine after a fat-containing meal is consumed. Inside the enterocyte, cholesterol is esterified and incorporated into triglyceride-rich lipoproteins known as *chylomicrons*, which enter the circulation.[6] As circulating chylomicrons become depleted of triglycerides, they become chylomicron remnants, which are taken up by the liver. In the liver, cholesterol from chylomicron remnants may be repackaged into other lipoproteins for transport throughout the circulation or, alternatively, secreted into bile, which is released into the small intestine.

Absorption and Metabolism of Dietary Phytosterols

Although varied diets typically contain similar amounts of phytosterols and cholesterol, serum phytosterol concentrations are usually several hundred times lower than serum cholesterol concentrations in humans.[7] Less than 10% of dietary phytosterols are systemically absorbed, in contrast to approximately 50%–60% of dietary cholesterol.[8] Like cholesterol, phytosterols must be incorporated into mixed micelles before they are taken up by enterocytes. Once inside the enterocyte, systemic absorption of phytosterols is inhibited by the activity of efflux transporters, consisting of a pair of ATP-binding cassette (ABC) proteins known as ABCG5 and ABCG8.[4] ABCG5 and ABCG8 each form one half of a transporter that secretes phytosterols and unesterified cholesterol from the enterocyte into the intestinal lumen. Phytosterols are secreted back into the intestine by ABCG5/G8 transporters at a much greater rate than cholesterol, resulting in much lower intestinal absorption of dietary phytosterols than of cholesterol. Within the enterocyte, phytosterols are not as readily esterified as cholesterol, so they are incorporated into chylomicrons at much lower concentrations. Those phytosterols that are incorporated into chylomicrons enter the circulation and are taken up by the liver. Once inside the liver, phytosterols are rapidly secreted into bile by hepatic ABCG5/G8 transporters. Although cholesterol may also be secreted into bile, the rate of phytosterol secretion into bile is much greater than the rate of cholesterol secretion.[9] Thus, the low serum concentrations of phytosterols relative to cholesterol can be explained by decreased intestinal absorption and increased excretion of phytosterols into bile.

Biological Activities

Effects on Cholesterol Absorption and Lipoprotein Metabolism

It is well established that high intakes of plant sterols or stanols can lower serum total and low-density lipoprotein (LDL) cholesterol concentrations in humans (see the Cardiovascular Disease section below).[10,11] In the intestinal lumen, phytosterols displace cholesterol from mixed micelles and inhibit cholesterol absorption.[12] In humans, the consumption of 1.5–1.8 g/day of plant sterols or stanols reduced cholesterol absorption by 30%–40%.[13,14] At higher doses (2.2 g/day of plant sterols), cholesterol absorption was reduced by 60%.[15] In response to decreased cholesterol absorption, tissue LDL-receptor expression was increased, resulting in increased clearance of circulating LDL.[16] Decreased cholesterol absorption is also associated with increased cholesterol synthesis, and increasing phytosterol intake has been found to increase endogenous cholesterol synthesis in humans.[13] Despite the increase in cholesterol synthesis induced by increasing phytosterol intake, the net result is a reduction in serum LDL cholesterol concentration.

Other Biological Activities

Experiments in cell culture and animal models suggest that phytosterols may have biological activities unrelated to cholesterol lowering. However, their significance in humans is not yet known.

Alterations in Cell Membrane Properties

Cholesterol is an important structural component of mammalian cell membranes.[17] Displacement of cholesterol with phytosterols has been found to alter the physical properties of cell membranes in vitro,[18] which could potentially affect signal transduction or membrane-bound enzyme activity.[19,20] Limited evidence from an animal model of hemorrhagic stroke suggested that very high intakes of plant sterols or stanols displaced cholesterol in red blood cell membranes, resulting in decreased deformability and potentially increased fragility.[21,22] However, daily phytosterol supplementation (1 g/1000 kcal) for 4 weeks did not alter red blood cell fragility in humans.[23]

Alterations in Testosterone Metabolism

Limited evidence from animal studies suggests that very high phytosterol intakes can alter testosterone metabolism by inhibiting 5-α-reductase, a membrane-bound enzyme that converts testosterone to dihydrotestosterone, a more potent metabolite.[24,25] It is not known whether phytosterol consumption alters testosterone metabolism in humans. No significant changes in free or total serum testosterone concentrations were

observed in men who consumed 1.6 g/day of plant sterol esters for 1 year.[26]

Induction of Apoptosis in Cancer Cells

Unlike normal cells, cancerous cells lose their ability to respond to death signals that initiate apoptosis (programmed cell death). Sitosterol has been found to induce apoptosis when added to cultured human prostate,[27] breast,[28] and colon cancer cells.[29]

Anti-inflammatory Effects

Limited data from cell-culture and animal studies suggest that phytosterols may attenuate the inflammatory activity of immune cells, including macrophages and neutrophils.[30,31]

Disease Prevention

Cardiovascular Disease

Foods Enriched with Plant Sterols or Stanols

LDL cholesterol. Numerous clinical trials have found that daily consumption of foods enriched with free or esterified forms of plant sterols or stanols lowers concentrations of serum total and LDL cholesterol.[10,32–35] A meta-analysis that combined the results of 18 controlled clinical trials found that the consumption of spreads providing an average of 2 g/day of plant sterols or stanols lowered serum LDL cholesterol concentrations by 9%–14%.[36] More recently, a meta-analysis that combined the results of 23 controlled clinical trials found that the consumption of plant foods providing an average of 3.4 g/day of plant sterols or stanols decreased LDL cholesterol concentrations by approximately 11%.[37] Another meta-analysis examined the results of 23 clinical trials of plant-sterol-enriched foods and 27 clinical trials of plant-stanol-enriched foods, separately.[11] At doses of at least 2 g/day, both plant sterols and stanols decreased LDL cholesterol concentrations by approximately 10%. Doses higher than 2 g/day did not substantially improve the cholesterol-lowering effects of plant sterols or stanols. Most recently, a meta-analysis that analyzed the results of 59 randomized controlled trials found that reductions in LDL cholesterol are greater in those with higher baseline levels of LDL cholesterol.[38] The results of studies providing lower doses of plant sterols or stanols suggest that 0.8–

1.0 g/day is the lowest dose that results in clinically significant LDL cholesterol reductions of at least 5%.[39–43] In general, trials that have compared the cholesterol-lowering efficacy of plant sterols with that of stanols have found them to be equivalent.[44–46] Few of these studies lasted longer than 4 weeks, but at least two studies have found that the cholesterol-lowering effects of plant sterols and stanols last for up to 1 year.[26,47] In addition to data from controlled clinical trials, a 5-year study that examined the customary use of phytosterol/stanol-enriched margarines under free-living conditions found beneficial effects on cholesterol levels.[48] Recently, concerns have been raised that plant sterols are not as effective as stanols in maintaining long-term reductions in LDL cholesterol.[49–51] Long-term trials that directly compare the efficacy of plant sterols and plant stanols are needed to address these concerns.[11]

Coronary heart disease risk. The effect of long-term use of foods enriched with plant sterols or stanols on coronary heart disease (CHD) risk is not known. The results of numerous intervention trials suggest that a 10% reduction in LDL cholesterol induced by medication or diet modification could decrease the risk of CHD by as much as 20%.[52] The National Cholesterol Education Program (NCEP) Adult Treatment Panel III has included the use of plant sterol or stanol esters (2 g/day) as a component of maximal dietary therapy for elevated LDL cholesterol.[53] The addition of plant-sterol- or stanol-enriched foods to a heart-healthy diet that is low in saturated fat and rich in fruits and vegetables, whole grains, and fiber offers the potential for additive effects in CHD risk reduction. For example, following a diet that substituted monounsaturated and polyunsaturated fats for saturated fat resulted in a 9% reduction in serum LDL cholesterol after 30 days, but the addition of 1.7 g/day of plant sterols to the same diet resulted in a 24% reduction.[54] More recently, 1-month adherence to a diet providing a portfolio of cholesterol-lowering foods, including plant sterols (1 g/1000 kcal), soy protein, almonds, and viscous fibers lowered serum LDL cholesterol concentrations by an average of 30%— a decrease that was not significantly different from that induced by statin therapy (drugs that inhibit the enzyme, 3-hydroxy-3-methyl-glutaryl-coenzyme A [HMG-CoA] reductase).[55] However, analysis of individuals on such a cholesterol-lowering diet for 1 year found that the average LDL cholesterol reduction was only 13%, but almost one-third of the participants experienced LDL cholesterol reductions that were greater than 20%.[56] Plant sterols are the major component in this diet responsible for the observed reductions in cholesterol concentrations.[57] The United States Food and Drug Administration (FDA) has authorized the use of health claims on food labels indicating that regular consumption of foods enriched with plant sterol or stanol esters may reduce the risk of heart disease.[58]

Dietary Phytosterols

Clinical trials finding daily consumption of foods enriched with plant sterols or stanols can significantly lower LDL cholesterol concentrations do not account for naturally occurring phytosterols in the diet.[59] Relatively few studies have considered the effects of dietary phytosterol intakes on serum LDL cholesterol concentrations. Dietary phytosterol intakes have been estimated to range from approximately 150 mg/day to 450 mg/day in various populations.[60] Limited evidence suggests that dietary phytosterols may play an important role in decreasing cholesterol absorption. A cross-sectional study in the United Kingdom found that dietary phytosterol intakes were inversely related to serum total and LDL cholesterol concentrations, even after adjusting for saturated fat and fiber intake.[61] Similarly, an analysis in a Swedish population found that dietary intake of phytosterols was inversely associated with total cholesterol in both men and women and with LDL cholesterol in women.[62] In single-meal tests, removal of 150 mg of phytosterols from corn oil increased cholesterol absorption by 38%,[63] and removal of 328 mg of phytosterols from wheat germ increased cholesterol absorption by 43%.[64] Although more research is needed, these findings suggest that dietary intakes of phytosterols from plant foods could have an important impact on cardiovascular health.

Cancer

Limited data from animal studies suggest that very high intakes of phytosterols, particularly sitosterol, may inhibit the growth of breast and prostate cancer.[65–67] Only a few epidemiological studies have examined associations between dietary phytosterol intakes and cancer risk in humans because databases providing information on the phytosterol content of commonly consumed foods have only recently been developed. A series of case–control studies in Uruguay found that dietary phytosterol intakes were lower in people diagnosed with stomach, lung, or breast cancer than in control groups of individuals who were cancer free.[68–70] Case–control studies in the United States found that women diagnosed with breast or endometrial (uterine) cancer had lower dietary phytosterol intakes than women who did not have cancer.[71,72] In contrast, another case–control study in the United States found that men diagnosed with prostate cancer had higher dietary campesterol intakes than men who did not have cancer, but total phytosterol consumption was not associated with prostate cancer risk.[73] Although some epidemiological studies have found that higher intakes of plant foods containing phytosterols are associated with decreased cancer risk, it is not clear whether the protective factors are phytosterols or other compounds in plant foods.

Disease Treatment

Benign Prostatic Hyperplasia

Benign prostatic hyperplasia (BPH) is the term used to describe a noncancerous enlargement of the prostate. The enlarged prostate may exert pressure on the urethra, resulting in difficulty urinating. Plant extracts that provide a mixture of phytosterols (marketed as β-sitosterol) are often included in herbal therapies for urinary symptoms related to BPH. However, relatively few controlled studies have examined the efficacy of phytosterol supplements in men with symptomatic BPH. In a 6-month study of 200 men with symptomatic BPH, 60 mg/day of a β-sitosterol preparation improved symptom scores, increased peak urinary flow, and decreased post-void residual urine volume compared with placebo.[74] A follow-up study reported that these improvements were maintained for up to 18 months in the 38 participants who continued β-sitosterol treatment.[75] Similarly, in a 6-month study of 177 men with symptomatic BPH, 130 mg/day of a different β-sitosterol preparation improved urinary symptom scores, increased peak urinary flow, and decreased post-void residual urine volume compared with pla-

cebo.[76] A systematic review that combined the results of these and two other controlled clinical trials found that β-sitosterol extracts increased peak urinary flow by an average of 3.9 mL/s and decreased post-void residual volume by an average of 29 mL.[77] Although the results of a few clinical trials suggest that relatively low doses of phytosterols can improve lower urinary tract symptoms related to BPH, further research is needed to confirm these findings.[78]

Sources

Food Sources

Unlike the typical diet in most developed countries today, the diets of our ancestors were rich in phytosterols, likely providing as much as 1000 mg/day.[1] Present-day dietary phytosterol intakes have been estimated to vary from 150 to 450 mg/day in different populations.[3] Vegetarians, particularly vegans, generally have the highest intakes of dietary phytosterols.[79] Phytosterols are found in all plant foods, but the highest concentrations are found in unrefined plant oils, including vegetable, nut, and olive oils.[3] Nuts, seeds, whole grains, and legumes are also good dietary sources of phytosterols.[5] The phytosterol contents of selected foods are presented in Table 18.1.

Foods Enriched with Plant Sterols and Plant Stanols

The majority of clinical trials that demonstrated a cholesterol-lowering effect used plant sterol or stanol esters solubilized in fat-containing foods, such as margarine or mayonnaise.[11] More recent studies indicate that low-fat or even nonfat foods can effectively deliver plant sterols or stanols if they are adequately solubilized.[10,59] Plant sterols or stanols added to low-fat yogurt,[43,84–86] low-fat milk,[87–89] low-fat cheese,[90] dark chocolate,[91] and orange juice[92,93] have been reported to lower LDL cholesterol in controlled clinical trials. A variety of foods containing added plant sterols or stanols, including margarines, mayonnaises, vegetable oils, salad dressings, yogurt, milk, soy milk, orange juice, snack bars, and meats, are available in the United States, Europe, Asia, Australia, and New Zealand.[10] A recent meta-analysis found that plant sterols/stanols added to fat spreads,

Table 18.1 Total phytosterol content of selected foods[80-83]

Food	Serving	Phytosterols (mg)
Wheat germ	½ cup	197
Rice bran oil	1 tbs	162
Sesame oil	1 tbs	118
Corn oil	1 tbs	102
Canola oil	1 tbs	92
Peanuts	1 oz	62
Wheat bran	½ cup	58
Almonds	1 oz	39
Brussels sprouts	½ cup	34
Rye bread	2 slices	33
Macadamia nuts	1 oz	33
Olive oil	1 tbs	22
Take Control[a] spread	1 tbs	1650 mg plant sterol esters (1000 mg free sterols)
Benecol spread	1 tbs	850 mg plant stanol esters (500 mg free stanols)

[a] Known as Flora in Europe.

mayonnaise, salad dressings, milk, or yogurt were more effective in reducing LDL cholesterol levels compared with plant sterols/stanols incorporated into other products, such as chocolate, orange juice, cheese, meats, and cereal bars.[38] Available research indicates that the maximum effective dose for lowering LDL cholesterol is approximately 2 g/day[11] and the minimum effective dose is 0.8–1.0 g/day.[10] In the majority of clinical trials that demonstrated a cholesterol-lowering effect, the daily dose of plant sterols or stanols was divided among two or three meals, which may be more effective in lowering LDL cholesterol.[38] However, consumption of the daily dose of plant sterols or stanols with a single meal has been found to lower LDL cholesterol in a few clinical trials.[43,85,86,94,95]

Supplements

Phytosterol supplements marketed as β-sitosterol are available without a prescription in the United States. Doses of 60–130 mg/day of β-sitosterol have been found to alleviate the symptoms of BPH in a few clinical trials (see Benign Prostatic Hyperplasia section above). Soft gel chews providing 0.5 g of plant stanols are being marketed for cholesterol lowering at a recommended dose of 2 g/day. Phytosterol supplements should be taken with meals that contain fat.

Safety

In the United States, plant sterols and stanols added to a variety of food products are generally recognized as safe (GRAS) by the FDA.[96] Additionally, the Scientific Committee on Foods of the European Union concluded that plant sterols and stanols added to various food products are safe for human use.[97] However, this committee recommended that intakes of plant sterols and stanols from food products should not exceed 3 g/day because there is no evidence of health benefits at higher intakes and there might be undesirable effects at high intakes.

Adverse Effects

Few adverse effects have been associated with regular consumption of plant sterols or stanols for up to 1 year. People who consumed a plant-sterol-enriched spread providing 1.6 g/day did not report any more adverse effects than those consuming a control spread for up to 1 year,[26] and people consuming a plant stanol-enriched spread providing 1.8–2.6 g/day for 1 year did not report any adverse effects.[47] Consumption of up to 8.6 g/day of phytosterols in margarine for 3–4 weeks was well tolerated by healthy men and women and did not adversely affect intestinal bacteria or female hormone levels.[98] Although phytosterols are usually well tolerated, nausea, indigestion, diarrhea, and constipation have occasionally been reported.[74,76]

Sitosterolemia (Phytosterolemia)

Sitosterolemia, also known as *phytosterolemia*, is a very rare hereditary disease that results from inheriting a mutation in both copies of the *ABCG5* or *ABCG8* gene.[99] Individuals who are homozygous for a mutation in either transporter protein have dramatically elevated serum phytosterol concentrations due to increased intestinal absorption and decreased biliary excretion of phytosterols. Although serum cholesterol concentrations may be normal or only mildly elevated, individuals with sitosterolemia are at high risk for premature atherosclerosis. People with sitos-terolemia should avoid foods or supplements with added plant sterols.[10] Two studies have examined the effect of plant sterol consumption in heterozygous carriers of sitosterolemia, a more common condition. Consumption of 3 g/day of plant sterols for 4 weeks by two heterozygous carriers,[100] and consumption of 2.2 g/day of plant sterols for 6–12 weeks by 12 heterozygous carriers did not result in abnormally elevated serum phytosterols.[101]

Pregnancy and Lactation

Plant sterols or stanols added to foods or supplements are not recommended for pregnant or breast-feeding women because their safety has not been studied.[10] At present, there is no evidence that high dietary intakes of naturally occurring phytosterols, such as those consumed by vegetarian women, adversely affect pregnancy or lactation.

Drug Interactions

The LDL-cholesterol-lowering effects of plant sterols or stanols may be additive to those of HMG-CoA reductase inhibitors (statins).[102,103] The results of controlled clinical trials suggest that consumption of 2–3 g/day of plant sterols or stanols by individuals on statin therapy may result in an additional 7%–11% reduction in LDL cholesterol, an effect comparable to doubling the statin dose.[50,104–106] Consumption of 4.5 g/day of stanol esters for 8 weeks did not affect prothrombin times (international normalized ratios—INRs) in patients on warfarin (Coumadin) for anticoagulation.[107]

Nutrient Interactions

Fat-Soluble Vitamins (Vitamins A, D, E, and K)

Because plant sterols and stanols decrease cholesterol absorption and serum LDL cholesterol concentrations, their effects on fat-soluble vitamin status have also been studied in clinical trials. Plasma vitamin A (retinol) concentrations were not affected by plant stanol or sterol ester consumption for up to 1 year.[11,26] Although the majority of studies found no changes in plasma vitamin D (25-hydroxyvitamin D_3) concentra-

tions, one placebo-controlled study in individuals consuming 1.6 g/day of sterol esters for 1 year observed a small (7%) but statistically significant decrease in plasma 25-hydroxyvitamin D_3 concentrations.[26] There is little evidence that plant sterol or stanol consumption adversely affects vitamin K status. Consumption of 1.6 g/day of sterol esters for 6 months was associated with a nonsignificant 14% decrease in plasma vitamin K_1 concentrations, but carboxylated osteocalcin, a functional indicator of vitamin K status, was unaffected.[26] In other studies of shorter duration, consumption of plant sterol and stanol esters did not significantly change plasma concentrations of vitamin K_1[108,109] or vitamin-K-dependent clotting factors.[110] Consumption of plant sterol or stanol-enriched foods has been found to decrease plasma vitamin E (α-tocopherol) concentrations in several studies.[11,109] However, those decreases generally do not persist when plasma α-tocopherol concentrations are standardized to LDL cholesterol concentrations. This suggests that observed reductions in plasma α-tocopherol are due in part to reductions in its carrier lipoprotein, LDL. In general, consumption of plant-sterol- and stanol-enriched foods at doses of 1.5 g/day or more have not been found to have adverse effects on fat-soluble vitamin status in well-nourished populations.

Carotenoids

Dietary carotenoids are fat-soluble phytochemicals that circulate in lipoproteins. Several studies have observed 10%–20% reductions in plasma carotenoids after short-term and long-term consumption of plant-sterol- or stanol-enriched foods.[11] Even when standardized to serum total or LDL cholesterol concentrations, decreases in α-carotene, β-carotene, and lycopene may persist, suggesting that phytosterols can inhibit the absorption of these carotenoids.[111] It is not clear whether reductions in plasma carotenoid concentrations confer any health risks, but several studies have found that increasing intakes of carotenoid-rich fruits and vegetables can prevent phytosterol-induced decreases in plasma carotenoids.[112] In one case, advice to consume five daily servings of fruits and vegetables, including one serving of carotenoid-rich vegetables, was enough to maintain plasma carotenoid levels in people consuming 2.5 g/day of plant sterol or stanol esters.[113]

Summary

- Phytosterols are plant-derived compounds that are similar in structure and function to cholesterol.
- Early human diets were rich in phytosterols, providing as much as 1 g/day; however, the typical Western diet today is relatively low in phytosterols.
- Phytosterols inhibit the intestinal absorption of cholesterol.
- Numerous clinical trials have demonstrated that daily consumption of foods enriched with at least 0.8 g of plant sterols or stanols lowers serum LDL cholesterol.
- Although some epidemiological studies have found that higher intakes of plant foods containing phytosterols are associated with decreased cancer risk, it is not clear whether phytosterols or other compounds in plant foods are the protective factors.
- The results of a few clinical trials suggest that phytosterol supplementation at relatively low doses can improve urinary tract symptoms related to benign prostatic hyperplasia, but further research is needed to confirm these findings.
- Foods rich in phytosterols include unrefined vegetable oils, whole grains, nuts, and legumes.
- Foods and beverages with added plant sterols or stanols are now available in many countries throughout the world, and many countries now allow health claims for such commercial products.

References

1. Jenkins DJ, Kendall CW, Marchie A, et al. The Garden of Eden—plant based diets, the genetic drive to conserve cholesterol and its implications for heart disease in the 21st century. Comp Biochem Physiol A Mol Integr Physiol 2003;136(1):141–151
2. Kendall CW, Jenkins DJ. A dietary portfolio: maximal reduction of low-density lipoprotein cholesterol with diet. Curr Atheroscler Rep 2004;6(6):492–498
3. Ostlund RE Jr. Phytosterols in human nutrition. Annu Rev Nutr 2002;22:533–549
4. Sudhop T, Lütjohann D, von Bergmann K. Sterol transporters: targets of natural sterols and new lipid lowering drugs. Pharmacol Ther 2005;105(3):333–341
5. de Jong A, Plat J, Mensink RP. Metabolic effects of plant sterols and stanols (Review). J Nutr Biochem 2003;14(7):362–369
6. Plat J, Mensink RP. Plant stanol and sterol esters in the control of blood cholesterol levels: mechanism and safety aspects. Am J Cardiol 2005; 96(1A, Suppl):15D–22D
7. von Bergmann K, Sudhop T, Lütjohann D. Cholesterol and plant sterol absorption: recent insights. Am J Cardiol 2005; 96(1A, Suppl):10D–14D
8. Ostlund RE Jr, McGill JB, Zeng CM, et al. Gastrointestinal absorption and plasma kinetics of soy Delta(5)-phytosterols and phytostanols in humans. Am J Physiol Endocrinol Metab 2002;282(4):E911–E916
9. Sudhop T, Sahin Y, Lindenthal B, et al. Comparison of the hepatic clearances of campesterol, sitosterol, and cholesterol in healthy subjects suggests that efflux transporters controlling intestinal sterol absorption also regulate biliary secretion. Gut 2002;51(6):860–863
10. Berger A, Jones PJ, Abumweis SS. Plant sterols: factors affecting their efficacy and safety as functional food ingredients. Lipids Health Dis 2004;3(1):5
11. Katan MB, Grundy SM, Jones P, Law M, Miettinen T, Paoletti R; Stresa Workshop Participants. Efficacy and safety of plant stanols and sterols in the management of blood cholesterol levels. Mayo Clin Proc 2003; 78(8):965–978
12. Nissinen M, Gylling H, Vuoristo M, Miettinen TA. Micellar distribution of cholesterol and phytosterols after duodenal plant stanol ester infusion. Am J Physiol Gastrointest Liver Physiol 2002;282(6):G1009–G1015
13. Jones PJ, Raeini-Sarjaz M, Ntanios FY, Vanstone CA, Feng JY, Parsons WE. Modulation of plasma lipid levels and cholesterol kinetics by phytosterol versus phytostanol esters. J Lipid Res 2000;41(5):697–705
14. Normén L, Dutta P, Lia A, Andersson H. Soy sterol esters and beta-sitostanol ester as inhibitors of cholesterol absorption in human small bowel. Am J Clin Nutr 2000;71(4):908–913
15. Richelle M, Enslen M, Hager C, et al. Both free and esterified plant sterols reduce cholesterol absorption and the bioavailability of beta-carotene and alpha-tocopherol in normocholesterolemic humans. Am J Clin Nutr 2004;80(1):171–177
16. Plat J, Mensink RP. Effects of plant stanol esters on LDL receptor protein expression and on LDL receptor and HMG-CoA reductase mRNA expression in mononuclear blood cells of healthy men and women. FASEB J 2002;16(2):258–260
17. Mouritsen OG, Zuckermann MJ. What's so special about cholesterol? Lipids 2004;39(11):1101–1113
18. Halling KK, Slotte JP. Membrane properties of plant sterols in phospholipid bilayers as determined by differential scanning calorimetry, resonance energy transfer and detergent-induced solubilization. Biochim Biophys Acta 2004;1664(2):161–171
19. Awad AB, Chen YC, Fink CS, Hennessey T. beta-Sitosterol inhibits HT-29 human colon cancer cell growth and alters membrane lipids. Anticancer Res 1996; 16(5A):2797–2804
20. Leikin AI, Brenner RR. Fatty acid desaturase activities are modulated by phytosterol incorporation in microsomes. Biochim Biophys Acta 1989;1005(2):187–191
21. Ratnayake WM, L'Abbé MR, Mueller R, et al. Vegetable oils high in phytosterols make erythrocytes less deformable and shorten the life span of stroke-prone spontaneously hypertensive rats. J Nutr 2000;130(5):1166–1178
22. Ratnayake WM, Plouffe L, L'Abbé MR, Trick K, Mueller R, Hayward S. Comparative health effects of margarines fortified with plant sterols and stanols on a rat

model for hemorrhagic stroke. Lipids 2003;38(12): 1237–1247

23. Jones PJ, Raeini-Sarjaz M, Jenkins DJ, et al. Effects of a diet high in plant sterols, vegetable proteins, and viscous fibers (dietary portfolio) on circulating sterol levels and red cell fragility in hypercholesterolemic subjects. Lipids 2005;40(2):169–174

24. Awad AB, Hartati MS, Fink CS. Phytosterol feeding induces alteration in testosterone metabolism in rat tissues. J Nutr Biochem 1998;9(12):712–717

25. Cabeza M, Bratoeff E, Heuze I, Ramírez E, Sánchez M, Flores E. Effect of beta-sitosterol as inhibitor of 5 alpha-reductase in hamster prostate. Proc West Pharmacol Soc 2003;46:153–155

26. Hendriks HF, Brink EJ, Meijer GW, Princen HM, Ntanios FY. Safety of long-term consumption of plant sterol esters-enriched spread. Eur J Clin Nutr 2003; 57(5):681–692

27. von Holtz RL, Fink CS, Awad AB. beta-Sitosterol activates the sphingomyelin cycle and induces apoptosis in LNCaP human prostate cancer cells. Nutr Cancer 1998;32(1):8–12

28. Awad AB, Roy R, Fink CS. Beta-sitosterol, a plant sterol, induces apoptosis and activates key caspases in MDA-MB-231 human breast cancer cells. Oncol Rep 2003;10(2):497–500

29. Choi YH, Kong KR, Kim YA, et al. Induction of Bax and activation of caspases during beta-sitosterol-mediated apoptosis in human colon cancer cells. Int J Oncol 2003;23(6):1657–1662

30. Awad AB, Toczek J, Fink CS. Phytosterols decrease prostaglandin release in cultured P388D1/MAB macrophages. Prostaglandins Leukot Essent Fatty Acids 2004;70(6):511–520

31. Navarro A, De las Heras B, Villar A. Anti-inflammatory and immunomodulating properties of a sterol fraction from Sideritis foetens Clem. Biol Pharm Bull 2001;24(5):470–473

32. St-Onge MP, Jones PJ. Phytosterols and human lipid metabolism: efficacy, safety, and novel foods. Lipids 2003;38(4):367–375

33. Moruisi KG, Oosthuizen W, Opperman AM. Phytosterols/stanols lower cholesterol concentrations in familial hypercholesterolemic subjects: a systematic review with meta-analysis. J Am Coll Nutr 2006; 25(1):41–48

34. Ellegård LH, Andersson SW, Normén AL, Andersson HA. Dietary plant sterols and cholesterol metabolism. Nutr Rev 2007;65(1):39–45

35. Van Horn L, McCoin M, Kris-Etherton PM, et al. The evidence for dietary prevention and treatment of cardiovascular disease. J Am Diet Assoc 2008;108(2):287–331

36. Law M. Plant sterol and stanol margarines and health. BMJ 2000;320(7238):861–864

37. Chen JT, Wesley R, Shamburek RD, Pucino F, Csako G. Meta-analysis of natural therapies for hyperlipidemia: plant sterols and stanols versus policosanol. Pharmacotherapy 2005;25(2):171–183

38. AbuMweis SS, Barake R, Jones P. Plant sterols/stanols as cholesterol lowering agents: A meta-analysis of randomized controlled trials. Food Nutr Res 2008; 52:doi:10.3402/fnr.v52i0.1811

39. Hendriks HF, Weststrate JA, van Vliet T, Meijer GW. Spreads enriched with three different levels of vegetable oil sterols and the degree of cholesterol lowering in normocholesterolaemic and mildly hypercholesterolaemic subjects. Eur J Clin Nutr 1999; 53(4): 319–327

40. Miettinen TA, Vanhanen H. Dietary sitostanol related to absorption, synthesis and serum level of cholesterol in different apolipoprotein E phenotypes. Atherosclerosis 1994;105(2):217–226

41. Pelletier X, Belbraouet S, Mirabel D, et al. A diet moderately enriched in phytosterols lowers plasma cholesterol concentrations in normocholesterolemic humans. Ann Nutr Metab 1995;39(5):291–295

42. Sierksma A, Weststrate JA, Meijer GW. Spreads enriched with plant sterols, either esterified 4,4-dimethylsterols or free 4-desmethylsterols, and plasma total- and LDL-cholesterol concentrations. Br J Nutr 1999;82(4):273–282

43. Volpe R, Niittynen L, Korpela R, et al. Effects of yoghurt enriched with plant sterols on serum lipids in patients with moderate hypercholesterolaemia. Br J Nutr 2001;86(2):233–239

44. Hallikainen MA, Sarkkinen ES, Gylling H, Erkkilä AT, Uusitupa MI. Comparison of the effects of plant sterol ester and plant stanol ester-enriched margarines in lowering serum cholesterol concentrations in hypercholesterolaemic subjects on a low-fat diet. Eur J Clin Nutr 2000;54(9):715–725

45. Vanstone CA, Raeini-Sarjaz M, Parsons WE, Jones PJ. Unesterified plant sterols and stanols lower LDL-cholesterol concentrations equivalently in hypercholesterolemic persons. Am J Clin Nutr 2002;76(6):1272–1278

46. Weststrate JA, Meijer GW. Plant sterol-enriched margarines and reduction of plasma total- and LDL-cholesterol concentrations in normocholesterolaemic and mildly hypercholesterolaemic subjects. Eur J Clin Nutr 1998;52(5):334–343

47. Miettinen TA, Puska P, Gylling H, Vanhanen H, Vartiainen E. Reduction of serum cholesterol with sitostanol-ester margarine in a mildly hypercholesterolemic population. N Engl J Med 1995;333(20):1308–1312

48. Wolfs M, de Jong N, Ocké MC, Verhagen H, Monique Verschuren WM. Effectiveness of customary use of phytosterol/-stanol enriched margarines on blood cholesterol lowering. Food Chem Toxicol 2006; 44(10):1682–1688

49. Miettinen TA, Gylling H. Plant stanol and sterol esters in prevention of cardiovascular diseases. Ann Med 2004;36(2):126–134

50. O'Neill FH, Brynes A, Mandeno R, et al. Comparison of the effects of dietary plant sterol and stanol esters on lipid metabolism. Nutr Metab Cardiovasc Dis 2004; 14(3):133–142

51. O'Neill FH, Sanders TA, Thompson GR. Comparison of efficacy of plant stanol ester and sterol ester: short-term and longer-term studies. Am J Cardiol 2005; 96(1A):29D–36D

52. National Cholesterol Education Program. Third Report of the National Cholesterol Education Program Expert Panel on Detection, Evaluation, and Treatment of High Blood Cholesterol in Adults (Adult Treatment Panel III). Bethesda, MD: National Heart Lung and Blood Institute, National Institutes of Health; 2002. Available at: http://www.nhlbi.nih.gov/guidelines/cholesterol/atp3_rpt.htm. Accessed May 7, 2012

53. Grundy SM. Stanol esters as a component of maximal dietary therapy in the National Cholesterol Education Program Adult Treatment Panel III report. Am J Cardiol 2005; 96(1A, Suppl):47D–50D

54. Jones PJ, Ntanios FY, Raeini-Sarjaz M, Vanstone CA. Cholesterol-lowering efficacy of a sitostanol-contain-

ing phytosterol mixture with a prudent diet in hyperlipidemic men. Am J Clin Nutr 1999;69(6):1144–1150

55. Jenkins DJ, Kendall CW, Marchie A, et al. Direct comparison of a dietary portfolio of cholesterol-lowering foods with a statin in hypercholesterolemic participants. Am J Clin Nutr 2005;81(2):380–387

56. Jenkins DJ, Kendall CW, Faulkner DA, et al. Assessment of the longer-term effects of a dietary portfolio of cholesterol-lowering foods in hypercholesterolemia. Am J Clin Nutr 2006;83(3):582–591

57. Jenkins DJ, Kendall CW, Nguyen TH, et al. Effect of plant sterols in combination with other cholesterol-lowering foods. Metabolism 2008;57(1):130–139

58. Food and Drug Administration. Federal Register 65-FR 54685-54739, September 8, 2000. Food Labeling: Health Claims; Plant Sterol/Stanol Esters and Coronary Heart Disease; Interim Final Rule. Available at: http://www.fda.gov/Food/LabelingNutrition/Label Claims/HealthClaimsMeetingSingnificantScientific AgreementSSA/ucm/74747.htm

59. Ostlund RE Jr. Phytosterols and cholesterol metabolism. Curr Opin Lipidol 2004;15(1):37–41

60. Ostlund RE Jr, Racette SB, Stenson WF. Effects of trace components of dietary fat on cholesterol metabolism: phytosterols, oxysterols, and squalene. Nutr Rev 2002;60(11):349–359

61. Andersson SW, Skinner J, Ellegård L, et al. Intake of dietary plant sterols is inversely related to serum cholesterol concentration in men and women in the EPIC Norfolk population: a cross-sectional study. Eur J Clin Nutr 2004;58(10):1378–1385

62. Klingberg S, Ellegård L, Johansson I, et al. Inverse relation between dietary intake of naturally occurring plant sterols and serum cholesterol in northern Sweden. Am J Clin Nutr 2008;87(4):993–1001

63. Ostlund RE Jr, Racette SB, Okeke A, Stenson WF. Phytosterols that are naturally present in commercial corn oil significantly reduce cholesterol absorption in humans. Am J Clin Nutr 2002;75(6):1000–1004

64. Ostlund RE Jr, Racette SB, Stenson WF. Inhibition of cholesterol absorption by phytosterol-replete wheat germ compared with phytosterol-depleted wheat germ. Am J Clin Nutr 2003;77(6):1385–1389

65. Ju YH, Clausen LM, Allred KF, Almada AL, Helferich WG. Beta-sitosterol, beta-sitosterol glucoside, and a mixture of beta-sitosterol and beta-sitosterol glucoside modulate the growth of estrogen-responsive breast cancer cells in vitro and in ovariectomized athymic mice. J Nutr 2004;134(5):1145–1151

66. Awad AB, Fink CS, Williams H, Kim U. In vitro and in vivo (SCID mice) effects of phytosterols on the growth and dissemination of human prostate cancer PC-3 cells. Eur J Cancer Prev 2001;10(6):507–513

67. Awad AB, Downie A, Fink CS, Kim U. Dietary phytosterol inhibits the growth and metastasis of MDA-MB-231 human breast cancer cells grown in SCID mice. Anticancer Res 2000;20(2A):821–824

68. De Stefani E, Boffetta P, Ronco AL, et al. Plant sterols and risk of stomach cancer: a case-control study in Uruguay. Nutr Cancer 2000;37(2):140–144

69. Mendilaharsu M, De Stefani E, Deneo-Pellegrini H, Carzoglio J, Ronco A. Phytosterols and risk of lung cancer: a case-control study in Uruguay. Lung Cancer 1998;21(1):37–45

70. Ronco A, De Stefani E, Boffetta P, Deneo-Pellegrini H, Mendilaharsu M, Leborgne F. Vegetables, fruits, and related nutrients and risk of breast cancer: a case-control study in Uruguay. Nutr Cancer 1999; 35(2): 111–119

71. McCann SE, Freudenheim JL, Marshall JR, Brasure JR, Swanson MK, Graham S. Diet in the epidemiology of endometrial cancer in Western New York (United States). Cancer Causes Control 2000;11(10):965–974

72. McCann SE, Freudenheim JL, Marshall JR, Graham S. Risk of human ovarian cancer is related to dietary intake of selected nutrients, phytochemicals and food groups. J Nutr 2003;133(6):1937–1942

73. Strom SS, Yamamura Y, Duphorne CM, et al. Phytoestrogen intake and prostate cancer: a case-control study using a new database. Nutr Cancer 1999; 33(1):20–25

74. Berges RR, Windeler J, Trampisch HJ, Senge T; Beta-sitosterol Study Group. Randomised, placebo-controlled, double-blind clinical trial of beta-sitosterol in patients with benign prostatic hyperplasia. Lancet 1995;345(8964):1529–1532

75. Berges RR, Kassen A, Senge T. Treatment of symptomatic benign prostatic hyperplasia with beta-sitosterol: an 18-month follow-up. BJU Int 2000;85(7):842–846

76. Klippel KF, Hiltl DM, Schipp B. A multicentric, place-bo-controlled, double-blind clinical trial of beta-sitosterol (phytosterol) for the treatment of benign prostatic hyperplasia. German BPH-Phyto Study group. Br J Urol 1997;80(3):427–432

77. Wilt TJ, MacDonald R, Ishani A. beta-sitosterol for the treatment of benign prostatic hyperplasia: a systematic review. BJU Int 1999;83(9):976–983

78. Dreikorn K. The role of phytotherapy in treating lower urinary tract symptoms and benign prostatic hyperplasia. World J Urol 2002;19(6):426–435

79. Nair PP, Turjman N, Kessie G, et al. Diet, nutrition intake, and metabolism in populations at high and low risk for colon cancer. Dietary cholesterol, beta-sitosterol, and stigmasterol. Am J Clin Nutr 1984; 40(4, Suppl):927–930

80. US Department of Agriculture, Agricultural Research Service. USDA Nutrient Database for Standard Reference, Release 20. 2007. Available at: http://www.nal.usda.gov/fnic/foodcomp/Data/SR20/nutrlist/sr20w430.pdf. Accessed July 24, 2008

81. Normén L, Bryngelsson S, Johnsson M, et al. The phytosterol content of some cereal foods commonly consumed in Sweden and in the Netherlands. J Food Compost Anal 2002;15(6):693–704

82. Normén L, Johnsson M, Andersson H, van Gameren Y, Dutta P. Plant sterols in vegetables and fruits commonly consumed in Sweden. Eur J Nutr 1999; 38(2):84–89

83. Phillips KM, Ruggio DM, Toivo JI, Swank MA, Simpkins AH. Free and esterified sterol composition of edible oils and fats. J Food Compost Anal 2002;15(2):123–142

84. Mensink RP, Ebbing S, Lindhout M, Plat J, van Heugten MM. Effects of plant stanol esters supplied in low-fat yoghurt on serum lipids and lipoproteins, non-cholesterol sterols and fat soluble antioxidant concentrations. Atherosclerosis 2002;160(1):205–213

85. Plana N, Nicolle C, Ferre R, et al; DANACOL group. Plant sterol-enriched fermented milk enhances the attainment of LDL-cholesterol goal in hypercholesterolemic subjects. Eur J Nutr 2008;47(1):32–39

86. Doornbos AM, Meynen EM, Duchateau GS, van der Knaap HC, Trautwein EA. Intake occasion affects the serum cholesterol lowering of a plant sterol-enriched single-dose yoghurt drink in mildly hypercholesterolaemic subjects. Eur J Clin Nutr 2006;60(3):325–333

87. Noakes M, Clifton PM, Doornbos AME, Trautwein EA. Plant sterol ester-enriched milk and yoghurt effectively reduce serum cholesterol in modestly hypercholesterolemic subjects. Eur J Nutr 2005;44(4):214–222

88. Thomsen AB, Hansen HB, Christiansen C, Green H, Berger A. Effect of free plant sterols in low-fat milk on serum lipid profile in hypercholesterolemic subjects. Eur J Clin Nutr 2004;58(6):860–870

89. Seppo L, Jauhiainen T, Nevala R, Poussa T, Korpela R. Plant stanol esters in low-fat milk products lower serum total and LDL cholesterol. Eur J Nutr 2007; 46(2):111–117

90. Jauhiainen T, Salo P, Niittynen L, Poussa T, Korpela R. Effects of low-fat hard cheese enriched with plant stanol esters on serum lipids and apolipoprotein B in mildly hypercholesterolaemic subjects. Eur J Clin Nutr 2006;60(11):1253–1257

91. Allen RR, Carson L, Kwik-Uribe C, Evans EM, Erdman JW Jr. Daily consumption of a dark chocolate containing flavanols and added sterol esters affects cardiovascular risk factors in a normotensive population with elevated cholesterol. J Nutr 2008;138(4):725–731

92. Devaraj S, Jialal I, Vega-López S. Plant sterol-fortified orange juice effectively lowers cholesterol levels in mildly hypercholesterolemic healthy individuals. Arterioscler Thromb Vasc Biol 2004;24(3):e25–e28

93. Devaraj S, Autret BC, Jialal I. Reduced-calorie orange juice beverage with plant sterols lowers C-reactive protein concentrations and improves the lipid profile in human volunteers. Am J Clin Nutr 2006;84(4):756–761

94. Matvienko OA, Lewis DS, Swanson M, et al. A single daily dose of soybean phytosterols in ground beef decreases serum total cholesterol and LDL cholesterol in young, mildly hypercholesterolemic men. Am J Clin Nutr 2002;76(1):57–64

95. Plat J, van Onselen EN, van Heugten MM, Mensink RP. Effects on serum lipids, lipoproteins and fat soluble antioxidant concentrations of consumption frequency of margarines and shortenings enriched with plant stanol esters. Eur J Clin Nutr 2000;54(9):671–677

96. Food and Drug Administration. Agency Response Letter. GRAS Notice No. GRN 000112. 2003. Available at: http://www.fda.gov/ohrms/dockets/dockets/95s0316/95s-0316-rpt000343-043-appx-E-Ref-31-GRAS-vol268.pdf. Accessed May 7, 2012

97. Scientific Committee on Food. Opinion on Applications for Approval of a Variety of Plant Sterol-Enriched Foods. Brussels: European Commission; 2003. Available at: http://ec.europa.eu/food/fs/sc/scf/out174_en.pdf. Accessed May 7, 2012

98. Ayesh R, Weststrate JA, Drewitt PN, Hepburn PA. Safety evaluation of phytosterol esters. Part 5. Faecal short-chain fatty acid and microflora content, faecal bacterial enzyme activity and serum female sex hormones in healthy normolipidaemic volunteers consuming a controlled diet either with or without a phytosterol ester-enriched margarine. Food Chem Toxicol 1999;37(12):1127–1138

99. Berge KE. Sitosterolemia: a gateway to new knowledge about cholesterol metabolism. Ann Med 2003;35(7):502–511

100. Stalenhoef AF, Hectors M, Demacker PN. Effect of plant sterol-enriched margarine on plasma lipids and sterols in subjects heterozygous for phytosterolaemia. J Intern Med 2001;249(2):163–166

101. Kwiterovich PO Jr, Chen SC, Virgil DG, Schweitzer A, Arnold DR, Kratz LE. Response of obligate heterozygotes for phytosterolemia to a low-fat diet and to a plant sterol ester dietary challenge. J Lipid Res 2003;44(6):1143–1155

102. Normén L, Holmes D, Frohlich J. Plant sterols and their role in combined use with statins for lipid lowering. Curr Opin Investig Drugs 2005;6(3):307–316

103. Thompson GR. Additive effects of plant sterol and stanol esters to statin therapy. Am J Cardiol 2005; 96(1A, Suppl):37D–39D

104. Blair SN, Capuzzi DM, Gottlieb SO, Nguyen T, Morgan JM, Cater NB. Incremental reduction of serum total cholesterol and low-density lipoprotein cholesterol with the addition of plant stanol ester-containing spread to statin therapy. Am J Cardiol 2000;86(1):46–52

105. Neil HA, Meijer GW, Roe LS. Randomised controlled trial of use by hypercholesterolaemic patients of a vegetable oil sterol-enriched fat spread. Atherosclerosis 2001;156(2):329–337

106. Simons LA. Additive effect of plant sterol-ester margarine and cerivastatin in lowering low-density lipoprotein cholesterol in primary hypercholesterolemia. Am J Cardiol 2002;90(7):737–740

107. Nguyen TT, Dale LC. Plant stanol esters and vitamin K. Mayo Clin Proc 1999;74(6):642–643

108. Raeini-Sarjaz M, Ntanios FY, Vanstone CA, Jones PJ. No changes in serum fat-soluble vitamin and carotenoid concentrations with the intake of plant sterol/stanol esters in the context of a controlled diet. Metabolism 2002;51(5):652–656

109. Korpela R, Tuomilehto J, Högström P, et al. Safety aspects and cholesterol-lowering efficacy of low fat dairy products containing plant sterols. Eur J Clin Nutr 2006;60(5):633–642

110. Plat J, Mensink RP. Vegetable oil based versus wood based stanol ester mixtures: effects on serum lipids and hemostatic factors in non-hypercholesterolemic subjects. Atherosclerosis 2000;148(1):101–112

111. Plat J, Mensink RP. Effects of diets enriched with two different plant stanol ester mixtures on plasma ubiquinol-10 and fat-soluble antioxidant concentrations. Metabolism 2001;50(5):520–529

112. Ntanios FY, Duchateau GS. A healthy diet rich in carotenoids is effective in maintaining normal blood carotenoid levels during the daily use of plant sterol-enriched spreads. Int J Vitam Nutr Res 2002; 72(1):32–39

113. Noakes M, Clifton P, Ntanios F, Shrapnel W, Record I, McInerney J. An increase in dietary carotenoids when consuming plant sterols or stanols is effective in maintaining plasma carotenoid concentrations. Am J Clin Nutr 2002;75(1):79–86

19 Resveratrol

Resveratrol (3,4′,5-trihydroxystilbene) belongs to a class of polyphenolic compounds called *stilbenes*.[1] Some types of plants produce resveratrol and other stilbenes in response to stress, injury, fungal infection, or ultraviolet radiation.[2] Resveratrol is a fat-soluble compound that occurs in a *trans* and a *cis* configuration (Fig. 19.1). Both *cis*- and *trans*-resveratrol also occur as glucosides (bound to a glucose molecule). Resveratrol-3-O-β-glucoside is called *piceid*.[3] Scientists became interested in exploring potential health benefits of resveratrol in 1992 when its presence was first reported in red wine,[4] leading to speculation that resveratrol might help explain the "French Paradox" (see the Cardiovascular Disease section be-

low). More recently, reports on the potential for resveratrol to inhibit the development of cancer[5] and extend lifespan[6] in cell culture and animal models have continued to generate scientific interest.

Bioavailability and Metabolism

Although *trans*-resveratrol appears to be well-absorbed by humans when taken orally, its bioavailability is relatively low due to its rapid metabolism and elimination.[7,8] Resveratrol metabolites are primarily detected upon oral exposure to *trans*-resveratrol. When six healthy men and

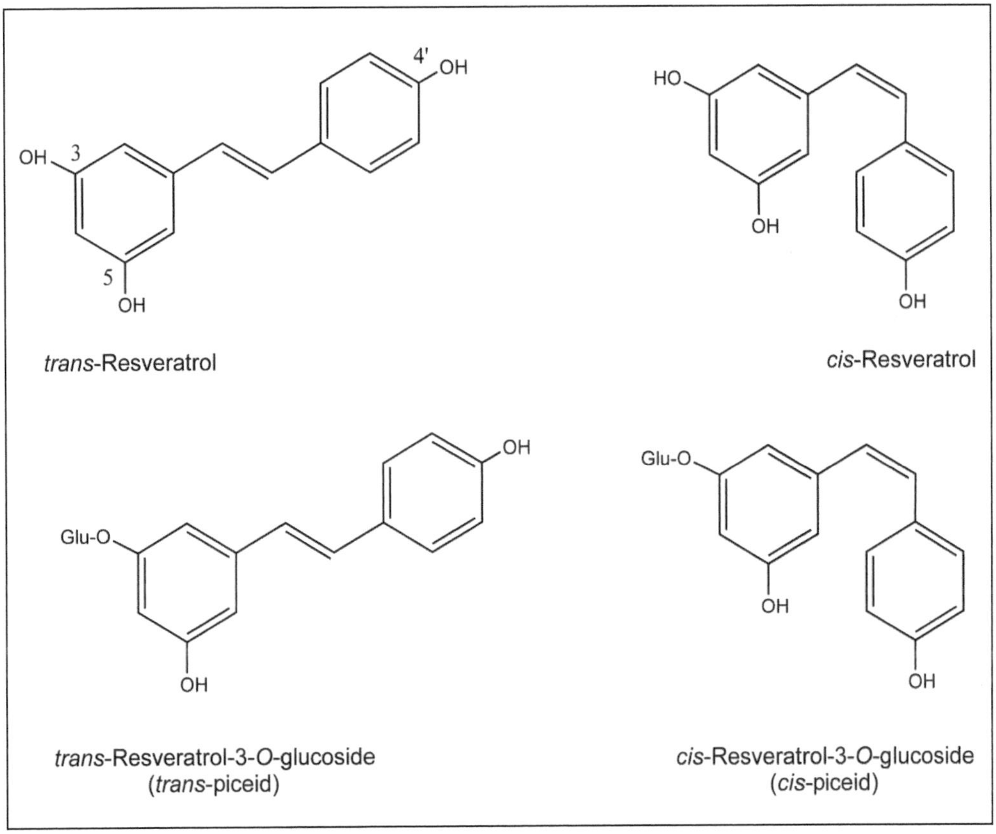

Fig. 19.1 Chemical structures of *trans*-resveratrol, *cis*-resveratrol, *trans*-resveratrol-3-O-glucoside (*trans*-piceid), and *cis*-3-O-glucoside (*cis*-piceid).

women took an oral dose of 25 mg of *trans*-resveratrol, only traces of the unchanged resveratrol were detected in plasma (blood). Plasma concentrations of resveratrol and metabolites peaked around 60 minutes later at concentrations around 2 µmol/L (491 µg/L).[7] A study in 12 healthy men administered an oral dose of 25 mg of *trans*-resveratrol per 70 kg of body weight reported that serum concentration of resveratrol and metabolites peaked at 30 minutes after administration. The concentration of total resveratrol (resveratrol and metabolites) ranged from 416 µg/L to 471 µg/L, depending on whether resveratrol was administered in wine, vegetable juice, or grape juice.[9] Results of another study suggested that the bioavailability of resveratrol from grape juice, which contains mostly glucosides of resveratrol (piceid), may be even lower than that of *trans*-resveratrol.[10] Additionally a study reported that bioavailability of *trans*-resveratrol from red wine did not differ when the wine was consumed with a meal (low- or high-fat) versus on an empty stomach.[11]

Information about the bioavailability of resveratrol in humans is important because much of the basic research on resveratrol has been conducted in cultured cells exposed to unmetabolized resveratrol at concentrations that are often 10 to 100 times greater than the peak concentrations observed in human plasma after oral consumption.[12] Although cells that line the digestive tract are exposed to unmetabolized resveratrol, research in humans suggests that other tissues are exposed primarily to resveratrol metabolites. Little is known about the biological activity of resveratrol metabolites, and it is not known whether some tissues are capable of converting resveratrol metabolites back to resveratrol.[7]

Biological Activities

Direct Antioxidant Activity

In the test tube, resveratrol effectively scavenges (neutralizes) free radicals and other oxidants[13] and inhibits low-density lipoprotein (LDL) oxidation.[14,15] However, there is little evidence that resveratrol is an important antioxidant in vivo.[16] Upon oral consumption of resveratrol, circulating and intracellular levels of resveratrol in humans are likely to be much lower than those of other important antioxidants, such as vitamin C, uric acid, vitamin E, and glutathione. Moreover, the antioxidant activity of resveratrol metabolites, which comprise most of the circulating resveratrol, may be lower than that of resveratrol.

Estrogenic and Antiestrogenic Activities

Endogenous estrogens are steroid hormones synthesized by humans and other mammals; these hormones bind to estrogen receptors within cells. The estrogen–receptor complex interacts with unique sequences in DNA (estrogen response elements—EREs) to modulate the expression of estrogen-responsive genes.[17] A compound that binds to estrogen receptors and elicits similar responses to endogenous estrogens is considered an estrogen agonist, while a compound that binds estrogen receptors but prevents or inhibits the response elicited by endogenous estrogens is considered an estrogen antagonist. The chemical structure of resveratrol is very similar to that of the synthetic estrogen agonist, diethylstilbestrol (Fig. 19.2), suggesting that resveratrol might also function as an estrogen agonist. However, in cell-culture experiments resveratrol acts as an estrogen agonist under some conditions and an estrogen antagonist under other conditions.[18,19] In estrogen receptor-positive breast cancer cells, resveratrol acted as an estrogen agonist in the absence of the endogenous estrogen, 17β-estradiol but acted as an estrogen antagonist in the presence of 17β-estradiol.[20,21] At present, it appears that resveratrol has the potential to act as an estrogen agonist or antagonist depending on such factors as cell type, estrogen receptor isoform (ERα or ERβ), and the presence of endogenous estrogens.[17]

Biological Activities Related to Cancer Prevention

Effects on Biotransformation Enzymes

Some compounds are not carcinogenic until they have been metabolized in the body by cytochrome P450 (CYP) enzymes.[2] By inhibiting the expression and activity of certain CYP enzymes,[22,23] resveratrol could help prevent cancer by decreasing exposure to these activated carcinogens. In contrast, increasing the activity of phase II biotransformation enzymes generally promotes the excretion of potentially toxic or

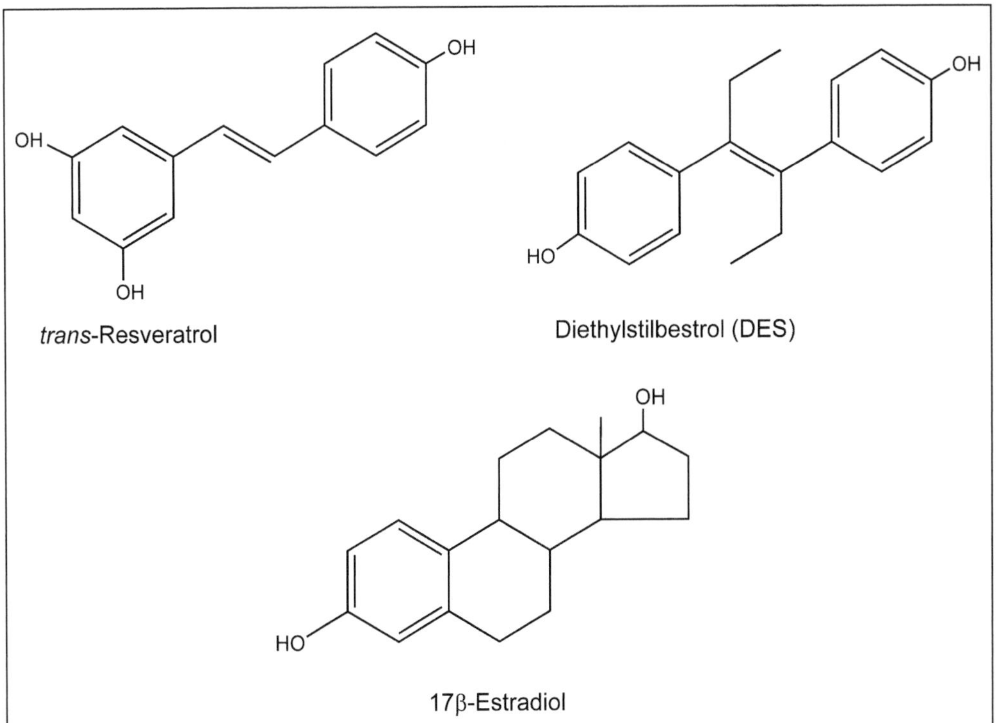

Fig. 19.2 Chemical structures of *trans*-resveratrol; diethylstilbestrol, a synthetic estrogen agonist; and 17β-estradiol, an endogenous estrogen.

carcinogenic chemicals. Resveratrol has been found to increase the expression and activity of the phase II enzyme NAD(P)H:quinone reductase in cultured cells.[5,24]

Preservation of Normal Cell-Cycle Regulation

Following DNA damage, the cell cycle can be transiently arrested to allow for DNA repair or activation of pathways leading to cell death (apoptosis) if the damage is irreparable.[25] Defective cell-cycle regulation may result in the propagation of mutations that contribute to the development of cancer. Resveratrol has been found to induce cell-cycle arrest when added to cancer cells grown in culture.[26]

Inhibition of Proliferation and Induction of Apoptosis

Unlike normal cells, cancer cells proliferate rapidly and are unable to respond to cell-death signals that initiate apoptosis. Resveratrol has been found to inhibit proliferation and induce apoptosis in several cancer cell lines.[2,27]

Inhibition of Tumor Invasion and Angiogenesis

Cancerous cells invade normal tissue aided by enzymes called *matrix metalloproteinases*. Resveratrol has been found to inhibit the activity of at least one type of matrix metalloproteinase.[28] To fuel their rapid growth, invasive tumors must also develop new blood vessels by a process known as *angiogenesis*. Resveratrol has been found to inhibit angiogenesis in vitro.[29–31]

Anti-inflammatory Effects

Inflammation promotes cellular proliferation and angiogenesis and inhibits apoptosis.[32] Resveratrol has been found to inhibit the activity of several inflammatory enzymes in vitro, including cyclooxygenase and lipoxygenase.[33,34] Resveratrol may also inhibit pro-inflammatory transcription factors, such as nuclear factor kappa B (NF-κB) or activator protein 1 (AP-1).[35,36]

Biological Activities Related to Cardiovascular Disease Prevention

Inhibition of Vascular Cell Adhesion Molecule Expression

Atherosclerosis is now recognized as an inflammatory disease, and several measures of inflammation are associated with increased risk of myocardial infarction (MI; heart attack).[37] One of the earliest events in the development of atherosclerosis is the recruitment of inflammatory white blood cells from the blood to the arterial wall by vascular cell adhesion molecules.[38] Resveratrol has been found to inhibit the expression of adhesion molecules in cultured endothelial cells.[39,40]

Inhibition of Vascular Smooth Muscle Cell Proliferation

The proliferation of vascular smooth muscle cells plays an important role in the progression of atherosclerosis.[41] Resveratrol has been found to inhibit the proliferation of vascular smooth muscle cells in culture.[42,43]

Stimulation of Endothelial Nitric Oxide Synthase Activity

Endothelial nitric oxide synthase (eNOS) is an enzyme that catalyzes the formation of nitric oxide (NO) by vascular endothelial cells. NO is needed to maintain arterial relaxation (vasodilation), and impaired NO-dependent vasodilation is associated with increased risk of cardiovascular disease.[44] Resveratrol has been found to stimulate eNOS activity in cultured endothelial cells.[45,46]

Inhibition of Platelet Aggregation

Platelet aggregation is one of the first steps in the formation of a blood clot that can occlude a coronary or cerebral artery, resulting in MI or stroke, respectively. Resveratrol has been found to inhibit platelet aggregation in vitro.[47,48]

It is important to keep in mind that many of the biological activities discussed above were observed in cells cultured in the presence of resveratrol at higher concentrations than those likely to be achieved in humans consuming resveratrol orally (see the Bioavailability and Metabolism section above).

Disease Prevention

Cardiovascular Disease

Red Wine Polyphenols

Significant reductions in cardiovascular disease risk have been associated with moderate consumption of alcoholic beverages.[49,50] The "French Paradox"—the observation that mortality from coronary heart disease (CHD) is relatively low in France despite relatively high levels of dietary saturated fat and cigarette smoking—led to the idea that regular consumption of red wine might provide additional protection from cardiovascular disease.[51,52] Red wine contains resveratrol and even higher levels of flavonoids. These polyphenolic compounds have antioxidant, anti-inflammatory, and other potentially anti-atherogenic effects in the test tube and in some animal models of atherosclerosis.[53] However, it is not yet known whether increased consumption of polyphenols from red wine provides any additional protection from cardiovascular disease beyond that associated with its alcohol content. The results of epidemiological studies addressing this question have been inconsistent. While some large prospective studies found that wine drinkers were at lower risk of cardiovascular disease than beer or liquor drinkers,[54–56] others found no difference.[57–59] Socioeconomic and lifestyle differences between people who prefer wine and those who prefer beer or liquor may explain part of the additional benefit observed in some studies. Several studies have found that people who prefer wine tend to have higher incomes, more education, smoke less, and eat more fruits and vegetables and less saturated fat than people who prefer other alcoholic beverages.[59–64] Although moderate alcohol consumption has been consistently associated with 20%–30% reductions in CHD risk, it is not yet clear whether red wine polyphenols confer any additional risk reduction. Interestingly, studies that administered alcohol-free red wine to rodents noted improvements in various parameters related to cardiovascular disease,[65,66] and a placebo-controlled human study found that heart disease patients administered red grape polyphenol extract experienced acute improvements in endothelial function.[67] However, more studies are needed to determine whether drinking red wine confers any cardiovascular benefit beyond that associated with its alcohol content.

Resveratrol

Resveratrol has been found to exert several potentially cardioprotective effects in vitro, including inhibition of platelet aggregation,[47,48,68] promotion of vasodilation by enhancing the production of NO,[46,69] and inhibition of inflammatory enzymes.[34,70,71] However, the concentrations of resveratrol required to produce these effects are often higher than those that have been measured in human plasma after oral consumption of resveratrol.[7] The results of some animal studies suggest that high oral doses of resveratrol could decrease the risk of thrombosis (clot formation) and atherosclerosis,[72,73] but at least one study found increased atherosclerosis in animals fed resveratrol.[74] Although its presence in red wine has stimulated a great deal of interest in the potential for resveratrol to prevent cardiovascular disease, there is currently no convincing evidence that resveratrol has cardioprotective effects in humans, particularly in the amounts present in 1–2 glasses of red wine (see the Sources section below).

Cancer

Resveratrol has been found to inhibit the proliferation of a variety of human cancer cell lines, including those from breast, prostate, stomach, colon, pancreatic, and thyroid cancers.[2] In animal models, oral administration of resveratrol inhibited the development of esophageal,[75] intestinal,[76] and mammary (breast) cancer[20,77] induced by chemical carcinogens. However, oral resveratrol was not effective in inhibiting the development of lung cancer induced by carcinogens in cigarette smoke.[78,79] The effects of oral resveratrol administration on mice that are genetically predisposed to colon cancer have been mixed,[80,81] and a few studies have documented that oral resveratrol protects against development of colon cancer in rats administered the carcinogen, 1,2-dimethylhydrazine.[82–84] It is not known whether high intakes of resveratrol can help prevent cancer in humans. Clinical trials are currently under way to address this question and to also determine whether resveratrol might be beneficial in cancer treatment.[85] Studies on human metabolism of resveratrol suggest that even very high dietary intakes of resveratrol may not result in tissue levels that are high enough to realize most of the protective effects demonstrated in cell culture studies.[7,12]

Longevity

Caloric restriction is known to extend the lifespans of several species, including mammals.[86] In yeast, caloric restriction stimulates the activity of an enzyme known as Sir2.[87] Providing resveratrol to yeast increased Sir2 activity in the absence of caloric restriction and extended the replicative lifespan of yeast by 70%.[6] Resveratrol feeding also extended the lifespans of worms (*C. elegans*) and fruit flies (*D. melanogaster*) by a similar mechanism.[88] Additionally, resveratrol dose-dependently increased the lifespan of a vertebrate fish (*N. furzeri*).[89] However, it is not known whether resveratrol will have similar effects in higher animals. One study reported that resveratrol extended the lifespan of mice on a high-calorie diet, such that their lifespan was similar to that of mice fed a standard diet.[90] Although resveratrol increased the activity of the homologous human enzyme (Sirt1) in the test tube,[6] it is not known whether resveratrol can extend the human lifespan. Moreover, the resveratrol concentrations required to increase human Sirt1 activity were considerably higher than concentrations that have been measured in human plasma after oral consumption. Interestingly, a recent aging study in mice found that a low dose of dietary resveratrol led to altered gene expression in heart, brain, and skeletal muscle similar to that induced by caloric restriction.[91] Like caloric restriction, resveratrol also blunted the age-related decline in heart function in this study. Clinical trials will be needed to determine if these findings are relevant to humans.

Sources

Food Sources

Resveratrol is found in grapes, wine, grape juice, peanuts, and berries of *Vaccinum* species, including blueberries, bilberries, and cranberries.[92–94] In grapes, resveratrol is found only in the skins.[95] The amount of resveratrol in grape skins varies with the grape cultivar, its geographic origin, and exposure to fungal infection.[96] The amount of

Table 19.1 Total resveratrol content of some white, rosé, and red wines and red (purple) grape juice[3,99,100]

Beverage	Total Resveratrol (mg/L)	Total Resveratrol in a 5-oz Glass (mg)
White wines (Spanish)	0.05–1.80	0.01–0.27
Rosé wines (Spanish)	0.43–3.52	0.06–0.53
Red wines (Spanish)	1.92–12.59	0.29–1.89
Red wines (global)	1.98–7.13	0.30–1.07
Red grape juice (Spanish)	1.14–8.69	0.17–1.30

Table 19.2 Total resveratrol content of selected foods[92,94,101]

Food	Serving	Total Resveratrol (mg)
Peanuts (raw)	1 cup	0.01–0.26
Peanuts (boiled)	1 cup	0.32–1.28
Peanut butter	1 cup	0.04–0.13
Red grapes	1 cup	0.24–1.25

fermentation time a wine spends in contact with grape skins is an important determinant of its resveratrol content. Consequently, white and rosé wines generally contain less resveratrol than red wines.[4] Red or purple grape juices may also be good sources of resveratrol.[3] The predominant form of resveratrol in grapes and grape juice is *trans*-resveratrol glucoside (*trans*-piceid), but wines also contain significant amounts of resveratrol aglycones, thought to be the result of sugar cleavage during fermentation.[92] Many wines also contain significant amounts of *cis*-resveratrol (Fig. 19.1), which may be produced during fermentation or released from viniferins (resveratrol polymers).[97] Red wine is a relatively rich source of resveratrol, but other polyphenols are present in red wine at considerably higher concentrations than resveratrol (see Chapter 11).[98] The total resveratrol content of some beverages and foods are listed in **Tables 19.1** and **19.2**, respectively. These values should be considered approximate, since the resveratrol content of foods and beverages can vary considerably.

Supplements

Most resveratrol supplements available in the United States contain extracts of the root of *Polygonum cuspidatum*, also known as *Hu Zhang* or *kojo-kon*.[102] Red wine extracts and red grape extracts containing resveratrol and other polyphenols are also available in the United States as dietary supplements. Resveratrol supplements may contain anywhere from 10–50 mg of resveratrol, but the effective doses for prevention of chronic disease in humans are not known.

Safety

Adverse Effects

Resveratrol is not known to be toxic or cause adverse effects in humans, but there have been only a few controlled clinical trials to date. A recent trial that evaluated the safety of oral resveratrol in 10 subjects found a single dose up to 5 g resulted in no serious adverse effects.[103] In rats, daily oral administration of *trans*-resveratrol at doses up to 300 mg/kg of body weight for 4 weeks resulted in no apparent adverse effects.[104,105]

Pregnancy and Lactation

The safety of resveratrol-containing supplements during pregnancy and lactation has not been established.[102] Since no safe level of alcohol consumption has been established at any stage of pregnancy,[106] pregnant women should avoid consuming wine as a source of resveratrol.

Estrogen-Sensitive Cancers

Until more is known about the estrogenic activity of resveratrol in humans, women with a history of estrogen-sensitive cancers, such as breast, ovarian, and uterine cancers, should avoid resveratrol supplements (see the Estrogenic and Antiestrogenic Activities section above).

Drug Interactions

Anticoagulant and Antiplatelet Drugs

Resveratrol has been found to inhibit human platelet aggregation in vitro.[48,107] Theoretically, high intakes of resveratrol (e.g., from supplements) could increase the risk of bleeding when taken with anticoagulant drugs, such as warfarin (Coumadin); antiplatelet drugs, such as clopidogrel (Plavix) and dipyridamole (Persantin); and nonsteroidal anti-inflammatory drugs, including aspirin, ibuprofen, and others.

Drugs Metabolized by Cytochrome P450 3A4

Resveratrol has been reported to inhibit the activity of CYP3A4 in vitro.[108,109] Although this interaction has not been reported in humans, high intakes of resveratrol (e.g., from supplements) could theoretically increase the bioavailability and toxicity of drugs that undergo extensive first-pass metabolism by CYP3A4. Drugs known to be metabolized by CYP3A4 include but are not limited to 3-hydroxy-3-methyl-glutaryl-coenzyme A reductase inhibitors (atorvastatin, lovastatin, and simvastatin), calcium channel antagonists (felodipine, nicardipine, nifedipine, nisoldipine, nitrendipine, nimodipine, and verapamil), antiarrhythmic agents (amiodarone), HIV protease inhibitors (saquinivir), immunosuppressants (ciclosporin and tacrolimus), antihistamines (terfenadine), benzodiazepines (midazolam and triazolam), and drugs used to treat erectile dysfunction (sildenafil).

Summary

- Resveratrol is a polyphenolic compound found in grapes, red wine, purple grape juice, peanuts, and some berries.
- When taken orally, resveratrol appears to be well absorbed by humans, but its bioavailability is relatively low because it is rapidly metabolized and eliminated.
- Scientists became interested in exploring potential health benefits of resveratrol when its presence was reported in red wine, leading to speculation that resveratrol might help explain the "French Paradox."
- Moderate alcohol consumption has been consistently associated with 20%–30% reductions in coronary heart disease risk, but it is not yet clear whether red wine polyphenols, such as resveratrol, confer any additional risk reduction.
- Although resveratrol can inhibit the growth of cancer cells in culture and in some animal

models, it is not known whether high intakes of resveratrol can prevent cancer in humans.
- Resveratrol administration has increased the lifespans of yeast, worms, fruit flies, fish, and mice fed a high-calorie diet, but it is not known whether resveratrol will have similar effects in humans.
- At present, relatively little is known about the effects of resveratrol in humans.

References

1. Soleas GJ, Diamandis EP, Goldberg DM. Resveratrol: a molecule whose time has come? And gone? Clin Biochem 1997;30(2):91–113
2. Aggarwal BB, Bhardwaj A, Aggarwal RS, Seeram NP, Shishodia S, Takada Y. Role of resveratrol in prevention and therapy of cancer: preclinical and clinical studies. Anticancer Res 2004;24(5A):2783–2840
3. Romero-Pérez AI, Ibern-Gómez M, Lamuela-Raventós RM, de La Torre-Boronat MC. Piceid, the major resveratrol derivative in grape juices. J Agric Food Chem 1999;47(4):1533–1536
4. Siemann EH, Creasey LL. Concentration of the phytoalexin resveratrol in wine. Am J Enol Vitic 1992; 43(1):49–52
5. Jang M, Cai L, Udeani GO, et al. Cancer chemopreventive activity of resveratrol, a natural product derived from grapes. Science 1997;275(5297):218–220
6. Howitz KT, Bitterman KJ, Cohen HY, et al. Small molecule activators of sirtuins extend Saccharomyces cerevisiae lifespan. Nature 2003;425(6954):191–196
7. Walle T, Hsieh F, DeLegge MH, Oatis JE Jr, Walle UK. High absorption but very low bioavailability of oral resveratrol in humans. Drug Metab Dispos 2004; 32(12):1377–1382
8. Wenzel E, Somoza V. Metabolism and bioavailability of trans-resveratrol. Mol Nutr Food Res 2005;49(5): 472–481
9. Goldberg DM, Yan J, Soleas GJ. Absorption of three wine-related polyphenols in three different matrices by healthy subjects. Clin Biochem 2003;36(1):79–87
10. Meng X, Maliakal P, Lu H, Lee MJ, Yang CS. Urinary and plasma levels of resveratrol and quercetin in humans, mice, and rats after ingestion of pure compounds and grape juice. J Agric Food Chem 2004;52(4):935–942
11. Vitaglione P, Sforza S, Galaverna G, et al. Bioavailability of trans-resveratrol from red wine in humans. Mol Nutr Food Res 2005;49(5):495–504
12. Gescher AJ, Steward WP. Relationship between mechanisms, bioavailibility, and preclinical chemopreventive efficacy of resveratrol: a conundrum. Cancer Epidemiol Biomarkers Prev 2003;12(10):953–957
13. Stojanović S, Sprinz H, Brede O. Efficiency and mechanism of the antioxidant action of trans-resveratrol and its analogues in the radical liposome oxidation. Arch Biochem Biophys 2001;391(1):79–89
14. Brito P, Almeida LM, Dinis TC. The interaction of resveratrol with ferrylmyoglobin and peroxynitrite; protection against LDL oxidation. Free Radic Res 2002; 36(6):621–631
15. Frankel EN, Waterhouse AL, Kinsella JE. Inhibition of human LDL oxidation by resveratrol. Lancet 1993; 341(8852):1103–1104

16. Bradamante S, Barenghi L, Villa A. Cardiovascular protective effects of resveratrol. Cardiovasc Drug Rev 2004;22(3):169–188
17. Tangkeangsirisin W, Serrero G. Resveratrol in the chemoprevention and chemotherapy of breast cancer. In: Bagchi D, Preuss HG, eds. Phytopharmaceuticals in Cancer Chemoprevention. Boca Raton, FL: CRC Press; 2005:449–463
18. Bowers JL, Tyulmenkov VV, Jernigan SC, Klinge CM. Resveratrol acts as a mixed agonist/antagonist for estrogen receptors alpha and beta. Endocrinology 2000;141(10):3657–3667
19. Gehm BD, McAndrews JM, Chien PY, Jameson JL. Resveratrol, a polyphenolic compound found in grapes and wine, is an agonist for the estrogen receptor. Proc Natl Acad Sci U S A 1997;94(25):14138–14143
20. Bhat KP, Lantvit D, Christov K, Mehta RG, Moon RC, Pezzuto JM. Estrogenic and antiestrogenic properties of resveratrol in mammary tumor models. Cancer Res 2001;61(20):7456–7463
21. Lu R, Serrero G. Resveratrol, a natural product derived from grape, exhibits antiestrogenic activity and inhibits the growth of human breast cancer cells. J Cell Physiol 1999;179(3):297–304
22. Chen ZH, Hurh YJ, Na HK, et al. Resveratrol inhibits TCDD-induced expression of CYP1A1 and CYP1B1 and catechol estrogen-mediated oxidative DNA damage in cultured human mammary epithelial cells. Carcinogenesis 2004;25(10):2005–2013
23. Ciolino HP, Yeh GC. Inhibition of aryl hydrocarbon-induced cytochrome P-450 1A1 enzyme activity and CYP1A1 expression by resveratrol. Mol Pharmacol 1999;56(4):760–767
24. Yang SH, Kim JS, Oh TJ, et al. Genome-scale analysis of resveratrol-induced gene expression profile in human ovarian cancer cells using a cDNA microarray. Int J Oncol 2003;22(4):741–750
25. Stewart ZA, Westfall MD, Pietenpol JA. Cell-cycle dysregulation and anticancer therapy. Trends Pharmacol Sci 2003;24(3):139–145
26. Joe AK, Liu H, Suzui M, Vural ME, Xiao D, Weinstein IB. Resveratrol induces growth inhibition, S-phase arrest, apoptosis, and changes in biomarker expression in several human cancer cell lines. Clin Cancer Res 2002;8(3):893–903
27. Fulda S, Debatin KM. Resveratrol modulation of signal transduction in apoptosis and cell survival: a minireview. Cancer Detect Prev 2006;30(3):217–223
28. Woo JH, Lim JH, Kim YH, et al. Resveratrol inhibits phorbol myristate acetate-induced matrix metalloproteinase-9 expression by inhibiting JNK and PKC delta signal transduction. Oncogene 2004; 23(10): 1845–1853
29. Igura K, Ohta T, Kuroda Y, Kaji K. Resveratrol and quercetin inhibit angiogenesis in vitro. Cancer Lett 2001;171(1):11–16
30. Lin MT, Yen ML, Lin CY, Kuo ML. Inhibition of vascular endothelial growth factor-induced angiogenesis by resveratrol through interruption of Src-dependent vascular endothelial cadherin tyrosine phosphorylation. Mol Pharmacol 2003;64(5):1029–1036
31. Chen Y, Tseng SH. Review. Pro- and anti-angiogenesis effects of resveratrol. In Vivo 2007;21(2):365–370
32. Steele VE, Hawk ET, Viner JL, Lubet RA. Mechanisms and applications of non-steroidal anti-inflammatory drugs in the chemoprevention of cancer. Mutat Res 2003;523–524:137–144
33. Donnelly LE, Newton R, Kennedy GE, et al. Anti-inflammatory effects of resveratrol in lung epithelial cells: molecular mechanisms. Am J Physiol Lung Cell Mol Physiol 2004;287(4):L774–L783
34. Pinto MC, García-Barrado JA, Macías P. Resveratrol is a potent inhibitor of the dioxygenase activity of lipoxygenase. J Agric Food Chem 1999;47(12):4842–4846
35. Shankar S, Singh G, Srivastava RK. Chemoprevention by resveratrol: molecular mechanisms and therapeutic potential. Front Biosci 2007;12:4839–4854
36. de la Lastra CA, Villegas I. Resveratrol as an anti-inflammatory and anti-aging agent: mechanisms and clinical implications. Mol Nutr Food Res 2005; 49(5):405–430
37. Blake GJ, Ridker PM. C-reactive protein and other inflammatory risk markers in acute coronary syndromes. J Am Coll Cardiol 2003; 41(4, Suppl S):37S–42S
38. Stocker R, Keaney JF Jr. Role of oxidative modifications in atherosclerosis. Physiol Rev 2004;84(4):1381–1478
39. Carluccio MA, Siculella L, Ancora MA, et al. Olive oil and red wine antioxidant polyphenols inhibit endothelial activation: antiatherogenic properties of Mediterranean diet phytochemicals. Arterioscler Thromb Vasc Biol 2003;23(4):622–629
40. Ferrero ME, Bertelli AE, Fulgenzi A, et al. Activity in vitro of resveratrol on granulocyte and monocyte adhesion to endothelium. Am J Clin Nutr 1998;68(6): 1208–1214
41. Faxon DP, Fuster V, Libby P, et al; American Heart Association. Atherosclerotic Vascular Disease Conference: Writing Group III: pathophysiology. Circulation 2004;109(21):2617–2625
42. Mnjoyan ZH, Fujise K. Profound negative regulatory effects by resveratrol on vascular smooth muscle cells: a role of p53-p21(WAF1/CIP1) pathway. Biochem Biophys Res Commun 2003;311(2):546–552
43. Haider UG, Sorescu D, Griendling KK, Vollmar AM, Dirsch VM. Resveratrol increases serine15-phosphorylated but transcriptionally impaired p53 and induces a reversible DNA replication block in serum-activated vascular smooth muscle cells. Mol Pharmacol 2003;63(4):925–932
44. Duffy SJ, Vita JA. Effects of phenolics on vascular endothelial function. Curr Opin Lipidol 2003;14(1):21–27
45. Klinge CM, Blankenship KA, Risinger KE, et al. Resveratrol and estradiol rapidly activate MAPK signaling through estrogen receptors alpha and beta in endothelial cells. J Biol Chem 2005;280(9):7460–7468
46. Wallerath T, Deckert G, Ternes T, et al. Resveratrol, a polyphenolic phytoalexin present in red wine, enhances expression and activity of endothelial nitric oxide synthase. Circulation 2002;106(13):1652–1658
47. Kirk RI, Deitch JA, Wu JM, Lerea KM. Resveratrol decreases early signaling events in washed platelets but has little effect on platelet in whole blood. Blood Cells Mol Dis 2000;26(2):144–150
48. Pace-Asciak CR, Hahn S, Diamandis EP, Soleas G, Goldberg DM. The red wine phenolics trans-resveratrol and quercetin block human platelet aggregation and eicosanoid synthesis: implications for protection against coronary heart disease. Clin Chim Acta 1995;235(2):207–219
49. Klatsky AL. Drink to your health? Sci Am 2003; 288(2):74–81
50. Corrao G, Rubbiati L, Bagnardi V, Zambon A, Poikolainen K. Alcohol and coronary heart disease: a meta-analysis. Addiction 2000;95(10):1505–1523

51. Criqui MH, Ringel BL. Does diet or alcohol explain the French paradox? Lancet 1994;344(8939–8940): 1719–1723
52. St Leger AS, Cochrane AL, Moore F. Factors associated with cardiac mortality in developed countries with particular reference to the consumption of wine. Lancet 1979;1(8124):1017–1020
53. German JB, Walzem RL. The health benefits of wine. Annu Rev Nutr 2000;20:561–593
54. Grønbæk M, Becker U, Johansen D, et al. Type of alcohol consumed and mortality from all causes, coronary heart disease, and cancer. Ann Intern Med 2000;133(6):411–419
55. Klatsky AL, Friedman GD, Armstrong MA, Kipp H. Wine, liquor, beer, and mortality. Am J Epidemiol 2003;158(6):585–595
56. Renaud SC, Guéguen R, Siest G, Salamon R. Wine, beer, and mortality in middle-aged men from eastern France. Arch Intern Med 1999;159(16):1865–1870
57. Mukamal KJ, Conigrave KM, Mittleman MA, et al. Roles of drinking pattern and type of alcohol consumed in coronary heart disease in men. N Engl J Med 2003;348(2):109–118
58. Rimm EB, Klatsky A, Grobbee D, Stampfer MJ. Review of moderate alcohol consumption and reduced risk of coronary heart disease: is the effect due to beer, wine, or spirits. BMJ 1996;312(7033):731–736
59. Wannamethee SG, Shaper AG. Type of alcoholic drink and risk of major coronary heart disease events and all-cause mortality. Am J Public Health 1999; 89(5):685–690
60. Barefoot JC, Grønbæk M, Feaganes JR, McPherson RS, Williams RB, Siegler IC. Alcoholic beverage preference, diet, and health habits in the UNC Alumni Heart Study. Am J Clin Nutr 2002;76(2):466–472
61. McCann SE, Sempos C, Freudenheim JL, et al. Alcoholic beverage preference and characteristics of drinkers and nondrinkers in Western New York (United States). Nutr Metab Cardiovasc Dis 2003;13(1):2–11
62. Mortensen EL, Jensen HH, Sanders SA, Reinisch JM. Better psychological functioning and higher social status may largely explain the apparent health benefits of wine: a study of wine and beer drinking in young Danish adults. Arch Intern Med 2001; 161(15):1844–1848
63. Johansen D, Friis K, Skovenborg E, Grønbæk M. Food buying habits of people who buy wine or beer: cross sectional study. BMJ 2006;332(7540):519–522
64. Ruidavets JB, Bataille V, Dallongeville J, et al. Alcohol intake and diet in France, the prominent role of lifestyle. Eur Heart J 2004;25(13):1153–1162
65. Stocker R, O'Halloran RA. Dealcoholized red wine decreases atherosclerosis in apolipoprotein E gene-deficient mice independently of inhibition of lipid peroxidation in the artery wall. Am J Clin Nutr 2004;79(1):123–130
66. De Curtis A, Murzilli S, Di Castelnuovo A, et al. Alcohol-free red wine prevents arterial thrombosis in dietary-induced hypercholesterolemic rats: experimental support for the 'French paradox'. J Thromb Haemost 2005;3(2):346–350
67. Lekakis J, Rallidis LS, Andreadou I, et al. Polyphenolic compounds from red grapes acutely improve endothelial function in patients with coronary heart disease. Eur J Cardiovasc Prev Rehabil 2005;12(6):596–600
68. Wang Z, Huang Y, Zou J, Cao K, Xu Y, Wu JM. Effects of red wine and wine polyphenol resveratrol on platelet aggregation in vivo and in vitro. Int J Mol Med 2002;9(1):77–79
69. Chen CK, Pace-Asciak CR. Vasorelaxing activity of resveratrol and quercetin in isolated rat aorta. Gen Pharmacol 1996;27(2):363–366
70. Szewczuk LM, Forti L, Stivala LA, Penning TM. Resveratrol is a peroxidase-mediated inactivator of COX-1 but not COX-2: a mechanistic approach to the design of COX-1 selective agents. J Biol Chem 2004; 279(21):22727–22737
71. Tsai SH, Lin-Shiau SY, Lin JK. Suppression of nitric oxide synthase and the down-regulation of the activation of NFkappaB in macrophages by resveratrol. Br J Pharmacol 1999;126(3):673–680
72. Fukao H, Ijiri Y, Miura M, et al. Effect of trans-resveratrol on the thrombogenicity and atherogenicity in apolipoprotein E-deficient and low-density lipoprotein receptor-deficient mice. Blood Coagul Fibrinolysis 2004;15(6):441–446
73. Wang Z, Zou J, Huang Y, Cao K, Xu Y, Wu JM. Effect of resveratrol on platelet aggregation in vivo and in vitro. Chin Med J (Engl) 2002;115(3):378–380
74. Wilson T, Knight TJ, Beitz DC, Lewis DS, Engen RL. Resveratrol promotes atherosclerosis in hypercholesterolemic rabbits. Life Sci 1996;59(1):PL15–PL21
75. Li ZG, Hong T, Shimada Y, et al. Suppression of N-nitrosomethylbenzylamine (NMBA)-induced esophageal tumorigenesis in F344 rats by resveratrol. Carcinogenesis 2002;23(9):1531–1536
76. Tessitore L, Davit A, Sarotto I, Caderni G. Resveratrol depresses the growth of colorectal aberrant crypt foci by affecting bax and p21(CIP) expression. Carcinogenesis 2000;21(8):1619–1622
77. Banerjee S, Bueso-Ramos C, Aggarwal BB. Suppression of 7,12-dimethylbenz(a)anthracene-induced mammary carcinogenesis in rats by resveratrol: role of nuclear factor-kappaB, cyclooxygenase 2, and matrix metalloprotease 9. Cancer Res 2002;62(17):4945–4954
78. Hecht SS, Kenney PM, Wang M, et al. Evaluation of butylated hydroxyanisole, myo-inositol, curcumin, esculetin, resveratrol and lycopene as inhibitors of benzo[a]pyrene plus 4-(methylnitrosamino)-1-(3-pyridyl)-1-butanone-induced lung tumorigenesis in A/J mice. Cancer Lett 1999;137(2):123–130
79. Berge G, Øvrebø S, Eilertsen E, Haugen A, Mollerup S. Analysis of resveratrol as a lung cancer chemopreventive agent in A/J mice exposed to benzo[a]pyrene. Br J Cancer 2004;91(7):1380–1383
80. Ziegler CC, Rainwater L, Whelan J, McEntee MF. Dietary resveratrol does not affect intestinal tumorigenesis in Apc(Min/+) mice. J Nutr 2004;134(1):5–10
81. Schneider Y, Duranton B, Gossé F, Schleiffer R, Seiler N, Raul F. Resveratrol inhibits intestinal tumorigenesis and modulates host-defense-related gene expression in an animal model of human familial adenomatous polyposis. Nutr Cancer 2001;39(1):102–107
82. Sengottuvelan M, Nalini N. Dietary supplementation of resveratrol suppresses colonic tumour incidence in 1,2-dimethylhydrazine-treated rats by modulating biotransforming enzymes and aberrant crypt foci development. Br J Nutr 2006;96(1):145–153
83. Sengottuvelan M, Senthilkumar R, Nalini N. Modulatory influence of dietary resveratrol during different phases of 1,2-dimethylhydrazine induced mucosal lipid-peroxidation, antioxidant status and aberrant crypt foci development in rat colon carcinogenesis. Biochim Biophys Acta 2006;1760(8):1175–1183

84. Sengottuvelan M, Viswanathan P, Nalini N. Chemopreventive effect of trans-resveratrol—a phytoalexin against colonic aberrant crypt foci and cell proliferation in 1,2-dimethylhydrazine induced colon carcinogenesis. Carcinogenesis 2006;27(5):1038–1046

85. Baur JA, Sinclair DA. Therapeutic potential of resveratrol: the in vivo evidence. Nat Rev Drug Discov 2006;5(6):493–506

86. Heilbronn LK, Ravussin E. Calorie restriction and aging: review of the literature and implications for studies in humans. Am J Clin Nutr 2003;78(3):361–369

87. Lin SJ, Defossez PA, Guarente L. Requirement of NAD and SIR2 for life-span extension by calorie restriction in Saccharomyces cerevisiae. Science 2000;289 (5487):2126–2128

88. Wood JG, Rogina B, Lavu S, et al. Sirtuin activators mimic caloric restriction and delay ageing in metazoans. Nature 2004;430(7000):686–689

89. Valenzano DR, Terzibasi E, Genade T, Cattaneo A, Domenici L, Cellerino A. Resveratrol prolongs lifespan and retards the onset of age-related markers in a short-lived vertebrate. Curr Biol 2006;16(3):296–300

90. Baur JA, Pearson KJ, Price NL, et al. Resveratrol improves health and survival of mice on a high-calorie diet. Nature 2006;444(7117):337–342

91. Barger JL, Kayo T, Vann JM, et al. A low dose of dietary resveratrol partially mimics caloric restriction and retards aging parameters in mice. PLoS ONE 2008; 3(6):e2264

92. Burns J, Yokota T, Ashihara H, Lean ME, Crozier A. Plant foods and herbal sources of resveratrol. J Agric Food Chem 2002;50(11):3337–3340

93. Rimando AM, Kalt W, Magee JB, Dewey J, Ballington JR. Resveratrol, pterostilbene, and piceatannol in vaccinium berries. J Agric Food Chem 2004;52(15):4713–4719

94. Sanders TH, McMichael RW Jr, Hendrix KW. Occurrence of resveratrol in edible peanuts. J Agric Food Chem 2000;48(4):1243–1246

95. Creasey LL, Coffee M. Phytoalexin production potential of grape berries. J Am Soc Hortic Sci 1988; 113(2):230–234

96. Frémont L. Biological effects of resveratrol. Life Sci 2000;66(8):663–673

97. Goldberg DM, Karumanchiri A, Ng E, Yan J, Eleftherios P, Soleas G. Direct gas chromatographic-mass spectrometric method to assay cis-resveratrol in wines: preliminary survey of its concentration in commercial wines. J Agric Food Chem 1995;43(5):1245–1250

98. Burns J, Gardner PT, Matthews D, Duthie GG, Lean ME, Crozier A. Extraction of phenolics and changes in antioxidant activity of red wines during vinification. J Agric Food Chem 2001;49(12):5797–5808

99. Moreno-Labanda JF, Mallavia R, Pérez-Fons L, Lizama V, Saura D, Micol V. Determination of piceid and resveratrol in Spanish wines deriving from Monastrell (Vitis vinifera L.) grape variety. J Agric Food Chem 2004;52(17):5396–5403

100. Romero-Pérez AI, Lamuela-Raventós RM, Waterhouse AL, de la Torre-Boronat MC. Levels of cis- and trans-resveratrol and their glucosides in white and rosé Vitis vinifera wines from Spain. J Agric Food Chem 1996;44(8):2124–2128

101. Sobolev VS, Cole RJ. trans-resveratrol content in commercial peanuts and peanut products. J Agric Food Chem 1999;47(4):1435–1439

102. Hendler SS, Rorvik DR, eds. PDR for Nutritional Supplements. Montvale, NJ: Medical Economics Company, Inc; 2001

103. Boocock DJ, Faust GE, Patel KR, et al. Phase I dose escalation pharmacokinetic study in healthy volunteers of resveratrol, a potential cancer chemopreventive agent. Cancer Epidemiol Biomarkers Prev 2007;16(6):1246–1252

104. Crowell JA, Korytko PJ, Morrissey RL, Booth TD, Levine BS. Resveratrol-associated renal toxicity. Toxicol Sci 2004;82(2):614–619

105. Juan ME, Vinardell MP, Planas JM. The daily oral administration of high doses of trans-resveratrol to rats for 28 days is not harmful. J Nutr 2002;132(2):257–260

106. American Academy of Pediatrics. Committee on Substance Abuse and Committee on Children With Disabilities. Fetal alcohol syndrome and alcohol-related neurodevelopmental disorders. Pediatrics 2000;106(2 Pt 1):358–361

107. Bertelli AA, Giovannini L, Giannessi D, et al. Antiplatelet activity of synthetic and natural resveratrol in red wine. Int J Tissue React 1995;17(1):1–3

108. Piver B, Berthou F, Dreano Y, Lucas D. Inhibition of CYP3A, CYP1A and CYP2E1 activities by resveratrol and other non volatile red wine components. Toxicol Lett 2001;125(1–3):83–91

109. Regev-Shoshani G, Shoseyov O, Kerem Z. Influence of lipophilicity on the interactions of hydroxy stilbenes with cytochrome P450 3A4. Biochem Biophys Res Commun 2004;323(2):668–673

20 Essential Fatty Acids (Omega-3 and Omega-6)

Omega-3 and omega-6 fatty acids are polyunsaturated fatty acids (PUFAs), meaning they contain more than one *cis* double bond.[1] In all omega-3 fatty acids, the first double bond is located between the third and fourth carbon atom counting from the methyl end of the fatty acid (*n*-3). Similarly, the first double bond in all omega-6 fatty acids is located between the sixth and seventh carbon atom from the methyl end of the fatty acid (*n*-6). Scientific abbreviations for fatty acids tell the reader something about their chemical structure. One scientific abbreviation for α-linolenic acid (ALA) is 18:3*n*-3. The first part (18:3) tells the reader that ALA is an 18-carbon fatty acid with three double bonds, while the second part (*n*-3) tells the reader that the first double bond is in the *n*-3 position, which defines it as an omega-3 fatty acid.

Although humans and other mammals can synthesize saturated fatty acids and some monounsaturated fatty acids from carbon groups in carbohydrates and proteins, they lack the enzymes necessary to insert a *cis* double bond at the *n*-6 or the *n*-3 position of a fatty acid.[1] Consequently, omega-6 and omega-3 fatty acids are essential nutrients. The parent fatty acid of the omega-6 series is linoleic acid (LA; 18:2*n*-6), and the parent fatty acid of the omega-3 series is ALA (**Fig. 20.1**). Humans can synthesize long-chain (20 carbons or more) omega-6 fatty acids, such as dihomo-γ-linolenic acid (DGLA; 20:3*n*-6) and arachidonic acid (AA; 20:4*n*-6) from LA and long-chain omega-3 fatty acids, such as eicosapentaenoic acid (EPA; 20:5*n*-3) and docosahexaenoic acid (DHA; 22:6*n*-3) from ALA (see the Bioavailability and Metabolism section below). It has been estimated that the ratio of omega-6 to omega-3 fatty acids in the diet of early humans was 1:1,[2] but the ratio in the typical Western diet is now almost 10:1 due to increased use of vegetable oils rich in LA, as well as reduced fish consumption.[3] A large body of scientific research suggests that increasing the relative abundance of dietary omega-3 fatty acids may have several health benefits.

Bioavailability and Metabolism

Prior to absorption in the small intestine, fatty acids must be hydrolyzed from dietary fats (triglycerides, phospholipids, and cholesterol) by pancreatic enzymes.[4] Bile salts must also be present in the small intestine to allow for the incorporation of fatty acids and other products of fat digestion into mixed micelles. Fat absorption from mixed micelles occurs throughout the small intestine and is 85%–95% efficient under normal conditions. Humans can synthesize longer omega-6 and omega-3 fatty acids from the essential fatty acids LA and ALA, respectively, through a series of desaturation (addition of a double bond) and elongation (addition of two carbon atoms) reactions (**Fig. 20.2**).[5] LA and ALA compete for the same elongase and desaturase enzymes in the synthesis of longer polyunsaturated fatty acids, such as AA and EPA. Although ALA is the preferred substrate of the Δ6 desaturase enzyme, the excess of dietary LA compared with ALA results in greater net formation of AA (20:4*n*-6) than EPA (20:5*n*-3).[6] The capacity for conversion of ALA to DHA is higher in women than men. Studies of ALA metabolism in healthy young men indicate that approximately 8% of dietary ALA is converted to EPA and 0%–4% is converted to DHA.[7] In healthy young women, approximately 21% of dietary ALA is converted to EPA and 9% is converted to DHA.[8] The better conversion efficiency of young women compared with men appears to be related to the effects of estrogen.[6,9] Although ALA is considered the essential omega-3 fatty acid because it cannot be synthesized by humans, evidence that human conversion of EPA and particularly DHA is relatively inefficient suggests that EPA and DHA may also be essential under some conditions.[10,11]

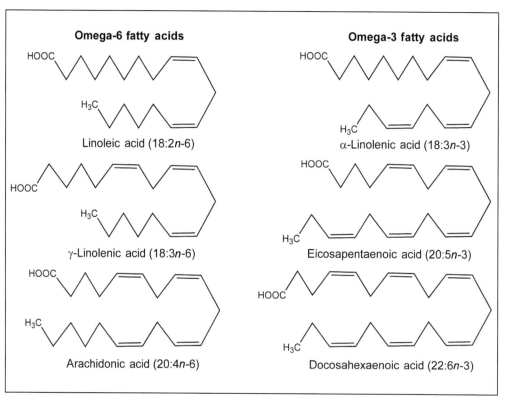

Fig. 20.1   Chemical structures of the omega-6 fatty acids, linoleic acid (LA, 18:2*n*-6), γ-linolenic acid (GLA, 18:3*n*-6), and arachidonic acid (AA, 20:4*n*-6), and the omega-3 fatty acids, α-linolenic acid (ALA, 18:3*n*-3), eicosapentaenoic acid (EPA, 20:5*n*-3), and docosahexaenoic acid (DHA, 22:6*n*-3).

Biological Activities

Membrane Structure and Function

Omega-6 and omega-3 PUFA are important structural components of cell membranes. When incorporated into phospholipids, they affect cell membrane properties such as fluidity, flexibility, permeability, and the activity of membrane-bound enzymes.[12] DHA is selectively incorporated into retinal cell membranes and postsynaptic neuronal cell membranes, suggesting it plays important roles in vision and nervous system function.

Vision

DHA is found at very high concentrations in the cell membranes of the retina; the retina conserves and recycles DHA even when omega-3 fatty acid intake is low.[13] Animal studies indicate that DHA is required for the normal development and function of the retina. Moreover, these studies suggest that there is a critical period during retinal development when inadequate DHA will result in permanent abnormalities in retinal function. Recent research indicates that DHA plays an important role in regeneration of the visual pigment rhodopsin, which plays a critical role in the visual transduction system that converts light hitting the retina to visual images in the brain.[14]

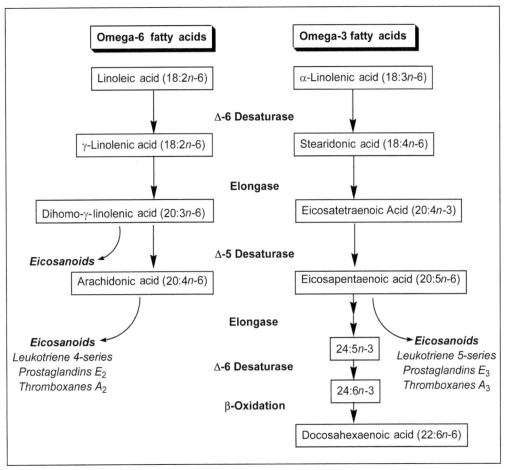

Fig. 20.2 Synthesis of long-chain omega-6 and omega-3 polyunsaturated fatty acids from the parent fatty acids, linoleic acid (LA, 18:2n-6) and α-linolenic acid (ALA, 18:3n-3), in humans.

Nervous System

The phospholipids of the brain's gray matter contain high proportions of DHA and AA, suggesting they are important to central nervous system function.[15] Brain DHA content may be particularly important, since animal studies have shown that depletion of DHA in the brain can result in learning deficits. It is not clear how DHA affects brain function, but changes in the DHA content of neuronal cell membranes could alter the function of ion channels or membrane-associated receptors, as well as the availability of neurotransmitters.[16]

Eicosanoid Synthesis

Eicosanoids, derived from 20-carbon PUFA, are potent chemical messengers that play critical roles in immune and inflammatory responses. During an inflammatory response, DGLA, AA, and EPA in cell membranes can be metabolized by enzymes known as *cyclooxygenases* and *lipoxygenases*, to form prostaglandins and leukotrienes, respectively (**Fig. 20.2**). In those who consume typical Western diets, the amount of AA in cell membranes is much greater than the amount of EPA, resulting in the formation of more eicosanoids derived from AA than from EPA. However, increasing omega-3 fatty acid intake increases the EPA content of cell membranes, resulting in higher proportions of eicosanoids derived from

EPA. Physiological responses to AA-derived eicosanoids differ from responses to EPA-derived eicosanoids. In general, eicosanoids derived from EPA are less potent inducers of inflammation, blood vessel constriction, and coagulation than eicosanoids derived from AA.[3,17]

Regulation of Gene Expression

The results of cell culture and animal studies indicate that omega-6 and omega-3 fatty acids can modulate the expression of several genes, including those involved with fatty acid metabolism and inflammation.[17,18] Although the mechanisms require further clarification, omega-6 and omega-3 fatty acids may regulate gene expression by interacting with specific transcription factors, including peroxisome proliferator-activated receptors (PPARs) and liver X receptors (LXRs).[19] Multiple mechanisms are involved in these regulatory schemes.[20] In many cases, PUFAs act like hydrophobic hormones (e.g., steroid hormones) to control gene expression. In this case, PUFAs bind directly to receptors like PPARs. These receptors bind to the promoters of genes and function to increase/decrease transcription of genes. In other cases, PUFAs regulate the abundance of transcription factors inside the cell's nucleus.[20] For these factors, the mechanism for PUFA control is less clear. Two examples include nuclear factor kappa B (NF-κB) and sterol regulatory element–binding protein 1 (SREBP-1). NF-κB is a transcription factor involved in regulating the expression of multiple genes involved in inflammation. Omega-3 PUFAs suppress NF-κB nuclear content, thus inhibiting the production of inflammatory eicosanoids and cytokines. SREBP-1 is a major transcription factor controlling fatty-acid synthesis—both de novo lipogenesis and PUFA synthesis.[21] Dietary PUFAs can suppress SREBP-1, which decreases the expression of enzymes involved in fatty acid synthesis and PUFA synthesis.[22,23] In this way, dietary PUFAs function as feedback inhibitors of all fatty acid synthesis.

Deficiency

Essential Fatty Acid Deficiency

Clinical signs of essential fatty acid deficiency include a dry scaly rash, decreased growth in infants and children, increased susceptibility to infection, and poor wound healing.[24] Omega-3, omega-6, and omega-9 fatty acids compete for the same desaturase enzymes. The desaturase enzymes show preference for the different series of fatty acids in the following order: omega-3 > omega-6 > omega-9. Consequently, synthesis of the omega-9 fatty acid eicosatrienoic acid ($20:3n-9$, mead acid, or $5,8,11$-eicosatrienoic acid) increases only when dietary intakes of omega-3 and omega-6 fatty acids are very low; therefore, mead acid is one marker of essential fatty acid deficiency.[25] A plasma eicosatrienoic acid:arachidonic acid (triene:tetraene) ratio greater than 0.2 is generally considered indicative of essential fatty acid deficiency.[24,26] In patients who were given total parenteral nutrition containing fat-free glucose-amino acid mixtures, biochemical signs of essential fatty acid deficiency developed in as little as 7–10 days.[27] In these cases, the continuous glucose infusion resulted in high circulating insulin levels, which inhibited the release of essential fatty acids stored in adipose tissue. When glucose-free amino acid solutions were used, parenteral nutrition up to 14 days did not result in biochemical signs of essential fatty acid deficiency. Essential fatty acid deficiency has also been found to occur in patients with chronic fat malabsorption[28] and in patients with cystic fibrosis.[29] Moreover, it has been proposed that essential fatty acid deficiency may play a role in the pathology of protein-energy malnutrition.[25]

Omega-3 Fatty Acid Deficiency

At least one case of isolated omega-3 fatty acid deficiency has been reported. A young girl who received intravenous lipid emulsions with very little ALA developed visual problems and sensory neuropathy; these conditions were resolved when she was administered an emulsion containing more ALA.[30] Plasma DHA concentrations decrease when omega-3 fatty acid intake is insufficient, but no cutoff values have been established. Isolated omega-3 fatty acid deficiency does not result in increased plasma triene:tetraene ratios.[1] Studies in rodents, however, have revealed significant impairment of learning and memory associated with *n*-3 PUFA deficiency.[31,32] These studies have prompted clinical trials in humans to assess the impact of omega-3 PUFA on cognitive development and cognitive decline.

Disease Prevention

Visual and Neurological Development

Because the last trimester of pregnancy is a critical period for the accumulation of DHA in the brain and retina, preterm infants are thought to be particularly vulnerable to adverse effects of insufficient DHA on visual and neurological development.[33] Human milk contains DHA in addition to ALA and EPA but, until recently, ALA was the only omega-3 fatty acid present in conventional infant formulas. Although preterm infants can synthesize DHA from ALA, they generally cannot synthesize enough to prevent declines in plasma and cellular DHA concentrations without additional dietary intake. Therefore, it was proposed that preterm infant formulas be supplemented with enough DHA to bring plasma and cellular DHA levels of formula-fed infants up to those of breast-fed infants.[34] Although formulas enriched with DHA raise plasma and red blood cell DHA concentrations in preterm and term infants, the results of randomized controlled trials examining measures of visual acuity and neurological development in infants fed formulas with or without added DHA have been mixed.[35–38] Although several controlled trials found that healthy preterm infants fed formulas with DHA added showed subtle but significant improvements in visual acuity at 2 months and 4 months of age compared with those fed DHA-free formulas,[39] most randomized controlled trials found no differences in visual acuity between healthy preterm infants fed formulas with or without DHA added.[36] Similarly, two randomized controlled trials that assessed general measures of infant development at 12 months and 24 months of age found no difference between preterm infants fed formula with or without DHA added.[40,41] However, two randomized controlled trials assessing infant development at 18 months of age reported

beneficial effects of DHA supplementation in preterm infants, but one of these trials found a significant effect only in boys.[42,43] Infant formulas enriched with DHA are also commercially available for term infants, but the results of randomized controlled trials of these formulas on visual acuity and development in term infants have also been mixed.[37,38,44–48] While DHA appears to be important for visual and neurological development, it is not yet clear whether feeding infants formula enriched with DHA enhances visual acuity or neurological development in preterm or term infants.[49]

Pregnancy and Lactation

Although infant requirements for DHA have been the subject of a great deal of research, there has been relatively little investigation of maternal requirements for omega-3 fatty acids, despite the fact that the mother is the sole source of omega-3 fatty acids for the fetus and exclusively breast-fed infant.[50] The results of randomized controlled trials during pregnancy suggest that omega-3 fatty acid supplementation does not decrease the incidence of gestational diabetes, pregnancy-induced hypertension, or preeclampsia[51–53] but may result in modest increases in the length of gestation, especially in women with low consumption of omega-3 fatty acid. In healthy Danish women, fish oil supplementation that provided 2.7 g/day of EPA + DHA increased the length of gestation by an average of 4 days.[52] More recently, consumption of only 0.13 g/day of DHA from enriched eggs during the last trimester of pregnancy increased the length of gestation by an average of 6 days in a low-income population in the United States.[53] A recent meta-analysis of six randomized controlled trials in women with low-risk pregnancies found that omega-3 PUFA supplementation during pregnancy resulted in an increased length of pregnancy by 1.6 days.[54] In European women with high-risk pregnancies, fish oil supplementation, which provided 2.7 g/day of EPA + DHA during the last trimester of pregnancy, lowered the risk of premature delivery from 33% to 21%.[55] However, a meta-analysis of randomized controlled trials in women with high-risk pregnancies found that supplementation with long-chain PUFAs did not affect the duration of pregnancy or the incidence of premature births but decreased the incidence of early premature births (<34 weeks of gestation).[56] The World Association of Perinatal Medicine, the Early Nutrition Academy, and the Child Health Foundation recommend that pregnant and lactating women consume an average of at least 200 mg DHA daily (approx. one to two servings of fish weekly).[57]

The effect of long-chain PUFA supplementation during pregnancy and/or lactation on neurodevelopmental outcomes in the offspring is an area of active investigation. In Norway, children born to mothers who were given supplements of cod liver oil (2 g/day of EPA + DHA) during pregnancy and during the first 3 months of lactation scored higher on mental processing tests at 4 years of age when compared with the children whose mothers were not given the supplements.[58] However, only 14% of the original study participants were available for testing when the children were aged 4 years. In a double-blind, randomized, placebo-controlled trial, children born to mothers who were given fish oil supplements (2.2 g DHA and 1.1 g EPA) during pregnancy (20 weeks' gestation until delivery) displayed higher scores of eye and hand coordination at 2½ years of age, compared with children whose mothers were given olive oil supplements.[59] A small trial that provided either DHA-containing cereal bars (300 mg DHA/bar, average of 5 bars/week) or placebo cereal bars to 29 pregnant women (from 24 weeks' gestation until delivery) associated maternal DHA supplementation with improvements in infant problem-solving skills at 9 months of age.[60] No differences in recognition memory tasks were observed between the two groups of infants. Results of randomized controlled trials assessing cognitive function in children whose mothers were provided omega-3 fatty acids only during lactation have been mixed.[38] Although some results are promising, more studies are needed to determine whether long-chain PUFA supplementation during pregnancy and/or lactation has beneficial effects on long-term cognitive development in children. At present, the potential benefits associated with obtaining long-chain omega-3 fatty acids through moderate consumption of fish (e.g., one to two servings weekly) during pregnancy and lactation outweigh any risks of contaminant exposure, but fish with high levels of methylmercury should be avoided.[61] For information about contaminants in fish and guidelines for fish consumption by women of childbearing age, see the Contaminants in Fish section below.

Cardiovascular Disease

Omega-6 Fatty Acids: Linoleic Acid

LA is the most abundant dietary PUFA. The results of prospective cohort studies examining the relationships between PUFA intake and the risk of coronary heart disease (CHD) have been somewhat inconsistent.[62] Some, but not all, prospective cohort studies have found that higher PUFA intakes are associated with significant reductions in CHD risk[63–65] or cardiovascular-related mortality.[66] The largest prospective cohort study to examine the effects of dietary fat intake on CHD risk is the Nurses' Health Study (NHS), which followed more than 78 000 women for 20 years. In that cohort, those with the highest intakes of total PUFA (7.4% of energy) and LA had a risk of CHD that was 25% lower than that of those with the lowest intakes of total PUFA (5% of energy) and LA.[64] Although saturated fatty acid (SFA) intake was not associated with CHD risk, the ratio of PUFA:SFA intake was inversely associated with CHD risk. In controlled feeding trials, replacing dietary SFA with PUFA consistently lowers serum total and low-density lipoprotein (LDL) cholesterol concentrations.[67] In fact, LA has been shown to be the most potent fatty acid for lowering serum total and LDL cholesterol when substituted for dietary SFA.[68] Several dietary intervention trials have compared the effects of diets high in SFA (18%–19% of energy) with diets low in SFA (8%–9% of energy) and high in PUFA (14%–21% of energy) on morbidity (illness) and mortality from CHD.[62] Although most of the increase in dietary PUFA was provided by LA, ALA intakes were also increased in these trials.[67] Several dietary intervention trials in men found that replacing dietary SFA with PUFA reduced morbidity or mortality from CHD.[69–72] However, two similar dietary intervention trials in women did not result in significant reductions in morbidity or mortality from CHD.[73,74] In a recently released scientific advisory, the American Heart Association concluded that obtaining 5%–10% of total caloric intake from omega-6 PUFAs is associated with a reduced risk of CHD.[75]

Omega-3 Fatty Acids: α-Linolenic Acid

Several prospective cohort studies have examined the relationship between dietary ALA intake and CHD risk. In a cohort of more than 45 000 US men followed for 14 years, each 1 g/day increase in dietary ALA intake was associated with a 16% reduction in the risk of CHD.[76] Moreover, in those who ate little or no seafood, each 1 g/day increase in dietary ALA intake was associated with a 47% reduction in the risk of CHD. In a cohort of more than 76 000 US women followed for 10 years, those with the highest ALA intakes (approx. 1.4 g/day) had a risk of fatal CHD that was 45% lower than in women with the lowest intakes (approx. 0.7 g/day).[77] Interestingly, oil and vinegar salad dressing was an important source of dietary ALA in this population. Women who consumed oil and vinegar salad dressing five to six times weekly had a risk of fatal CHD that was 54% lower than that of those who rarely consumed it, even after adjusting the analysis for vegetable intake. In a smaller cohort of more than 6000 US men, those with the highest intakes of ALA had a risk of death from CHD over the next 10 years that was 40% lower than in those with the lowest intakes.[78] In contrast, two studies in Europe found no association between dietary ALA intake and CHD risk.[79,80] Additionally, in the NHS (76 763 women followed for 18 years), dietary intake of ALA was not associated with fatal CHD or nonfatal myocardial infarction (MI) but was inversely associated with sudden cardiac death (see the section on Sudden Cardiac Death below).[81] Although not as consistent as the evidence supporting higher intakes of long-chain omega-3 fatty acids from seafood, the results of most prospective studies suggest that higher dietary ALA intakes (2–3 g/day) are associated with significant reductions in CHD risk, especially in populations with low levels of fish consumption.[82] Unlike LA, the cardioprotective effects of higher ALA intakes do not appear to be related to changes in serum lipid profiles. A meta-analysis of 14 randomized controlled trials concluded that ALA supplementation had no effect on total cholesterol, LDL cholesterol, or triglyceride levels.[83] However, several controlled clinical trials found that increasing ALA intake decreased serum concentrations of C-reactive protein, a marker of inflammation that is strongly associated with the risk of cardiovascular events such as MI and stroke.[84–86]

Long-Chain Omega-3 Fatty Acids: Eicosapentaenoic Acid and Docosahexaenoic Acid

Evidence is accumulating that increasing intakes of long-chain omega-3 fatty acids (EPA and DHA) can decrease the risk of cardiovascular disease by (1) preventing arrhythmias that can lead to sudden cardiac death, (2) decreasing the risk of thrombosis (a clot) that can lead to MI or stroke, (3) decreasing serum triglyceride levels, (4) slowing the growth of atherosclerotic plaque, (5) improving vascular endothelial function, (6) lowering blood pressure slightly, and (7) decreasing inflammation.[87] A recent systematic review of randomized controlled trials found that consumption of EPA and DHA from fish or fish oil supplements was associated with reductions in all-cause mortality, cardiac death, and sudden death.[88] Yet, another systematic review and meta-analysis of randomized controlled trials and prospective cohort studies concluded that long-chain omega-3 fatty acids do not significantly reduce the risk of total mortality or cardiovascular events.[89]

Coronary heart disease. Several prospective cohort studies have found that men who eat fish at least once weekly have lower mortality from CHD than men who do not eat fish.[90–92] One such study followed 1822 men for 30 years and found that mortality from CHD was 38% lower in men who consumed an average of at least 35 g (1.2 oz) of fish daily than in men who did not eat fish, while mortality from MI was 67% lower in the group that ate fish.[93] The cardioprotective effects of fish consumption may not be confined to those consuming a typical Western diet. A study in China that followed more than 18 000 men for 10 years found that those who consumed more than 200 g (approx. 7 oz) of fish or shellfish weekly had a risk of fatal MI that was 59% lower than that of men who consumed less than 50 g (approx. 2 oz) weekly.[94] Less information is available regarding the effects of higher omega-3 fatty acid and fish intakes in women. In the NHS, which followed more than 84 000 women for 16 years, CHD mortality was 29%–34% lower in women who ate fish at least once a week compared with women who ate fish less than once a month.[95] In a prospective study in 2445 Finnish women, those in the highest quintile of fish intake (≥41 g/day; mean 70 g/day) had a 41% lower risk of CHD compared with those in the lowest quintile (≤8 g/day; mean 4.2 g/day).[96]

A large prospective study in a cohort of 41 478 Japanese men and women found that higher intakes of fish are associated with further reductions in the risk of CHD. In this study, those who consumed fish eight times weekly had a 57% lower risk of nonfatal coronary events and a 56% lower risk of MI compared with those who consumed fish only once weekly.[97] Yet, a smaller prospective study in 8879 Japanese men and women found that consumption of fish twice daily did not lower the risk of all-cause mortality or CHD mortality compared with eating fish once or twice weekly.[98]

Sudden cardiac death. Sudden cardiac death (SCD) is the result of a fatal ventricular arrhythmia, which usually occurs in people with CHD. Studies in cell culture indicate that long-chain omega-3 fatty acids decrease the excitability of cardiac muscle cells (myocytes) by modulating ion-channel conductance.[99] The results of epidemiological studies suggest that regular fish consumption is inversely associated with the risk of SCD. In a large prospective cohort study that followed more than 20 000 men for 11 years, those who ate fish at least once a week had a risk of SCD that was 52% lower than that of those who ate fish less than once a month.[100] Plasma levels of EPA and DHA were also inversely related to the risk of SCD, supporting the idea that omega-3 fatty acids are at least partially responsible for the beneficial effect of fish consumption on SCD.[101] More recently, a prospective study that followed more than 45 000 men for 14 years found that the risk of SCD was approximately 40%–50% lower in those who consumed an average of at least 250 mg/day of dietary EPA + DHA (the equivalent of 1–2 meals of oily fish weekly) than those who consumed less than 250 mg/day.[76] Dietary EPA + DHA intake was not related to the risk of nonfatal MI or total CHD events, suggesting the antiarrhythmic effects of long-chain omega-3 fatty acids may be important at usual dietary intake levels. Thus, several observational studies and clinical trials have found that including fish or fish oils in the diet lowers the risk of SCD.[102] Fewer studies have looked at whether consumption of ALA, a shorter-chain omega-3 fatty acid, affects the risk of SCD. In the NHS, which included 76 763 women, higher dietary intakes of ALA were associated with a 38%–40% lower risk of SCD.[81] No association between dietary ALA intake and sudden death was found in the Health Professionals Follow-up Study, which included 45 722 men.[76] It is also not clear whether omega-3 supplementation reduces the risk of ventricular arrhythmias. A recent meta-analysis of three clinical trials[103–105] concluded that supplementation with fish oil did not help prevent ventricular arrhythmias in patients with implantable cardioverter defibrillators, but these patients had existing cardiac problems.[106] More epidemiological and clinical research is needed to determine whether omega-3 fatty acid status influences the risk of ventricular arrhythmias.[107]

Stroke. Ischemic strokes, which comprise 87% of all strokes, are the result of insufficient blood flow to an area of the brain and may occur when an artery supplying the brain becomes occluded by a clot. Hemorrhagic strokes occur when a blood vessel ruptures and bleeds into the brain.[108] Some prospective studies that have examined the relationship between fish or omega-3 fatty acid intake and total stroke incidence have found increased fish intake to be beneficial,[109,110] while others have found no beneficial effect.[111–113] More recently, two large prospective studies found that increased fish and omega-3 fatty acid intakes were associated with significantly lower risks of ischemic stroke but not hemorrhagic stroke. In a study that followed more than 79 000 women for 14 years, those who ate fish at least twice weekly had a risk of thrombotic (ischemic) stroke that was 52% lower than that of those who ate fish less than once a month.[114] Similarly, in a study that followed more than 43 000 men for 12 years, those who ate fish at least once a month had a risk of ischemic stroke that was 43% lower than that of those who ate fish less than once a month.[115] Although the effects of long-chain omega-3 fatty acid intake on the incidence of stroke have not been studied as thoroughly as the effects on CHD, a meta-analysis of available evidence suggests that increased fish intake may decrease the risk of ischemic stroke but not hemorrhagic stroke.[116] Results of a recent study indicate that high-dose EPA supplementation may be beneficial in the secondary prevention of stroke, that is, preventing recurrent stroke in individuals with a prior history.[117]

Serum triglycerides. A meta-analysis of 17 prospective studies found hypertriglyceridemia (serum triglycerides >200 mg/dL) to be an independent risk factor for cardiovascular disease.[118] Numerous controlled clinical trials in humans have demonstrated that increasing intakes of EPA and DHA significantly lower serum triglyceride concentrations.[119] The triglyceride-lowering effects of EPA and DHA increase with dose,[120] but clinically meaningful reductions in serum triglyceride concentrations have been demonstrated at doses of 2 g/day of EPA + DHA.[3] In its recommendations regarding omega-3 fatty acids and cardiovascular disease (see the section on Intake Recommendations below), the American Heart Association indicates that an EPA + DHA supplement may be useful in patients with hypertriglyceridemia.[87]

Summary: Omega-3 and Omega-6 PUFA and Prevention of Cardiovascular Disease

The results of epidemiological studies and randomized controlled trials suggest that replacing dietary SFA with omega-6 and omega-3 PUFA lowers LDL cholesterol and decreases the risk of cardiovascular disease. Additionally, the results of epidemiological studies provide strong evidence that increasing dietary omega-3 fatty acid intake is associated with significant reductions in the risk of cardiovascular disease, through mechanisms other than lowering LDL cholesterol. In particular, increasing EPA and DHA intake from seafood has been associated with significant reductions in SCD, suggesting that long-chain omega-3 fatty acids have antiarrhythmic effects at intake levels equivalent to the amount in two small servings of oily fish per week. This amount of fish would provide approximately 400–500 mg/day of EPA + DHA.[121] Thus, some researchers have proposed that the US Institute of Medicine should establish a dietary reference intake for EPA + DHA.[122]

Alzheimer Disease and Dementia

Alzheimer disease is the most common cause of dementia in older adults. It is characterized by the formation of amyloid plaque in the brain and nerve cell degeneration. Disease symptoms, including memory loss and confusion, worsen over time.[123] Some epidemiological studies have associated high intake of fish with decreased risk of impaired cognitive function,[124] dementia,[125] and Alzheimer disease.[125,126] DHA, the major omega-3 fatty acid in the brain, appears to be protective against Alzheimer disease.[127] Observational studies have found that lower DHA status is associated with increased risk of Alzheimer disease,[128–130] as well as other types of dementia.[129] In a cohort of the Framingham Heart Study, men and women in the highest quartile of plasma phosphatidylcholine DHA content had a 47% decreased risk of developing all-cause dementia and a 39% decreased risk of developing Alzheimer disease when compared with those in the lower three quartiles.[131] Individuals in the top quartile consumed an average of three servings of fish weekly (0.18 g/day of DHA).[131] Thus, low DHA status may be a risk factor for Alzheimer disease, other types of dementia, and cognitive impairment associated with aging.

Disease Treatment

Coronary Heart Disease

Dietary Intervention Trials

Total mortality and fatal MI decreased by 29% in male MI survivors advised to increase their weekly intake of oily fish to 200–400 g (7–14 oz)—an amount estimated to provide an additional 500–800 mg/day of long-chain omega-3 fatty acids (EPA + DHA).[132] In another dietary intervention trial, patients who survived a first MI were randomly assigned to usual care or advised to adopt a Mediterranean diet that was higher in omega-3 fatty acids (especially ALA) and lower in omega-6 fatty acids than the standard Western-style diet. After almost 4 years, those on the Mediterranean diet had a risk of cardiac death and nonfatal MI that was 38% lower than in the group that was assigned to usual care.[133] Although higher plasma ALA levels were associated with better outcomes, the benefit of the Mediterranean diet cannot be attributed entirely to increased ALA intakes, since intakes of monounsaturated fatty acids and fruits and vegetables also increased. A recent intervention trial compared survival in MI survivors who followed a Mediterranean-style diet or a low-fat diet for an average of 46 months; total mortality and cardiovascular-related mortality did not differ between the two groups.[134]

Supplementation Trials

In the largest randomized controlled trial of supplemental omega-3 fatty acids to date, CHD patients who received supplements providing 850 mg/day of EPA + DHA for 3.5 years had a risk of sudden death that was 45% lower than that of those who did not take supplements; supplement users also experienced a 20% lower risk of death from all causes compared with non-supplement users.[135] Interestingly, it took only 3 months of supplementation to demonstrate a significant decrease in total mortality and 4 months to demonstrate a significant decrease in sudden death.[136] In another supplementation trial, patients admitted to hospital with an acute MI were randomized to receive capsules containing fish oil (1.8 g/day of EPA + DHA), mustard oil (2.9 g/day of ALA), or a placebo.[137] After 1 year, total cardiac events, including nonfatal MI, were significantly lower in the groups that received fish oil or mustard oil compared with the groups that received a placebo. In contrast, patients with acute MI did not realize any additional benefit from supplementation with 3.5 g/day of EPA + DHA compared with corn oil in a region of Norway where fish intakes are relatively high.[138] The results of a meta-analysis that pooled the findings of 11 randomized controlled trials of dietary or supplementary omega-3 fatty acids indicated that increased omega-3 fatty acid intakes significantly decreased overall mortality, mortality due to MI, and SCD in patients with CHD.[139]

Two randomized controlled trials have examined the effect of fish oil supplementation on the progression of coronary artery atherosclerosis measured by coronary angiography. Although a study of 59 patients with coronary artery disease found no benefit after 2 years of supplementation with fish oil, providing 6 g/day of EPA + DHA, compared with olive oil,[140] a larger trial of 223 patients found that supplementation with 3.3 g/day of EPA + DHA for 3 months and 1.65 g/day for an additional 21 months resulted in a modest decrease in the progression of coronary atherosclerosis compared with a placebo.[141] Numerous randomized controlled trials have examined the effect of fish oil supplementation on coronary artery restenosis after percutaneous transluminal coronary angioplasty. A meta-analysis that combined the results of 12 randomized controlled trials found that fish oil supplementation resulted in a 14% reduction of coronary restenosis, but

this reduction did not quite reach statistical significance.[142] Supplemental fish oil doses in the coronary artery restenosis trials ranged from 2.6 g/day to 6.0 g/day.

Summary: Long-Chain Omega-3 Fatty Acids in Treatment of Coronary Heart Disease

The results of randomized controlled trials in individuals with documented CHD suggest a beneficial effect of dietary and supplemental omega-3 fatty acids. Based on the results of these trials, the American Heart Association recommends that individuals with documented CHD consume approximately 1 g/day of EPA + DHA (see the section on Intake Recommendations below).[143]

Diabetes Mellitus

Cardiovascular diseases are the leading causes of death in individuals with diabetes mellitus (DM). Hypertriglyceridemia (serum triglycerides >200 mg/dL) is a common lipid abnormality in individuals with type 2 DM, and several randomized controlled trials have found that fish oil supplementation significantly lowers serum triglyceride levels in individuals with diabetes (see the section on serum triglycerides above).[144] Although early, uncontrolled, studies raised concerns that fish oil supplementation adversely affected blood glucose (glycemic) control,[145,146] randomized controlled trials have not generally found adverse effects of fish oil supplementation on long-term glycemic control.[147] A systematic review that pooled the results of 18 randomized controlled trials, including more than 800 patients with diabetes, found that fish oil supplementation significantly lowered serum triglycerides, especially in those with hypertriglyceridemia.[144] A meta-analysis that combined the results of 18 randomized controlled trials in individuals with type 2 DM or metabolic syndrome found that fish oil supplementation decreased serum triglycerides by 31 mg/dL compared with placebo but had no effect on serum cholesterol, fasting glucose, or hemoglobin A_{1c} concentrations.[147] A more recent meta-analysis of randomized controlled trials in patients with type 2 DM found that omega-3 fatty acid supplementation lowered serum triglyceride levels by 25%.[148] However, fish oil supplementation has been associated with a slight increase in LDL cholesterol levels.[144,148,149] Although few controlled trials have examined the effect of fish oil supplementation on cardiovascular disease outcomes in patients with diabetes, a prospective study that followed 5103 women diagnosed with type 2 DM, but free of cardiovascular disease or cancer at the start of the study, found that higher fish intakes were associated with significantly decreased risks of CHD over a 16-year follow-up period.[150] Thus, increasing EPA and DHA intakes may be beneficial to individuals with diabetes, especially those with elevated serum triglycerides.[151] Moreover, there is little evidence that daily EPA + DHA intakes of less than 3 g/day adversely affect long-term glycemic control in individuals with diabetes.[144,152] The American Diabetes Association recommends that individuals with diabetes increase their consumption of omega-3 fatty acid, by consuming two to three 3-oz servings of fish weekly.[153]

Inflammatory Diseases

Rheumatoid Arthritis

Three meta-analyses of randomized controlled trials in patients with rheumatoid arthritis found that fish oil supplementation significantly decreased the number of painful and/or tender joints on physical examination.[147,154,155] The most recent of these meta-analyses also associated omega-3 PUFA supplementation with improvements in the intensity of pain and the duration of morning stiffness.[155] In general, clinical benefits were observed at a minimum dose of 2.7 g/day of EPA + DHA and were not apparent until at least 12 weeks from the start of supplementation.[155] Two of these meta-analyses assessed the effect of fish-oil supplementation on erythrocyte sedimentation rate (ESR), a measure of inflammation.[147,154] Neither found a significant effect of fish oil supplementation on ESR. Six out of seven studies that examined the effect of long-chain omega-3 fatty acid supplementation on nonsteroidal anti-inflammatory drug or corticosteroid use in patients with rheumatoid arthritis demonstrated a reduced requirement for anti-inflammatory medication.[147]

Inflammatory Bowel Disease

Clinical trials of long-chain omega-3 fatty acid supplementation have demonstrated beneficial effects less consistently in patients with inflammatory bowel disease than in patients with rheumatoid arthritis. Although two randomized controlled trials of fish oil supplementation in patients with Crohn disease reported no benefit,[156,157] one randomized controlled trial found that a significantly higher proportion of patients with Crohn disease given supplements of 2.7 g/day of EPA + DHA remained in remission over a 12-month period than those given a placebo.[158] A randomized controlled trial in 38 children (aged 5–16 years) with Crohn disease found that supplementation with omega-3 PUFA (1.2 g/day of EPA and 0.6 g/day of DHA), in addition to standard therapy with 5-aminosalicylic acid, significantly reduced the 1-year relapse rate.[159] Three randomized controlled trials of EPA + DHA supplementation (4.2–5.4 g/day for 3–12 months) in patients with ulcerative colitis reported significant improvement in at least one outcome measure, including weight gain, decreased corticosteroid use, improved disease activity scores, and improved histology scores.[160–162] In contrast, giving supplements of 5.1 g/day of EPA + DHA to patients with ulcerative colitis who were in remission did not significantly alter the incidence of relapse over a 2-year period.[163] More research is necessary to determine whether long-chain omega-3 fatty acid supplementation has any therapeutic benefit in ulcerative colitis.[164]

Asthma

Inflammatory eicosanoids (leukotrienes) derived from AA ($20{:}4n{-}6$) are thought to play an important role in the pathology of asthma.[17] Since increasing omega-3 fatty acid intake has been found to decrease the formation of AA-derived leukotrienes, several clinical trials have examined the effects of supplementation with long-chain omega-3 fatty acid on asthma. Although there is some evidence that omega-3 fatty acid supplementation can decrease the production of inflammatory mediators in patients with asthma,[165,166] evidence that omega-3 fatty acid supplementation decreases the clinical severity of asthma in controlled trials has been inconsistent.[167] Three systematic reviews of randomized controlled trials of long-chain omega-3 fatty acid supplementation in adults and children with asthma found no consistent effects on clinical outcome measures, including pulmonary function tests, symptoms of asthma, medication use, or bronchial hyperreactivity.[168–170]

Immunoglobulin A Nephropathy

Immunoglobulin A (IgA) nephropathy is a kidney disorder that results from the deposition of IgA in the glomeruli of the kidney. The cause of IgA nephropathy is not clear, but progressive renal failure may eventually develop in 15%–40% of patients.[171] Since glomerular IgA deposition results in increased production of inflammatory mediators, omega-3 fatty acid supplementation could potentially modulate the inflammatory response and preserve renal function. In a multicenter, randomized controlled trial, giving supplements of fish oil to patients with IgA nephropathy (1.8 g/day of EPA + 1.2 g/day of DHA) for 2 years significantly slowed declines in renal function.[172] Over the 2-year treatment period, 33% of the placebo group experienced a 50% increase in serum creatinine (i.e., evidence of declining renal function) compared with only 6% in the group given fish oil supplements. These results were sustained over an average of 6 years of follow-up,[173] but improvements were not observed with higher doses of fish oil.[174] A much smaller 2-year trial found that a low dose of omega-3 fatty acids (0.85 g/day of EPA + 0.57 g/day of DHA) slowed the progression of renal disease in high-risk IgA nephropathy patients.[175] In contrast, several studies have failed to find a significant benefit of omega-3 PUFA supplementation in patients with IgA nephropathy.[176-179] Interestingly, fish-oil treatment (3 g/day of EPA + DHA) for 6 months did not decrease the urinary excretion of inflammatory mediators in patients with IgA nephropathy.[180] Two meta-analyses of randomized controlled trials of fish oil supplementation did not find evidence of a statistically significant benefit in patients with IgA nephropathy overall.[181,182] Due to the inconsistent results of available randomized controlled trials, it is not clear whether fish oil supplementation will prevent the progression of IgA nephropathy in children or adults.[147]

Major Depression and Bipolar Disorder

Data from ecological studies across different countries suggest an inverse association between seafood consumption and national rates of major depression[183] and bipolar disorder.[184] Several small studies have found omega-3 fatty acid concentrations to be lower in the plasma[185-187] and adipose tissue (fat)[188] of individuals suffering from depression compared with controls. Although it is not known how omega-3 fatty acid intake affects the incidence of depression, modulation of neuronal signaling pathways and eicosanoid production have been proposed as possible mechanisms.[189] The results of randomized controlled trials examining the effect of supplementation with long-chain omega-3 fatty acids on depression have been mixed. Adding fish oil supplements (8 g/day) to existing therapy in people who were being treated for depression was not significantly more effective than adding the same amount of olive oil for 12 weeks.[190] In patients with diagnosed major depression, fish oil supplementation (2.2 g/day of DHA + 0.6 g/day of EPA) for 4 months did not provide any therapeutic benefit beyond that associated with standard therapy.[191] In patients with mild to moderate depression, a lower dose (0.85 g/day of DHA + 0.63 g of EPA) was not effective when taken for 12 weeks.[192] Supplementation with 2 g/day of DHA for 6 weeks was not significantly more effective than a placebo in the treatment of major depression.[193] However, a small randomized controlled trial in Chinese patients diagnosed with major depression found that supplementation with 6.6 g/day of EPA + DHA for 8 weeks improved scores on the Hamilton Rating Scale for Depression compared with placebo.[194] Another small randomized controlled trial in 30 women diagnosed with borderline personality disorder found that the 20 women randomized to treatment with 1 g/day of ethyl-EPA for 8 weeks experienced less severe depressive symptoms than the 10 women randomized to treatment with a placebo.[195] Additionally, results of a recent pilot study suggest that omega-3 fatty acid supplementation may have utility in treating children with major depression.[196]

Unipolar depression and bipolar disorder are considered distinct psychiatric conditions, although major depression occurs in both. A randomized controlled trial that assessed the effects of high doses of EPA (6.2 g/day) + DHA (3.4 g/day) in patients with bipolar disorder found that those given EPA + DHA supplements had a significantly longer period of remission than those on an olive oil placebo over a 4-month period.[197] Patients who took the EPA + DHA supplements also experienced less depression than those who took the placebo. However, one study found that patients who took 6 g/day of ethyl-EPA for 4 weeks did not experience any relief from bipolar depression.[198] Lower doses of EPA may be more efficacious in treating bipolar disorder. A small study found that patients taking 1.5 g/day or 2 g/day of EPA for 6 months had some relief of depression associated with bipolar disorder.[199] A 12-week, double-blind, placebo-controlled trial in individuals with bipolar depression found those who took either 1 g/day or 2 g/day of ethyl-EPA experienced significant improvements in symptoms of depression, but measures of mania were not significantly different in either group compared with the placebo group.[200] Further, some recent meta-analyses of randomized controlled trials have concluded that omega-3 PUFA supplementation is beneficial in treating unipolar and bipolar depressive disorders.[201,202] However, another systematic review and meta-analysis concluded that there is little indication for using omega-3 PUFA supplementation in depression.[203] Large, long-term randomized controlled trials are required to determine the efficacy of long-chain omega-3 fatty acid supplementation on major depression and bipolar disorder.

Schizophrenia

Findings of decreased levels of omega-3 fatty acid in the red blood cells[204,205] and brains[206] of a limited number of patients with schizophrenia, together with the results of uncontrolled supplementation studies,[207] have created interest in the use of long-chain omega-3 fatty acid supplements as an adjunct to conventional regimens of antipsychotic therapy for schizophrenia. A pilot study in 45 patients with schizophrenia found that the addition of 2 g/day of EPA to standard antipsychotic therapy was superior to the addition of 2 g/day of DHA or placebo in decreasing residual symptoms.[208] When EPA supplementation was used as the sole treatment for patients with schizophrenia experiencing a relapse, eight out of 14 patients given 2 g/day of EPA supplements required antipsychotic medication by the end of the 12-week study period, compared with 12 out of 12 of those on the placebo.[208] Results of randomized controlled trials using ethyl-EPA as an adjunct to standard antipsychotic therapy in patients with schizophrenia have been somewhat contradictory. In one trial, the addition of 3 g/day of ethyl-EPA to standard antipsychotic

treatment for 12 weeks improved symptom scores and decreased dyskinesia scores[209]; a similar 12-week trial found that 2 g/day of ethyl-EPA did not benefit patients with schizophrenia and dyskinesia.[210] In another trial, supplementation with 3 g/day of ethyl-EPA for 16 weeks was not different than placebo in improving symptoms, mood, or cognition.[211] In a placebo-controlled trial comparing the addition of 1, 2, or 4 g/day of ethyl-EPA to different medication regimens, ethyl-EPA supplementation improved the symptoms of patients with schizophrenia on the antipsychotic medication clozapine but not those on other medications.[212] Although limited evidence suggests that EPA supplementation may be a useful adjunct to antipsychotic therapy in patients with schizophrenia, larger long-term studies addressing clinically relevant outcomes are needed.[213]

Alzheimer Disease and Dementia

Some epidemiological studies have associated decreased DHA status with Alzheimer disease and other types of dementia (see the Alzheimer Disease and Dementia section in the Disease Prevention section above). Although the results of studies in animal models have been promising,[214] it is not known whether DHA supplementation can help treat Alzheimer disease in humans. Recently, a randomized, double-blind, placebo-controlled trial in 295 patients with mild to moderate Alzheimer disease found that 2 g/day of DHA for 18 months had no cognitive benefit compared with placebo.[215]

Sources

Food Sources

Omega-6 Fatty Acids

Linoleic acid. Food sources of LA include vegetable oils, such as soybean, safflower, and corn oil, nuts, seeds, and some vegetables. Dietary surveys in the United States indicate that the average adult intake of LA ranges from 12 g/day to 17 g/day for men and 9 g/day to 11 g/day for women.[1] Some foods that are rich in LA are listed in **Table 20.1**.[216]

Arachidonic acid. Animals, but not plants, can convert LA to AA. Therefore, AA is present in small amounts in meat, poultry, and eggs.

Omega-3 Fatty Acids

α-Linolenic acid. Flaxseeds, walnuts, and their oils are among the richest dietary sources of ALA. Canola oil is also an excellent source of ALA. Dietary surveys in the United States indicate that average adult intakes for ALA range from 1.2 g/day to 1.6 g/day for men and from 0.9 g/day to 1.1 g/day for women.[1] Some foods that are rich in ALA are listed in **Table 20.2**.[216]

Eicosapentaenoic acid and docosahexaenoic acid. Oily fish are the major dietary source of EPA and DHA. Dietary surveys in the United States indicate that average adult intakes of EPA range from 0.04 g/day to 0.07 g/day and average adult intakes of DHA range from 0.05 g/day to 0.09 g/day.[1] Eggs enriched with omega-3 fatty acid are also available in the United States. Some foods that are rich in EPA and DHA are listed in Table 20.3.[216]

Biosynthesis

Humans can synthesize AA from LA and EPA and DHA from ALA through a series of desaturation and elongation reactions (see the Bioavailability and Metabolism section above).

Supplements

Omega-6 Fatty Acids

Borage seed oil, evening primrose oil, and blackcurrant seed oil are rich in γ-linolenic acid (GLA) and are often marketed as GLA or essential fatty acid (EFA) supplements.[217]

Omega-3 Fatty Acids

Flaxseed oil (also known as *flax oil* or *linseed oil*) is available as an ALA supplement. Several fish oils are marketed as omega-3 fatty acid supplements. Ethyl esters of EPA and DHA (ethyl-EPA and ethyl-DHA) are concentrated sources of long-chain omega-3 fatty acids. Since EPA and DHA content will vary in fish-oil and ethyl-ester preparations, it is necessary to read the label to determine the EPA and DHA content of a particular supplement. DHA supplements derived from algal and fungal sources are also available. All omega-3 fatty acid supplements are absorbed more efficiently with meals. Dividing one's daily dose into two or three smaller doses throughout the day will decrease the risk of gastrointestinal side

Table 20.1 Some food sources of linoleic acid $(18:2n\text{-}6)$[216]

Food	Serving	Linoleic Acid (g)
Safflower oil	1 tbs	10.1
Sunflower seeds, oil roasted	1 oz	9.7
Pine nuts	1 oz	9.4
Sunflower oil	1 tbs	8.9
Corn oil	1 tbs	7.3
Soybean oil	1 tbs	6.9
Pecans, oil roasted	1 oz	6.4
Brazil nuts	1 oz	5.8
Sesame oil	1 tbs	5.6

Table 20.2 Some food sources of α-linolenic acid $(18:3n\text{-}3)$[216]

Food	Serving	α-Linolenic Acid (g)
Flaxseed oil	1 tbs	7.3
Walnuts, English	1 oz	2.6
Flaxseeds, ground	1 tbs	1.6
Walnut oil	1 tbs	1.4
Canola oil	1 tbs	1.3
Soybean oil	1 tbs	0.9
Mustard oil	1 tbs	0.8
Tofu, firm	½ cup	0.7
Walnuts, black	1 oz	0.6

Table 20.3   Some food sources of eicosapentaenoic acid (EPA; 20:5n-3) and docosahexaenoic acid (DHA; 22:6n-3)[3]

Food	Serving	EPA (g)	DHA (g)	Amount Providing 1 g of EPA + DHA
Herring, Pacific	3 oz[a]	1.06	0.75	1.5 oz
Salmon, Chinook	3 oz	0.86	0.62	2 oz
Salmon, Atlantic	3 oz	0.28	0.95	2.5 oz
Oysters, Pacific	3 oz	0.75	0.43	2.5 oz
Salmon, sockeye	3 oz	0.45	0.60	3 oz
Trout, rainbow	3 oz	0.40	0.44	3.5 oz
Tuna, canned, white	3 oz	0.20	0.54	4 oz
Crab, Dungeness	3 oz	0.24	0.10	9 oz
Tuna, canned, light	3 oz	0.04	0.19	12 oz

[a] A 3-oz serving of fish is about the size of a deck of cards.

effects (see the Safety section below). Cod liver oil is a rich source of EPA and DHA, but some cod liver oil preparations may contain excessive amounts of preformed vitamin A (retinol).[217]

Infant Formula

In 2001, the US Food and Drug Administration (FDA) began permitting the addition of DHA and AA to infant formula in the United States.[218] At present, manufacturers are not required to list the amounts of DHA and AA added to infant formula on the label. However, most manufacturers of infant formula provide this information. The amounts added to formulas in the United States range from 8 mg to 17 mg DHA/100 calories (5 fl oz) and from 16 mg to 34 mg AA/100 calories. For example, an infant drinking 20 fl oz of DHA-enriched formula daily would receive 32–68 mg/day of DHA and 64–136 mg/day of AA.

Safety

Adverse Effects

γ-Linolenic Acid (18:3n-6)

Supplemental GLA is generally well tolerated, and serious adverse side effects have not been observed at doses up to 2.8 g/day for 12 months.[219] High doses of borage seed oil, evening primrose oil, or blackcurrant seed oil may cause gastrointestinal upset, loose stools, or diarrhea.[217] Because of case reports that supplementation with evening primrose oil induced seizure activity in people with undiagnosed temporal lobe epilep-

sy,[220] people with a history of seizures or seizure disorder are generally advised to avoid evening primrose oil and other GLA-rich oils.[217]

α-Linolenic Acid (18:3n-3)

Although flaxseed oil is generally well tolerated, high doses may cause loose stools or diarrhea.[221] Allergic and anaphylactic reactions have been reported with ingestion of flaxseed and flaxseed oil.[222]

Eicosapentaenoic Acid (20:5n-3) and Docosahexaenoic Acid (22:6n-3)

Serious adverse reactions have not been reported in those using fish-oil or other EPA and DHA supplements. The most common adverse effect of fish oil or EPA and DHA supplements is a fishy aftertaste. Belching and heartburn have also been reported. Additionally, high doses may cause nausea and loose stools.

Potential for excessive bleeding. The potential for high omega-3 fatty acid intakes, especially EPA and DHA, to prolong bleeding times has been well studied and may play a role in the cardioprotective effects of omega-3 fatty acids. Although excessively long bleeding times and increased incidence of hemorrhagic stroke have been observed in Greenland Eskimos with very high intakes of EPA + DHA (6.5 g/day), it is not known whether high intakes of EPA and DHA are the only factor responsible for these observations.[1] The FDA has ruled that intakes up to 3 g/day of long-chain omega-3 fatty acids (EPA and DHA) are generally recognized as safe (GRAS) for inclusion in the diet, and available evidence suggests that intakes below 3 g/day are unlikely to result in clinically significant bleeding.[3] Although the Institute of Medicine did not establish a tolerable upper intake level for omega-3 fatty acids, caution was advised with the use of supplemental EPA and DHA, especially in those who are at increased risk of excessive bleeding (see the Drug Interactions and Nutrient Interactions sections below).[1]

Potential for suppression of the immune system. Although the suppression of inflammatory responses resulting from increased omega-3 fatty acid intakes may benefit individuals with inflammatory or autoimmune diseases, anti-inflammatory doses of omega-3 fatty acids could decrease the potential of the immune system to destroy pathogens.[223] Studies comparing measures of immune-cell function outside the body (ex vivo) at baseline and after giving supplements of omega-3 fatty acids, mainly EPA and DHA, have demonstrated immunosuppressive effects at doses as low as 0.9 g/day for EPA and 0.6 g/day for DHA.[1] Although it is not clear if these findings translate to impaired immune responses in vivo, caution should be observed when considering omega-3 fatty acid supplementation in individuals with compromised immune systems.

Infant Formula

In early studies of DHA-enriched infant formula, EPA- and DHA-rich fish oil was used as a source of DHA. However, some preterm infants receiving formula enriched with fish oil had decreased plasma AA concentrations, which were associated with decreased growth.[224] This effect was attributed to the potential for high concentrations of EPA to interfere with the synthesis of AA, which is essential for normal growth. Consequently, EPA was removed and AA was added to DHA-enriched formula. Currently available infant formulas in the United States contain only AA and DHA derived from algal or fungal sources, rather than from fish oil. Randomized controlled trials have not found any adverse effects on growth in infants fed formulas enriched with AA and DHA for up to 1 year.[36,37]

Pregnancy and Lactation

The safety of supplemental omega-3 and omega-6 fatty acids, including borage seed oil, evening primrose oil, blackcurrant seed oil, and flaxseed oil, has not been established in pregnant or lactating women.[217] Studies of fish oil supplementation during pregnancy and lactation have not reported any serious adverse effects (see the Contaminants in Fish and Contaminants in Supplements sections below).

Contaminants in Fish

Some species of fish may contain significant levels of methylmercury, polychlorinated biphenyls (PCBs), or other environmental contaminants.[61] In general, larger predatory fish, such as swordfish, tend to contain the highest levels of these contaminants. Removing the skin, fat, and internal organs of the fish prior to cooking and allowing the fat to drain from the fish while it cooks will decrease exposure to several fat-soluble pollutants, such as PCBs.[225] However, methylmercury is found throughout the muscle of fish, so these cooking precautions will not reduce exposure to methylmercury. Organic mercury compounds are toxic, and excessive exposure can cause brain and kidney damage. The developing fetus, infants, and young children are especially vulnerable to the toxic effects of mercury on the brain. To limit their exposure to methylmercury, the US Department of Health and Human Services (DHHS) and Environmental Protection Agency (EPA) have made the following joint recommendations for women who may become pregnant, pregnant women, and breast-feeding women[170]:

1. Do not eat shark, swordfish, king mackerel, or tile fish (also known as *golden bass* or *golden snapper*) because they contain high methylmercury levels.
2. Eat up to 12 oz (two average meals) per week of a variety of fish that are lower in mercury.
   a) The five most commonly consumed fish that are low in mercury include canned light tuna, shrimp, salmon, catfish, and pollock.
   b) Limit the consumption of canned white (albacore) tuna and tuna steak to 6 oz (one average meal) per week.

3. Check local advisories regarding the safety of fish caught by friends or family in local lakes, rivers, and coastal areas.

When feeding fish to young children, the DHHS and the EPA advise following the above guidelines but serving smaller portions, such as 3 oz, for an average meal.

Contaminants in Supplements

Although concerns have been raised regarding the potential for omega-3 fatty acid supplements derived from fish oil to contain methylmercury, PCBs, and dioxins, several independent laboratory analyses in the United States have found commercially available omega-3 fatty acid supplements to be free of methylmercury, PCBs, and dioxins.[226–228] The absence of methylmercury in omega-3 fatty acid supplements can be explained by the fact that mercury accumulates in the muscle, rather than the fat of fish.[3] In general, fish body oils contain lower levels of PCBs and other fat-soluble contaminants than fish liver oils. Additionally, fish oils that have been more highly refined and deodorized also contain lower levels of PCBs.[229] Pyrrolizidine alkaloids, potentially hepatotoxic and carcinogenic compounds, are found in various parts of the borage plant. People who take borage oil supplements should use products that are certified free of pyrrolizidine alkaloids.[217]

Drug Interactions

γ-Linolenic acid supplements, such as evening primrose oil or borage seed oil, may increase the risk of seizures in people on phenothiazines, such as chlorpromazine.[220] High doses of blackcurrant seed oil, borage seed oil, evening primrose oil, flaxseed oil, and fish oil may inhibit platelet aggregation; therefore, these supplements should be used with caution in people on anticoagulant medications. In particular, people taking supplements of fish oil or long-chain omega-3 fatty acid (EPA and DHA) supplementation in combination with anticoagulant drugs, including aspirin, clopidogrel (Plavix), dalteparin (Fragmin), dipyridamole (Persantin), enoxaparin (Lovenox), heparin, ticlopidine (Ticlid), and warfarin (Coumadin), should have their coagulation status monitored using a standardized prothrombin time assay (international normalized ratio—INR). One small study found that 3 g/day or 6 g/day of fish oil did not affect INR values in 10 patients on warfarin over a 4-week period.[230] However, a case report described an individual who required a reduction of her warfarin dose when she doubled her dose of fish oil from 1 g/day to 2 g/day.[231]

Nutrient Interactions

Vitamin E

Outside the body, PUFAs become rancid (oxidized) more easily than SFAs. Fat-soluble antioxidants, such as vitamin E, play an important role in preventing the oxidation of PUFAs. Inside the body, results of animal studies and limited data in humans suggest that the amount of vitamin E required to prevent lipid peroxidation increases with the amount of PUFA consumed.[232] One widely used recommendation for vitamin E intake is 0.6 mg of α-tocopherol per gram of dietary PUFA. This recommendation was based on a small study in men and the ratio of α-tocopherol to LA in the US diet, and has not been verified in more comprehensive studies. Although EPA and DHA are easily oxidized outside the body, it is presently unclear whether EPA and DHA are more susceptible to oxidative damage within the body.[233] High vitamin E intakes have not been found to decrease biomarkers of oxidative damage when EPA and DHA intakes are increased,[234,235] but some experts believe that an increase in PUFA intake, particularly omega-3 PUFA intake, should be accompanied by an increase in vitamin E intake.[1]

Intake Recommendations

US Institute of Medicine

In 2002, the Food and Nutrition Board of the US Institute of Medicine established adequate intakes (AIs) for omega-6 and omega-3 fatty acids, which are listed in **Tables 20.4** and **20.5**, respectively.[1]

International Recommendations

The European Commission recommends an omega-6 fatty acid intake of 4%–8% of energy and an omega-3 fatty acid intake of 2 g/day of ALA and 200 mg/day of long-chain omega-3 fatty acids

Table 20.4   Adequate intakes for omega-6 fatty acids[1]

Life Stage	Age	Source	Males (g/day)	Females (g/day)
Infants	0–6 months	Omega-6 PUFA[a]	4.4	4.4
Infants	7–12 months	Omega-6 PUFA[a]	4.6	4.6
Children	1–3 years	LA	7	7
Children	4–8 years	LA	10	10
Children	9–13 years	LA	12	10
Adolescents	14–18 years	LA	16	11
Adults	19–50 years	LA	17	12
Adults	51 years or older	LA	14	11
Pregnancy	All ages	LA	–	13
Lactation	All ages	LA	–	13

[a] The various omega-6 fatty polyunsaturated fatty acids (PUFAs) present in human milk can contribute to the adequate intake for infants.
LA, linoleic acid.

Table 20.5   Adequate intakes for omega-3 fatty acids[1]

Life Stage	Age	Source	Males (g/day)	Females (g/day)
Infants	0–6 months	ALA, EPA, DHA	0.5	0.5
Infants	7–12 months	ALA, EPA, DHA	0.5	0.5
Children	1–3 years	ALA	0.7	0.7
Children	4–8 years	ALA	0.9	0.9
Children	9–13 years	ALA	1.2	1.0
Adolescents	14–18 years	ALA	1.6	1.1
Adults	19 years and older	ALA	1.6	1.1
Pregnancy	All ages	ALA	–	1.4
Lactation	All ages	ALA	–	1.3

ALA, α-linolenic acid; DHA, docosahexaenoic acid; EPA, eicosapentaenoic acid.

(EPA and DHA).[236] The World Health Organization recommends an omega-6 fatty acid intake of 5%–8% of energy and an omega-3 fatty acid intake of 1%–2% of energy.[147] However, the Japan Society for Lipid Nutrition has recommended that LA intake be reduced to 3%–4% of energy in Japanese people whose omega-3 fatty acid intakes average 2.6 g/day, including approximately 1 g/day of EPA + DHA.[237]

American Heart Association

The American Heart Association recommends that people without documented CHD eat a variety of fish (preferably oily) at least twice weekly, in addition to consuming oils and foods rich in ALA.[143] Pregnant women and children should avoid fish that typically have higher levels of methylmercury (see the Contaminants in Fish section above). People with documented CHD are advised to consume approximately 1 g/day of EPA + DHA, preferably from oily fish, or to consider EPA + DHA supplements in consultation with a physician. Patients who need to lower their serum triglycerides may take 2–4 g/day of EPA + DHA supplements under a physician's care.[143]

Summary

• α-Linolenic acid (ALA), an omega-3 fatty acid, and linoleic acid (LA), an omega-6 fatty acid, are considered essential fatty acids because they cannot be synthesized by humans.

- The long-chain omega-6 fatty acid, arachidonic acid (AA), can be synthesized from LA.
- The long-chain omega-3 fatty acids, eicosapentaenoic acid (EPA) and docosahexaenoic acid (DHA), can be synthesized from ALA, but synthesis of EPA and DHA may be insufficient under certain conditions.
- Typical Western diets tend to be much higher in omega-6 fatty acids than omega-3 fatty acids.
- While DHA appears to be important for visual and neurological development, it is not yet clear whether feeding infants formula enriched with DHA and AA enhances visual acuity or neurological development in preterm or term infants.
- A large body of scientific research suggests that higher dietary omega-3 fatty acid intakes are associated with reductions in cardiovascular disease risk. Thus, the American Heart Association recommends that all adults eat fish, particularly oily fish, at least twice a week.
- The results of randomized controlled trials indicate that increasing omega-3 fatty acid intake can decrease the risk of myocardial infarction (heart attack) and sudden cardiac death in individuals with coronary heart disease.
- Low DHA status may be a risk factor for Alzheimer disease and other types of dementia, but it is not yet known whether DHA supplementation can help prevent or treat such cognitive disorders.
- Increasing EPA and DHA intake may be beneficial in individuals with type 2 diabetes, especially those with elevated serum triglycerides.
- Randomized controlled trials have found that fish oil supplementation decreases joint tenderness and reduces the requirement for anti-inflammatory medication in patients with rheumatoid arthritis.
- Although limited preliminary data suggest that omega-3 fatty acid supplementation may be beneficial in the therapy of depression, bipolar disorder, and schizophrenia, larger controlled clinical trials are needed to determine the therapeutic efficacy.

References

1. Food and Nutrition Board, Institute of Medicine. Dietary Fats: Total Fat and Fatty Acids. Dietary Reference Intakes for Energy, Carbohydrate, Fiber, Fat, Fatty Acids, Cholesterol, Protein, and Amino Acids. Washington, DC: National Academies Press; 2002: 422–541
2. Simopoulos AP, Leaf A, Salem N Jr. Workshop statement on the essentiality of and recommended dietary intakes for Omega-6 and Omega-3 fatty acids. Prostaglandins Leukot Essent Fatty Acids 2000; 63(3):119–121
3. Kris-Etherton PM, Harris WS, Appel LJ; American Heart Association. Nutrition Committee. Fish consumption, fish oil, omega-3 fatty acids, and cardiovascular disease. Circulation 2002;106(21):2747–2757
4. Lichtenstein AH, Jones PJ. Lipids: absorption and transport. In: Bowman BA, Russel RM, eds. Present Knowledge in Nutrition. 8th ed. Washington, DC: ILSI Press; 2001:93–103
5. Nakamura MT, Nara TY. Structure, function, and dietary regulation of delta6, delta5, and delta9 desaturases. Annu Rev Nutr 2004;24:345–376
6. Burdge G. Alpha-linolenic acid metabolism in men and women: nutritional and biological implications. Curr Opin Clin Nutr Metab Care 2004;7(2):137–144
7. Burdge GC, Jones AE, Wootton SA. Eicosapentaenoic and docosapentaenoic acids are the principal products of alpha-linolenic acid metabolism in young men*. Br J Nutr 2002;88(4):355–363
8. Burdge GC, Wootton SA. Conversion of alpha-linolenic acid to eicosapentaenoic, docosapentaenoic and docosahexaenoic acids in young women. Br J Nutr 2002;88(4):411–420
9. Giltay EJ, Gooren LJ, Toorians AW, Katan MB, Zock PL. Docosahexaenoic acid concentrations are higher in women than in men because of estrogenic effects. Am J Clin Nutr 2004;80(5):1167–1174
10. Muskiet FA, Fokkema MR, Schaafsma A, Boersma ER, Crawford MA. Is docosahexaenoic acid (DHA) essential? Lessons from DHA status regulation, our ancient diet, epidemiology and randomized controlled trials. J Nutr 2004;134(1):183–186
11. Cunnane SC. Problems with essential fatty acids: time for a new paradigm? Prog Lipid Res 2003;42(6):544–568
12. Stillwell W, Wassall SR. Docosahexaenoic acid: membrane properties of a unique fatty acid. Chem Phys Lipids 2003;126(1):1–27
13. Jeffrey BG, Weisinger HS, Neuringer M, Mitchell DC. The role of docosahexaenoic acid in retinal function. Lipids 2001;36(9):859–871
14. SanGiovanni JP, Chew EY. The role of omega-3 long-chain polyunsaturated fatty acids in health and disease of the retina. Prog Retin Eye Res 2005;24(1):87–138
15. Innis SM. Perinatal biochemistry and physiology of long-chain polyunsaturated fatty acids. J Pediatr 2003; 143(4, Suppl):S1–S8
16. Chalon S, Vancassel S, Zimmer L, Guilloteau D, Durand G. Polyunsaturated fatty acids and cerebral function: focus on monoaminergic neurotransmission. Lipids 2001;36(9):937–944
17. Calder PC. Dietary modification of inflammation with lipids. Proc Nutr Soc 2002;61(3):345–358

18. Price PT, Nelson CM, Clarke SD. Omega-3 polyunsaturated fatty acid regulation of gene expression. Curr Opin Lipidol 2000;11(1):3–7

19. Sampath H, Ntambi JM. Polyunsaturated fatty acid regulation of gene expression. Nutr Rev 2004;62(9): 333–339

20. Jump DB. Fatty acid regulation of gene transcription. Crit Rev Clin Lab Sci 2004;41(1):41–78

21. Jump DB, Botolin D, Wang Y, Xu J, Demeure O, Christian B. Docosahexaenoic acid (DHA) and hepatic gene transcription. Chem Phys Lipids 2008;153(1):3–13

22. Jump DB. N-3 polyunsaturated fatty acid regulation of hepatic gene transcription. Curr Opin Lipidol 2008; 19(3):242–247

23. Jump DB, Botolin D, Wang Y, Xu J, Christian B, Demeure O. Fatty acid regulation of hepatic gene transcription. J Nutr 2005;135(11):2503–2506

24. Jeppesen PB, Høy CE, Mortensen PB. Essential fatty acid deficiency in patients receiving home parenteral nutrition. Am J Clin Nutr 1998;68(1):126–133

25. Smit EN, Muskiet FA, Boersma ER. The possible role of essential fatty acids in the pathophysiology of malnutrition: a review. Prostaglandins Leukot Essent Fatty Acids 2004;71(4):241–250

26. Mascioli EA, Lopes SM, Champagne C, Driscoll DF. Essential fatty acid deficiency and home total parenteral nutrition patients. Nutrition 1996;12(4):245–249

27. Steginck LD, Freeman JB, Wispe J, Connor WE. Absence of the biochemical symptoms of essential fatty acid deficiency in surgical patients undergoing protein sparing therapy. Am J Clin Nutr 1977;30(3):388–393

28. Jeppesen PB, Høy CE, Mortensen PB. Deficiencies of essential fatty acids, vitamin A and E and changes in plasma lipoproteins in patients with reduced fat absorption or intestinal failure. Eur J Clin Nutr 2000; 54(8):632–642

29. Lepage G, Levy E, Ronco N, Smith L, Galéano N, Roy CC. Direct transesterification of plasma fatty acids for the diagnosis of essential fatty acid deficiency in cystic fibrosis. J Lipid Res 1989;30(10):1483–1490

30. Holman RT, Johnson SB, Hatch TF. A case of human linolenic acid deficiency involving neurological abnormalities. Am J Clin Nutr 1982;35(3):617–623

31. Fedorova I, Hussein N, Baumann MH, Di Martino C, Salem N Jr. An n-3 fatty acid deficiency impairs rat spatial learning in the Barnes maze. Behav Neurosci 2009;123(1):196–205

32. Fedorova I, Salem N Jr. Omega-3 fatty acids and rodent behavior. Prostaglandins Leukot Essent Fatty Acids 2006;75(4–5):271–289

33. Uauy R, Hoffman DR, Peirano P, Birch DG, Birch EE. Essential fatty acids in visual and brain development. Lipids 2001;36(9):885–895

34. Larque E, Demmelmair H, Koletzko B. Perinatal supply and metabolism of long-chain polyunsaturated fatty acids: importance for the early development of the nervous system. Ann N Y Acad Sci 2002;967:299–310

35. Uauy R, Hoffman DR, Mena P, Llanos A, Birch EE. Term infant studies of DHA and A.R.A supplementation on neurodevelopment: results of randomized controlled trials. J Pediatr 2003; 143(4, Suppl):S17–S25

36. Simmer K, Patole S. Longchain polyunsaturated fatty acid supplementation in preterm infants. Cochrane Database Syst Rev 2004; (1):CD000375

37. Simmer K. Longchain polyunsaturated fatty acid supplementation in infants born at term. Cochrane Database Syst Rev 2001; (4):CD000376

38. Eilander A, Hundscheid DC, Osendarp SJ, Transler C, Zock PL. Effects of n-3 long chain polyunsaturated fatty acid supplementation on visual and cognitive development throughout childhood: a review of human studies. Prostaglandins Leukot Essent Fatty Acids 2007;76(4):189–203

39. SanGiovanni JP, Parra-Cabrera S, Colditz GA, Berkey CS, Dwyer JT. Meta-analysis of dietary essential fatty acids and long-chain polyunsaturated fatty acids as they relate to visual resolution acuity in healthy preterm infants. Pediatrics 2000;105(6):1292–1298

40. O'Connor DL, Hall R, Adamkin D, et al; Ross Preterm Lipid Study. Growth and development in preterm infants fed long-chain polyunsaturated fatty acids: a prospective, randomized controlled trial. Pediatrics 2001;108(2):359–371

41. Fewtrell MS, Morley R, Abbott RA, et al. Double-blind, randomized trial of long-chain polyunsaturated fatty acid supplementation in formula fed to preterm infants. Pediatrics 2002;110(1 Pt 1):73–82

42. Fewtrell MS, Abbott RA, Kennedy K, et al. Randomized, double-blind trial of long-chain polyunsaturated fatty acid supplementation with fish oil and borage oil in preterm infants. J Pediatr 2004;144(4):471–479

43. Clandinin MT, Van Aerde JE, Merkel KL, et al. Growth and development of preterm infants fed infant formulas containing docosahexaenoic acid and arachidonic acid. J Pediatr 2005;146(4):461–468

44. Birch EE, Castañeda YS, Wheaton DH, Birch DG, Uauy RD, Hoffman DR. Visual maturation of term infants fed long-chain polyunsaturated fatty acid-supplemented or control formula for 12 mo. Am J Clin Nutr 2005;81(4):871–879

45. Auestad N, Scott DT, Janowsky JS, et al. Visual, cognitive, and language assessments at 39 months: a follow-up study of children fed formulas containing long-chain polyunsaturated fatty acids to 1 year of age. Pediatrics 2003;112(3 Pt 1):e177–e183

46. Gibson RA, Chen W, Makrides M. Randomized trials with polyunsaturated fatty acid interventions in preterm and term infants: functional and clinical outcomes. Lipids 2001;36(9):873–883

47. Birch EE, Garfield S, Castañeda Y, Hughbanks-Wheaton D, Uauy R, Hoffman D. Visual acuity and cognitive outcomes at 4 years of age in a double-blind, randomized trial of long-chain polyunsaturated fatty acid-supplemented infant formula. Early Hum Dev 2007;83(5):279–284

48. McCann JC, Ames BN. Is docosahexaenoic acid, an n-3 long-chain polyunsaturated fatty acid, required for development of normal brain function? An overview of evidence from cognitive and behavioral tests in humans and animals. Am J Clin Nutr 2005;82(2):281–295

49. Koo WW. Efficacy and safety of docosahexaenoic acid and arachidonic acid addition to infant formulas: can one buy better vision and intelligence? J Am Coll Nutr 2003;22(2):101–107

50. Makrides M, Gibson RA. Long-chain polyunsaturated fatty acid requirements during pregnancy and lactation. Am J Clin Nutr 2000; 71(1, Suppl):307S–311S

51. Onwude JL, Lilford RJ, Hjartardottir H, Staines A, Tuffnell D. A randomised double blind placebo controlled trial of fish oil in high risk pregnancy. Br J Obstet Gynaecol 1995;102(1):95–100

52. Olsen SF, Sørensen JD, Secher NJ, et al. Randomised controlled trial of effect of fish-oil supplementation

on pregnancy duration. Lancet 1992;339(8800):1003–1007

53. Smuts CM, Huang M, Mundy D, Plasse T, Major S, Carlson SE. A randomized trial of docosahexaenoic acid supplementation during the third trimester of pregnancy. Obstet Gynecol 2003;101(3):469–479

54. Szajewska H, Horvath A, Koletzko B. Effect of n-3 long-chain polyunsaturated fatty acid supplementation of women with low-risk pregnancies on pregnancy outcomes and growth measures at birth: a meta-analysis of randomized controlled trials. Am J Clin Nutr 2006;83(6):1337–1344

55. Olsen SF, Secher NJ, Tabor A, Weber T, Walker JJ, Gluud C; Fish Oil Trials In Pregnancy (FOTIP) Team. Randomised clinical trials of fish oil supplementation in high risk pregnancies. BJOG 2000;107(3):382–395

56. Horvath A, Koletzko B, Szajewska H. Effect of supplementation of women in high-risk pregnancies with long-chain polyunsaturated fatty acids on pregnancy outcomes and growth measures at birth: a meta-analysis of randomized controlled trials. Br J Nutr 2007;98(2):253–259

57. Koletzko B, Lien E, Agostoni C, et al; World Association of Perinatal Medicine Dietary Guidelines Working Group. The roles of long-chain polyunsaturated fatty acids in pregnancy, lactation and infancy: review of current knowledge and consensus recommendations. J Perinat Med 2008;36(1):5–14

58. Helland IB, Smith L, Saarem K, Saugstad OD, Drevon CA. Maternal supplementation with very-long-chain n-3 fatty acids during pregnancy and lactation augments children's I.Q. at 4 years of age. Pediatrics 2003;111(1):e39–e44

59. Dunstan JA, Simmer K, Dixon G, Prescott SL. Cognitive assessment of children at age 2(1/2) years after maternal fish oil supplementation in pregnancy: a randomised controlled trial. Arch Dis Child Fetal Neonatal Ed 2008;93(1):F45–F50

60. Judge MP, Harel O, Lammi-Keefe CJ. Maternal consumption of a docosahexaenoic acid-containing functional food during pregnancy: benefit for infant performance on problem-solving but not on recognition memory tasks at age 9 mo. Am J Clin Nutr 2007;85(6):1572–1577

61. Mozaffarian D, Rimm EB. Fish intake, contaminants, and human health: evaluating the risks and the benefits. JAMA 2006;296(15):1885–1899

62. Kris-Etherton PM, Hecker KD, Binkoski AE. Polyunsaturated fatty acids and cardiovascular health. Nutr Rev 2004;62(11):414–426

63. Shekelle RB, Shryock AM, Paul O, et al. Diet, serum cholesterol, and death from coronary heart disease. The Western Electric study. N Engl J Med 1981;304(2):65–70

64. Oh K, Hu FB, Manson JE, Stampfer MJ, Willett WC. Dietary fat intake and risk of coronary heart disease in women: 20 years of follow-up of the nurses' health study. Am J Epidemiol 2005;161(7):672–679

65. Ascherio A, Rimm EB, Giovannucci EL, Spiegelman D, Stampfer M, Willett WC. Dietary fat and risk of coronary heart disease in men: cohort follow up study in the United States. BMJ 1996;313(7049):84–90

66. Laaksonen DE, Nyyssönen K, Niskanen L, Rissanen TH, Salonen JT. Prediction of cardiovascular mortality in middle-aged men by dietary and serum linoleic and polyunsaturated fatty acids. Arch Intern Med 2005;165(2):193–199

67. Sacks FM, Katan M. Randomized clinical trials on the effects of dietary fat and carbohydrate on plasma li-poproteins and cardiovascular disease. Am J Med 2002;113(Suppl 9B):13S–24S

68. Mensink RP, Katan MB. Effect of dietary fatty acids on serum lipids and lipoproteins. A meta-analysis of 27 trials. Arterioscler Thromb 1992;12(8):911–919

69. Lewis B, Krikler D. Controlled trial of soya-bean oil in myocardial infarction. Lancet 1968;2(7570):693–699

70. Dayton S, Pearce ML, Goldman H, et al. Controlled trial of a diet high in unsaturated fat for prevention of atherosclerotic complications. Lancet 1968;2(7577):1060–1062

71. Leren P. The Oslo diet-heart study. Eleven-year report. Circulation 1970;42(5):935–942

72. Turpeinen O, Karvonen MJ, Pekkarinen M, Miettinen M, Elosuo R, Paavilainen E. Dietary prevention of coronary heart disease: the Finnish Mental Hospital Study. Int J Epidemiol 1979;8(2):99–118

73. Frantz ID Jr, Dawson EA, Ashman PL, et al. Test of effect of lipid lowering by diet on cardiovascular risk. The Minnesota Coronary Survey. Arteriosclerosis 1989;9(1):129–135

74. Miettinen M, Turpeinen O, Karvonen MJ, Pekkarinen M, Paavilainen E, Elosuo R. Dietary prevention of coronary heart disease in women: the Finnish mental hospital study. Int J Epidemiol 1983;12(1):17–25

75. Harris WS, Mozaffarian D, Rimm E, et al. Omega-6 fatty acids and risk for cardiovascular disease: a science advisory from the American Heart Association Nutrition Subcommittee of the Council on Nutrition, Physical Activity, and Metabolism; Council on Cardiovascular Nursing; and Council on Epidemiology and Prevention. Circulation 2009;119(6):902–907

76. Mozaffarian D, Ascherio A, Hu FB, et al. Interplay between different polyunsaturated fatty acids and risk of coronary heart disease in men. Circulation 2005;111(2):157–164

77. Hu F.B., Stampfer MJ, Manson J.E., et al. Dietary intake of alpha-linolenic acid and risk of fatal ischemic heart disease among women. Am J Clin Nutr 1999;69(5):890–897

78. Dolecek TA. Epidemiological evidence of relationships between dietary polyunsaturated fatty acids and mortality in the multiple risk factor intervention trial. Proc Soc Exp Biol Med 1992;200(2):177–182

79. Pietinen P, Ascherio A, Korhonen P, et al. Intake of fatty acids and risk of coronary heart disease in a cohort of Finnish men. The Alpha-Tocopherol, Beta-Carotene Cancer Prevention Study. Am J Epidemiol 1997;145(10):876–887

80. Oomen CM, Ocké MC, Feskens EJ, Kok FJ, Kromhout D. alpha-Linolenic acid intake is not beneficially associated with 10-y risk of coronary artery disease incidence: the Zutphen Elderly Study. Am J Clin Nutr 2001;74(4):457–463

81. Albert CM, Oh K, Whang W, et al. Dietary alpha-linolenic acid intake and risk of sudden cardiac death and coronary heart disease. Circulation 2005;112(21):3232–3238

82. Mozaffarian D. Does alpha-linolenic acid intake reduce the risk of coronary heart disease? A review of the evidence. Altern Ther Health Med 2005;11(3):24–30, quiz 31, 79

83. Wendland E, Farmer A, Glasziou P, Neil A. Effect of alpha linolenic acid on cardiovascular risk markers: a systematic review. Heart 2006;92(2):166–169

84. Bemelmans WJ, Lefrandt JD, Feskens EJ, et al. Increased alpha-linolenic acid intake lowers C-reactive protein, but has no effect on markers of atherosclerosis. Eur J Clin Nutr 2004;58(7):1083–1089

85. Rallidis LS, Paschos G, Liakos GK, Velissaridou AH, Anastasiadis G, Zampelas A. Dietary alpha-linolenic acid decreases C-reactive protein, serum amyloid A and interleukin-6 in dyslipidaemic patients. Atherosclerosis 2003;167(2):237–242

86. Zhao G, Etherton TD, Martin KR, West SG, Gillies PJ, Kris-Etherton PM. Dietary alpha-linolenic acid reduces inflammatory and lipid cardiovascular risk factors in hypercholesterolemic men and women. J Nutr 2004;134(11):2991–2997

87. Kris-Etherton PM, Harris WS, Appel LJ; AHA Nutrition Committee. American Heart Association. Omega-3 fatty acids and cardiovascular disease: new recommendations from the American Heart Association. Arterioscler Thromb Vasc Biol 2003;23(2):151–152

88. Wang C, Harris WS, Chung M, et al. n-3 Fatty acids from fish or fish-oil supplements, but not alpha-linolenic acid, benefit cardiovascular disease outcomes in primary- and secondary-prevention studies: a systematic review. Am J Clin Nutr 2006;84(1):5–17

89. Hooper L, Thompson RL, Harrison RA, et al. Risks and benefits of omega 3 fats for mortality, cardiovascular disease, and cancer: systematic review. BMJ 2006; 332(7544):752–760

90. Kromhout D, Bosschieter EB, de Lezenne Coulander C. The inverse relation between fish consumption and 20-year mortality from coronary heart disease. N Engl J Med 1985;312(19):1205–1209

91. Kromhout D, Feskens EJ, Bowles CH. The protective effect of a small amount of fish on coronary heart disease mortality in an elderly population. Int J Epidemiol 1995;24(2):340–345

92. Dolecek TA, Granditis G. Dietary polyunsaturated fatty acids and mortality in the Multiple Risk Factor Intervention Trial (MRFIT). World Rev Nutr Diet 1991;66:205–216

93. Daviglus ML, Stamler J, Orencia AJ, et al. Fish consumption and the 30-year risk of fatal myocardial infarction. N Engl J Med 1997;336(15):1046–1053

94. Yuan JM, Ross RK, Gao YT, Yu MC. Fish and shellfish consumption in relation to death from myocardial infarction among men in Shanghai, China. Am J Epidemiol 2001;154(9):809–816

95. Hu FB, Bronner L, Willett WC, et al. Fish and omega-3 fatty acid intake and risk of coronary heart disease in women. JAMA 2002;287(14):1815–1821

96. Järvinen R, Knekt P, Rissanen H, Reunanen A. Intake of fish and long-chain n-3 fatty acids and the risk of coronary heart mortality in men and women. Br J Nutr 2006;95(4):824–829

97. Iso H, Kobayashi M, Ishihara J, et al; JPHC. Study Group. Intake of fish and n3 fatty acids and risk of coronary heart disease among Japanese: the Japan Public Health Center-Based (JPHC.) Study Cohort I. Circulation 2006;113(2):195–202

98. Nakamura Y, Ueshima H, Okamura T, et al; NIPPON DATA80 Research Group. Association between fish consumption and all-cause and cause-specific mortality in Japan: NIPPON DATA80, 1980–99. Am J Med 2005;118(3):239–245

99. Leaf A, Xiao YF, Kang JX, Billman GE. Prevention of sudden cardiac death by n-3 polyunsaturated fatty acids. Pharmacol Ther 2003;98(3):355–377

100. Albert C.M., Hennekens C.H., O'Donnell C.J., et al. Fish consumption and risk of sudden cardiac death. JAMA 1998;279(1):23–28

101. Albert C.M., Campos H, Stampfer MJ, et al. Blood levels of long-chain n-3 fatty acids and the risk of sudden death. N Engl J Med 2002;346(15):1113–1118

102. Mozaffarian D. Fish and n-3 fatty acids for the prevention of fatal coronary heart disease and sudden cardiac death. Am J Clin Nutr 2008;87(6):1991S–1996S

103. Leaf A, Albert CM, Josephson M, et al; Fatty Acid Antiarrhythmia Trial Investigators. Prevention of fatal arrhythmias in high-risk subjects by fish oil n-3 fatty acid intake. Circulation 2005;112(18):2762–2768

104. Raitt MH, Connor WE, Morris C, et al. Fish oil supplementation and risk of ventricular tachycardia and ventricular fibrillation in patients with implantable defibrillators: a randomized controlled trial. JAMA 2005;293(23):2884–2891

105. Brouwer IA, Zock PL, Camm AJ, et al; SOFA Study Group. Effect of fish oil on ventricular tachyarrhythmia and death in patients with implantable cardioverter defibrillators: the Study on Omega-3 Fatty Acids and Ventricular Arrhythmia (SOFA) randomized trial. JAMA 2006;295(22):2613–2619

106. Jenkins DJ, Josse AR, Beyene J, et al. Fish-oil supplementation in patients with implantable cardioverter defibrillators: a meta-analysis. CMAJ 2008; 178(2): 157–164

107. London B, Albert C, Anderson ME, et al. Omega-3 fatty acids and cardiac arrhythmias: prior studies and recommendations for future research: a report from the National Heart, Lung, and Blood Institute and Office Of Dietary Supplements Omega-3 Fatty Acids and their Role in Cardiac Arrhythmogenesis Workshop. Circulation 2007;116(10):e320–e335

108. American Stroke Association. Types of Stroke. Available at: http://www.strokeassociation.org/STROKE-ORG/AboutStroke/Types-of-Stroke_UCM_308531_SubHomePage.jsp. Accessed May 8, 2012

109. Keli SO, Feskens EJ, Kromhout D. Fish consumption and risk of stroke. The Zutphen Study. Stroke 1994;25(2):328–332

110. Gillum R.F., Mussolino ME, Madans JH; The NHANES I Epidemiologic Follow-up Study (National Health and Nutrition Examination Survey). The relationship between fish consumption and stroke incidence. Arch Intern Med 1996;156(5):537–542

111. Morris MC, Manson JE, Rosner B, Buring JE, Willett WC, Hennekens CH. Fish consumption and cardiovascular disease in the physicians' health study: a prospective study. Am J Epidemiol 1995;142(2):166–175

112. Orencia AJ, Daviglus ML, Dyer AR, Shekelle RB, Stamler J. Fish consumption and stroke in men. 30-year findings of the Chicago Western Electric Study. Stroke 1996;27(2):204–209

113. Myint PK, Welch AA, Bingham SA, et al. Habitual fish consumption and risk of incident stroke: the European Prospective Investigation into Cancer (EPIC)-Norfolk prospective population study. Public Health Nutr 2006;9(7):882–888

114. Iso H, Rexrode KM, Stampfer MJ, et al. Intake of fish and omega-3 fatty acids and risk of stroke in women. JAMA 2001;285(3):304–312

115. He K, Rimm EB, Merchant A, et al. Fish consumption and risk of stroke in men. JAMA 2002;288(24):3130–3136

116. He K, Song Y, Daviglus ML, et al. Fish consumption and incidence of stroke: a meta-analysis of cohort studies. Stroke 2004;35(7):1538–1542

117. Tanaka K, Ishikawa Y, Yokoyama M, et al; JELIS Investigators, Japan. Reduction in the recurrence of stroke by eicosapentaenoic acid for hypercholesterolemic

patients: subanalysis of the JELIS trial. Stroke 2008;39(7):2052–2058

118. Austin MA, Hokanson JE, Edwards KL. Hypertriglyceridemia as a cardiovascular risk factor. Am J Cardiol 1998;81(4A):7B–12B

119. Harris WS. n-3 fatty acids and serum lipoproteins: human studies. Am J Clin Nutr 1997; 65(5, Suppl):1645S–1654S

120. Balk EM, Lichtenstein AH, Chung M, Kupelnick B, Chew P, Lau J. Effects of omega-3 fatty acids on serum markers of cardiovascular disease risk: a systematic review. Atherosclerosis 2006;189(1):19–30

121. Harris WS, Kris-Etherton PM, Harris KA. Intakes of long-chain omega-3 fatty acid associated with reduced risk for death from coronary heart disease in healthy adults. Curr Atheroscler Rep 2008;10(6): 503–509

122. Harris WS, Mozaffarian D, Lefevre M, et al. Towards establishing dietary reference intakes for eicosapentaenoic and docosahexaenoic acids. J Nutr 2009; 139(4):804S–819S

123. Maccioni RB, Muñoz JP, Barbeito L. The molecular bases of Alzheimer's disease and other neurodegenerative disorders. Arch Med Res 2001;32(5):367–381

124. Kalmijn S, van Boxtel MP, Ocké M, Verschuren WM, Kromhout D, Launer LJ. Dietary intake of fatty acids and fish in relation to cognitive performance at middle age. Neurology 2004;62(2):275–280

125. Kalmijn S, Launer LJ, Ott A, Witteman JC, Hofman A, Breteler MM. Dietary fat intake and the risk of incident dementia in the Rotterdam Study. Ann Neurol 1997;42(5):776–782

126. Morris MC, Evans DA, Bienias JL, et al. Consumption of fish and n-3 fatty acids and risk of incident Alzheimer disease. Arch Neurol 2003;60(7):940–946

127. van Marum RJ. Current and future therapy in Alzheimer's disease. Fundam Clin Pharmacol 2008; 22(3):265–274

128. Kyle DJ, Schaefer E, Patton G, Beiser A. Low serum docosahexaenoic acid is a significant risk factor for Alzheimer's dementia. Lipids 1999;34(Suppl):S245

129. Conquer JA, Tierney MC, Zecevic J, Bettger WJ, Fisher RH. Fatty acid analysis of blood plasma of patients with Alzheimer's disease, other types of dementia, and cognitive impairment. Lipids 2000;35(12):1305–1312

130. Tully AM, Roche HM, Doyle R, et al. Low serum cholesteryl ester-docosahexaenoic acid levels in Alzheimer's disease: a case-control study. Br J Nutr 2003;89(4):483–489

131. Schaefer EJ, Bongard V, Beiser AS, et al. Plasma phosphatidylcholine docosahexaenoic acid content and risk of dementia and Alzheimer disease: the Framingham Heart Study. Arch Neurol 2006;63(11):1545–1550

132. Burr ML, Fehily AM, Gilbert JF, et al. Effects of changes in fat, fish, and fibre intakes on death and myocardial reinfarction: diet and reinfarction trial (DART). Lancet 1989;2(8666):757–761

133. de Lorgeril M, Salen P, Martin JL, Monjaud I, Delaye J, Mamelle N. Mediterranean diet, traditional risk factors, and the rate of cardiovascular complications after myocardial infarction: final report of the Lyon Diet Heart Study. Circulation 1999;99(6):779–785

134. Tuttle KR, Shuler LA, Packard DP, et al. Comparison of low-fat versus Mediterranean-style dietary intervention after first myocardial infarction (from The Heart Institute of Spokane Diet Intervention and Evaluation Trial). Am J Cardiol 2008;101(11):1523–1530

135. Dietary supplementation with n-3 polyunsaturated fatty acids and vitamin E after myocardial infarction: results of the GISSI-Prevenzione trial. Gruppo Italiano per lo Studio della Sopravvivenza nell'Infarto miocardico. Lancet 1999;354(9177):447–455

136. Marchioli R, Barzi F, Bomba E, et al; GISSI-Prevenzione Investigators. Early protection against sudden death by n-3 polyunsaturated fatty acids after myocardial infarction: time-course analysis of the results of the Gruppo Italiano per lo Studio della Sopravvivenza nell'Infarto Miocardico (GISSI)-Prevenzione. Circulation 2002;105(16):1897–1903

137. Singh RB, Niaz MA, Sharma JP, Kumar R, Rastogi V, Moshiri M. Randomized, double-blind, placebo-controlled trial of fish oil and mustard oil in patients with suspected acute myocardial infarction: the Indian experiment of infarct survival—4. Cardiovasc Drugs Ther 1997;11(3):485–491

138. Nilsen DW, Albrektsen G, Landmark K, Moen S, Aarsland T, Woie L. Effects of a high-dose concentrate of n-3 fatty acids or corn oil introduced early after an acute myocardial infarction on serum triacylglycerol and HDL cholesterol. Am J Clin Nutr 2001;74(1):50–56

139. Bucher HC, Hengstler P, Schindler C, Meier G. N-3 polyunsaturated fatty acids in coronary heart disease: a meta-analysis of randomized controlled trials. Am J Med 2002;112(4):298–304

140. Sacks FM, Stone PH, Gibson CM, Silverman DI, Rosner B, Pasternak RC; HARP Research Group. Controlled trial of fish oil for regression of human coronary atherosclerosis. J Am Coll Cardiol 1995;25(7):1492–1498

141. von Schacky C, Angerer P, Kothny W, Theisen K, Mudra H. The effect of dietary omega-3 fatty acids on coronary atherosclerosis. A randomized, double-blind, placebo-controlled trial. Ann Intern Med 1999;130(7):554–562

142. Balk E, Chung M, Lichtenstein A, et al. Effects of omega-3 fatty acids on cardiovascular risk factors and intermediate markers of cardiovascular disease. Evid Rep Technol Assess (Summ) 2004; (93):1–6

143. Lichtenstein AH, Appel LJ, Brands M, et al; American Heart Association Nutrition Committee. Diet and lifestyle recommendations revision 2006: a scientific statement from the American Heart Association Nutrition Committee. Circulation 2006;114(1):82–96

144. Montori VM, Farmer A, Wollan PC, Dinneen SF. Fish oil supplementation in type 2 diabetes: a quantitative systematic review. Diabetes Care 2000;23(9):1407–1415

145. Glauber H, Wallace P, Griver K, Brechtel G. Adverse metabolic effect of omega-3 fatty acids in non-insulin-dependent diabetes mellitus. Ann Intern Med 1988;108(5):663–668

146. Friday KE, Childs MT, Tsunehara CH, Fujimoto WY, Bierman EL, Ensinck JW. Elevated plasma glucose and lowered triglyceride levels from omega-3 fatty acid supplementation in type I.I. diabetes. Diabetes Care 1989;12(4):276–281

147. MacLean CH, Mojica WA, Morton SC, et al. Effects of omega-3 fatty acids on lipids and glycemic control in type II diabetes and the metabolic syndrome and on inflammatory bowel disease, rheumatoid arthritis, renal disease, systemic lupus erythematosus, and

osteoporosis. Evid Rep Technol Assess (Summ) 2004; (89):1–4

148. Hartweg J, Farmer AJ, Perera R, Holman RR, Neil HA. Meta-analysis of the effects of n-3 polyunsaturated fatty acids on lipoproteins and other emerging lipid cardiovascular risk markers in patients with type 2 diabetes. Diabetologia 2007;50(8):1593–1602

149. Farmer A, Montori V, Dinneen S, Clar C. Fish oil in people with type 2 diabetes mellitus. Cochrane Database Syst Rev 2001;(3):CD003205

150. Hu FB, Cho E, Rexrode KM, Albert CM, Manson JE. Fish and long-chain omega-3 fatty acid intake and risk of coronary heart disease and total mortality in diabetic women. Circulation 2003;107(14):1852–1857

151. Nettleton JA, Katz R. n-3 long-chain polyunsaturated fatty acids in type 2 diabetes: a review. J Am Diet Assoc 2005;105(3):428–440

152. Friedberg CE, Janssen MJ, Heine RJ, Grobbee DE. Fish oil and glycemic control in diabetes. A meta-analysis. Diabetes Care 1998;21(4):494–500

153. Franz MJ, Bantle JP, Beebe CA, et al; American Diabetes Association. Evidence-based nutrition principles and recommendations for the treatment and prevention of diabetes and related complications. Diabetes Care 2003;26(Suppl 1):S51–S61

154. Fortin PR, Lew RA, Liang MH, et al. Validation of a meta-analysis: the effects of fish oil in rheumatoid arthritis. J Clin Epidemiol 1995;48(11):1379–1390

155. Goldberg RJ, Katz J. A meta-analysis of the analgesic effects of omega-3 polyunsaturated fatty acid supplementation for inflammatory joint pain. Pain 2007;129(1–2):210–223

156. Lorenz R, Weber PC, Szimnau P, Heldwein W, Strasser T, Loeschke K. Supplementation with n-3 fatty acids from fish oil in chronic inflammatory bowel disease—a randomized, placebo-controlled, double-blind cross-over trial. J Intern Med Suppl 1989;731: 225–232

157. Lorenz-Meyer H, Bauer P, Nicolay C, et al; Study Group Members (German Crohn's Disease Study Group). Omega-3 fatty acids and low carbohydrate diet for maintenance of remission in Crohn's disease. A randomized controlled multicenter trial. Scand J Gastroenterol 1996;31(8):778–785

158. Belluzzi A, Brignola C, Campieri M, Pera A, Boschi S, Miglioli M. Effect of an enteric-coated fish-oil preparation on relapses in Crohn's disease. N Engl J Med 1996;334(24):1557–1560

159. Romano C, Cucchiara S, Barabino A, Annese V, Sferlazzas C. Usefulness of omega-3 fatty acid supplementation in addition to mesalazine in maintaining remission in pediatric Crohn's disease: a double-blind, randomized, placebo-controlled study. World J Gastroenterol 2005;11(45):7118–7121

160. Aslan A, Triadafilopoulos G. Fish oil fatty acid supplementation in active ulcerative colitis: a double-blind, placebo-controlled, crossover study. Am J Gastroenterol 1992;87(4):432–437

161. Hawthorne AB, Daneshmend TK, Hawkey CJ, et al. Treatment of ulcerative colitis with fish oil supplementation: a prospective 12 month randomised controlled trial. Gut 1992;33(7):922–928

162. Stenson WF, Cort D, Rodgers J, et al. Dietary supplementation with fish oil in ulcerative colitis. Ann Intern Med 1992;116(8):609–614

163. Loeschke K, Ueberschaer B, Pietsch A, et al. n-3 fatty acids only delay early relapse of ulcerative colitis in remission. Dig Dis Sci 1996;41(10):2087–2094

164. De Ley M, de Vos R, Hommes DW, Stokkers P. Fish oil for induction of remission in ulcerative colitis. Cochrane Database Syst Rev 2007; (4):CD005986

165. Hodge L, Salome CM, Hughes JM, et al. Effect of dietary intake of omega-3 and omega-6 fatty acids on severity of asthma in children. Eur Respir J 1998; 11(2):361–365

166. Okamoto M, Mitsunobu F, Ashida K, et al. Effects of dietary supplementation with n-3 fatty acids compared with n-6 fatty acids on bronchial asthma. Intern Med 2000;39(2):107–111

167. Wong KW. Clinical efficacy of n-3 fatty acid supplementation in patients with asthma. J Am Diet Assoc 2005;105(1):98–105

168. Schachter HM, Reisman J, Tran K, et al. Health effects of omega-3 fatty acids on asthma. Evid Rep Technol Assess (Summ) 2004; (91):1–7

169. Woods RK, Thien FC, Abramson MJ. Dietary marine fatty acids (fish oil) for asthma in adults and children. Cochrane Database Syst Rev 2002;(3):CD001283

170. Reisman J, Schachter HM, Dales RE, et al. Treating asthma with omega-3 fatty acids: where is the evidence? A systematic review. BMC Complement Altern Med 2006;6:26

171. Donadio JV, Grande JP. IgA nephropathy. N Engl J Med 2002;347(10):738–748

172. Donadio JV Jr, Bergstralh EJ, Offord KP, Spencer DC, Holley KE; Mayo Nephrology Collaborative Group. A controlled trial of fish oil in IgA nephropathy. N Engl J Med 1994;331(18):1194–1199

173. Donadio JV Jr, Grande JP, Bergstralh EJ, Dart RA, Larson TS, Spencer DC; Mayo Nephrology Collaborative Group. The long-term outcome of patients with IgA nephropathy treated with fish oil in a controlled trial. J Am Soc Nephrol 1999;10(8):1772–1777

174. Donadio JV Jr, Larson TS, Bergstralh EJ, Grande JP. A randomized trial of high-dose compared with low-dose omega-3 fatty acids in severe IgA nephropathy. J Am Soc Nephrol 2001;12(4):791–799

175. Alexopoulos E, Stangou M, Pantzaki A, Kirmizis D, Memmos D. Treatment of severe IgA nephropathy with omega-3 fatty acids: the effect of a "very low dose" regimen. Ren Fail 2004;26(4):453–459

176. Bennett WM, Walker RG, Kincaid-Smith P. Treatment of IgA nephropathy with eicosapentanoic acid (EPA): a two-year prospective trial. Clin Nephrol 1989; 31(3):128–131

177. Cheng IK, Chan PC, Chan MK. The effect of fish-oil dietary supplement on the progression of mesangial IgA glomerulonephritis. Nephrol Dial Transplant 1990;5(4):241–246

178. Pettersson EE, Rekola S, Berglund L, et al. Treatment of IgA nephropathy with omega-3-polyunsaturated fatty acids: a prospective, double-blind, randomized study. Clin Nephrol 1994;41(4):183–190

179. Hogg RJ, Lee J, Nardelli N, et al; Southwest Pediatric Nephrology Study Group. Clinical trial to evaluate omega-3 fatty acids and alternate day prednisone in patients with IgA nephropathy: report from the Southwest Pediatric Nephrology Study Group. Clin J Am Soc Nephrol 2006;1(3):467–474

180. Branten AJ, Klasen IS, Wetzels JF. Short-term effects of fish oil treatment on urinary excretion of high- and low-molecular weight proteins in patients with IgA nephropathy. Clin Nephrol 2002;58(4):267–274

181. Dillon JJ. Fish oil therapy for IgA nephropathy: efficacy and interstudy variability. J Am Soc Nephrol 1997;8(11):1739–1744

182. Strippoli GF, Manno C, Schena FP. An "evidence-based" survey of therapeutic options for IgA nephropathy: assessment and criticism. Am J Kidney Dis 2003;41(6):1129–1139

183. Hibbeln JR.. Fish consumption and major depression. Lancet 1998;351(9110):1213

184. Noaghiul S, Hibbeln JR. Cross-national comparisons of seafood consumption and rates of bipolar disorders. Am J Psychiatry 2003;160(12):2222–2227

185. Maes M, Christophe A, Delanghe J, Altamura C, Neels H, Meltzer HY. Lowered omega3 polyunsaturated fatty acids in serum phospholipids and cholesteryl esters of depressed patients. Psychiatry Res 1999; 85(3):275–291

186. Peet M, Murphy B, Shay J, Horrobin D. Depletion of omega-3 fatty acid levels in red blood cell membranes of depressive patients. Biol Psychiatry 1998;43(5):315–319

187. Tiemeier H, van Tuijl HR, Hofman A, Kiliaan AJ, Breteler MM. Plasma fatty acid composition and depression are associated in the elderly: the Rotterdam Study. Am J Clin Nutr 2003;78(1):40–46

188. Mamalakis G, Tornaritis M, Kafatos A. Depression and adipose essential polyunsaturated fatty acids. Prostaglandins Leukot Essent Fatty Acids 2002; 67(5):311–318

189. Locke CA, Stoll AL. Omega-3 fatty acids in major depression. World Rev Nutr Diet 2001;89:173–185

190. Silvers KM, Woolley CC, Hamilton FC, Watts PM, Watson RA. Randomised double-blind placebo-controlled trial of fish oil in the treatment of depression. Prostaglandins Leukot Essent Fatty Acids 2005; 72(3):211–218

191. Grenyer BF, Crowe T, Meyer B, et al. Fish oil supplementation in the treatment of major depression: a randomised double-blind placebo-controlled trial. Prog Neuropsychopharmacol Biol Psychiatry 2007; 31(7):1393–1396

192. Rogers PJ, Appleton KM, Kessler D, et al. No effect of n-3 long-chain polyunsaturated fatty acid (EPA and DHA) supplementation on depressed mood and cognitive function: a randomised controlled trial. Br J Nutr 2008;99(2):421–431

193. Marangell LB, Martinez JM, Zboyan HA, Kertz B, Kim HF, Puryear LJ. A double-blind, placebo-controlled study of the omega-3 fatty acid docosahexaenoic acid in the treatment of major depression. Am J Psychiatry 2003;160(5):996–998

194. Su KP, Huang SY, Chiu CC, Shen WW. Omega-3 fatty acids in major depressive disorder. A preliminary double-blind, placebo-controlled trial. Eur Neuropsychopharmacol 2003;13(4):267–271

195. Zanarini MC, Frankenburg FR. omega-3 Fatty acid treatment of women with borderline personality disorder: a double-blind, placebo-controlled pilot study. Am J Psychiatry 2003;160(1):167–169

196. Nemets H, Nemets B, Apter A, Bracha Z, Belmaker RH. Omega-3 treatment of childhood depression: a controlled, double-blind pilot study. Am J Psychiatry 2006;163(6):1098–1100

197. Stoll AL, Severus WE, Freeman MP, et al. Omega 3 fatty acids in bipolar disorder: a preliminary double-blind, placebo-controlled trial. Arch Gen Psychiatry 1999;56(5):407–412

198. Keck PE Jr, Mintz J, McElroy SL, et al. Double-blind, randomized, placebo-controlled trials of ethyl-eicosapentanoate in the treatment of bipolar depression and rapid cycling bipolar disorder. Biol Psychiatry 2006;60(9):1020–1022

199. Osher Y, Bersudsky Y, Belmaker RH. Omega-3 eicosapentaenoic acid in bipolar depression: report of a small open-label study. J Clin Psychiatry 2005; 66(6):726–729

200. Frangou S, Lewis M, McCrone P. Efficacy of ethyl-eicosapentaenoic acid in bipolar depression: randomised double-blind placebo-controlled study. Br J Psychiatry 2006;188:46–50

201. Lin PY, Su KP. A meta-analytic review of double-blind, placebo-controlled trials of antidepressant efficacy of omega-3 fatty acids. J Clin Psychiatry 2007;68(7):1056–1061

202. Freeman MP, Hibbeln JR, Wisner KL, et al. Omega-3 fatty acids: evidence basis for treatment and future research in psychiatry. J Clin Psychiatry 2006; 67(12):1954–1967

203. Appleton KM, Hayward RC, Gunnell D, et al. Effects of n-3 long-chain polyunsaturated fatty acids on depressed mood: systematic review of published trials. Am J Clin Nutr 2006;84(6):1308–1316

204. Assies J, Lieverse R, Vreken P, Wanders RJ, Dingemans PM, Linszen DH. Significantly reduced docosahexaenoic and docosapentaenoic acid concentrations in erythrocyte membranes from schizophrenic patients compared with a carefully matched control group. Biol Psychiatry 2001;49(6):510–522

205. Kemperman RF, Veurink M, van der Wal T, et al. Low essential fatty acid and B-vitamin status in a subgroup of patients with schizophrenia and its response to dietary supplementation. Prostaglandins Leukot Essent Fatty Acids 2006;74(2):75–85

206. Horrobin DF, Manku MS, Hillman H, Iain A, Glen M. Fatty acid levels in the brains of schizophrenics and normal controls. Biol Psychiatry 1991;30(8):795–805

207. Laugharne JD, Mellor JE, Peet M. Fatty acids and schizophrenia. Lipids 1996;31(Suppl):S163–S165

208. Peet M, Brind J, Ramchand CN, Shah S, Vankar GK. Two double-blind placebo-controlled pilot studies of eicosapentaenoic acid in the treatment of schizophrenia. Schizophr Res 2001;49(3):243–251

209. Emsley R, Myburgh C, Oosthuizen P, van Rensburg SJ. Randomized, placebo-controlled study of ethyl-eicosapentaenoic acid as supplemental treatment in schizophrenia. Am J Psychiatry 2002;159(9):1596–1598

210. Emsley R, Niehaus DJ, Koen L, et al. The effects of eicosapentaenoic acid in tardive dyskinesia: a randomized, placebo-controlled trial. Schizophr Res 2006;84(1):112–120

211. Fenton WS, Dickerson F, Boronow J, Hibbeln JR, Knable M. A placebo-controlled trial of omega-3 fatty acid (ethyl eicosapentaenoic acid) supplementation for residual symptoms and cognitive impairment in schizophrenia. Am J Psychiatry 2001; 158(12):2071–2074

212. Peet M, Horrobin DF; E-E Multicentre Study Group. A dose-ranging exploratory study of the effects of ethyl-eicosapentaenoate in patients with persistent schizophrenic symptoms. J Psychiatr Res 2002; 36(1):7–18

213. Joy CB, Mumby-Croft R, Joy LA. Polyunsaturated fatty acid (fish or evening primrose oil) for schizophrenia. Cochrane Database Syst Rev 2003;(2):CD001257

214. Hooijmans CR, Kiliaan AJ. Fatty acids, lipid metabolism and Alzheimer pathology. Eur J Pharmacol 2008;585(1):176–196

215. Quinn JF, Raman R, Thomas RG, et al. Docosahexaenoic acid supplementation and cognitive decline in

Alzheimer disease: a randomized trial. JAMA 2010;304(17):1903–1911

216. US Department of Agriculture, Agricultural Research Service. USDA National Nutrient Database for Standard Reference, Release 21. 2008. Available at: http://www.nal.usda.gov/fnic/foodcomp/search/. Accessed May 8, 2012

217. Hendler SS, Rorvik DR, eds. PDR for Nutritional Supplements. Montvale, NJ: Medical Economics Company, Inc; 2001

218. US Food and Drug Administration, Center for Food Safety and Applied Nutrition. Agency Response Letter: GRAS Notice No. GRN 000080. 2001. Available at: http://www.fda.gov/ohrms/dockets/dockets/95s0316/95s-0316-rpt0354-061-Ref-F-FDA-Response-Ltr-g80-vol273.pdf. Accessed May 8, 2012

219. Zurier RB, Rossetti RG, Jacobson EW, et al. gamma-Linolenic acid treatment of rheumatoid arthritis. A randomized, placebo-controlled trial. Arthritis Rheum 1996;39(11):1808–1817

220. Vaddadi KS. The use of gamma-linolenic acid and linoleic acid to differentiate between temporal lobe epilepsy and schizophrenia. Prostaglandins Med 1981;6(4):375–379

221. Nordström DC, Honkanen VE, Nasu Y, Antila E, Friman C, Konttinen YT. Alpha-linolenic acid in the treatment of rheumatoid arthritis. A double-blind, placebo-controlled and randomized study: flaxseed vs. safflower seed. Rheumatol Int 1995;14(6):231–234

222. Alonso L, Marcos ML, Blanco JG, et al. Anaphylaxis caused by linseed (flaxseed) intake. J Allergy Clin Immunol 1996;98(2):469–470

223. Harbige LS. Fatty acids, the immune response, and autoimmunity: a question of n-6 essentiality and the balance between n-6 and n-3. Lipids 2003;38(4):323–341

224. Carlson SE, Cooke RJ, Werkman SH, Tolley EA. First year growth of preterm infants fed standard compared to marine oil n-3 supplemented formula. Lipids 1992;27(11):901–907

225. Environmental Protection Agency. Fish Consumption Advisories. Available at: http://www.epa.gov/waterscience/fish/. Accessed May 8, 2012

226. Omega-3 oil: fish or pills? Consum Rep 2003; 68(7):30–32

227. ConsumerLab. Product Review: Omega-3 Fatty Acids (EPA and DHA) from Fish, Algae, and Krill. 2010. Available at: http://www.consumerlab.com/results/omega3.asp. Accessed May 8, 2012

228. Melanson SF, Lewandrowski EL, Flood JG, Lewandrowski KB. Measurement of organochlorines in commercial over-the-counter fish oil preparations: implications for dietary and therapeutic recommendations for omega-3 fatty acids and a review of the literature. Arch Pathol Lab Med 2005;129(1):74–77

229. Hilbert G, Lillemark L, Balchen S, Højskov CS. Reduction of organochlorine contaminants from fish oil during refining. Chemosphere 1998;37(7):1241–1252

230. Bender NK, Kraynak MA, Chiquette E, Linn WD, Clark GM, Bussey HI. Effects of marine fish oils on the anticoagulation status of patients receiving chronic warfarin therapy. J Thromb Thrombolysis 1998;5(3):257–261

231. Buckley MS, Goff AD, Knapp WE. Fish oil interaction with warfarin. Ann Pharmacother 2004;38(1):50–52

232. Valk EE, Hornstra G. Relationship between vitamin E requirement and polyunsaturated fatty acid intake in man: a review. Int J Vitam Nutr Res 2000;70(2):31–42

233. Higdon JV, Liu J, Du SH, Morrow JD, Ames BN, Wander RC. Supplementation of postmenopausal women with fish oil rich in eicosapentaenoic acid and docosahexaenoic acid is not associated with greater in vivo lipid peroxidation compared with oils rich in oleate and linoleate as assessed by plasma malondialdehyde and F(2)-isoprostanes. Am J Clin Nutr 2000;72(3):714–722

234. Wander RC, Du SH, Ketchum SO, Rowe KE. alpha-Tocopherol influences in vivo indices of lipid peroxidation in postmenopausal women given fish oil. J Nutr 1996;126(3):643–652

235. Wander RC, Du SH. Oxidation of plasma proteins is not increased after supplementation with eicosapentaenoic and docosahexaenoic acids. Am J Clin Nutr 2000;72(3):731–737

236. European Commission Directorate General for Health and Consumer Protection. Eurodiet: Nutrition and Diet for Healthy Lifestyles in Europe. 2001. Available at: http://ec.europa.eu/health/archive/ph_determinants/life_style/nutrition/report01_en.pdf. Accessed May 8, 2012

237. Hamazaki T, Okuyama H. The Japan Society for Lipid Nutrition recommends to reduce the intake of linoleic acid. A review and critique of the scientific evidence. World Rev Nutr Diet 2003;92:109–132

21 Choline

Although choline is not by strict definition a vitamin, it is an essential nutrient. Despite the fact that humans can synthesize it in small amounts, choline must be consumed in the diet to maintain health.[1] The majority of the body's choline is found in specialized fat molecules known as *phospholipids*, the most common of which is called *phosphatidylcholine* or *lecithin*.[2]

Function

Choline and compounds derived from choline (i.e., metabolites) serve several vital biological functions.[2–4]

Structural Integrity of Cell Membranes

Choline is used in the synthesis of the phospholipids, phosphatidylcholine and sphingomyelin, which are structural components of all human cell membranes.

Cell Signaling

The choline-containing phospholipids, phosphatidylcholine and sphingomyelin, are precursors for the intracellular messenger molecules, diacylglycerol and ceramide. Two other choline metabolites, platelet-activating factor and sphingophosphorylcholine, are also known to be cell-signaling molecules.

Nerve Impulse Transmission

Choline is a precursor for acetylcholine, an important neurotransmitter involved in muscle control, memory, and many other functions.

Lipid Transport and Metabolism

Fat and cholesterol consumed in the diet are transported to the liver by lipoproteins called *chylomicrons*. In the liver, fat and cholesterol are packaged into lipoproteins called *very low-density lipoproteins* (VLDLs) for transport through the blood to tissues that require them. Phosphatidylcholine is a required component of VLDL particles. Without adequate phosphatidylcholine, fat and cholesterol accumulate in the liver (see the Deficiency section below).

Major Source of Methyl Groups

Choline may be oxidized in the body to form a metabolite called *betaine*. Betaine is a source of methyl (CH_3) groups required for methylation reactions. Methyl groups from betaine may be used to convert homocysteine to methionine. Elevated levels of homocysteine in the blood have been associated with increased risk of cardiovascular diseases.[5]

Deficiency

Symptoms

Men and women fed intravenously with solutions that contained adequate methionine and folate but lacked choline have developed a condition called *"fatty liver"* and signs of liver damage that resolved when choline was provided.[3] Choline is required to form the phosphatidylcholine portion of VLDL particles. VLDL particles transport fat from the liver to the tissues (see the Function section above). When the supply of choline is inadequate, VLDL particles cannot be synthesized and fat accumulates in the liver, ultimately resulting in liver damage. Because low-density lipoprotein (LDL) particles are formed from VLDL particles, choline-deficient individuals also have reduced blood levels of LDL cholesterol.[6] Healthy male volunteers with adequate folate and vitamin B_{12} nutrition developed elevated blood levels of a liver enzyme called *alanine aminotransferase* (ALT) when fed a choline-deficient diet. Elevated ALT activity is a sign of liver damage. More recently, a study in 57 adults who were fed choline-deficient diets under controlled conditions found that 77% of men, 80% of postmenopausal women, and 44% of premeno-

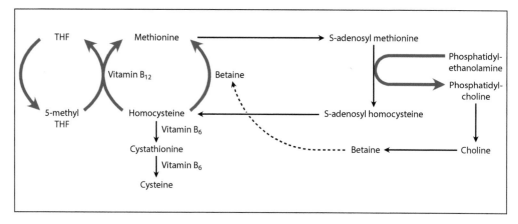

Fig. 21.1   Nutrient interactions: tetrahydrofolate (THF), vitamin B_{12}, methionine, and choline.

pausal women developed fatty liver, liver damage, and/or muscle damage.[7] These signs of organ dysfunction resolved when choline was replaced in the diet. Premenopausal women may be relatively resistant to choline deficiency, because estrogen induces endogenous synthesis of choline via the phosphatidylethanolamine N-methyltransferase (PEMT) enzyme.[8] Further, recent studies have identified a small number of very common genetic polymorphisms that predict the risk for developing symptoms of organ dysfunction when deprived of dietary choline.[9,10] In choline deficiency, liver damage appears to be the result of increased liver cell death, because cell-culture studies have shown liver cells initiate programmed cell death (apoptosis) when deprived of choline.[3] A recent study in 51 men and women reported that a choline-deficient diet induced DNA damage and apoptosis in peripheral lymphocytes.[11]

Nutrient Interactions

The human requirement for choline is affected by its relationships with other methyl-group donors, such as folate and S-adenosyl methionine (SAM) (**Fig. 21.1**). SAM is synthesized from the amino acid, methionine. Three molecules of SAM are required for the three methylations of phosphatidylethanolamine needed to synthesize phosphatidylcholine. Once SAM donates a methyl group it becomes S-adenosyl homocysteine, which is metabolized to homocysteine. Homocysteine can be converted to methionine in a reaction that requires 5-methyl tetrahydrofolate (THF) and a vitamin B_{12}-dependent enzyme. Alternately, betaine (a metabolite of choline) may be used as the methyl donor for the conversion of homocysteine to methionine.[2]

A study of 21 men and women fed diets with varied folate and choline content indicated that choline is used as a methyl-group donor when folate intake is low, and that the de novo synthesis of phosphatidylcholine is not sufficient to maintain adequate choline nutritional status when dietary folate and choline intakes are low.[12]

Adequate Intake

In 1998, the Food and Nutrition Board (FNB) of the Institute of Medicine established a dietary reference intake (DRI) for choline (**Table 21.1**).[4] The FNB felt the existing scientific evidence was insufficient to calculate a recommended dietary allowance (RDA) for choline, so they set an adequate intake (AI). The main criterion for establishing the AI for choline was the prevention of liver damage (see the Deficiency section above). Recent studies have found that polymorphisms in genes involved in choline[9] or folate[10] metabolism alter an individual's susceptibility to choline deficiency and thus may affect dietary requirements for choline.

Table 21.1 Adequate intake for choline[4]

Life Stage	Age	Males (mg/day)	Females (mg/day)
Infants	0–6 months	125	125
Infants	7–12 months	150	150
Children	1–3 years	200	200
Children	4–8 years	250	250
Children	9–13 years	375	375
Adolescents	14–18 years	550	400
Adults	19 years and older	550	425
Pregnancy	All ages	–	450
Breast-feeding	All ages	–	550

Disease Prevention

Cardiovascular Diseases

A large body of research indicates that even moderately elevated levels of homocysteine in the blood increase the risk of cardiovascular diseases.[5] When oxidized in the body to form betaine, choline provides a methyl group for the conversion of homocysteine to methionine by the enzyme, betaine-homocysteine methyltransferase (BHMT) (**Fig. 21.1**). Despite its relevance, the relationship of betaine and choline to homocysteine metabolism has been only lightly investigated in humans. Methodological problems make betaine and BHMT difficult to measure. One study found higher urinary excretion of betaine and its metabolites in patients with vascular disease and elevated homocysteine levels compared with control subjects, suggesting that elevated blood homocysteine levels were not related to reduced intake of choline or betaine or diminished activity of BHMT.[13] In preliminary studies, pharmacologic doses of betaine (1.7–6 g/day) were found to reduce blood levels of homocysteine in a small number of patients with vascular disease and elevated homocysteine levels. Additionally, a small study in 26 healthy men reported that choline supplementation decreased plasma homocysteine concentrations.[14] However, a prospective cohort study in 14 430 middle-aged men and women participating in the Atherosclerosis Risk in Communities study found that dietary choline, or dietary choline and dietary betaine together, was not associated with coronary heart disease.[15] Although further research is indicated, convincing evidence that increased dietary intake or blood levels of choline or betaine affect homocysteine levels and cardiovascular disease risk in humans is presently lacking.

Cancer

In rats, dietary choline deficiency is associated with an increased incidence of spontaneous liver cancer and increased sensitivity to carcinogenic chemicals. Several mechanisms have been proposed to explain the cancer-promoting effects of choline deficiency: (a) choline deficiency causes liver damage and regenerating liver cells are more sensitive to the effects of carcinogenic chemicals; (b) choline deficiency results in decreased methylation of DNA, resulting in abnormal DNA repair; (c) choline deficiency results in increased oxidative stress in the liver, increasing the likelihood of DNA damage; (d) choline deficiency may stimulate changes in the programmed cell death (apoptosis) of liver cells, contributing to the development of liver cancer; and (e) choline deficiency activates the potent cell-signaling molecule, protein kinase C, which creates a cascade of effects that is still being investigated.[2,3] The implications for the effect of choline deficiency on human susceptibility to cancer remain unclear.

Pregnancy Complications

Neural Tube Defects

It is known that folate is critical for normal embryonic development, and maternal supplementation with folic acid decreases the incidence of neural tube defects (NTDs).[16] NTDs result in either anencephaly or spina bifida, which are devastating and sometimes fatal birth defects. These defects occur between the 21st and 27th days after conception, a time when many women do not realize that they are pregnant.[17] While folate's protective effect against NTDs is well recognized, the effects of other methyl-group donors, including choline and betaine, are not known. A case–control study (424 NTD cases and 440 controls) found that women in the highest quartiles of choline and betaine intake, in combination, had a 72% lower risk of an NTD-affected pregnancy.[18] More recently, a case–control study (80 NTD-affected pregnancy and 409 controls) in US women found that the lowest levels of serum choline during mid-pregnancy were associated with a 2.4-fold higher risk of NTDs.[19] However, more research is needed to determine whether choline is involved in the etiology of NTDs.

Cognitive Function (Memory)

Increased dietary intake of choline very early in life can diminish the severity of memory deficits in aged rats. Choline supplementation of the mothers of unborn rats, as well as rat pups during the first month of life, leads to improved performance in spatial memory tests months after choline supplementation has been discontinued.[2] A recent review by McCann et al discusses the experimental evidence from rodent studies regarding the availability of choline during prenatal development and cognitive function in the offspring.[20] It is not clear whether findings in rodent studies are applicable to humans. More research is needed to determine the role of choline in the developing brain and whether choline intake is useful in the prevention of memory loss or dementia in humans.

Disease Treatment

Alzheimer Disease

Alzheimer disease has been associated with a deficit of the neurotransmitter, acetylcholine, in the brain.[21] One possible cause for the acetylcholine deficit is a decrease in the expression of an enzyme that converts choline into acetylcholine in the brain. Large doses of lecithin (phosphatidylcholine) have been used to treat patients with dementia associated with Alzheimer disease in the hope of raising the amount of acetylcholine available in the brain. However, a systematic review of the randomized trials did not find leci-

thin to be more beneficial than placebo in the treatment of patients with dementia or cognitive impairment.[22]

Sources

Biosynthesis

Humans can synthesize choline in small amounts by converting the phospholipid, phosphatidylethanolamine, to phosphatidylcholine. This is referred to as *de novo synthesis* of choline. Three methylation reactions are required, each using the compound SAM as a methyl-group donor. Because phosphatidylcholine can be synthesized and metabolized to provide choline, choline was not previously considered an essential nutrient.[3] However, more recent research indicates that humans cannot synthesize enough choline to meet their metabolic needs (see the Deficiency section above).

Food Sources

Very little information is available on the choline content of foods.[4] Most choline in foods is found in the form of phosphatidylcholine. Milk, eggs, liver, and peanuts are especially rich in choline. Phosphatidylcholine, also known as *lecithin*, contains approximately 13% choline by weight. Presently, national surveys do not provide any information on the dietary intake of choline, but it has been estimated that the average intake by adults is between 730 mg/day and 1040 mg/day.[2] Lecithins added during food processing may increase the daily consumption of choline by approximately 115 mg/day.[4] Strict vegetarians who consume no milk or eggs may be at risk of inadequate choline intake. The total choline contents of some choline-rich foods are listed in milligrams in **Table 21.2**.[23]

Supplements

Choline salts, such as choline chloride and choline bitartrate, are available as supplements. Phosphatidylcholine supplements also provide choline; however, they are only 13% choline by weight. Therefore, a supplement providing 4230 mg (4.23 g) of phosphatidylcholine would provide 550 mg of choline. Although the chemical term "*lecithin*" is synonymous with phosphatidylcholine, commercial lecithin preparations may contain anywhere from 20% to 90% phosphatidylcholine. Thus, lecithin supplements may contain even less than 13% choline.[24]

Safety

Toxicity

High doses (10–16 g/day) of choline have been associated with a fishy body odor, vomiting, salivation, and increased sweating. The fishy body odor results from excessive production and excretion of trimethylamine, a metabolite of choline. Taking large doses of choline in the form of phosphatidylcholine (lecithin) does not generally result in fishy body odor, because its metabolism results in little trimethylamine. A dose of 7.5 g of choline per day was found to have a slight blood-pressure-lowering (hypotensive) effect, which could result in dizziness or fainting. Choline magnesium trisalicylate at doses of 3 g/day has resulted in impaired liver function, generalized itching, and ringing of the ears (tinnitus). However, it is likely that these effects were a result of the salicylate, rather than the choline in the preparation.[4]

In 1998, the FNB established the tolerable upper intake level (UL) for choline at 3.5 g/day for adults (**Table 21.3**). This recommendation was based primarily on preventing hypotension (low blood pressure) and secondarily on preventing the fishy body odor due to increased excretion of trimethylamine. The UL was established for generally healthy people, and the FNB noted that individuals with liver or kidney disease, Parkinson disease, depression, or a genetic disorder known as *trimethylaminuria* might be at increased risk of adverse effects when consuming choline at levels near the UL.[4]

Drug Interactions

Methotrexate, a medication used in the treatment of cancer, psoriasis, and rheumatoid arthritis, inhibits the enzyme dihydrofolate reductase and therefore limits the availability of methyl groups donated from folate derivatives. Rats given methotrexate have shown evidence of diminished nutritional status of choline, including fatty liver, which can be reversed by choline supplementation.[2] Thus, individuals taking methotrexate may have an increased choline requirement.

Table 21.2 Choline content of selected foods[23]

Food	Serving	Total Choline (mg)
Beef liver, pan fried	3 oz[a]	355
Wheat germ, toasted	1 cup	172
Egg	1 large	126
Atlantic cod, cooked	3 oz	71
Beef, trim cut, cooked	3 oz	67
Brussel sprouts, cooked	1 cup	63
Broccoli, cooked	1 cup, chopped	62
Shrimp, canned	3 oz	60
Salmon	3 oz	56
Milk, skim	8 fl oz	38
Peanut butter, smooth	2 tbs	20
Milk chocolate	1.5-oz bar	20

[a] A 3-oz serving of meat or fish is about the size of a deck of cards.

Table 21.3 Tolerable upper intake level (UL) for choline[4]

Life Stage	Age	UL (g/d)
Infants	0–12 months	Not possible to establish[a]
Children	1–8 years	1.0
Children	9–13 years	2.0
Adolescents	14–18 years	3.0
Adults	≥19 years	3.5

[a] Source of intake should be food and formula only.

Summary

- Humans can synthesize choline endogenously but not in sufficient amounts; therefore, choline is considered an essential nutrient.
- Choline contributes to the structural integrity of cell membranes, modulates cell signaling, nerve impulse transmission, and lipid transport and metabolism, and is the precursor for the methyl group donor, betaine.
- Choline deficiency leads to fat accumulation in the liver and to liver damage.
- Choline is needed by the developing brain, but more research is needed to determine whether sufficient intake of choline during pregnancy is helpful in the prevention of neural tube defects or memory loss in humans.

References

1. Blusztajn JK. Choline, a vital amine. Science 1998; 281(5378):794–795
2. Zeisel SH. Choline and phosphatidylcholine. In: Shils M, Olson JA, Shike M, Ross AC, eds. Modern Nutrition in Health and Disease, 9th ed. Baltimore, MD: Williams & Wilkins; 1999:513–523
3. Zeisel SH. Choline: an essential nutrient for humans. Nutrition 2000;16(7–8):669–671
4. Food and Nutrition Board, Institute of Medicine. Choline. In: Dietary Reference Intakes for Thiamin, Riboflavin, Niacin, Vitamin B$_6$, Vitamin B$_{12}$, Pantothenic Acid, Biotin, and Choline. Washington, DC: National Academy Press; 1998:390–422
5. Gerhard GT, Duell PB. Homocysteine and atherosclerosis. Curr Opin Lipidol 1999;10(5):417–428
6. Zeisel SH, Blusztajn JK. Choline and human nutrition. Annu Rev Nutr 1994;14:269–296
7. Fischer LM, daCosta KA, Kwock L, et al. Sex and menopausal status influence human dietary requirements for the nutrient choline. Am J Clin Nutr 2007; 85(5): 1275–1285
8. Resseguie M, Song J, Niculescu MD, da Costa KA, Randall TA, Zeisel SH. Phosphatidylethanolamine N-methyltransferase (PEMT) gene expression is induced by estrogen in human and mouse primary hepatocytes. FASEB J 2007;21(10):2622–2632
9. da Costa KA, Kozyreva OG, Song J, Galanko JA, Fischer LM, Zeisel SH. Common genetic polymorphisms affect the human requirement for the nutrient choline. FASEB J 2006;20(9):1336–1344
10. Kohlmeier M, da Costa KA, Fischer LM, Zeisel SH. Genetic variation of folate-mediated one-carbon transfer pathway predicts susceptibility to choline deficiency in humans. Proc Natl Acad Sci U S A 2005; 102(44):16025–16030
11. da Costa KA, Niculescu MD, Craciunescu CN, Fischer LM, Zeisel SH. Choline deficiency increases lymphocyte apoptosis and DNA damage in humans. Am J Clin Nutr 2006;84(1):88–94
12. Jacob RA, Jenden DJ, Allman-Farinelli MA, Swendseid ME. Folate nutriture alters choline status of women and men fed low choline diets. J Nutr 1999; 129(3): 712–717
13. Lundberg P, Dudman NP, Kuchel PW, Wilcken DE. 1H NMR determination of urinary betaine in patients with premature vascular disease and mild homocysteinemia. Clin Chem 1995;41(2):275–283
14. Olthof MR, Brink EJ, Katan MB, Verhoef P. Choline supplemented as phosphatidylcholine decreases fasting and postmethionine-loading plasma homocysteine concentrations in healthy men. Am J Clin Nutr 2005;82(1):111–117
15. Bidulescu A, Chambless LE, Siega-Riz AM, Zeisel SH, Heiss G. Usual choline and betaine dietary intake and incident coronary heart disease: the Atherosclerosis Risk in Communities (ARIC) study. BMC Cardiovasc Disord 2007;7:20
16. Pitkin RM. Folate and neural tube defects. Am J Clin Nutr 2007;85(1):285S–288S
17. Eskes TK. Open or closed? A world of difference: a history of homocysteine research. Nutr Rev 1998; 56(8):236–244
18. Shaw GM, Carmichael SL, Yang W, Selvin S, Schaffer DM. Periconceptional dietary intake of choline and betaine and neural tube defects in offspring. Am J Epidemiol 2004;160(2):102–109
19. Shaw GM, Finnell RH, Blom HJ, et al. Choline and risk of neural tube defects in a folate-fortified population. Epidemiology 2009;20(5):714–719
20. McCann JC, Hudes M, Ames BN. An overview of evidence for a causal relationship between dietary availability of choline during development and cognitive function in offspring. Neurosci Biobehav Rev 2006; 30(5):696–712
21. Whitehouse PJ. The cholinergic deficit in Alzheimer's disease. J Clin Psychiatry 1998;59(Suppl 13):19–22
22. Higgins JP, Flicker L. Lecithin for dementia and cognitive impairment. Cochrane Database Syst Rev 2000; (2):CD001015
23. Zeisel SH, Mar MH, Howe JC, Holden JM. Concentrations of choline-containing compounds and betaine in common foods. J Nutr 2003;133(5):1302–1307
24. Hendler SS, Rorvik DR, eds. PDR for Nutritional Supplements. Montvale, NJ: Medical Economics Company, Inc; 2001

22 Coenzyme Q$_{10}$

Coenzyme Q$_{10}$ is a member of the ubiquinone family of compounds. All animals, including humans, can synthesize ubiquinones, hence coenzyme Q$_{10}$ cannot be considered a vitamin.[1] The name ubiquinone refers to the ubiquitous presence of these compounds in living organisms and their chemical structure, which contains a functional group known as a *benzoquinone*. Ubiquinones are fat-soluble molecules with anywhere from one to 12 isoprene (5-carbon) units. The ubiquinone found in humans, ubidecaquinone or coenzyme Q$_{10}$, has a "tail" of 10 isoprene units (a total of 50 carbon atoms) attached to its benzoquinone "head" (**Fig. 22.1**).[2]

Function

Coenzyme Q$_{10}$ is soluble in lipids (fats) and is found in virtually all cell membranes, as well as lipoprotein.[2] The ability of the benzoquinone head group of coenzyme Q$_{10}$ to accept and donate electrons is a critical feature in its biochemical functions. Coenzyme Q$_{10}$ can exist in three oxidation states (**Fig. 22.1**): (1) the fully reduced ubiquinol form (CoQ$_{10}$H$_2$), (2) the radical semiquinone intermediate (CoQ$_{10}$H·), and (3) the fully oxidized ubiquinone form (CoQ$_{10}$).

Mitochondrial ATP Synthesis

The conversion of energy from carbohydrates and fats to adenosine triphosphate (ATP), the form of energy used by cells, requires the presence of coenzyme Q$_{10}$ in the inner mitochondrial membrane. As part of the mitochondrial electron transport chain, coenzyme Q$_{10}$ accepts electrons from reducing equivalents generated during fatty acid and glucose metabolism and then transfers them to electron acceptors. At the same time, coenzyme Q$_{10}$ transfers protons outside the inner mitochondrial membrane, creating a proton gradient across that membrane. The energy released when the protons flow back into the mitochondrial interior is used to form ATP.[2]

Lysosomal Function

Lysosomes are organelles within cells that are specialized for the digestion of cellular debris. The digestive enzymes within lysosomes function optimally at an acidic pH, meaning they require a permanent supply of protons. The lysosomal membranes that separate those digestive enzymes from the rest of the cell contain relatively high concentrations of coenzyme Q$_{10}$. Research suggests that coenzyme Q$_{10}$ plays an important role in the transport of protons across lysosomal membranes to maintain the optimal pH.[2,3]

Antioxidant Functions

In its reduced form, CoQ$_{10}$H$_2$ is an effective fat-soluble antioxidant. The presence of a significant amount of CoQ$_{10}$H$_2$ in cell membranes, along with enzymes that are capable of reducing oxidized CoQ$_{10}$ back to CoQ$_{10}$H$_2$, supports the idea that CoQ$_{10}$H$_2$ is an important cellular antioxidant.[2] CoQ$_{10}$H$_2$ has been found to inhibit lipid peroxidation when cell membranes and low-density lipoproteins (LDL) are exposed to oxidizing conditions outside the body (ex vivo). When LDL is oxidized ex vivo, CoQ$_{10}$H$_2$ is the first antioxidant consumed. Moreover, the formation of oxidized lipids and the consumption of α-tocopherol (α-TOH, biologically the most active form of vitamin E) are suppressed while CoQ$_{10}$H$_2$ is present.[4] In isolated mitochondria, coenzyme Q$_{10}$ can protect membrane proteins and DNA from the oxidative damage that accompanies lipid peroxidation.[1] In addition to neutralizing free radicals directly, CoQ$_{10}$H$_2$ is capable of regenerating α-TOH from its one-electron oxidation product, α-tocopheroxyl radical (α-TO·).

Nutrient Interactions

Vitamin E

α-Tocopherol (vitamin E) and coenzyme Q$_{10}$ are the principal fat-soluble antioxidants in membranes and lipoproteins. When α-TOH neutraliz-

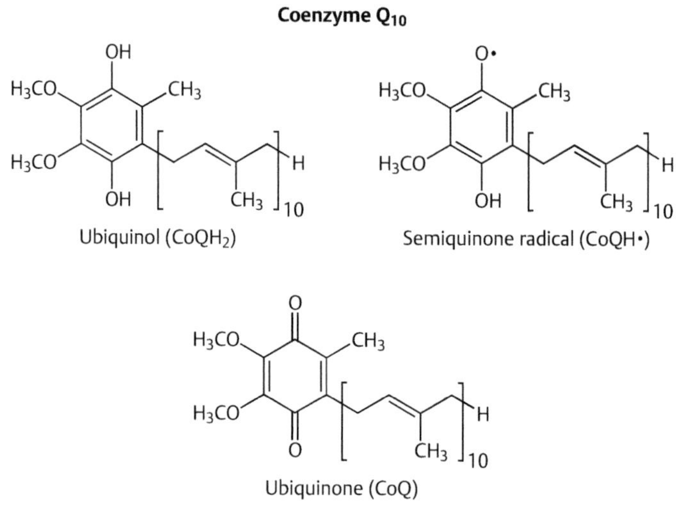

Coenzyme Q$_{10}$

Ubiquinol (CoQH$_2$)

Semiquinone radical (CoQH·)

Ubiquinone (CoQ)

Fig. 22.1 Chemical structure of coenzyme Q$_{10}$. Coenzyme Q$_{10}$ can exist in three oxidation states: the fully reduced ubiquinol form (CoQH$_2$), the radical semiquinone intermediate (CoQH·), and the fully oxidized ubiquinone form (CoQ).

es a free radical, such as a lipid peroxyl radical (LOO·), it becomes oxidized itself, forming α-TO·, which can promote the oxidation of lipoprotein lipids under certain conditions in the test tube. When the reduced form of coenzyme Q$_{10}$ (Co-Q$_{10}$H$_2$) reacts with α-TO·, α-TOH is regenerated and the semiquinone radical (CoQ$_{10}$H·) is formed. It is possible for CoQ$_{10}$H· to react with oxygen (O$_2$) to produce superoxide anion radical (O$_2$·⁻), which is a much less oxidizing radical than LOO·. However, CoQ$_{10}$H· can also reduce α-TO· back to α-TOH, resulting in the formation of fully oxidized coenzyme Q$_{10}$ (CoQ$_{10}$), which does not react with O$_2$ to form O$_2$·⁻ (**Fig. 22.2**).[4,5]

Deficiency

Symptoms of coenzyme Q$_{10}$ deficiency have not been reported in the general population, so it is generally assumed that normal biosynthesis and a varied diet provide sufficient coenzyme Q$_{10}$ for healthy individuals.[6] It has been estimated that dietary consumption contributes approximately 25% of plasma coenzyme Q$_{10}$, but there are currently no specific dietary intake recommendations for coenzyme Q$_{10}$ from the Institute of Medicine or other agencies.[7] The extent to which dietary consumption contributes to tissue coenzyme Q$_{10}$ levels is not clear.

Primary coenzyme Q$_{10}$ deficiency is a rare, autosomal recessive disorder caused by genetic defects in coenzyme Q$_{10}$ biosynthesis. The resultant low tissue levels of coenzyme Q$_{10}$ severely compromise neuronal and muscular function. Oral coenzyme Q$_{10}$ supplementation has been shown to improve neurological and muscular symptoms in some patients with primary coenzyme Q$_{10}$ deficiency.[8]

Coenzyme Q$_{10}$ levels have been found to decline gradually with age in several different tissues,[1,9] but it is unclear whether this age-associated decline constitutes a deficiency (see the Disease Prevention section below). Decreased plasma levels of coenzyme Q$_{10}$ have been observed in individuals with diabetes, cancer, and congestive heart failure (see the Disease Treatment section below). Lipid-lowering medications that inhibit the activity of 3-hydroxy-3-methyl-glutaryl-coenzyme A (HMG-CoA) reductase, a critical enzyme in both cholesterol and coenzyme Q$_{10}$ biosynthesis, decrease plasma coenzyme Q$_{10}$ levels (see the section on Drug Interactions below), although it remains unclear whether this has clinical or symptomatic implications.

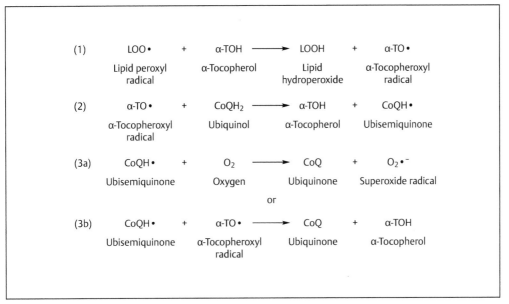

Fig. 22.2 Potential interactions between coenzyme Q_{10} and α-tocopherol. When α-tocopherol (α-TOH) neutralizes a free radical, such as a lipid hydroperoxyl radical (LOO·), it becomes oxidized itself, forming the α-tocopheroxyl radical (α-TO·), which can promote the oxidation of lipoproteins under certain conditions in the test tube (Reaction 1). When the reduced form of coenzyme Q_{10} ($CoQH_2$) reacts with α-TO·, α-TOH is regenerat- ed and the semiquinone radical (CoQH·) is formed (Reaction 2). It is possible for CoQH· to react with oxygen (O_2) to produce superoxide (O_2·⁻), which is a much less-oxidizing radical than LOO· (Reaction 3a). However, CoQH· can also reduce α-TO· back to α-TOH, resulting in the formation of fully oxidized coenzyme Q_{10} (CoQ), which does not react with O_2 to form O_2·⁻ (Reaction 3b).

Disease Prevention

Aging

According to the free radical and mitochondrial theories of aging, oxidative damage of cell structures by reactive oxygen species (ROS) plays an important role in the functional declines that accompany aging.[10] ROS are generated by mitochondria as a by-product of ATP production. If not neutralized by antioxidants, ROS may damage mitochondria over time, causing them to function less efficiently and to generate more damaging ROS in a self-perpetuating cycle. Coenzyme Q_{10} plays an important role in mitochondrial ATP synthesis and functions as an antioxidant in mitochondrial membranes. Moreover, tissue levels of coenzyme Q_{10} have been reported to decline with age.[9] One of the hallmarks of aging is a decline in energy metabolism in many tissues, especially liver, heart, and skeletal muscle. It has been proposed that age-associated declines in tissue coenzyme Q_{10} levels may play a role in this decline.[11] In recent studies, lifelong dietary supplementation with coenzyme Q_{10} increased tissue concentrations of coenzyme Q_{10} but did not increase the lifespans of rats or mice[12,13]; however, one study showed that coenzyme Q_{10} supplementation attenuates the age-related increase in DNA damage.[14] Presently, there is no scientific evidence that coenzyme Q_{10} supplementation prolongs life or prevents age-related functional decline in humans.

Cardiovascular Disease

Oxidative modification of LDL in arterial walls is thought to represent an early event leading to the development of atherosclerosis. Reduced coenzyme Q_{10} ($CoQ_{10}H_2$) inhibits the oxidation of LDL in the test tube (in vitro) and works together with α-TOH to inhibit LDL oxidation by reducing the α-TO· back to α-TOH. In the absence of a co-antioxidant, such as $CoQ_{10}H_2$ (or vitamin C), α-TOH can, under certain conditions, promote the oxidation of LDL in vitro.[4] Supplementation with coenzyme Q_{10} increases the concentration of Co-$Q_{10}H_2$ in human LDL.[15] Studies in apolipoprotein-E-deficient mice, an animal model of atherosclerosis, found that coenzyme Q_{10} supplementation with suprapharmacological amounts of coenzyme Q_{10} significantly inhibited the formation of atherosclerotic lesions.[16] Interestingly, co-supplementation of these mice with α-TOH and co-enzyme Q_{10} was more effective in inhibiting atherosclerosis than supplementation with either α-TOH or coenzyme Q_{10} alone.[17] Another important step in the development of atherosclerosis is the recruitment of immune cells known as *monocytes* into the blood vessel walls. This recruitment is dependent in part on monocyte expression of cell adhesion molecules (integrins). Giving supplements of 200 mg/day of coenzyme Q_{10} to 10 healthy men and women for 10 weeks resulted in significant decreases in monocyte expression of integrins, suggesting another potential mechanism for the inhibition of atherosclerosis by coenzyme Q_{10}.[18] Although coenzyme Q_{10} supplementation shows promise as an inhibitor of LDL oxidation and atherosclerosis, more research is needed to determine whether coenzyme Q_{10} supplementation can inhibit the development or progression of atherosclerosis in humans.

Disease Treatment

Mitochondrial Encephalomyopathies

Mitochondrial encephalomyopathies represent a diverse group of genetic disorders resulting from numerous inherited abnormalities in the function of the mitochondrial electron transport chain. Coenzyme Q_{10} supplementation has resulted in clinical and metabolic improvement in some patients with various types of mitochondrial encephalomyopathies.[19] Neuromuscular and widespread tissue coenzyme Q_{10} deficiencies have been found in a very small subpopulation of individuals with mitochondrial encephalomyopathies.[20,21] In those rare individuals with genetic defects in coenzyme Q_{10} biosynthesis, coenzyme Q_{10} supplementation has resulted in substantial improvement.[22,23] It is not clear whether coenzyme Q_{10} supplementation might have therapeutic benefit in patients with other mitochondrial disorders; a phase III clinical trial investigating that question is currently under way.[24]

Cardiovascular Diseases

Congestive Heart Failure

Impairment of the heart's ability to pump enough blood for all of the body's needs is known as *congestive heart failure*. In coronary artery disease, accumulation of atherosclerotic plaque in the coronary arteries may prevent parts of the heart muscle from getting adequate blood supply, ultimately resulting in cardiac damage and impaired pumping ability. Myocardial infarction (MI) may also damage the heart muscle, leading to heart failure. Because physical exercise increases the demand on the weakened heart, measures of exercise tolerance are frequently used to monitor the severity of heart failure. Echocardiography is also used to determine the left ventricular ejection fraction, an objective measure of the heart's pumping ability.[25] The finding that myocardial coenzyme Q_{10} levels were lower in patients with more severe versus milder heart failure led to several clinical trials of coenzyme Q_{10} supplementation in patients with heart failure.[26] Several small intervention trials that administered supplemental coenzyme Q_{10} (100–300 mg/day of coenzyme Q_{10} for 1–3 months) to patients with congestive heart failure, in conjunction with conventional medical therapy, have demonstrated improvements in some cardiac function measures.[27–29] However, other researchers have found that supplementing the diet with 100–200 mg/day of coenzyme Q_{10}, along with conventional medical therapy, did not significantly improve left ventricular ejection fraction or exercise performance in patients with heart failure.[30,31] A 2006 meta-analysis of 10 randomized controlled trials found that coenzyme Q_{10} supplementation (99–200 mg/day for 1–6 months) in patients with heart failure resulted in a significant, 3.7% improvement in left ventricular ejection fraction; the effect was stronger in patients not taking angiotensin-converting enzyme inhibitors.[32] A slight increase in cardiac output (0.28 L/min) was also found with coenzyme Q_{10} supplementation, but this analysis only included two trials (60 mg/day for 1 month or 200 mg/day for 3 months).[32] A recent study in 236 patients with heart failure found that lower plasma coenzyme Q_{10} levels were associated with a heightened risk of mortality;[33] however, a larger study of 1191 patients with heart failure found that plasma coenzyme Q_{10} level was a biomarker of advanced heart disease and not an independent predictor of clinical outcomes in patients with heart failure.[34] Although there is some evidence that coenzyme Q_{10} supplementation may be of benefit, large well-designed intervention trials are needed to determine whether coenzyme Q_{10} supplementation has value as an adjunct to conventional medical therapy in the treatment of congestive heart failure. One such large trial is presently being conducted.

Myocardial Infarction and Cardiac Surgery

The heart muscle may become oxygen deprived (ischemic) as the result of MI or during cardiac surgery. Increased generation of ROS when the heart muscle's oxygen supply is restored (reperfusion) is thought to be an important contributor to myocardial damage occurring during ischemia–reperfusion. Pretreatment of animals with coenzyme Q_{10} has been found to decrease myocardial damage due to ischemia–reperfusion.[35] Another potential source of ischemia–reperfusion injury is aortic clamping during some types of cardiac surgery, such as coronary artery bypass graft (CABG) surgery. Three out of four placebo-controlled trials found that coenzyme Q_{10} pretreatment (100–300 mg/day for 7–14 days prior to surgery) provided some benefit in short-term outcome measures after CABG surgery.[36,37] In the placebo-controlled trial that did not find preoperative coenzyme Q_{10} supplementation to be of benefit, patients were treated with 600 mg of coenzyme Q_{10} 12 hours prior to surgery,[38] suggesting that preoperative coenzyme Q_{10} treatment may need to commence at least 1 week prior to CABG surgery to realize any benefit. Although the results are promising, these trials have included relatively few people and have only examined outcomes shortly after CABG surgery.

Angina Pectoris

Myocardial ischemia may also lead to chest pain known as *angina pectoris*. People with angina pectoris often experience symptoms when the demand for oxygen exceeds the capacity of the coronary circulation to deliver it to the heart muscle, for example, during exercise. Five small placebo-controlled studies have examined the effects of oral coenzyme Q_{10} supplementation (60–600 mg/day) in addition to conventional medical therapy in patients with chronic stable angina.[28] In most of the studies, coenzyme Q_{10} supplementation improved exercise tolerance and reduced or delayed electrocardiographic changes associated with myocardial ischemia compared with placebo. However, only two of the studies found significant decreases in symptom frequency and nitroglycerin consumption with coenzyme Q_{10} supplementation. Presently, there is only limited evidence suggesting that coenzyme Q_{10} supplementation would be a useful adjunct to conventional angina therapy.

Hypertension

The results of several small, uncontrolled studies in humans suggest that coenzyme Q_{10} supplementation could be beneficial in the treatment of hypertension.[37] More recently, two short-term placebo-controlled trials found that coenzyme Q_{10} supplementation resulted in moderate decreases in blood pressure in hypertensive individuals. The addition of 120 mg/day of coenzyme Q_{10} to conventional medical therapy for 8 weeks in patients with hypertension and coronary artery disease decreased systolic blood pressure by an average of 12 mmHg and diastolic blood pressure by an average of 6 mmHg, in comparison to a placebo containing B-complex vitamins.[39] In patients with isolated systolic hypertension, supplementation with both coenzyme Q_{10} (120 mg/day) and vitamin E (300 IU/day) for 12 weeks resulted in an average decrease of 17 mmHg in systolic blood pressure compared with 300 IU/day of vitamin E alone.[40] A 2007 meta-analysis of 12 clinical trials, including 362 hypertensive patients, found that supplemental coenzyme Q_{10} reduces systolic blood pressure by 11–17 mmHg and diastolic blood pressure by 8–10 mmHg.[41] The four randomized controlled trials included in this meta-analysis used doses of 100–120 mg/day of coenzyme Q_{10}.

Vascular Endothelial Function (Blood Vessel Dilation)

Normal function of the inner lining of blood vessels, known as the *vascular endothelium*, plays an important role in preventing cardiovascular diseases.[42] Atherosclerosis is associated with impairment of vascular endothelial function, thereby compromising the ability of blood vessels to relax and permit normal blood flow. Endothelium-dependent blood vessel relaxation (vasodilation) is impaired in individuals with elevated serum cholesterol levels as well as in patients with coronary artery disease or diabetes. One placebo-controlled trial found that coenzyme Q$_{10}$ supplementation (200 mg/day) for 12 weeks improved endothelium-dependent vasodilation in patients with diabetes and abnormal serum lipid profiles, although it did not restore vasodilation to levels seen in individuals who did not have diabetes.[43] Another placebo-controlled study in 23 individuals with type 2 diabetes taking statins (HMG-CoA reductase inhibitors) found that 200 mg/day of coenzyme Q$_{10}$ for 12 weeks improved flow-mediated dilatation, but not nitrate-mediated dilatation, of the brachial artery.[44] However, a placebo-controlled trial in 80 individuals with type 2 diabetes found that this supplementation protocol did not improve endothelial function.[45]

In a study of 12 individuals with high serum cholesterol levels and endothelial dysfunction who were otherwise healthy, supplementation with 150 mg/day of coenzyme Q$_{10}$ did not affect endothelium-dependent vasodilation.[46] A prospective, randomized crossover study of 25 men with endothelial dysfunction found that coenzyme Q$_{10}$ supplementation (150 mg/day) significantly improved endothelial function, similar to that of a lipid-lowering medication.[47] Yet, it is important to mention that this study was not placebo-controlled and, importantly, the authors reported that the subjects' mean baseline for flow-mediated vasodilation was below zero. A randomized, double-blind, placebo-controlled trial in 22 patients with coronary artery disease found that 300 mg/day of coenzyme Q$_{10}$ for 1 month improved endothelium-dependent vasodilation.[48] Another randomized, double-blind, placebo-controlled trial in 56 patients with ischemic left ventricular systolic dysfunction reported that 300 mg/day of coenzyme Q$_{10}$ for 8 weeks significantly improved measures of endothelial dysfunction.[49] A 2011 meta-analysis examining the results of five randomized controlled trials, including 194 subjects, found that supplemental coenzyme Q$_{10}$ (150–300 mg/day for 4–12 weeks) resulted in a clinically significant, 1.7% increase in flow-dependent endothelial-mediated dilatation.[50] Large-scale studies are needed to further elucidate the therapeutic role of coenzyme Q$_{10}$ in endothelial dysfunction.

Diabetes Mellitus

Diabetes mellitus is a condition of increased oxidative stress and impaired energy metabolism. Plasma levels of reduced coenzyme Q$_{10}$ (CoQ$_{10}$H$_2$) have been found to be lower in patients with diabetes than in healthy controls, when normalized to plasma cholesterol levels.[51,52] However, supplementation with 100 mg/day of coenzyme Q$_{10}$ for 3 months neither improved glycemic (blood glucose) control nor decreased insulin requirements in patients with type 1 (insulin-dependent) diabetes compared with placebo.[53] Similarly, 200 mg/day of coenzyme Q$_{10}$ supplementation for 12 weeks or 6 months did not improve glycemic control or serum lipid profiles in individuals with type 2 (noninsulin-dependent) diabetes.[44,54] Because coenzyme Q$_{10}$ supplementation did not influence glycemic control in either study, the authors of both studies concluded that coenzyme Q$_{10}$ supplements could be used safely in patients with diabetes as adjunct therapy for cardiovascular diseases.

Maternally inherited diabetes mellitus and deafness is the result of a mutation in mitochondrial DNA, which is inherited exclusively from one's mother. Although mitochondrial diabetes accounts for less than 1% of all diabetes, there is some evidence that long-term supplementation with coenzyme Q$_{10}$ (150 mg/day) may improve insulin secretion and prevent progressive hearing loss in these patients.[55,56]

Neurodegenerative Diseases

Parkinson Disease

Parkinson disease is a degenerative neurological disorder characterized by tremors, muscular rigidity, and slow movements. It is estimated to affect approximately 1% of Americans over the age of 65 years. Although the causes of Parkinson disease are not all known, decreased activity of complex I of the mitochondrial electron transport chain and increased oxidative stress in a part of the brain called the *substantia nigra* are thought to play a role. Coenzyme Q$_{10}$ is the electron acceptor for complex I as well as an antioxidant, and decreased ratios of reduced to oxidized coenzyme Q$_{10}$ have been found in platelets of individuals with Parkinson disease.[57,58] One study also found higher concentrations of oxidized coenzyme Q$_{10}$ in the cerebrospinal fluid of patients with untreated Parkinson disease compared with healthy controls.[59] Additionally, a study of coenzyme Q_{10} levels in postmortem Parkinson disease patients found lower levels of total coenzyme Q_{10} in the cortex region of the brain compared with age-matched controls, but no differences were seen in other brain areas, including the striatum, substantia nigra, and cerebellum.[60] A 16-month randomized placebo-controlled trial evaluated the safety and efficacy of 300, 600, or 1200 mg/day of coenzyme Q_{10} in 80 people with early Parkinson disease.[61] Coenzyme Q_{10} supplementation was well tolerated at all doses and was associated with slower deterioration of function in patients with Parkinson disease compared with placebo. However, the difference was statistically significant only in the group taking 1200 mg/day. A smaller placebo-controlled trial showed that oral administration of 360 mg/day of coenzyme Q_{10} for 4 weeks moderately benefited patients with Parkinson disease.[62] More recently, a randomized, double-blind, placebo-controlled trial in 106 patients with midstage Parkinson disease reported that 300 mg/day of nanoparticular coenzyme Q_{10} for 3 months had no therapeutic benefit.[63] Another trial found that 2400 mg/day of coenzyme Q_{10} for 12 months was not effective in early Parkinson disease.[64] A phase III clinical trial of coenzyme Q_{10} (1200–2400 mg/day) and vitamin E (1200 IU/day) supplementation in patients with Parkinson disease was recently terminated because it was unlikely that such a treatment was effective in treating Parkinson disease.[65]

Huntington Disease

Huntington disease is an inherited neurodegenerative disorder characterized by selective degeneration of nerve cells known as *striatal spiny neurons*. Symptoms, such as movement disorders and impaired cognitive function, typically develop in the fourth decade of life and progressively deteriorate over time. Animal models indicate that impaired mitochondrial function and glutamate-mediated neurotoxicity may play roles in the pathology of Huntington disease. Coenzyme Q_{10} supplementation has been found to decrease brain lesion size in animal models of Huntington disease and to decrease brain lactate levels in patients with Huntington disease.[66,67] Feeding a combination of coenzyme Q_{10} (0.2% of diet) and remacemide (0.007% of diet) to transgenic mice

that express the Huntington disease protein (HD-N171-82Q mice) resulted in improved motor performance and/or survival.[68,69] Remacemide is an antagonist of the neuronal receptor that is activated by glutamate.

It was recently shown that the R6/2 mouse model of Huntington disease exhibits a progressive decline in behavioral and neurological symptoms similar to that of the human condition.[70] Thus, R6/2 mice may be an ideal model to investigate potential therapies for Huntington disease. Some, but not all, studies employing these mice have shown that dietary supplementation with coenzyme Q_{10} (0.2% of diet) improves motor performance and overall survival and helps prevent loss of body weight; coenzyme Q_{10} supplementation has also been associated with reductions in the various hallmarks of Huntington disease (i.e., brain atrophy, ventricular enlargement, and striatal neuronal atrophy).[68,71] Interestingly, co-administration of coenzyme Q_{10} with remacemide, the antibiotic minocycline, or creatine has been shown to result in even greater improvements in most measured parameters.[68,71,72]

To date, only one clinical trial has examined whether coenzyme Q_{10} might be efficacious in human patients with Huntington disease. A 30-month, randomized, placebo-controlled trial of coenzyme Q_{10} (600 mg/day), remacemide, or both in 347 patients with early Huntington disease found that neither coenzyme Q_{10} nor remacemide significantly altered the decline in total functional capacity, although coenzyme Q_{10} supplementation (with or without remacemide) resulted in a nonsignificant 13% decrease in the decline.[73] A recent 20-week pilot trial examined the safety and tolerability of increasing dosages of coenzyme Q_{10} (1200 mg/day, 2400 mg/day, and 3600 mg/day) in eight healthy subjects and in 20 patients with Huntington disease; 22 of the subjects completed the study.[74] All dosages were generally well tolerated, with gastrointestinal symptoms being the most frequently reported adverse effect. Blood levels of coenzyme Q_{10} at the end of the study were not higher than the levels resulting from the intermediate dose, suggesting that the 2400 mg/day dose effectively maximizes blood coenzyme Q_{10} levels and potentially avoids any side effects with higher dosages.[74] A phase III clinical trial administering 2400 mg/day of coenzyme Q_{10} or placebo for 5 years is currently recruiting participants with Huntington disease.[75] At present, there is insufficient evidence to recommend coenzyme Q$_{10}$ supplements to patients with Huntington disease.

Friedreich Ataxia

Friedreich ataxia (FRDA) is an inherited, autosomal recessive neurodegenerative disease caused by mutations in the gene that encodes frataxin, a protein of unknown function that is primarily located in the mitochondria. Decreased expression of frataxin is associated with accumulation of iron within the mitochondria, thereby resulting in increased oxidative stress; imbalances in iron-sulfur proteins, including mitochondrial aconitase; and reduced activities of the mitochondrial respiratory chain.[76] Clinically, FRDA is a progressive disease characterized by limb ataxia and abnormalities of the central nervous system that result from sensory nerve degeneration.[77,78] In addition, FRDA patients experience symptoms of hypertrophic cardiomyopathy and diabetes.[79] A pilot study administering coenzyme Q$_{10}$ (200 mg/day) and vitamin E (2100 IU/day) to 10 FDRA patients found that energy metabolism of cardiac and skeletal muscle was improved after only 3 months of therapy.[80] Follow-up assessments at 47 months indicated that cardiac and skeletal muscle improvements were maintained and that patients with FRDA showed significant increases in fractional shortening, a measure of cardiac function. Moreover, the therapy was effective at preventing the progressive decline of neurological function.[81] A recent study reported that deficiencies of both coenzyme Q$_{10}$ and vitamin E are quite common among FRDA patients and that co-supplementation with both compounds, at doses as low as 30 mg/day of coenzyme Q$_{10}$ and 4 IU/day of vitamin E, may improve disease symptoms.[82] Large-scale, randomized clinical trials are necessary to determine whether coenzyme Q$_{10}$, in conjunction with vitamin E, has therapeutic benefit in FRDA.

Cancer

Interest in coenzyme Q$_{10}$ as a potential therapeutic agent in cancer was stimulated by an observational study that found that individuals with lung, pancreas, and especially breast cancer were more likely to have low plasma coenzyme Q$_{10}$ levels than healthy controls.[83] Although a few case reports and an uncontrolled trial suggest that coenzyme Q$_{10}$ supplementation may be beneficial as an adjunct to conventional therapy for breast cancer,[84] the lack of controlled clinical trials makes it impossible to determine the effects, if any, of coenzyme Q$_{10}$ supplementation in patients with cancer.

Performance

Athletic Performance

Although coenzyme Q$_{10}$ supplementation has improved exercise tolerance in some individuals with mitochondrial encephalomyopathies (see the Deficiency section above),[19] there is little evidence that it improves athletic performance in healthy individuals. At least seven placebo-controlled trials have examined the effects of 100–150 mg/day of coenzyme Q$_{10}$ supplementation for 3–8 weeks on physical performance in trained and untrained men. Most found no significant differences between groups taking coenzyme Q$_{10}$ and groups taking placebos with respect to measures of aerobic exercise performance, such as maximal oxygen consumption and exercise time to exhaustion.[85–89] One study found the maximal cycling workload to be slightly (4%) increased after 8 weeks of coenzyme Q$_{10}$ supplementation compared with placebo, although measures of aerobic power were not increased.[90] Two studies actually found significantly greater improvement in measures of anaerobic[86] and aerobic[85] exercise performance after supplementation with a placebo compared with coenzyme Q$_{10}$. Studies on the effect of supplementation on physical performance in women are lacking, but there is little reason to suspect a sex difference in the response to coenzyme Q$_{10}$ supplementation.

Sources

Biosynthesis

Coenzyme Q$_{10}$ is synthesized in most human tissues. The biosynthesis of coenzyme Q$_{10}$ involves three major steps: (1) synthesis of the benzoquinone structure from either tyrosine or phenylalanine, two amino acids; (2) synthesis of the isoprene side chain from acetyl-coenzyme A (CoA) via the mevalonate pathway; and (3) the joining or condensation of these two structures. The enzyme HMG-CoA reductase plays a critical role in the regulation of coenzyme Q_{10} synthesis, as well as the regulation of cholesterol synthesis.[1,6]

The first step in benzoquinone biosynthesis (the conversion of tyrosine to 4-hydroxyphenyl-pyruvic acid) requires vitamin B_6 in the form of pyridoxal 5'-phosphate. Thus, adequate vitamin B_6 nutrition is essential for coenzyme Q_{10} biosynthesis. A pilot study in 29 patients and healthy volunteers found significant positive correlations between blood levels of coenzyme Q_{10} and measures of vitamin B_6 nutritional status.[91] However, further research is required to determine the clinical significance of this association.

Food Sources

Based on food frequency studies, the average dietary intake of coenzyme Q_{10} in Denmark was estimated to be 3–5 mg/day.[6,7] Most people probably have a dietary intake of less than 10 mg/day of coenzyme Q_{10}. Rich sources of dietary coenzyme Q_{10} include mainly meat, poultry, and fish. Other relatively rich sources include soybean and canola oils, and nuts. Fruits, vegetables, eggs, and dairy products are moderate sources of coenzyme Q_{10}. Approximately 14%–32% of coenzyme Q_{10} was lost during frying of vegetables and eggs, but the coenzyme Q_{10} content of these foods did not change when they were boiled. Some relatively rich dietary sources and their coenzyme Q_{10} content in milligrams are listed in Table 22.1.[92–94]

Supplements

Coenzyme Q_{10} is available without a prescription as a dietary supplement in the United States. Supplemental doses for adults range from 30–100 mg/day, which is considerably higher than normal dietary coenzyme Q_{10} intake. Therapeutic doses for adults generally range from 100–300 mg/day, although doses as high as 3000 mg/day have been used to treat early Parkinson disease under medical supervision.[95] Absorption of coenzyme Q_{10} decreases with increasing supplemental dose; total intestinal absorption is likely less than 10% in humans. Coenzyme Q_{10} is fat soluble and best absorbed with fat in a meal. Doses higher than 100 mg/day are generally divided into two or three doses throughout the day.[7,96]

Table 22.1 Coenzyme Q_{10} content of selected foods[92–94]

Food	Serving	Coenzyme Q_{10} (mg)
Beef, fried	3 oz[a]	2.6
Herring, marinated	3 oz	2.3
Chicken, fried	3 oz	1.4
Soybean oil	1 tbsp	1.3
Canola oil	1 tbsp	1.0
Rainbow trout, steamed	3 oz	0.9
Peanuts, roasted	1 oz	0.8
Sesame seeds, roasted	1 oz	0.7
Pistachio nuts, roasted	1 oz	0.6
Broccoli, boiled	½ cup, chopped	0.5
Cauliflower, boiled	½ cup, chopped	0.4
Orange	1 medium	0.3
Strawberries	½ cup	0.1
Egg, boiled	1 medium	0.1

[a] A 3-oz serving of meat or fish is about the size of a deck of cards.

Does Oral Coenzyme Q_{10} Supplementation Increase Tissue Levels?

Oral supplementation with coenzyme Q_{10} is known to increase blood and lipoprotein concentrations of coenzyme Q_{10} in humans.[2,12,15] However, it is not clear whether oral supplementation increases coenzyme Q_{10} concentrations in other tissues of individuals with normal endogenous coenzyme Q_{10} biosynthesis. Oral coenzyme Q_{10} supplementation of young healthy animals has not generally resulted in increased tissue concentrations, other than in the liver, spleen, and blood vessels.[97,98] Giving supplements of 120 mg/day for 3 weeks to healthy men did not increase skeletal muscle concentrations of coenzyme Q_{10}.[99] However, supplementation may increase coenzyme Q_{10} levels in tissues that are deficient. For example, oral supplementation of aged rats increased brain coenzyme Q_{10} concentrations,[100] and a study of 24 older adults given supplements of 300 mg/day of coenzyme Q_{10} or placebo for at least 7 days prior to cardiac surgery found that the coenzyme Q_{10} content of atrial tissue was significantly increased in those taking coenzyme Q_{10}, especially in those aged over 70 years.[36] Additionally, in a study of patients with left ventricular dysfunction, supplementation with 150 mg/day of coenzyme Q$_{10}$ for 4 weeks before cardiac surgery increased coenzyme Q$_{10}$ levels in the heart but not in skeletal muscle.[101] Clearly, this is an area of research that requires further investigation.

Safety

Toxicity

There have been no reports of significant adverse side effects of oral coenzyme Q$_{10}$ supplementation at doses as high as 1200 mg/day for up to 16 months[61] and 600 mg/day for up to 30 months.[73] In fact, 1200 mg/day has recently been proposed as the observed safe level (OSL) for coenzyme Q$_{10}$.[102] Some people have experienced gastrointestinal symptoms, such as nausea, diarrhea, appetite suppression, heartburn, and abdominal discomfort. These adverse effects may be minimized if daily doses higher than 100 mg are divided into two or three daily doses. Because controlled safety studies in pregnant and lactating women are not available, the use of coenzyme Q$_{10}$ supplements by pregnant or breast-feeding women should be avoided.[96,103]

Drug Interactions

Warfarin

Concomitant use of warfarin (Coumadin) and coenzyme Q$_{10}$ supplements has been reported to decrease the anticoagulant effect of warfarin in at least four cases.[104] An individual on warfarin should not begin taking coenzyme Q$_{10}$ supplements without consulting the health-care provider who is managing his or her anticoagulant therapy. If warfarin and coenzyme Q$_{10}$ are to be used concomitantly, blood tests to assess clotting time (prothrombin time international normalized ratio [INR]) should be monitored frequently, especially in the first 2 weeks.

HMG-CoA Reductase Inhibitors (Statins)

HMG-CoA reductase is an enzyme that plays a critical role in the regulation of cholesterol synthesis, as well as coenzyme Q$_{10}$ synthesis, although it is now recognized that there are additional rate-limiting steps in the biosynthesis of cholesterol and coenzyme Q$_{10}$. HMG-CoA reduc-

tase inhibitors, also known as *statins*, are widely used cholesterol-lowering medications that may also decrease the endogenous synthesis of coenzyme Q$_{10}$. Therapeutic use of statins, including simvastatin (Zocor), pravastatin (Pravachol), lovastatin (Mevacor, Altocor, Altoprev), rosuvastatin (Crestor), and atorvastatin (Lipitor), has been shown to decrease blood plasma or serum levels of coenzyme Q$_{10}$.[105–114] However, it has been suggested that blood coenzyme Q$_{10}$ concentrations should be reported only after normalizing to total lipid or cholesterol levels, because coenzyme Q$_{10}$ circulates with lipoproteins and levels of coenzyme Q$_{10}$ are highly dependent upon levels of circulating lipids.[115,116] Given the lipid-lowering effects of statins, it is therefore unclear whether these drugs actually decrease coenzyme Q$_{10}$ levels independent of a reduction in circulating lipids. Also, very few studies have examined coenzyme Q$_{10}$ content in target organs; thus, it is not clear whether statin therapy affects coenzyme Q$_{10}$ concentrations in the body's tissues.[111,113,117] At present, more research is needed to determine whether coenzyme Q$_{10}$ supplementation might be beneficial for those taking HMG-CoA reductase inhibitors.

Summary

- Coenzyme Q$_{10}$ is a fat-soluble compound primarily synthesized by the body and also consumed in the diet.
- Coenzyme Q$_{10}$ is required for mitochondrial ATP synthesis and functions as an antioxidant in cell membranes and lipoproteins.
- Endogenous synthesis and dietary intake appear to provide sufficient coenzyme Q$_{10}$ to prevent deficiency in healthy people, although tissue levels of coenzyme Q$_{10}$ decline with age.
- Oral supplementation of coenzyme Q$_{10}$ increases plasma, lipoprotein, and blood vessel levels, but it is unclear whether tissue coenzyme Q$_{10}$ levels are increased, especially in healthy individuals.
- Coenzyme Q$_{10}$ supplementation has resulted in clinical and metabolic improvement in some patients with hereditary mitochondrial disorders.
- Although coenzyme Q$_{10}$ supplementation may be a useful adjunct to conventional medical

therapy for congestive heart failure, additional research is needed.

- Roles for coenzyme Q_{10} supplementation in cardiovascular diseases, neurodegenerative diseases, cancer, and diabetes require further research.
- Coenzyme Q_{10} supplementation does not appear to improve athletic performance.
- Although coenzyme Q_{10} supplements are relatively safe, they may decrease the anticoagulant efficacy of warfarin.
- Although use of the cholesterol-lowering medications known as HMG-CoA reductase inhibitors (statins) decreases circulating levels of coenzyme Q_{10}, it is unclear whether coenzyme Q_{10} supplementation provides any health benefit to patients taking these drugs.

References

1. Ernster L, Dallner G. Biochemical, physiological and medical aspects of ubiquinone function. Biochim Biophys Acta 1995;1271(1):195–204
2. Crane FL. Biochemical functions of coenzyme Q10. J Am Coll Nutr 2001;20(6):591–598
3. Nohl H, Gille L. The role of coenzyme Q in lysosomes. In: Kagan VEQ, Quinn PJ, eds. Coenzyme Q: Molecular Mechanisms in Health and Disease. Boca Raton, FL: CRC Press; 2001:99–106
4. Thomas SR, Stocker R. Mechanisms of antioxidant action of ubiquinol-10 for low-density lipoprotein. In: Kagan VE, Quinn PJ, eds. Coenzyme Q: Molecular Mechanisms in Health and Disease. Boca Raton, FL: CRC Press; 2001:131–150
5. Kagan VE, Fabisak JP, Tyurina YY. Independent and concerted antioxidant functions of coenzyme Q. In: Kagan VE, Quinn PJ, eds. Coenzyme Q: Molecular Mechanisms in Health and Disease. Boca Raton, FL: CRC Press; 2001:119–130
6. Overvad K, Diamant B, Holm L, Holmer G, Mortensen SA, Stender S. Coenzyme Q10 in health and disease. Eur J Clin Nutr 1999;53(10):764–770
7. Weber C. Dietary intake and absorption of coenzyme Q. In: Kagan VE, Quinn PJ, eds. Coenzyme Q: Molecular Mechanisms in Health and Disease. Boca Raton, FL: CRC Press; 2001:209–215
8. Rustin P, Munnich A, Rötig A. Mitochondrial respiratory chain dysfunction caused by coenzyme Q deficiency. Methods Enzymol 2004;382:81–88
9. Kalén A, Appelkvist EL, Dallner G. Age-related changes in the lipid compositions of rat and human tissues. Lipids 1989;24(7):579–584
10. Beckman KB, Ames BN. Mitochondrial aging: open questions. Ann N Y Acad Sci 1998;854:118–127
11. Alho H, Lonnrot K. Coenzyme Q supplementation and longevity. In: Kagan VE, Quinn PJ, eds. Coenzyme Q: Molecular Mechanisms in Health and Disease. Boca Raton, FL: CRC Press; 2001:371–380
12. Singh RB, Niaz MA, Kumar A, Sindberg CD, Moesgaard S, Littarru GP. Effect on absorption and oxidative stress of different oral Coenzyme Q10 dosages and intake strategy in healthy men. Biofactors 2005;25(1–4):219–224
13. Sohal RS, Kamzalov S, Sumien N, et al. Effect of coenzyme Q10 intake on endogenous coenzyme Q content, mitochondrial electron transport chain, antioxidative defenses, and life span of mice. Free Radic Biol Med 2006;40(3):480–487
14. Quiles JL, Ochoa JJ, Battino M, et al. Life-long supplementation with a low dosage of coenzyme Q10 in the rat: effects on antioxidant status and DNA damage. Biofactors 2005;25(1–4):73–86
15. Mohr D, Bowry VW, Stocker R. Dietary supplementation with coenzyme Q10 results in increased levels of ubiquinol-10 within circulating lipoproteins and increased resistance of human low-density lipoprotein to the initiation of lipid peroxidation. Biochim Biophys Acta 1992;1126(3):247–254
16. Witting PK, Pettersson K, Letters J, Stocker R. Anti-atherogenic effect of coenzyme Q10 in apolipoprotein E gene knockout mice. Free Radic Biol Med 2000;29(3–4):295–305
17. Thomas SR, Leichtweis SB, Pettersson K, et al. Dietary cosupplementation with vitamin E and coenzyme Q(10) inhibits atherosclerosis in apolipoprotein E gene knockout mice. Arterioscler Thromb Vasc Biol 2001;21(4):585–593
18. Turunen M, Wehlin L, Sjöberg M, et al. beta2-Integrin and lipid modifications indicate a non-antioxidant mechanism for the anti-atherogenic effect of dietary coenzyme Q10. Biochem Biophys Res Commun 2002;296(2):255–260
19. Shoffner JM. Oxidative phosphorylation diseases. In: Scriver CR, Beaudet AL, Sly WS, Valle D, eds. The metabolic and molecular bases of inherited disease. 8th ed. New York: McGraw-Hill; 2001:2367–2392
20. Rötig A, Appelkvist EL, Geromel V, et al. Quinone-responsive multiple respiratory-chain dysfunction due to widespread coenzyme Q10 deficiency. Lancet 2000;356(9227):391–395
21. Boitier E, Degoul F, Desguerre I, et al. A case of mitochondrial encephalomyopathy associated with a muscle coenzyme Q10 deficiency. J Neurol Sci 1998;156(1):41–46
22. Munnich A, Rotig A, Cormier-Daire V, Rustin P. Clinical presentation of respiratory chain deficiency. In: Scriver CR, Beaudet AL, Sly WS, Valle D, eds. The metabolic and molecular bases of inherited disease. 8th ed. New York: McGraw-Hill; 2001:2261–2274
23. Horvath R, Gorman G, Chinnery PF. How can we treat mitochondrial encephalomyopathies? Approaches to therapy. Neurotherapeutics 2008;5(4):558–568
24. National Institutes of Health. Phase III Trial of Coenzyme Q10 in Mitochondrial Disease. ClinicalTrials. gov. Available at: http://www.clinicaltrials.gov/ct2/show/NCT00432744?term=coenzyme+Q10+AND+mitochondrial&rank=1. Accessed May 9, 2012
25. Trupp RJ, Abraham WT. Congestive heart failure. In: Rakel RE, Bope ET, eds. Conn's Current Therapy 2002. 54th ed. New York: WB Saunders Company; 2002:306–313
26. Folkers K, Vadhanavikit S, Mortensen SA. Biochemical rationale and myocardial tissue data on the effective therapy of cardiomyopathy with coenzyme Q10. Proc Natl Acad Sci U S A 1985;82(3):901–904
27. Belardinelli R, Muçaj A, Lacalaprice F, et al. Coenzyme Q10 and exercise training in chronic heart failure. Eur Heart J 2006;27(22):2675–2681
28. Tran MT, Mitchell TM, Kennedy DT, Giles JT. Role of coenzyme Q10 in chronic heart failure, angina, and

hypertension. Pharmacotherapy 2001;21(7):797–806

29. Belardinelli R, Muçaj A, Lacalaprice F, et al. Coenzyme Q10 improves contractility of dysfunctional myocardium in chronic heart failure. Biofactors 2005;25(1–4):137–145

30. Khatta M, Alexander BS, Krichten CM, et al. The effect of coenzyme Q10 in patients with congestive heart failure. Ann Intern Med 2000;132(8):636–640

31. Watson PS, Scalia GM, Galbraith A, Burstow DJ, Bett N, Aroney CN. Lack of effect of coenzyme Q on left ventricular function in patients with congestive heart failure. J Am Coll Cardiol 1999;33(6):1549–1552

32. Sander S, Coleman CI, Patel AA, Kluger J, White CM. The impact of coenzyme Q10 on systolic function in patients with chronic heart failure. J Card Fail 2006;12(6):464–472

33. Molyneux SL, Florkowski CM, George PM, et al. Coenzyme Q10: an independent predictor of mortality in chronic heart failure. J Am Coll Cardiol 2008;52(18):1435–1441

34. McMurray JJ, Dunselman P, Wedel H, et al; CORONA Study Group. Coenzyme Q10, rosuvastatin, and clinical outcomes in heart failure: a pre-specified substudy of CORONA (controlled rosuvastatin multinational study in heart failure). J Am Coll Cardiol 2010;56(15):1196–1204

35. Lönnrot K, Tolvanen JP, Pörsti I, Ahola T, Hervonen A, Alho H. Coenzyme Q10 supplementation and recovery from ischemia in senescent rat myocardium. Life Sci 1999;64(5):315–323

36. Rosenfeldt FL, Pepe S, Linnane A, et al. The effects of ageing on the response to cardiac surgery: protective strategies for the ageing myocardium. Biogerontology 2002;3(1–2):37–40

37. Langsjoen PH, Langsjoen AM. Overview of the use of CoQ10 in cardiovascular disease. Biofactors 1999;9(2–4):273–284

38. Taggart DP, Jenkins M, Hooper J, et al. Effects of short-term supplementation with coenzyme Q10 on myocardial protection during cardiac operations. Ann Thorac Surg 1996;61(3):829–833

39. Singh RB, Niaz MA, Rastogi SS, Shukla PK, Thakur AS. Effect of hydrosoluble coenzyme Q10 on blood pressures and insulin resistance in hypertensive patients with coronary artery disease. J Hum Hypertens 1999;13(3):203–208

40. Burke BE, Neuenschwander R, Olson RD. Randomized, double-blind, placebo-controlled trial of coenzyme Q10 in isolated systolic hypertension. South Med J 2001;94(11):1112–1117

41. Rosenfeldt FL, Haas SJ, Krum H, et al. Coenzyme Q10 in the treatment of hypertension: a meta-analysis of the clinical trials. J Hum Hypertens 2007;21(4):297–306

42. Ross R. Atherosclerosis—an inflammatory disease. N Engl J Med 1999;340(2):115–126

43. Watts GF, Playford DA, Croft KD, Ward NC, Mori TA, Burke V. Coenzyme Q(10) improves endothelial dysfunction of the brachial artery in Type II diabetes mellitus. Diabetologia 2002;45(3):420–426

44. Hamilton SJ, Chew GT, Watts GF. Coenzyme Q10 improves endothelial dysfunction in statin-treated type 2 diabetic patients. Diabetes Care 2009;32(5):810–812

45. Lim SC, Lekshminarayanan R, Goh SK, et al. The effect of coenzyme Q10 on microcirculatory endothelial function of subjects with type 2 diabetes mellitus. Atherosclerosis 2008;196(2):966–969

46. Raitakari OT, McCredie RJ, Witting P, et al. Coenzyme Q improves LDL resistance to ex vivo oxidation but does not enhance endothelial function in hypercholesterolemic young adults. Free Radic Biol Med 2000;28(7):1100–1105

47. Kuettner A, Pieper A, Koch J, Enzmann F, Schroeder S. Influence of coenzyme Q(10) and cerivastatin on the flow-mediated vasodilation of the brachial artery: results of the ENDOTACT study. Int J Cardiol 2005;98(3):413–419

48. Tiano L, Belardinelli R, Carnevali P, Principi F, Seddaiu G, Littarru GP. Effect of coenzyme Q10 administration on endothelial function and extracellular superoxide dismutase in patients with ischaemic heart disease: a double-blind, randomized controlled study. Eur Heart J 2007;28(18):2249–2255

49. Dai YL, Luk TH, Yiu KH, et al. Reversal of mitochondrial dysfunction by coenzyme Q10 supplement improves endothelial function in patients with ischaemic left ventricular systolic dysfunction: a randomized controlled trial. Atherosclerosis 2011;216(2):395–401

50. Gao L, Mao Q, Cao J, Wang Y, Zhou X, Fan L. Effects of coenzyme Q10 on vascular endothelial function in humans: A meta-analysis of randomized controlled trials. Atherosclerosis 2012;221(2):311–316

51. McDonnell MG, Archbold GP. Plasma ubiquinol/cholesterol ratios in patients with hyperlipidaemia, those with diabetes mellitus and in patients requiring dialysis. Clin Chim Acta 1996;253(1–2):117–126

52. Lim SC, Tan HH, Goh SK, et al. Oxidative burden in prediabetic and diabetic individuals: evidence from plasma coenzyme Q(10). Diabet Med 2006;23(12):1344–1349

53. Henriksen JE, Andersen CB, Hother-Nielsen O, Vaag A, Mortensen SA, Beck-Nielsen H. Impact of ubiquinone (coenzyme Q10) treatment on glycaemic control, insulin requirement and well-being in patients with Type 1 diabetes mellitus. Diabet Med 1999;16(4):312–318

54. Eriksson JG, Forsén TJ, Mortensen SA, Rohde M. The effect of coenzyme Q10 administration on metabolic control in patients with type 2 diabetes mellitus. Biofactors 1999;9(2–4):315–318

55. Alcolado JC, Laji K, Gill-Randall R. Maternal transmission of diabetes. Diabet Med 2002;19(2):89–98

56. Suzuki S, Hinokio Y, Ohtomo M, et al. The effects of coenzyme Q10 treatment on maternally inherited diabetes mellitus and deafness, and mitochondrial DNA 3243 (A to G) mutation. Diabetologia 1998;41(5):584–588

57. Götz ME, Gerstner A, Harth R, et al. Altered redox state of platelet coenzyme Q10 in Parkinson's disease. J Neural Transm 2000;107(1):41–48

58. Shults CW, Haas RH, Passov D, Beal MF. Coenzyme Q10 levels correlate with the activities of complexes I and II/III in mitochondria from parkinsonian and nonparkinsonian subjects. Ann Neurol 1997;42(2):261–264

59. Isobe C, Abe T, Terayama Y. Levels of reduced and oxidized coenzyme Q-10 and 8-hydroxy-2'-deoxyguanosine in the cerebrospinal fluid of patients with living Parkinson's disease demonstrate that mitochondrial oxidative damage and/or oxidative DNA damage contributes to the neurodegenerative process. Neurosci Lett 2010;469(1):159–163

60. Hargreaves IP, Lane A, Sleiman PM. The coenzyme Q10 status of the brain regions of Parkinson's disease patients. Neurosci Lett 2008;447(1):17–19

61. Shults CW, Oakes D, Kieburtz K, et al; Parkinson Study Group. Effects of coenzyme Q10 in early Parkinson disease: evidence of slowing of the functional decline. Arch Neurol 2002;59(10):1541–1550
62. Müller T, Büttner T, Gholipour AF, Kuhn W. Coenzyme Q10 supplementation provides mild symptomatic benefit in patients with Parkinson's disease. Neurosci Lett 2003;341(3):201–204
63. Storch A, Jost WH, Vieregge P, et al; German Coenzyme Q(10) Study Group. Randomized, double-blind, placebo-controlled trial on symptomatic effects of coenzyme Q(10) in Parkinson disease. Arch Neurol 2007;64(7):938–944
64. NINDS NET-PD Investigators. A randomized clinical trial of coenzyme Q10 and GPI-1485 in early Parkinson disease. Neurology 2007;68(1):20–28
65. National Institutes of Health. Effects of Coenzyme Q10 (CoQ) in Parkinson Disease (QE3). ClinicalTrials. gov. Available at: http://www.clinicaltrials.gov/ct2/show/NCT00740714?term=coenzyme+Q&rank=2. Accessed May 9, 2012
66. Koroshetz WJ, Jenkins BG, Rosen BR, Beal MF. Energy metabolism defects in Huntington's disease and effects of coenzyme Q10. Ann Neurol 1997;41(2):160–165
67. Beal MF. Coenzyme Q10 as a possible treatment for neurodegenerative diseases. Free Radic Res 2002; 36(4):455–460
68. Ferrante RJ, Andreassen OA, Dedeoglu A, et al. Therapeutic effects of coenzyme Q10 and remacemide in transgenic mouse models of Huntington's disease. J Neurosci 2002;22(5):1592–1599
69. Schilling G, Coonfield ML, Ross CA, Borchelt DR. Coenzyme Q10 and remacemide hydrochloride ameliorate motor deficits in a Huntington's disease transgenic mouse model. Neurosci Lett 2001;315(3):149–153
70. Stack EC, Kubilus JK, Smith K, et al. Chronology of behavioral symptoms and neuropathological sequela in R6/2 Huntington's disease transgenic mice. J Comp Neurol 2005;490(4):354–370
71. Stack EC, Smith KM, Ryu H, et al. Combination therapy using minocycline and coenzyme Q10 in R6/2 transgenic Huntington's disease mice. Biochim Biophys Acta 2006;1762(3):373–380
72. Yang L, Calingasan NY, Wille EJ, et al. Combination therapy with coenzyme Q10 and creatine produces additive neuroprotective effects in models of Parkinson's and Huntington's diseases. J Neurochem 2009;109(5):1427–1439
73. Huntington Study Group. A randomized, placebo-controlled trial of coenzyme Q10 and remacemide in Huntington's disease. Neurology 2001;57(3):397–404
74. Hyson HC, Kieburtz K, Shoulson I, et al; Huntington Study Group Pre2CARE Investigators. Safety and tolerability of high-dosage coenzyme Q10 in Huntington's disease and healthy subjects. Mov Disord 2010;25(12):1924–1928
75. National Institutes of Health. Coenzyme Q10 in Huntington's Disease (HD) (2CARE). ClinicalTrials.gov. Available at: http://www.clinicaltrials.gov/ct2/show/NCT00608881?term=coenzyme+Q10+and+huntington&rank=1 Accessed 2/15/12. Accessed May 9, 2012
76. Gatchel JR, Zoghbi HY. Diseases of unstable repeat expansion: mechanisms and common principles. Nat Rev Genet 2005;6(10):743–755
77. Cooper JM, Schapira AH. Friedreich's Ataxia: disease mechanisms, antioxidant and Coenzyme Q10 therapy. Biofactors 2003;18(1–4):163–171
78. Taroni F, DiDonato S. Pathways to motor incoordination: the inherited ataxias. Nat Rev Neurosci 2004; 5(8):641–655
79. Lodi R, Tonon C, Calabrese V, Schapira AH. Friedreich's ataxia: from disease mechanisms to therapeutic interventions. Antioxid Redox Signal 2006;8(3–4):438–443
80. Lodi R, Hart PE, Rajagopalan B, et al. Antioxidant treatment improves in vivo cardiac and skeletal muscle bioenergetics in patients with Friedreich's ataxia. Ann Neurol 2001;49(5):590–596
81. Hart PE, Lodi R, Rajagopalan B, et al. Antioxidant treatment of patients with Friedreich's ataxia: four-year follow-up. Arch Neurol 2005;62(4):621–626
82. Cooper JM, Korlipara LV, Hart PE, Bradley JL, Schapira AH. Coenzyme Q10 and vitamin E deficiency in Friedreich's ataxia: predictor of efficacy of vitamin E and coenzyme Q10 therapy. Eur J Neurol 2008; 15(12): 1371–1379
83. Folkers K, Osterborg A, Nylander M, Morita M, Mellstedt H. Activities of vitamin Q10 in animal models and a serious deficiency in patients with cancer. Biochem Biophys Res Commun 1997;234(2):296–299
84. Hodges S, Hertz N, Lockwood K, Lister R. CoQ10: could it have a role in cancer management? Biofactors 1999;9(2–4):365–370
85. Laaksonen R, Fogelholm M, Himberg JJ, Laakso J, Salorinne Y. Ubiquinone supplementation and exercise capacity in trained young and older men. Eur J Appl Physiol Occup Physiol 1995;72(1–2):95–100
86. Malm C, Svensson M, Ekblom B, Sjödin B. Effects of ubiquinone-10 supplementation and high intensity training on physical performance in humans. Acta Physiol Scand 1997;161(3):379–384
87. Weston SB, Zhou S, Weatherby RP, Robson SJ. Does exogenous coenzyme Q10 affect aerobic capacity in endurance athletes? Int J Sport Nutr 1997;7(3):197–206
88. Porter DA, Costill DL, Zachwieja JJ, et al. The effect of oral coenzyme Q10 on the exercise tolerance of middle-aged, untrained men. Int J Sports Med 1995; 16(7):421–427
89. Braun B, Clarkson PM, Freedson PS, Kohl RL. Effects of coenzyme Q10 supplementation on exercise performance, VO2max, and lipid peroxidation in trained cyclists. Int J Sport Nutr 1991;1(4):353–365
90. Bonetti A, Solito F, Carmosino G, Bargossi AM, Fiorella PL. Effect of ubidecarenone oral treatment on aerobic power in middle-aged trained subjects. J Sports Med Phys Fitness 2000;40(1):51–57
91. Willis R, Anthony M, Sun L, Honse Y, Qiao G. Clinical implications of the correlation between coenzyme Q10 and vitamin B6 status. Biofactors 1999;9(2–4):359–363
92. Mattila P, Kumpulainen J. Coenzymes Q9 and Q10: Contents in foods and dietary intake. J Food Compost Anal 2001;14(4):409–417
93. Kamei M, Fujita T, Kanbe T, et al. The distribution and content of ubiquinone in foods. Int J Vitam Nutr Res 1986;56(1):57–63
94. Weber C, Bysted A, Hølmer G. Coenzyme Q10 in the diet—daily intake and relative bioavailability. Mol Aspects Med 1997;18(Suppl):S251–S254
95. Shults CW, Flint Beal M, Song D, Fontaine D. Pilot trial of high dosages of coenzyme Q10 in patients with Parkinson's disease. Exp Neurol 2004;188(2):491–494

96. Hendler SS, Rorvik DR, eds. PDR for Nutritional Supplements. Montvale, NJ: Medical Economics Company, Inc; 2001

97. Lönnrot K, Holm P, Lagerstedt A, Huhtala H, Alho H. The effects of lifelong ubiquinone Q10 supplementation on the Q9 and Q10 tissue concentrations and life span of male rats and mice. Biochem Mol Biol Int 1998;44(4):727–737

98. Zhang Y, Aberg F, Appelkvist EL, Dallner G, Ernster L. Uptake of dietary coenzyme Q supplement is limited in rats. J Nutr 1995;125(3):446–453

99. Svensson M, Malm C, Tonkonogi M, Ekblom B, Sjödin B, Sahlin K. Effect of Q10 supplementation on tissue Q10 levels and adenine nucleotide catabolism during high-intensity exercise. Int J Sport Nutr 1999; 9(2):166–180

100. Matthews RT, Yang L, Browne S, Baik M, Beal MF. Coenzyme Q10 administration increases brain mitochondrial concentrations and exerts neuroprotective effects. Proc Natl Acad Sci U S A 1998;95(15):8892–8897

101. Keith M, Mazer CD, Mikhail P, Jeejeebhoy F, Briet F, Errett L. Coenzyme Q10 in patients undergoing CABG: Effect of statins and nutritional supplementation. Nutr Metab Cardiovasc Dis 2008;18(2):105–111

102. Hathcock JN, Shao A. Risk assessment for coenzyme Q10 (Ubiquinone). Regul Toxicol Pharmacol 2006; 45(3):282–288

103. Jellin JM. Natural Medicines Comprehensive Database. Therapeutic Research Faculty. Available at: http://www.naturaldatabase.com. Accessed May 9, 2012

104. Heck AM, DeWitt BA, Lukes AL. Potential interactions between alternative therapies and warfarin. Am J Health Syst Pharm 2000;57(13):1221–1227, quiz 1228–1230

105. Folkers K, Langsjoen P, Willis R, et al. Lovastatin decreases coenzyme Q levels in humans. Proc Natl Acad Sci U S A 1990;87(22):8931–8934

106. Colquhoun DM, Jackson R, Walters M, et al. Effects of simvastatin on blood lipids, vitamin E, coenzyme Q10 levels and left ventricular function in humans. Eur J Clin Invest 2005;35(4):251–258

107. Mabuchi H, Higashikata T, Kawashiri M, et al. Reduction of serum ubiquinol-10 and ubiquinone-10 levels by atorvastatin in hypercholesterolemic patients. J Atheroscler Thromb 2005;12(2):111–119

108. Bargossi AM, Battino M, Gaddi A, et al. Exogenous CoQ10 preserves plasma ubiquinone levels in patients treated with 3-hydroxy-3-methylglutaryl coenzyme A reductase inhibitors. Int J Clin Lab Res 1994;24(3):171–176

109. Watts GF, Castelluccio C, Rice-Evans C, Taub NA, Baum H, Quinn PJ. Plasma coenzyme Q (ubiquinone) concentrations in patients treated with simvastatin. J Clin Pathol 1993;46(11):1055–1057

110. Ghirlanda G, Oradei A, Manto A, et al. Evidence of plasma CoQ10-lowering effect by HMG-CoA reductase inhibitors: a double-blind, placebo-controlled study. J Clin Pharmacol 1993;33(3):226–229

111. Laaksonen R, Jokelainen K, Laakso J, et al. The effect of simvastatin treatment on natural antioxidants in low-density lipoproteins and high-energy phosphates and ubiquinone in skeletal muscle. Am J Cardiol 1996;77(10):851–854

112. Laaksonen R, Ojala JP, Tikkanen MJ, Himberg JJ. Serum ubiquinone concentrations after short- and long-term treatment with HMG-CoA reductase inhibitors. Eur J Clin Pharmacol 1994;46(4):313–317

113. Elmberger PG, Kalén A, Lund E, et al. Effects of pravastatin and cholestyramine on products of the mevalonate pathway in familial hypercholesterolemia. J Lipid Res 1991;32(6):935–940

114. Ashton E, Windebank E, Skiba M, et al. Why did high-dose rosuvastatin not improve cardiac remodeling in chronic heart failure? Mechanistic insights from the UNIVERSE study. Int J Cardiol 2011;146(3):404–407

115. Hughes K, Lee BL, Feng X, Lee J, Ong CN. Coenzyme Q10 and differences in coronary heart disease risk in Asian Indians and Chinese. Free Radic Biol Med 2002;32(2):132–138

116. Hargreaves IP, Duncan AJ, Heales SJ, Land JM. The effect of HMG-CoA reductase inhibitors on coenzyme Q10: possible biochemical/clinical implications. Drug Saf 2005;28(8):659–676

117. Laaksonen R, Jokelainen K, Sahi T, Tikkanen MJ, Himberg JJ. Decreases in serum ubiquinone concentrations do not result in reduced levels in muscle tissue during short-term simvastatin treatment in humans. Clin Pharmacol Ther 1995;57(1):62–66

23 L-Carnitine

L-carnitine is a derivative of the amino acid, lysine. Its name is derived from the fact that it was first isolated from meat (*carnus*) in 1905. Only the L-isomer of carnitine (**Fig. 23.1**) is biologically active.[1] L-carnitine appeared to act as a vitamin in the mealworm (*Tenebrio molitor*) and was therefore termed vitamin B_T.[2] Vitamin B_T, however, is actually a misnomer because humans and other higher organisms can synthesize L-carnitine (see the Bioavailability and Metabolism section below). Under certain conditions, the demand for L-carnitine may exceed an individual's capacity to synthesize it, making it a conditionally essential micronutrient.[3,4]

Bioavailability and Metabolism

In healthy people, carnitine homeostasis (balance) is maintained through endogenous biosynthesis of L-carnitine, absorption of carnitine from dietary sources, and elimination and reabsorption of carnitine by the kidneys.[5]

Endogenous Biosynthesis

Humans can synthesize L-carnitine from the amino acids lysine and methionine in a multistep process. Specifically, protein-bound lysine is enzymatically methylated to form epsilon-N-trimethyllysine; three molecules of methionine provide the methyl groups for the reaction. Epsilon-N-trimethyllysine is released for carnitine synthesis by protein hydrolysis.[5,6] Several enzymes are involved in endogenous L-carnitine biosynthesis. The enzyme γ-butyrobetaine hydroxylase, however, is absent from cardiac and skeletal muscle but highly expressed in human liver, testes, and kidney.[7] The rate of L-carnitine biosynthesis in humans was studied in vegetarians and is estimated to be 1.2 µmol/kg of body weight per day.[8] Changes in dietary carnitine intake or renal reabsorption do not appear to affect the rate of endogenous carnitine synthesis.[1]

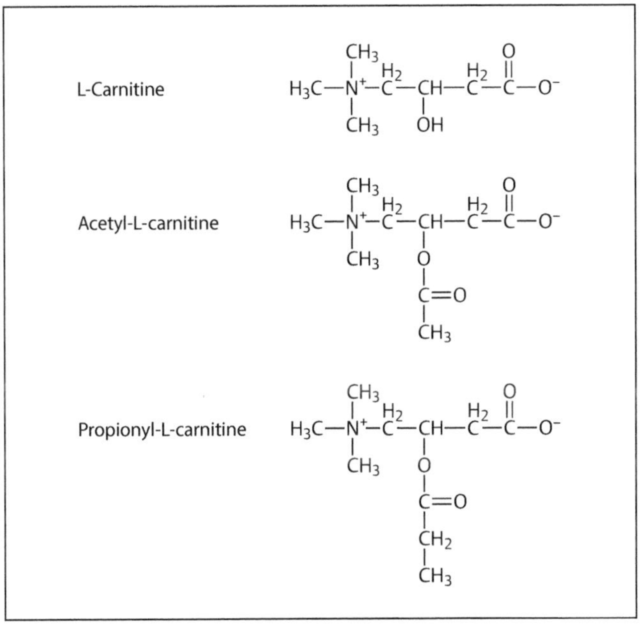

Fig. 23.1 Chemical structures of L-carnitine, acetyl-L-carnitine, and propionyl L-carnitine.

Absorption of Exogenous L-Carnitine

Dietary L-Carnitine

The bioavailability of L-carnitine from food can vary, depending on dietary composition. For instance, one study reported that bioavailability of L-carnitine in individuals adapted to low-carnitine diets (i.e., vegetarians; 66%–86%) is higher than those in adapted to high-carnitine diets (i.e., regular red meat eaters; 54%–72%).[9]

L-Carnitine Supplements

While the bioavailability of L-carnitine from the diet is quite high (see the Dietary L-Carnitine section above), absorption from oral L-carnitine supplements is considerably lower. According to one study, the bioavailability of L-carnitine from oral supplements (0.5–6 g dosage) ranges from 14% to 18% of the total dose.[5] Less is known regarding the metabolism of the acetylated form of L-carnitine, acetyl-L-carnitine (ALCAR); however, the bioavailability of ALCAR is thought to be higher than that of L-carnitine. The results of in vitro experiments suggest that ALCAR is partially hydrolyzed upon intestinal absorption.[10] In humans, administration of 2 g of ALCAR per day for 50 days increased plasma ALCAR levels by 43%, suggesting that some ALCAR is absorbed without hydrolysis or that L-carnitine is reacetylated in the enterocyte.[5]

Elimination and Reabsorption

L-Carnitine and short-chain acylcarnitines (esters of L-carnitine), such as ALCAR, are excreted by the kidneys. Renal reabsorption of L-carnitine is normally very efficient; in fact, an estimated 95% is thought to be reabsorbed by the kidneys.[1] Therefore, carnitine excretion by the kidney is normally very low. However, several conditions can decrease the efficiency of carnitine reabsorption and, correspondingly, increase carnitine excretion. Such conditions include high-fat (low-carbohydrate) diets, high-protein diets, pregnancy, and certain disease states (see the section on Primary Systemic Carnitine Deficiency below).[11] In addition, when circulating L-carnitine levels increase, as in the case of oral supplementation, renal reabsorption of L-carnitine becomes saturated, resulting in increased urinary excretion of L-carnitine.[5] Dietary or supplemental L-carnitine that is not absorbed by enterocytes is degraded by colonic bacteria to form two principal products, trimethylamine and γ-butyrobetaine. γ-Butyrobetaine is eliminated in the feces; trimethylamine is efficiently absorbed and metabolized to trimethylamine-N-oxide, which is excreted in the urine.[9]

Biological Activities

Mitochondrial Oxidation of Long-Chain Fatty Acids

L-Carnitine is synthesized primarily in the liver but also in the kidneys and then transported to other tissues. It is most concentrated in tissues that use fatty acids as their primary fuel, such as skeletal and cardiac (heart) muscle. In this regard, L-carnitine plays an important role in energy production by conjugating to fatty acids for transport into the mitochondria.[1]

L-Carnitine is required for mitochondrial β-oxidation of long-chain fatty acids for energy production.[1] Long-chain fatty acids must be in the form of esters of L-carnitine (acylcarnitines) to enter the mitochondrial matrix where β-oxidation occurs (**Fig. 23.2**). Proteins of the carnitine acyltransferase family transport acylcarnitines into the mitochondrial matrix. On the outer mitochondrial membrane, carnitine-palmitoyltransferase 1 (CPT1) catalyzes the transfer of long-chain fatty acids into the cytosol from coenzyme A (CoA) to L-carnitine, the rate-limiting step in fatty acid oxidation.[12] A transport protein called *carnitine:acylcarnitine translocase* (CACT) facilitates the transport of acylcarnitine esters across the inner mitochondrial membrane. On the inner mitochondrial membrane, carnitine-palmitoyltransferase 2 (CPT2) catalyzes the transfer of fatty acids from L-carnitine to free CoA in the mitochondrial matrix, where they are metabolized through β-oxidation, ultimately yielding propionyl-CoA and acetyl-CoA.[1]

Regulation of Energy Metabolism through Modulation of Acyl CoA:CoA Ratio

CoA is required as a cofactor for numerous cellular reactions.[1] Within the mitochondrial matrix, carnitine-acetyl transferase (CAT) catalyzes the trans-esterification (transfer) of short- and medium-chain fatty acids from CoA to carnitine (**Fig.

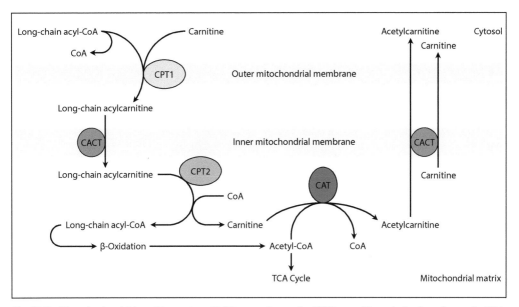

Fig. 23.2 The mitochondrial carnitine system. CACT, carnitine:acylcarnitine translocase; CAT, carnitine-acetyltransferase; CoA, coenzyme A; CPT1, carnitine-palmitoyltrans-ferase 1; CPT2, carnitine-palmitoyltransferase 2; TCA, tricarboxylic acid.

23.2). The acylcarnitine esters can then be exported from the mitochondria via CACT, and the resulting free CoA can participate in other reactions. For example, pyruvate dehydrogenase (PDH) catalyzes the formation of acetyl CoA from pyruvate and free CoA.[13] Acetyl-CoA, in turn, can be oxidized to produce energy (adenosine triphosphate—ATP) in the tricarboxylic acid (TCA) cycle. Carnitine facilitates the oxidation of glucose by removing acyl groups generated by fatty acid β-oxidation and freeing CoA to participate in the PDH reaction.[1]

Deficiency

Nutritional carnitine deficiencies have not been identified in healthy individuals without metabolic disorders, suggesting that most people can synthesize enough L-carnitine.[1] Even strict vegetarians (vegans) show no signs of carnitine deficiency, despite the fact that most dietary carnitine is derived from animal sources.[8] Infants, particularly premature infants, are born with low stores of L-carnitine, which could put them at risk of deficiency, given their rapid rate of growth. One study reported that infants fed carnitine-free, soy-based formulas grew normally and

showed no signs of a clinically relevant carnitine deficiency; however, some biochemical measures related to lipid metabolism differed significantly from those of infants fed the same formula supplemented with L-carnitine.[14] Soy-based infant formulas are now fortified with the amount of L-carnitine normally found in human milk.[15]

Primary Systemic Carnitine Deficiency

Primary systemic carnitine deficiency is a rare, autosomal recessive disorder caused by mutations in the gene for the carnitine transporter protein OCTN2.[16,17] Afflicted individuals have poor intestinal absorption of dietary L-carnitine and impaired L-carnitine reabsorption by the kidneys (i.e., increased urinary loss of L-carnitine)[4] The disorder usually presents in early childhood and is characterized by low plasma carnitine, progressive cardiomyopathy, skeletal myopathy, hypoglycemia, and hypoammonemia.[1,4,16] Without treatment, primary systemic carnitine deficiency is fatal. Treatment consists of pharmacological doses of L-carnitine; such therapy corrects the cardiomyopathy and muscle weakness.[17]

Myopathic Carnitine Deficiency

Primary myopathic carnitine deficiency is a rare genetic disorder in which the carnitine deficiency is limited to skeletal and cardiac muscle. Symptoms, including muscle pain and progressive muscle weakness, begin in childhood or adolescence.[4] Serum carnitine levels, however, are usually normal.[18] In general, the myopathic form of primary carnitine deficiency is less severe than the systemic form.[4]

Secondary Carnitine Deficiency or Depletion

Secondary carnitine deficiency or depletion may result from either genetic or acquired conditions. Hereditary causes include genetic defects in amino acid degradation (e.g., propionic aciduria) and lipid metabolism (e.g., medium chain acyl-CoA dehydrogenase deficiency).[19] Such inherited disorders can lead to a build-up of organic acids, which are subsequently removed from the body via urinary excretion of acylcarnitine esters. Increased urinary losses of carnitine can lead to a systemic depletion of carnitine.[1] Systemic carnitine depletion can also occur in disorders of impaired renal reabsorption. For instance, Fanconi syndrome is a hereditary or acquired condition in which the proximal tubular reabsorption function of the kidneys is impaired.[20] Malfunction of the kidney consequently results in increased urinary losses of carnitine. One example of an exclusively acquired carnitine deficiency involves chronic use of pivalate-conjugated antibiotics. Pivalate is a branched-chain fatty acid that is metabolized to form an acyl-CoA ester that is transesterified to carnitine and subsequently excreted in the urine as pivaloyl carnitine. Urinary losses of carnitine via this route can be 10-fold greater than the sum of daily carnitine intake and biosynthesis (see the Safety section below); thus, systemic carnitine depletion can result.[17] Further, patients with renal disease who undergo hemodialysis are at risk for secondary carnitine deficiency because hemodialysis removes carnitine from the blood (see the section on End-Stage Renal Disease/Hemodialysis below).[21]

Regardless of etiology, a secondary carnitine deficiency is characterized clinically by low plasma concentrations of free carnitine ($<20\,\mu M$) and increased acylcarnitine/free carnitine ratios (>0.4).[19,22] Secondary deficiencies are more common than the rare, primary carnitine disorders.

Nutrient Interactions

Endogenous biosynthesis of L-carnitine is catalyzed by the concerted action of five different enzymes. This process requires two essential amino acids (lysine and methionine), iron (Fe^{2+}), vitamin B_6, and niacin in the form of nicotinamide adenine dinucleotide (NAD), and may also require vitamin C.[4] One of the earliest symptoms of vitamin C deficiency is fatigue, thought to be related to decreased synthesis of L-carnitine.[23]

Disease Prevention

Aging

Age-related declines in mitochondrial function and increases in mitochondrial oxidant production are thought to be important contributors to the adverse effects of aging. Tissue L-carnitine levels have been found to decline with age in humans and animals.[24] One study found that feeding aged rats ALCAR reversed the age-related declines in tissue L-carnitine levels and also reversed several age-related changes in liver mitochondrial function; however, high doses of ALCAR increased liver mitochondrial oxidant production.[25] ALCAR supplementation in rats has also been shown to improve or reverse age-related mitochondrial declines in skeletal and cardiac muscle.[26,27] Studies have found that supplementing aged rats with either ALCAR or α-lipoic acid, a mitochondrial cofactor and antioxidant, improved mitochondrial energy metabolism, decreased oxidative stress, and improved memory.[28,29] Interestingly, co-supplementation of ALCAR and α-lipoic acid resulted in even greater improvements than seen with either compound administered alone. Likewise, several studies have reported that giving rats supplements of both L-carnitine and α-lipoic acid blunts the age-related increases in reactive oxygen species (ROS), lipid peroxidation, protein carbonylation, and DNA-strand breaks in a variety of tissues (heart, skeletal muscle, and brain). Improvements in mitochondrial enzyme and respiratory chain activities and decreased apoptosis have also been observed.[30–39] While these findings are very exciting, it is important to realize that these studies used relatively high doses of the compounds and only for a short time. Co-supplementation of aged rats with ALCAR and α-lipoic acid for a longer time period (3 months) improved both the number of total and intact mitochondria and the mitochondrial ultrastructure of neurons in the hippocampus.[39] It is not yet known whether taking relatively high doses of these two naturally occurring substances will have similar effects in humans. Clinical trials in humans are planned, but it will be several years before the results are available.

Disease Treatment

Cardiovascular Disease

In the studies discussed below, it is important to note that treatment with L-carnitine or propionyl-L-carnitine was used as an adjunct (in addition) to appropriate medical therapy, not in place of it.

Myocardial Infarction (Heart Attack)

Myocardial infarction (MI) occurs when an atherosclerotic plaque in a coronary artery ruptures. The resultant clot can obstruct the blood supply to the heart muscle, causing injury or damage to the heart. In several animal models, treatment with L-carnitine has been found to reduce the injury to heart muscle resulting from ischemia.[40] In humans, L-carnitine administration immediately after MI diagnosis has improved clinical outcomes in several small clinical trials. In one trial, half of 160 men and women diagnosed with a recent MI were randomly assigned to receive 4 g/day of oral L-carnitine in addition to standard pharmacological treatment. After 1 year of treatment, mortality was significantly lower in the group given L-carnitine supplements compared with the control group (1.2% versus 12.5%), and angina attacks were less frequent.[41] In a controlled clinical trial in 96 cardiac patients, treatment with intravenous L-carnitine (5 g bolus followed by 10 g/day for 3 days) following an MI resulted in lower levels of creatine kinase-MB and troponin-I, two markers of cardiac injury.[42] However, not all clinical trials have found L-carnitine supplementation to be beneficial after MI. In a randomized, double-blind, placebo-controlled trial, 60 men and women diagnosed with an acute MI were treated with either intravenous L-carnitine (6 g/day) for 7 days followed by oral L-carnitine (3 g/day) for 3 months, or placebo.[43] After 3 months, mortality did not differ between the two groups, nor did echocardiographic measures of cardiac function. In a larger placebo-controlled trial, 472 patients treated in an intensive care unit within 24 hours of having their first MI were randomly assigned to either intravenous L-carnitine therapy (9 g/day) for 5 days followed by oral L-carnitine (6 g/day) for 12 months, or a placebo; both groups also received standard medical therapy.[44,45] Although there were no significant differences in mortality or the incidence of congestive heart failure, left ventricular volumes were significantly lower in the L-carnitine-treated group at the end of 1 year, suggesting that L-carnitine therapy may limit the adverse effects of acute MI on the heart muscle. Based on these findings, a randomized placebo-controlled trial in 2330 patients with acute MI was undertaken to determine the effect of L-carnitine therapy on the incidence of heart failure 6 months after MI. L-Carnitine therapy (9 g/day intravenously for 5 days, then 4 g/day orally for 6 months) did not affect the incidence of heart failure and death in this study.[46]

Heart Failure

Heart failure is described as the heart's inability to pump enough blood for all of the body's needs. In coronary artery disease, accumulation of atherosclerotic plaque in the coronary arteries may prevent heart regions from getting adequate circulation, ultimately resulting in cardiac damage and impaired pumping ability. MI may also damage the heart muscle, which could potentially lead to heart failure. Because physical exercise increases the demand on the weakened heart, measures of exercise tolerance are frequently used to monitor the severity of heart failure. Echocardiography is also used to determine the left ventricular ejection fraction (LVEF), an objective measure of the heart's pumping ability. An LVEF of less than 40% is indicative of systolic heart failure.[47]

Addition of L-carnitine to standard medical therapy for heart failure has been evaluated in several clinical trials. A randomized, placebo-controlled study in 70 patients with heart failure found that 3-year survival was significantly higher in the group receiving oral L-carnitine (2 g/day) compared with the group receiving placebo.[48] In a randomized, single-blind, placebo-controlled trial in 30 patients with heart failure, oral administration of 1.5 g/day of propionyl-L-carnitine for 1 month resulted in significantly improved measures of exercise tolerance and a slight but significant decrease in left ventricular size compared with placebo.[49] A larger randomized, double-blind, placebo-controlled trial compared the addition of propionyl-L-carnitine (1.5 g/day for 6 months) to the treatment regimen of 271 patients with heart failure to a placebo group consisting of 266 patients.[50] Overall, exercise tolerance was not different between the two groups. However, in patients with higher LVEF values (>30%), exercise tolerance was significantly improved in the propionyl-L-carnitine versus placebo group, suggesting that propionyl-L-carnitine may help improve exercise tolerance in higher-functioning patients with heart failure. A recent study in 29 patients with mild diastolic heart failure (LVEF > 45%) found that 1.5 g/day of oral L-carnitine for 3 months improved some measures of diastolic function compared with baseline.[51]

Angina Pectoris

Angina pectoris is chest pain that occurs when the coronary blood supply is insufficient to meet the metabolic needs of the heart muscle (ischemia). The addition of oral L-carnitine or propionyl-L-carnitine to pharmacological therapy for chronic stable angina has been found to modestly improve exercise tolerance and decrease electrocardiographic signs of ischemia during exercise testing in a limited number of angina patients. One randomized, placebo-controlled study in 200 patients with exercise-induced stable angina found that supplementing conventional medical therapy with 2 g/day of L-carnitine for 6 months significantly reduced the incidence of premature ventricular contractions at rest and also improved exercise tolerance.[52] In addition, a randomized, placebo-controlled crossover trial in 44 men with chronic stable angina found that administering 2 g/day of L-carnitine for 4 weeks significantly increased the exercise workload tolerated prior to the onset of angina and decreased ST-segment depression (electrocardiographic evidence of ischemia) during exercise compared with placebo.[53] In a more recent randomized, placebo-controlled trial in 47 men and women with chronic stable angina, the addition of 2 g/

day of L-carnitine for 3 months significantly improved exercise duration and decreased the time required for exercise-induced ST-segment changes to return to baseline compared with placebo.[54] One study examined the effect of propionyl-L-carnitine on ischemia in men with myocardial dysfunction and angina pectoris by measuring hemodynamic and angiographic variables before, during, and after administering intravenous propionyl-L-carnitine (15 mg/kg body weight). In this study, propionyl-L-carnitine decreased myocardial ischemia, evidenced by significant reductions in ST-segment depression and left ventricular end-diastolic pressure.[55] Although these results are promising, large-scale studies are needed to determine whether L-carnitine or propionyl-L-carnitine is a beneficial therapy for angina pectoris.

Intermittent Claudication in Peripheral Arterial Disease

In peripheral arterial disease (PAD), atherosclerosis of the arteries that supply the lower extremities may diminish blood flow to the point that the metabolic needs of exercising muscles are not sufficiently met, thereby leading to ischemic leg or hip pain known as *claudication*.[56] Several clinical trials have found that treatment with propionyl-L-carnitine improves exercise tolerance in some patients with intermittent claudication (IC). In a double-blind, placebo-controlled, dose-titration study, 1–3 g/day of oral propionyl-L-carnitine for 24 weeks was well tolerated and improved maximal walking distance in patients with IC.[57] In a randomized, placebo-controlled study of 495 patients with IC, 2 g/day of propionyl-L-carnitine for 12 months significantly increased maximal walking distance and the distance walked prior to the onset of claudication in patients whose initial maximal walking distance was less than 250 m.[58] However, no significant response to propionyl-L-carnitine treatment was observed in more mildly affected patients whose initial maximal walking distance was greater than 250 m. In a double-blind, randomized, placebo-controlled trial of 155 patients in the United States and Russia with disabling claudication, administration of 2 g/day of propionyl-L-carnitine for 6 months significantly improved walking distance and claudication-onset time compared with placebo.[59] More recently, a clinical trial in 74 patients with PAD associated with type 2 diabetes found that 2 g/day of oral propionyl-L-carnitine for 12 months improved pain-free walking distance and the ankle–brachial index, a diagnostic measure of PAD.[60]

One study compared the efficacy of L-carnitine and propionyl-L-carnitine administered intravenously for the treatment of IC and concluded that propionyl-L-carnitine was more effective than L-carnitine when the same amount of carnitine was provided.[61] Moreover, propionyl-L-carnitine has been reported to be a vasodilator,[62] thus, the results mentioned above may in part be due to this compound's ability to affect endothelial function. In fact, a recent double-blind, placebo-controlled, crossover study in 21 patients with PAD found that intravenous infusion of propionyl-L-carnitine (6 g/day) increased flow-mediated dilatation of the brachial artery.[63]

End-Stage Renal Disease/ Hemodialysis

L-Carnitine and many of its precursors are removed from the circulation during hemodialysis. Impaired synthesis of L-carnitine by the kidneys may also contribute to the potential for carnitine deficiency in patients with end-stage renal disease undergoing hemodialysis. The US Food and Drug Administration has approved the use of L-carnitine in hemodialysis patients for the prevention and treatment of carnitine deficiency.[64] Carnitine depletion may lead to several conditions observed in dialysis patients, including muscle weakness and fatigue, plasma lipid abnormalities, and refractory anemia. A systematic review that examined the results of 18 randomized trials, including a total of 482 dialysis patients, found that L-carnitine treatment improved hemoglobin levels in studies performed before recombinant erythropoietin (EPO) was routinely used to treat anemia in dialysis patients, and that L-carnitine treatment decreased the EPO dose required and resistance to EPO in studies performed when patients routinely received EPO.[65] Although some uncontrolled studies found that treatment with L-carnitine improved blood lipid profiles in hemodialysis patients,[66] a 2002 systematic review of randomized controlled trials found no evidence that L-carnitine improved lipid profiles.[65] Moreover, two recent studies associated carnitine therapy by hemodialysis with reduced hospitalization.[67,68] The

National Kidney Foundation (NKF) does not recommend routine administration of L-carnitine to all dialysis patients.[69] However, the NKF and other consensus groups suggest a trial of L-carnitine for hemodialysis patients with selected symptoms that do not respond to standard therapy. Those symptoms include persistent muscle cramps or hypotension (low blood pressure) during dialysis, severe fatigue, skeletal muscle weakness or myopathy, cardiomyopathy, and anemia requiring large doses of EPO.[69] In general, intravenous L-carnitine therapy (20 mg/kg body weight) at the end of a dialysis session has been recommended for patients on hemodialysis.[70] Oral carnitine is not advised for hemodialysis patients due to the possible accumulation of potentially toxic metabolites (see the Safety section below).[71]

Alzheimer Disease (Dementia)

Several small, controlled clinical trials conducted in the 1990s suggested that ALCAR treatment (2–3 g/day for 6–12 months) might slow the cognitive decline in patients clinically diagnosed with Alzheimer disease.[72–74] However, a larger multicenter, randomized controlled trial involving 417 patients with Alzheimer disease found that ALCAR treatment (3 g/day for 12 months) was no different than placebo with respect to cognitive decline.[75] Subsequent statistical analyses of the data from that study suggested that patients with early-onset Alzheimer disease (65 years and younger) experienced a more rapid cognitive decline that was significantly slowed by ALCAR treatment.[76,77] However, a multicenter, randomized controlled trial involving 167 patients aged between 45 and 65 years, with early-onset Alzheimer disease, found that ALCAR treatment (3 g/day for 12 months) had no effect on most measures of cognitive decline, although ALCAR treatment was associated with a nonsignificant reduction in the attention-related decline compared with placebo.[76]

HIV/AIDS

One of the hallmarks of infection with the human immunodeficiency virus (HIV) is a progressive decline in the numbers of critical immune cells known as *CD4 T lymphocytes* (CD4 cells), ultimately leading to the development of acquired immunodeficiency syndrome (AIDS). Lymphocytes of HIV-infected individuals inappropriately undergo programmed cell death (apoptosis). Limited evidence in cell-culture experiments and in humans suggests that L-carnitine supplementation may help slow or prevent HIV-induced lymphocyte apoptosis. In an uncontrolled trial, 11 asymptomatic HIV-infected patients, who had refused antiretroviral treatment despite progressively declining CD4 cell counts, were treated with 6 g/day of L-carnitine intravenously for 4 months.[78] After 4 months of L-carnitine therapy, CD4 cell counts increased significantly and markers of lymphocyte apoptosis decreased, although there was no significant change in plasma levels of the HIV virus. Long-term outcomes were not reported in these patients. In a more recent study, 20 HIV-infected individuals were randomly assigned to receive the antiretroviral agents, zidovudine and didanosine, with or without supplemental L-carnitine.[79] Although CD4 cell counts and plasma HIV levels were not different between the two groups after 7 months of therapy, indicators of CD4 cell apoptosis were significantly lower in the group taking L-carnitine.

Some antiretroviral agents (nucleoside analogues) used to treat HIV infection appear to cause a secondary L-carnitine deficiency that may lead to some of their toxic side effects (see the Drug Interactions section below).[80] A small cross-sectional study found that nerve concentrations of ALCAR were significantly lower in patients with HIV who developed peripheral neuropathy while taking nucleoside analogues than in control subjects.[79] Ten out of 16 HIV patients with painful neuropathies reported improvement after 3 weeks of intravenous or intramuscular ALCAR treatment.[81] In a small study of 20 patients with antiretroviral-induced neuropathy, oral ALCAR (2 g/day) for 4 weeks significantly reduced the subjects' mean pain-intensity score but did not affect any of the measured neurophysiological parameters.[82] In a double-blind, placebo-controlled trial in 90 HIV patients with symptomatic distal symmetrical polyneuropathy, intramuscular injection of 1000 mg/day of ALCAR for 2 weeks had no benefit compared with placebo in the intention-to-treat analysis, but ALCAR provided some pain relief in the group of 66 patients who completed the trial.[83] Results from two recent trials suggest that long-term ALCAR supplementation (2–4 years) may be a beneficial

adjunct to antiretroviral therapy in some HIV-infected individuals.[84,85] However, large-scale, controlled studies are needed before any conclusions can be drawn.

Decreased Sperm Motility

L-Carnitine is concentrated in the epididymis, where spermatozoa mature and acquire their motility.[86] Two uncontrolled trials of L-carnitine supplementation in more than 100 men diagnosed with decreased sperm motility found that oral L-carnitine supplementation (3 g/day) for 3–4 months significantly improved sperm motility.[87,88] However, no information on subsequent fertility was reported. A cross-sectional study of 101 fertile and infertile men found that L-carnitine concentrations in semen were positively correlated with the number of spermatozoa, the percentage of motile spermatozoa, and the percentage of normal-appearing spermatozoa in the sample,[89] suggesting that L-carnitine levels in semen may be useful in evaluating male infertility. More recently, a placebo-controlled, double-blind, crossover trial in 86 patients with male infertility found that L-carnitine (2 g/day) supplementation for 2 months led to significant improvements in sperm quality, evidenced by increases in sperm concentration and motility.[90] Similar improvements in sperm motility were observed in a subsequent placebo-controlled, double-blind, randomized study conducted by the same group, but the patients received combination therapy consisting of L-carnitine (2 g/day) and ALCAR (1 g/day) for 6 months.[91] Interestingly, in both studies, the most dramatic carnitine-induced improvements were noted in patients with the lowest baseline sperm motility measures (i.e., the most severe cases).[90,91] Another group of researchers also reported improved sperm motility following combined carnitine therapy. In this placebo-controlled, double-blind, randomized study, 44 patients with idiopathic asthenozoospermia (reduced sperm motility) received placebo, L-carnitine (3 g/day), ALCAR (3 g/day), or a combination of L-carnitine (2 g/day) and ALCAR (1 g/day). The combination therapy, as well as ALCAR alone, resulted in significant increases in sperm motility.[92] Together, these data suggest that carnitine therapy may be useful in disorders of sperm motility and male infertility;

however, large-scale clinical trials are undoubtedly necessary.

Performance

Physical Performance

Interest in the potential of L-carnitine supplementation to improve athletic performance is related to its important roles in energy metabolism. Several small, uncontrolled studies have reported that either acute (dose given 1 hour before exercise bout) or short-term (2–3 weeks') L-carnitine supplementation (2–4 g/day) was associated with increases in maximal oxygen uptake and decreases in plasma lactate.[93–96] Most studies to date have shown no effect of L-carnitine supplementation on physical performance.[97] However, conclusions that can be drawn from this research are limited due to small numbers of participants, short duration of supplementation, and lack of appropriate control groups in most studies. In a recent double-blind, placebo-controlled trial in 32 healthy adults, propionyl-L-carnitine (1 g/day or 3 g/day) for 8 weeks did not improve aerobic or anaerobic exercise performance.[98] Several studies have shown that carnitine supplementation increases plasma carnitine levels,[99–103] but other studies have failed to demonstrate that carnitine supplementation increases levels of carnitine within skeletal or cardiac muscle.[27,98,104] Thus, while carnitine supplementation in theory might work, the available data suggest that it does not affect athletic performance in healthy individuals.

Sources

Biosynthesis

The normal rate of L-carnitine biosynthesis in humans ranges from 0.16 mg/kg of body weight/day to 0.48 mg/kg of body weight/day.[4] Thus, a 70 kg (154 lb) person would synthesize between 11 mg and 34 mg of carnitine per day. This rate of synthesis combined with efficient (95%) L-carnitine reabsorption by the kidneys is sufficient to prevent deficiency in generally healthy people, including strict vegetarians.[105]

Table 23.1 L-Carnitine content of selected foods[105]

Food	Serving	L-Carnitine (mg)
Beef steak	3 oz[a]	81
Ground beef	3 oz	80
Pork	3 oz	24
Canadian bacon	3 oz	20
Milk (whole)	8 fl oz (1 cup)	8
Fish (cod)	3 oz	5
Chicken breast	3 oz	3
Ice cream	4 oz (½ cup)	3
Avocado	1 medium	2
American cheese	1 oz	1
Whole-wheat bread	2 slices	0.2
Asparagus	6 spears (½ cup)	0.2

[a] A 3-oz serving of meat or fish is about the size of a deck of cards.

Food Sources

Meat, poultry, fish, and dairy products are the richest sources of L-carnitine, while fruits, vegetables, and grains contain relatively little L-carnitine. Some L-carnitine-rich foods and their L-carnitine content in milligrams are listed in **Table 23.1**.[105] Omnivorous diets have been found to provide 20–200 mg/day of L-carnitine for a 70 kg person, while strict vegetarian diets may provide as little as 1 mg/day for a 70 kg person. Between 63% and 75% of L-carnitine from food is absorbed, compared with 14%–20% from oral supplements.[1,105,106]

Supplements

- **Intravenous L-carnitine** is available by prescription only for the treatment of primary and secondary L-carnitine deficiencies.
- **Oral L-carnitine** is available by prescription for the treatment of primary and secondary L-carnitine deficiencies. It is also available without a prescription as a nutritional supplement; supplemental doses usually range from 500 mg/day to 2000 mg/day.
- **ALCAR** is available without a prescription as a nutritional supplement. In addition to providing L-carnitine, it provides acetyl groups, which may be used in the formation of the neurotransmitter, acetylcholine. Supplemental

doses usually range from 500 mg/day to 2000 mg/day.[107]

- **Propionyl-L-carnitine** is available in Europe but has not been approved for use in the United States. It provides L-carnitine as well as propionate, which may be utilized as an intermediate during energy metabolism.[106]

Safety

Adverse Effects

In general, L-carnitine appears to be well tolerated; toxic effects related to high-dose L-carnitine have not been reported. L-carnitine supplementation may cause mild gastrointestinal symptoms, including nausea, vomiting, abdominal cramps, and diarrhea. Supplements providing more than 3000 mg/day may cause a "fishy" body odor. ALCAR has been reported to increase agitation in some patients with Alzheimer disease and to increase seizure frequency and/or severity in some individuals with seizure disorders.[107] Only the L-isomer of carnitine is biologically active, and the D-isomer may actually compete with L-carnitine for absorption and transport, thereby increasing the risk of L-carnitine deficiency.[4] Supplements containing a mixture of the D- and L-isomers (D,L-carnitine) have been associated with muscle weakness in patients with kidney disease. Controlled studies examining the safety of L-carnitine supplementation in pregnant and breast-feeding women are lacking.[107]

Drug Interactions

The anticonvulsant, valproic acid, and nucleoside analogues used in the treatment of HIV infection, including zidovudine, didanosine, zalcitabine, and stavudine, may produce a secondary L-carnitine deficiency. Antibiotics used in Europe containing pivalic acid (pivampicillin, pivmecillinam, and pivcephalexin) may also produce a secondary L-carnitine deficiency.[105,107] Additionally, two cancer chemotherapy agents, ifosfamide and cisplatin, may increase the risk of secondary L-carnitine deficiency. Further, there is limited evidence that L-carnitine supplementation may help prevent cardiomyopathy induced by doxorubicin (Adriamycin) therapy.[80]

Summary

- L-carnitine supplementation is indicated for the treatment of primary and secondary carnitine deficiencies.
- Healthy individuals, including strict vegetarians, generally synthesize enough L-carnitine to prevent deficiency.
- Hemodialysis patients with selected symptoms that do not respond to standard therapy may benefit from a trial of L-carnitine supplementation.
- Propionyl-L-carnitine supplementation appears promising as a treatment for intermittent claudication in peripheral arterial disease.
- The roles of L-carnitine supplementation as an adjunct to standard medical therapy in myocardial infarction, heart failure, angina pectoris, Alzheimer disease, and HIV infection require further research.
- Although studies in rats suggest acetyl-L-carnitine supplementation may be beneficial in preventing age-related declines in energy metabolism and memory, it is not known whether acetyl-L-carnitine supplementation will help prevent such age-related declines in humans.
- There is little evidence that L-carnitine supplementation improves athletic performance in healthy people.

References

1. Rebouche CJ. Carnitine. In: Shils ME, Shike M, Ross AC, Caballero B, Cousins RJ, eds. Modern Nutrition in Health and Disease. 10th ed. Philadelphia: Lippincott, Williams and Wilkins; 2006:537–544
2. Fraenkel G, Friedman S. Carnitine. Vitam Horm 1957;15:73–118
3. De Grandis D, Minardi C. Acetyl-L-carnitine (levacecarnine) in the treatment of diabetic neuropathy. A long-term, randomised, double-blind, placebo-controlled study. Drugs R D 2002;3(4):223–231
4. Seim H, Eichler K, Kleber HL. (–)-Carnitine and its precursor, gamma-butyrobetaine. In: Kramer K, Hoppe P, Packer L, eds. Nutraceuticals in Health and Disease Prevention. New York: Marcel Dekker, Inc; 2001:217–256
5. Rebouche CJ. Kinetics, pharmacokinetics, and regulation of L-carnitine and acetyl-L-carnitine metabolism. Ann N Y Acad Sci 2004;1033:30–41
6. Rebouche CJ. Carnitine function and requirements during the life cycle. FASEB J 1992;6(15):3379–3386
7. Rebouche CJ. Ascorbic acid and carnitine biosynthesis. Am J Clin Nutr 1991; 54(6, Suppl):1147S–1152S
8. Lombard KA, Olson AL, Nelson SE, Rebouche CJ. Carnitine status of lactoovovegetarians and strict vegetar-

ian adults and children. Am J Clin Nutr 1989; 50(2): 301–306

9. Rebouche CJ, Chenard CA. Metabolic fate of dietary carnitine in human adults: identification and quantification of urinary and fecal metabolites. J Nutr 1991;121(4):539–546

10. Gross CJ, Henderson LM, Savaiano DA. Uptake of L-carnitine, D-carnitine and acetyl-L-carnitine by isolated guinea-pig enterocytes. Biochim Biophys Acta 1986;886(3):425–433

11. Rebouche CJ, Lombard KA, Chenard CA. Renal adaptation to dietary carnitine in humans. Am J Clin Nutr 1993;58(5):660–665

12. Foster DW. The role of the carnitine system in human metabolism. Ann N Y Acad Sci 2004;1033:1–16

13. McGrane MM. Carbohydrate metabolism–synthesis and oxidation. In: Stipanuk MH, ed. Biochemical and Physiological Aspects of Human Nutrition. Philadelphia: WB Saunders Company; 2000:158–210

14. Olson AL, Nelson SE, Rebouche CJ. Low carnitine intake and altered lipid metabolism in infants. Am J Clin Nutr 1989;49(4):624–628

15. American Academy of Pediatrics. Committee on Nutrition. Soy protein-based formulas: recommendations for use in infant feeding. Pediatrics 1998;101(1 Pt 1):148–153

16. Nezu J, Tamai I, Oku A, et al. Primary systemic carnitine deficiency is caused by mutations in a gene encoding sodium ion-dependent carnitine transporter. Nat Genet 1999;21(1):91–94

17. Stanley CA. Carnitine deficiency disorders in children. Ann N Y Acad Sci 2004;1033:42–51

18. Kerner J, Hoppel C. Genetic disorders of carnitine metabolism and their nutritional management. Annu Rev Nutr 1998;18:179–206

19. Pons R, De Vivo DC. Primary and secondary carnitine deficiency syndromes. J Child Neurol 1995;10(Suppl 2):S8–S24

20. Gregory MJ, Schwartz GJ. Diagnosis and treatment of renal tubular disorders. Semin Nephrol 1998;18(3): 317–329

21. Calvani M, Benatti P, Mancinelli A, et al. Carnitine replacement in end-stage renal disease and hemodialysis. Ann N Y Acad Sci 2004;1033:52–66

22. Winter SC, Szabo-Aczel S, Curry CJ, Hutchinson HT, Hogue R, Shug A. Plasma carnitine deficiency. Clinical observations in 51 pediatric patients. Am J Dis Child 1987;141(6):660–665

23. Food and Nutrition Board, Institute of Medicine. Vitamin C. Dietary Reference Intakes for Vitamin C, Vitamin E, Selenium, and Carotenoids. Washington DC: National Academy Press; 2000:95–185

24. Costell M, O'Connor JE, Grisolía S. Age-dependent decrease of carnitine content in muscle of mice and humans. Biochem Biophys Res Commun 1989; 161(3): 1135–1143

25. Hagen TM, Ingersoll RT, Wehr CM, et al. Acetyl-L-carnitine fed to old rats partially restores mitochondrial function and ambulatory activity. Proc Natl Acad Sci U S A 1998;95(16):9562–9566

26. Pesce V, Fracasso F, Cassano P, Lezza AM, Cantatore P, Gadaleta MN. Acetyl-L-carnitine supplementation to old rats partially reverts the age-related mitochondrial decay of soleus muscle by activating peroxisome proliferator-activated receptor gamma coactivator-1alpha-dependent mitochondrial biogenesis. Rejuvenation Res 2010;13(2–3):148–151

27. Gómez LA, Heath SH, Hagen TM. Acetyl-L-carnitine supplementation reverses the age-related decline in

carnitine palmitoyltransferase 1 (CPT1) activity in interfibrillar mitochondria without changing the L-carnitine content in the rat heart. Mech Ageing Dev 2012;133(2–3):99–106

28. Hagen TM, Liu J, Lykkesfeldt J, et al. Feeding acetyl-L-carnitine and lipoic acid to old rats significantly improves metabolic function while decreasing oxidative stress. Proc Natl Acad Sci U S A 2002;99(4):1870–1875

29. Liu J, Head E, Gharib AM, et al. Memory loss in old rats is associated with brain mitochondrial decay and RNA/DNA oxidation: partial reversal by feeding acetyl-L-carnitine and/or R-alpha -lipoic acid. Proc Natl Acad Sci U S A 2002;99(4):2356–2361

30. Muthuswamy AD, Vedagiri K, Ganesan M, Chinnakannu P. Oxidative stress-mediated macromolecular damage and dwindle in antioxidant status in aged rat brain regions: role of L-carnitine and DL-alpha-lipoic acid. Clin Chim Acta 2006;368(1–2):84–92

31. Kumaran S, Panneerselvam KS, Shila S, Sivarajan K, Panneerselvam C. Age-associated deficit of mitochondrial oxidative phosphorylation in skeletal muscle: role of carnitine and lipoic acid. Mol Cell Biochem 2005;280(1–2):83–89

32. Kumaran S, Subathra M, Balu M, Panneerselvam C. Supplementation of L-carnitine improves mitochondrial enzymes in heart and skeletal muscle of aged rats. Exp Aging Res 2005;31(1):55–67

33. Savitha S, Panneerselvam C. Mitochondrial membrane damage during aging process in rat heart: potential efficacy of L-carnitine and DL alpha lipoic acid. Mech Ageing Dev 2006;127(4):349–355

34. Savitha S, Sivarajan K, Haripriya D, Kokilavani V, Panneerselvam C. Efficacy of levo carnitine and alpha lipoic acid in ameliorating the decline in mitochondrial enzymes during aging. Clin Nutr 2005;24(5):794–800

35. Sethumadhavan S, Chinnakannu P. Carnitine and lipoic acid alleviates protein oxidation in heart mitochondria during aging process. Biogerontology 2006;7(2):101–109

36. Sundaram K, Panneerselvam KS. Oxidative stress and DNA single strand breaks in skeletal muscle of aged rats: role of carnitine and lipoicacid. Biogerontology 2006;7(2):111–118

37. Sethumadhavan S, Chinnakannu P. L-carnitine and alpha-lipoic acid improve age-associated decline in mitochondrial respiratory chain activity of rat heart muscle. J Gerontol A Biol Sci Med Sci 2006;61(7):650–659

38. Tamilselvan J, Jayaraman G, Sivarajan K, Panneerselvam C. Age-dependent upregulation of p53 and cytochrome c release and susceptibility to apoptosis in skeletal muscle fiber of aged rats: role of carnitine and lipoic acid. Free Radic Biol Med 2007;43(12): 1656–1669

39. Aliev G, Liu J, Shenk JC, et al. Neuronal mitochondrial amelioration by feeding acetyl-L-carnitine and lipoic acid to aged rats. J Cell Mol Med 2009;13(2):320–333

40. Lopaschuk G. Regulation of carbohydrate metabolism in ischemia and reperfusion. Am Heart J 2000;139(2 Pt 3):S115–S119

41. Davini P, Bigalli A, Lamanna F, Boem A. Controlled study on L-carnitine therapeutic efficacy in post-infarction. Drugs Exp Clin Res 1992;18(8):355–365

42. Xue YZ, Wang LX, Liu HZ, Qi XW, Wang XH, Ren HZ. L-carnitine as an adjunct therapy to percutaneous coronary intervention for non-ST elevation myocardial infarction. Cardiovasc Drugs Ther 2007;21(6): 445–448

43. Iyer R, Gupta A, Khan A, Hiremath S, Lokhandwala Y. Does left ventricular function improve with L-carnitine after acute myocardial infarction? J Postgrad Med 1999;45(2):38–41

44. Colonna P, Iliceto S. Myocardial infarction and left ventricular remodeling: results of the CEDIM trial. Carnitine Ecocardiografia Digitalizzata Infarto Miocardico. Am Heart J 2000;139(2 Pt 3):S124–S130

45. Iliceto S, Scrutinio D, Bruzzi P, et al. Effects of L-carnitine administration on left ventricular remodeling after acute anterior myocardial infarction: the L-Carnitine Ecocardiografia Digitalizzata Infarto Miocardico (CEDIM) Trial. J Am Coll Cardiol 1995;26(2):380–387

46. Tarantini G, Scrutinio D, Bruzzi P, Boni L, Rizzon P, Iliceto S. Metabolic treatment with L-carnitine in acute anterior ST segment elevation myocardial infarction. A randomized controlled trial. Cardiology 2006; 106(4):215–223

47. Trupp RJ, Abraham WT. Congestive heart failure. In: Rakel RE, Bope ET, eds. Conn's Current Therapy. 54th ed. New York: WB Saunders Company; 2002:306–313

48. Rizos I. Three-year survival of patients with heart failure caused by dilated cardiomyopathy and L-carnitine administration. Am Heart J 2000;139(2 Pt 3): S120–S123

49. Anand I, Chandrashekhan Y, De Giuli F, et al. Acute and chronic effects of propionyl-L-carnitine on the hemodynamics, exercise capacity, and hormones in patients with congestive heart failure. Cardiovasc Drugs Ther 1998;12(3):291–299

50. Study on propionyl-L-carnitine in chronic heart failure. Eur Heart J 1999;20(1):70–76

51. Serati AR, Motamedi MR, Emami S, Varedi P, Movahed MR. L-carnitine treatment in patients with mild diastolic heart failure is associated with improvement in diastolic function and symptoms. Cardiology 2010; 116(3):178–182

52. Cacciatore L, Cerio R, Ciarimboli M, et al. The therapeutic effect of L-carnitine in patients with exercise-induced stable angina: a controlled study. Drugs Exp Clin Res 1991;17(4):225–235

53. Cherchi A, Lai C, Angelino F, et al. Effects of L-carnitine on exercise tolerance in chronic stable angina: a multicenter, double-blind, randomized, placebo controlled crossover study. Int J Clin Pharmacol Ther Toxicol 1985;23(10):569–572

54. Iyer RN, Khan AA, Gupta A, Vajifdar BU, Lokhandwala YY. L-carnitine moderately improves the exercise tolerance in chronic stable angina. J Assoc Physicians India 2000;48(11):1050–1052

55. Bartels GL, Remme WJ, Pillay M, Schönfeld DH, Kruijssen DA. Effects of L-propionylcarnitine on ischemia-induced myocardial dysfunction in men with angina pectoris. Am J Cardiol 1994;74(2):125–130

56. Mills JL. Peripheral arterial disease. In: Rakel RE, Bope ET, eds. Conn's Current Therapy. 54th ed. New York: WB Saunders Company; 2002:340–343

57. Brevetti G, Perna S, Sabbá C, Martone VD, Condorelli M. Propionyl-L-carnitine in intermittent claudication: double-blind, placebo-controlled, dose titration, multicenter study. J Am Coll Cardiol 1995;26(6):1411–1416

58. Brevetti G, Diehm C, Lambert D. European multicenter study on propionyl-L-carnitine in intermittent claudication. J Am Coll Cardiol 1999;34(5):1618–1624

59. Hiatt WR. Carnitine and peripheral arterial disease. Ann N Y Acad Sci 2004;1033:92–98

60. Santo SS, Sergio N, Luigi DP, et al. Effect of PLC on functional parameters and oxidative profile in type 2 diabetes-associated PAD. Diabetes Res Clin Pract 2006;72(3):231–237

61. Brevetti G, Perna S, Sabbà C, et al. Superiority of L-propionylcarnitine vs L-carnitine in improving walking capacity in patients with peripheral vascular disease: an acute, intravenous, double-blind, cross-over study. Eur Heart J 1992;13(2):251–255

62. Cipolla MJ, Nicoloff A, Rebello T, Amato A, Porter JM. Propionyl-L-carnitine dilates human subcutaneous arteries through an endothelium-dependent mechanism. J Vasc Surg 1999;29(6):1097–1103

63. Loffredo L, Marcoccia A, Pignatelli P, et al. Oxidative-stress-mediated arterial dysfunction in patients with peripheral arterial disease. Eur Heart J 2007;28(5): 608–612

64. Guarnieri G, Situlin R, Biolo G. Carnitine metabolism in uremia. Am J Kidney Dis 2001;38(4, Suppl 1):S63–S67

65. Hurot JM, Cucherat M, Haugh M, Fouque D. Effects of L-carnitine supplementation in maintenance hemodialysis patients: a systematic review. J Am Soc Nephrol 2002;13(3):708–714

66. Veselá E, Racek J, Trefil L, Jankovy'ch V, Pojer M. Effect of L-carnitine supplementation in hemodialysis patients. Nephron 2001;88(3):218–223

67. Kazmi WH, Obrador GT, Sternberg M, et al. Carnitine therapy is associated with decreased hospital utilization among hemodialysis patients. Am J Nephrol 2005;25(2):106–115

68. Weinhandl ED, Rao M, Gilbertson DT, Collins AJ, Pereira BJ. Protective effect of intravenous levocarnitine on subsequent-month hospitalization among prevalent hemodialysis patients, 1998 to 2003. Am J Kidney Dis 2007;50(5):803–812

69. Clinical practice guidelines for nutrition in chronic renal failure. K/DOQI, National Kidney Foundation. Am J Kidney Dis 2000;35(6, Suppl 2):S1–S140

70. Eknoyan G, Latos DL, Lindberg J; National Kidney Foundation Carnitine Consensus Conference. Practice recommendations for the use of L-carnitine in dialysis-related carnitine disorder. Am J Kidney Dis 2003;41(4):868–876

71. Schreiber B. Safety of oral carnitine in dialysis patients. Semin Dial 2002;15(1):71–72

72. Pettegrew JW, Klunk WE, Panchalingam K, Kanfer JN, McClure RJ. Clinical and neurochemical effects of acetyl-L-carnitine in Alzheimer's disease. Neurobiol Aging 1995;16(1):1–4

73. Spagnoli A, Lucca U, Menasce G, et al. Long-term acetyl-L-carnitine treatment in Alzheimer's disease. Neurology 1991;41(11):1726–1732

74. Sano M, Bell K, Cote L, et al. Double-blind parallel design pilot study of acetyl levocarnitine in patients with Alzheimer's disease. Arch Neurol 1992;49(11): 1137–1141

75. Thal LJ, Carta A, Clarke WR, et al. A 1-year multicenter placebo-controlled study of acetyl-L-carnitine in patients with Alzheimer's disease. Neurology 1996; 47(3):705–711

76. Thal LJ, Calvani M, Amato A, Carta A. A 1-year controlled trial of acetyl-l-carnitine in early-onset AD. Neurology 2000;55(6):805–810

77. Brooks JO III, Yesavage JA, Carta A, Bravi D. Acetyl L-carnitine slows decline in younger patients with Alzheimer's disease: a reanalysis of a double-blind,

placebo-controlled study using the trilinear approach. Int Psychogeriatr 1998;10(2):193–203

78. Moretti S, Alesse E, Di Marzio L, et al. Effect of L-carnitine on human immunodeficiency virus-1 infection-associated apoptosis: a pilot study. Blood 1998; 91(10):3817–3824

79. Moretti S, Famularo G, Marcellini S, et al. L-carnitine reduces lymphocyte apoptosis and oxidant stress in HIV-1-infected subjects treated with zidovudine and didanosine. Antioxid Redox Signal 2002;4(3):391–403

80. Arrigoni-Martelli E, Caso V. Carnitine protects mitochondria and removes toxic acyls from xenobiotics. Drugs Exp Clin Res 2001;27(1):27–49

81. Scarpini E, Sacilotto G, Baron P, Cusini M, Scarlato G. Effect of acetyl-L-carnitine in the treatment of painful peripheral neuropathies in HIV+ patients. J Peripher Nerv Syst 1997;2(3):250–252

82. Osio M, Muscia F, Zampini L, et al. Acetyl-l-carnitine in the treatment of painful antiretroviral toxic neuropathy in human immunodeficiency virus patients: an open label study. J Peripher Nerv Syst 2006; 11(1):72–76

83. Youle M, Osio M; ALCAR Study Group. A double-blind, parallel-group, placebo-controlled, multicentre study of acetyl L-carnitine in the symptomatic treatment of antiretroviral toxic neuropathy in patients with HIV-1 infection. HIV Med 2007;8(4):241–250

84. Hart AM, Wilson AD, Montovani C, et al. Acetyl-l-carnitine: a pathogenesis based treatment for HIV-associated antiretroviral toxic neuropathy. AIDS 2004; 18(11):1549–1560

85. Herzmann C, Johnson MA, Youle M. Long-term effect of acetyl-L-carnitine for antiretroviral toxic neuropathy. HIV Clin Trials 2005;6(6):344–350

86. Jeulin C, Lewin LM. Role of free L-carnitine and acetyl-L-carnitine in post-gonadal maturation of mammalian spermatozoa. Hum Reprod Update 1996; 2(2):87–102

87. Vitali G, Parente R, Melotti C. Carnitine supplementation in human idiopathic asthenospermia: clinical results. Drugs Exp Clin Res 1995;21(4):157–159

88. Costa M, Canale D, Filicori M, D'Iddio S, Lenzi A; Italian Study Group on Carnitine and Male Infertility. L-carnitine in idiopathic asthenozoospermia: a multicenter study. Andrologia 1994;26(3):155–159

89. Matalliotakis I, Koumantaki Y, Evageliou A, Matalliotakis G, Goumenou A, Koumantakis E. L-carnitine levels in the seminal plasma of fertile and infertile men: correlation with sperm quality. Int J Fertil Womens Med 2000;45(3):236–240

90. Lenzi A, Lombardo F, Sgrò P, et al. Use of carnitine therapy in selected cases of male factor infertility: a double-blind crossover trial. Fertil Steril 2003; 79(2):292–300

91. Lenzi A, Sgrò P, Salacone P, et al. A placebo-controlled double-blind randomized trial of the use of combined l-carnitine and l-acetyl-carnitine treatment in men with asthenozoospermia. Fertil Steril 2004;81(6):1578–1584

92. Balercia G, Regoli F, Armeni T, Koverech A, Mantero F, Boscaro M. Placebo-controlled double-blind randomized trial on the use of L-carnitine, L-acetylcarnitine, or combined L-carnitine and L-acetylcarnitine in men with idiopathic asthenozoospermia. Fertil Steril 2005;84(3):662–671

93. Siliprandi N, Di Lisa F, Pieralisi G, et al. Metabolic changes induced by maximal exercise in human subjects following L-carnitine administration. Biochim Biophys Acta 1990;1034(1):17–21

94. Vecchiet L, Di Lisa F, Pieralisi G, et al. Influence of L-carnitine administration on maximal physical exercise. Eur J Appl Physiol Occup Physiol 1990;61(5–6):486–490

95. Drăgan GI, Vasiliu A, Georgescu E, Dumas I. Studies concerning chronic and acute effects of L-carnitine on some biological parameters in elite athletes. Physiologie 1987;24(1):23–28

96. Marconi C, Sassi G, Carpinelli A, Cerretelli P. Effects of L-carnitine loading on the aerobic and anaerobic performance of endurance athletes. Eur J Appl Physiol Occup Physiol 1985;54(2):131–135

97. Brass EP. Supplemental carnitine and exercise. Am J Clin Nutr 2000;72(2, Suppl):618S–623S

98. Smith WA, Fry AC, Tschume LC, Bloomer RJ. Effect of glycine propionyl-L-carnitine on aerobic and anaerobic exercise performance. Int J Sport Nutr Exerc Metab 2008;18(1):19–36

99. Natali A, Santoro D, Brandi LS, et al. Effects of acute hypercarnitinemia during increased fatty substrate oxidation in man. Metabolism 1993;42(5):594–600

100. Barnett C, Costill DL, Vukovich MD, et al. Effect of L-carnitine supplementation on muscle and blood carnitine content and lactate accumulation during high-intensity sprint cycling. Int J Sport Nutr 1994; 4(3):280–288

101. Vukovich MD, Costill DL, Fink WJ. Carnitine supplementation: effect on muscle carnitine and glycogen content during exercise. Med Sci Sports Exerc 1994;26(9):1122–1129

102. Trappe SW, Costill DL, Goodpaster B, Vukovich MD, Fink WJ. The effects of L-carnitine supplementation on performance during interval swimming. Int J Sports Med 1994;15(4):181–185

103. Brass EP, Hoppel CL, Hiatt WR. Effect of intravenous L-carnitine on carnitine homeostasis and fuel metabolism during exercise in humans. Clin Pharmacol Ther 1994;55(6):681–692

104. Brass EP. Carnitine and sports medicine: use or abuse? Ann N Y Acad Sci 2004;1033:67–78

105. Rebouche CJ. Carnitine. In: Shils ME, Olson JA, Shike M, Ross AC, eds. Nutrition in Health and Disease. 9th ed. Baltimore, MD: Lippincott Williams and Wilkins; 1999:505–512

106. Brass EP, Hiatt WR. The role of carnitine and carnitine supplementation during exercise in man and in individuals with special needs. J Am Coll Nutr 1998;17(3):207–215

107. Hendler SS, Rorvik DR, eds. PDR for Nutritional Supplements. Montvale, NJ: Medical Economics Company, Inc; 2001

24 Lipoic Acid

α-Lipoic acid (LA), also known as *thioctic acid*, is a naturally occurring compound that is synthesized in small amounts by plants and animals, including humans.[1,2] Endogenously synthesized LA is covalently bound to specific proteins, which function as cofactors for several important mitochondrial enzyme complexes (see the Biological Activities section below). In addition to the physiological functions of protein-bound LA, there is increasing scientific and medical interest in potential therapeutic uses of pharmacological doses of free LA.[3] LA contains two thiol (sulfur) groups, which may be oxidized or reduced (**Fig. 24.1**). The reduced form is known as *dihydrolipoic acid* (DHLA), while the oxidized form is known as LA.[4] LA also contains an asymmetric carbon, meaning there are two possible optical isomers that are mirror images of each other (*R*-LA and *S*-LA). Only the *R*-isomer is endogenously synthesized and bound to protein; *R*-LA occurs naturally in foods (see the Food Sources section below). Free LA supplements may contain either *R*-LA or a 50/50 (racemic) mixture of *R*-LA and *S*-LA (see the Supplements section below).

Bioavailability and Metabolism

Endogenous Biosynthesis

LA is synthesized de novo from an eight-carbon fatty acid (octanoic acid) in mitochondria, where protein-bound LA functions as an enzyme cofactor. Evidence suggests that LA can be synthesized "on site" from octanoic acid that is already covalently bound to LA-dependent enzymes.[5,6] The final step in LA synthesis is the insertion of two sulfur atoms into octanoic acid. This reaction is catalyzed by lipoyl synthase, an enzyme that contains iron–sulfur clusters, which are thought to act as sulfur donors to LA.[7,8]

Dietary and Supplemental α-Lipoic Acid

Exogenous LA from the diet can be activated with adenosine triphosphate (ATP) or guanosine triphosphate (GTP) by lipoate-activating enzyme, and transferred to LA-dependent enzymes by lipoyltransferase.[9,10] Consumption of LA from food has not yet been found to result in detectable increases of free LA in human plasma or cells.[3,11] In contrast, high oral doses of free LA (>50 mg) result in significant but transient increases in free LA in plasma and cells. Pharmacokinetic studies in humans have found that approximately 30%–40% of an oral dose of racemic LA is absorbed.[11,12]

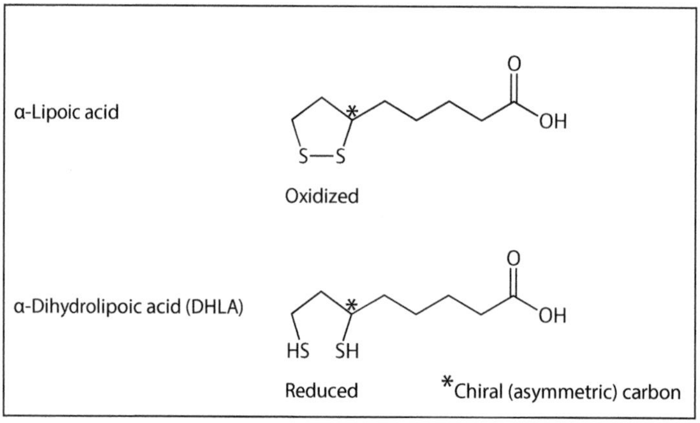

Fig. 24.1 Chemical structure of lipoic acid. *Lipoic acid has a chiral center, which means it can be found in two mirror image forms (*S*- and *R*-alpha-lipoic acid) that cannot be superimposed on each other.

Oral LA supplements are better absorbed on an empty stomach than with food: taking racemic LA with food decreased peak plasma LA concentrations by approximately 30% and total plasma LA concentrations by approximately 20% compared with fasting.[13] Additionally, the sodium salt of *R*-LA may be better absorbed than free LA, presumably because of its higher aqueous solubility.[14]

There may also be differences in the bioavailability of the two isomers of LA. After oral dosing with racemic LA (a 50/50 mixture of *R*-LA and *S*-LA), peak plasma concentrations of *R*-LA were found to be 40%–50% higher than those of *S*-LA, suggesting that *R*-LA is better absorbed than *S*-LA.[12,14,15] Following oral administration, both isomers are rapidly metabolized and excreted. Plasma LA concentrations generally peak in 1 hour or less and decline rapidly.[11,12,15,16] In cells, LA is quickly reduced to DHLA, and in vitro studies indicate that DHLA is rapidly exported from cells.[3]

Biological Activities

Protein-Bound α-Lipoic Acid

Enzyme Cofactor

R-LA is an essential cofactor for several mitochondrial enzyme complexes that catalyze critical reactions related to energy production and the catabolism of α-keto acids and amino acids.[17] In each case, *R*-LA is covalently bound to a specific lysine residue in one of the proteins of the enzyme complex. The pyruvate dehydrogenase complex catalyzes the conversion of pyruvate to acetyl-coenzyme A (CoA), an important substrate for energy production via the tricarboxylic acid (TCA) cycle. The α-ketoglutarate dehydrogenase complex catalyzes the conversion of α-ketoglutarate to succinyl CoA, another important intermediate of the TCA cycle. The activity of the branched-chain α-ketoacid dehydrogenase complex results in the catabolism of the branched-chain amino acids: leucine, isoleucine, and valine.[18] The glycine cleavage system is a multi-enzyme complex that catalyzes the oxidation of glycine to form 5,10-methylene tetrahydrofolate, an important cofactor in the synthesis of nucleic acids.[19]

Free α-Lipoic Acid

When considering the biological activities of supplemental free LA, it is important to keep in mind the limited and transient nature of the increases in plasma and tissue LA (see the Bioavailability and Metabolism section above).[3]

Antioxidant Activities

Scavenging reactive oxygen and nitrogen species. Reactive oxygen species (ROS) and reactive nitrogen species (RNS) are highly reactive compounds with the potential to damage DNA, proteins, and lipids (fats) in cell membranes. Both LA and DHLA can directly scavenge (neutralize) physiologically relevant ROS and RNS in the test tube.[3] However, it is not clear whether LA acts directly to scavenge ROS and RNS in vivo. The highest tissue concentrations of free LA likely to be achieved through oral supplementation are at least 10 times lower than those of other intracellular antioxidants, such as vitamin C and glutathione. Moreover, free LA is rapidly eliminated from cells, so any increases in direct radical-scavenging activity are unlikely to be sustained.

Regeneration of other antioxidants. When an antioxidant scavenges a free radical, it becomes oxidized itself and is not able to scavenge additional ROS or RNS until it has been reduced. DHLA is a potent reducing agent with the capacity to reduce the oxidized forms of several important antioxidants, including vitamin C and glutathione.[20] DHLA may also reduce the oxidized form of α-tocopherol (the α-tocopheroxyl radical), directly or indirectly, by reducing the oxidized form of vitamin C (dehydroascorbate), which is able to reduce the α-tocopheroxyl radical.[21] Coenzyme Q_{10}, an important component of the mitochondrial electron transport chain, also has antioxidant activity. DHLA can reduce oxidized forms of coenzyme Q_{10},[22] which may reduce the α-tocopheroxyl radical.[23] Although DHLA has been found to regenerate oxidized antioxidants in the test tube, it is not known whether DHLA effectively regenerates other antioxidants under physiological conditions.[3]

Metal chelation. Redox-active metal ions, such as free iron and copper, can induce oxidative damage by catalyzing reactions that generate highly reactive free radicals.[24] Compounds that chelate (bind) free metal ions in a way that prevents them from generating free radicals offer promise in the treatment of neurodegenerative diseases and other chronic diseases in which metal-induced oxidative damage may play a pathogenic role.[25] Both LA and DHLA have been found to inhibit copper- and iron-mediated oxidative damage in the test tube[26,27] and excess iron and copper accumulation in animal models.[28,29]

Induction of glutathione synthesis. Glutathione is an important intracellular antioxidant that also plays a role in the detoxification and elimination of potential carcinogens and toxins. Studies in rodents have found that glutathione synthesis and tissue glutathione levels are significantly lower in aged animals compared with younger animals, leading to decreased ability of aged animals to respond to oxidative stress or toxin exposure.[30] LA has been found to increase glutathione levels in cultured cells and in the tissues of aged animals fed LA.[31,32] Research suggests that LA may increase glutathione synthesis in aged rats by increasing the expression of γ-glutamylcysteine ligase (GCL), the rate-limiting enzyme in glutathione synthesis[33] and by increasing cellular uptake of cysteine, an amino acid required for glutathione synthesis.[34]

Modulation of Signal Transduction

Insulin signaling. The binding of insulin to the insulin receptor (IR) triggers the autophosphorylation of several tyrosine residues on the IR. Activation of the IR in this manner stimulates a cascade of protein phosphorylations, resulting in the translocation of glucose transporters (GLUT4) to the cell membrane and thus increased cellular glucose uptake.[3,35] LA has been found to activate the insulin signaling cascade in cultured cells,[3,35,36] increase GLUT4 translocation to cell membranes, and increase glucose uptake in cultured adipose (fat) and muscle cells.[37,38] A computer modeling study showed that LA binds to the tyrosine kinase domain of the IR and may stabilize the active form of the enzyme.[36]

PKB/Akt-dependent signaling. In addition to insulin signaling, phosphorylation and dephosphorylation of other cell-signaling molecules affect a variety of cellular processes, including metabolism, stress responses, proliferation, and survival.[3] One such molecule is protein kinase B,

also known as *Akt* (PKB/Akt). LA has been found to activate PKB/Akt-dependent signaling in vitro[36,39–41] and in vivo,[41] inhibit apoptosis in cultured hepatocytes,[36] and increase survival of cultured neurons.[39] LA has also been shown to improve nitric oxide–dependent vasodilation in aged rats by increasing PKB/Akt-dependent phosphorylation of endothelial nitric oxide synthase (eNOS), which increases eNOS-catalyzed production of nitric oxide.[42]

Redox-sensitive transcription factors. Transcription factors are proteins that bind to specific sequences of DNA and promote or repress the transcription of selected genes. Some transcription factors are sequestered outside the nucleus until some sort of signal induces their translocation to the nucleus. Oxidative stress or changes in the balance between oxidation and reduction (redox status) in a cell can trigger the translocation of redox-sensitive transcription factors to the nucleus. One such redox-sensitive transcription factor, known as *nuclear factor kappa B* (NF-κB), regulates several genes related to inflammation and cell-cycle control, that are involved in the pathology of diabetes, atherosclerosis, and cancer.[19] Physiologically relevant concentrations of LA added to cultured cells have been found to inhibit NF-κB nuclear translocation.[43] Another redox-sensitive transcription factor known as Nrf2 enhances the transcription of genes that contain specific DNA sequences known as antioxidant response elements (AREs). LA has been found to enhance the nuclear translocation of Nrf2 and the transcription of genes containing AREs in vivo, including genes for GCL, the rate-limiting enzyme in glutathione synthesis.[33]

Deficiency

LA deficiency has not been described, suggesting that humans are able to synthesize enough to meet their needs for enzyme cofactors.[44]

Disease Treatment

Diabetes Mellitus

Chronically elevated blood glucose levels are the hallmark of diabetes mellitus (DM). In type 1 DM, insulin production is insufficient due to autoimmune destruction of the insulin-producing β-cells of the pancreas. Type 1 DM is also known as insulin-dependent DM because exogenous insulin is required to maintain normal blood glucose levels. In contrast, impaired cellular glucose uptake in response to insulin (insulin resistance) plays a key role in the development of type 2 DM.[45] Although individuals with type 2 DM may eventually require insulin, type 2 DM is known as *noninsulin-dependent DM* because interventions that enhance insulin sensitivity may be used to maintain normal blood glucose levels.

Glucose Utilization

There is limited evidence that high doses of LA can improve glucose utilization in individuals with type 2 DM. A small clinical trial in 13 patients with type 2 DM found that a single intravenous infusion of 1000 mg of racemic LA improved insulin-stimulated glucose disposal (insulin sensitivity) by 50% compared with a placebo infusion.[46] In an uncontrolled pilot study of 20 patients with type 2 DM, intravenous infusion of 500 mg/day of racemic LA for 10 days also improved insulin sensitivity when measured 24 hours after the last infusion.[47] A placebo-controlled study of 72 patients with type 2 DM found that oral administration of racemic LA at doses of 600 mg/day, 1200 mg/day, or 1800 mg/day improved insulin sensitivity by 25% after 4 weeks of treatment.[48] There were no significant differences among the three doses of LA, suggesting that 600 mg/day may be the maximum effective dose.[45] Data from animal studies suggest that the *R*-isomer of LA may be more effective in improving insulin sensitivity than the *S*-isomer,[38,49] but this possibility has not been tested in any published human trials.

The effect of LA supplementation on long-term blood glucose (glycemic) control has not been well studied. In an uncontrolled pilot study of a controlled-release form of oral racemic LA, 15 patients with type 2 DM took 900 mg/day for 6 weeks and 1200 mg/day for another 6 weeks, in addition to their current medications.[15] At the end of 12 weeks, plasma fructosamine concentrations decreased by approximately 10% from baseline, but glycosylated hemoglobin (HbA$_{1c}$) levels did not change. Plasma fructosamine levels reflect blood glucose control over the past 2–3 weeks, while HbA$_{1c}$ values reflect blood glucose control over the past 2–4 months. At pres-

ent, it is not clear whether oral or intravenous LA therapy improves long-term glycemic control in individuals with type 2 DM.

Vascular Disease

The inner lining of blood vessels, known as the *endothelium*, plays an important role in vascular disease. Endothelial function is often impaired in patients with diabetes, who are at high risk for vascular disease.[50] Intra-arterial infusion of racemic LA improved endothelium-dependent vasodilation in 39 patients with diabetes but not in 11 healthy controls.[51] In addition, a randomized, double-blind, placebo-controlled study in 30 patients with type 2 diabetes found that intravenous infusion of 600 mg of LA improved the response to the endothelium-dependent vasodilator acetylcholine, but not to the endothelium-independent vasodilator, glycerol trinitrate.[52] Endothelial function can be assessed noninvasively by using ultrasound to measure flow-mediated vasodilation, which is endothelium dependent.[53] Using ultrasound, intravenous LA has also been shown to improve endothelial function in patients with impaired fasting glucose[54] or impaired glucose tolerance,[55] which are prediabetic conditions.

A few studies have investigated whether oral administration of LA might improve vascular function in patients with diabetes or metabolic syndrome. A randomized controlled trial assessed the effect of oral LA supplementation on flow-mediated vasodilation in 58 patients diagnosed with metabolic syndrome, a condition characterized by abnormal glucose and lipid (fat) metabolism.[56] Oral supplementation with 300 mg/day of LA for 4 weeks improved flow-mediated vasodilation by 44% compared with placebo. Patients with diabetes are also at high risk for microvascular disease, which may contribute to diabetic neuropathy.[45] In an uncontrolled study, oral supplementation with 1200 mg/day of racemic LA for 6 weeks improved a measure of capillary perfusion in the fingers of eight patients with diabetes who had peripheral neuropathy.[57] While these results are encouraging, long-term randomized controlled trials are needed to determine whether LA supplementation can reduce the risk of vascular complications in individuals with diabetes.

Diabetic Neuropathy

More than 20% of patients with diabetes develop peripheral neuropathy, a type of nerve damage that may result in pain, loss of sensation, and weakness, particularly in the lower extremities.[45] Peripheral neuropathy is also a leading cause of lower-limb amputation in patients with diabetes.[58] Chronic hyperglycemia has been linked to peripheral nerve damage; several mechanisms have been proposed to explain the glucose-induced nerve damage, such as intracellular accumulation of sorbitol, glycation reactions, and oxidative and nitrosative stress.[59] The results of several large randomized controlled trials indicate that maintaining blood glucose at near normal levels is the most important step in decreasing the risk of diabetic neuropathy.[60,61] However, such intensive blood glucose control may not be achievable in all patients with diabetes.

Intravenous and oral LA are approved for the treatment of diabetic neuropathy in Germany.[4] A meta-analysis that combined the results of four randomized controlled trials, including 1258 patients with diabetes, found that treatment with 600 mg/day of intravenous racemic LA for 3 weeks significantly reduced the symptoms of diabetic neuropathy to a clinically meaningful degree.[62]

The efficacy of oral LA in the treatment of diabetic neuropathy is less clear. A short-term study of 24 patients with type 2 DM found that the symptoms of peripheral neuropathy were improved in those who took 1800 mg/day of oral racemic LA for 3 weeks compared with those who took a placebo.[63] More recently, a randomized, double-blind, placebo-controlled trial in 181 patients with diabetic neuropathy found that oral supplementation with 600 mg/day, 1200 mg/day, or 1800 mg/day of racemic LA for 5 weeks significantly improved neuropathic symptoms.[64] In this study, the 600 mg/day dose was as effective as the higher doses. A much larger clinical trial randomly assigned more than 500 patients with type 2 DM and symptomatic peripheral neuropathy to one of the following treatments: (1) 600 mg/day of intravenous racemic LA for 3 weeks, followed by 1800 mg/day of oral racemic LA for 6 months; (2) 600 mg/day of intravenous racemic LA for 3 weeks followed by oral placebo for 6 months; or (3) intravenous placebo for 3 weeks followed by oral placebo for 6 months.[65] Although symptom scores did not

differ significantly from baseline in any of the groups, physician assessments of sensory and motor deficits improved significantly after 3 weeks of intravenous LA therapy. Motor and sensory deficits were also somewhat improved at the end of 6 months of oral LA therapy, but the trend did not reach statistical significance. In another trial of oral LA therapy, 299 patients with diabetic peripheral neuropathy were randomly assigned to treatment with 1200 mg/day of racemic LA, 600 mg/day of racemic LA, or a placebo.[66] However, after 2 years of treatment, only 65 of the original participants were included in the final analysis. In that subgroup, those who took either 1200 mg/day or 600 mg/day of LA showed significant improvement in electrophysiological tests of nerve conduction compared with those who took the placebo. In the longest clinical trial of oral LA therapy, 421 patients with diabetes and distal symmetric sensorimotor polyneuropathy took either 600 mg/day of racemic LA or a placebo for 4 years.[67] No difference between the two groups was seen for the primary endpoint, a composite score that assessed neuropathic impairment of the lower limbs and nerve conduction; however, some measures of neuropathic impairment improved with LA supplementation.

Another neuropathic complication of diabetes is cardiovascular autonomic neuropathy (CAN), which occurs in as many as 25% of patients with diabetes.[45] CAN is characterized by reduced heart-rate variability (HRV; variability in the time interval between heartbeats) and is associated with increased risk of mortality in patients with diabetes. In a randomized controlled trial of 72 patients with type 2 DM and reduced HRV, oral supplementation with 800 mg/day of racemic LA for 4 months resulted in significant improvement in two out of four measures of HRV compared with placebo.[68]

Overall, the available research suggests that treatment with 600 mg/day of intravenous LA for 3 weeks significantly reduces the symptoms of diabetic peripheral neuropathy. Although the benefit of long-term oral LA supplementation is less clear, there is some evidence to suggest that oral LA may be beneficial in the treatment of diabetic peripheral neuropathy (600–1800 mg/day) and cardiovascular autonomic neuropathy (800 mg/day).

Multiple Sclerosis

Feeding high doses of LA to mice with experimental autoimmune encephalomyelitis, a model of multiple sclerosis (MS), has been found to slow disease progression.[69,70] LA treatment through subcutaneous injection also reduced clinical signs of the disease in a rat model of MS.[71] LA treatment has been shown to inhibit the migration of leukocytes (inflammatory T cells, monocytes, and macrophages) into the brain and spinal cord, possibly by decreasing endothelial expression of cell adhesion molecules, inhibiting enzymes called *matrix metalloproteinases* (MMPs), and reducing the permeability of the blood–brain barrier.[69,71–73] More recently, LA has been found to reduce the production of proinflammatory cytokines[74] and stimulate the production of cyclic adenosine monophosphate (AMP) and cell signaling in certain immune cells,[74,75] which may also modulate the effects of LA in MS.

Although the results of animal studies are promising, human research is needed to determine whether oral LA supplementation might be efficacious in MS. A small pilot study designed to evaluate the safety of LA in 30 people with relapsing or progressive MS found that treatment with 1200–2400 mg/day of oral LA for 2 weeks was generally well tolerated (see the Safety section below), and that higher peak serum levels of LA were associated with greater decreases in serum MMP-9 levels.[76] A pharmacokinetic study showed that an oral dose of 1200 mg of racemic LA can result in similar serum levels in MS patients as those found to be therapeutic in mice.[77] However, large-scale, long-term clinical trials are needed to assess the safety and efficacy of LA in the treatment of MS.[78]

Cognitive Decline and Dementia

LA, alone or in combination with other antioxidants or L-carnitine, has been found to improve measures of memory in aged animals or in animal models of age-associated cognitive decline, including rats,[79,80] mice,[81–84] and dogs.[85] Memory assessments were done at the end of the LA treatment period, and it is not known whether LA treatment might have lasting memory effects in these animal models. It is also not clear whether oral LA supplementation can slow cognitive decline related to aging or pathological conditions in humans. An uncontrolled, open-label trial in nine patients with probable Alzheimer disease and related dementias, who were taking acetylcholinesterase inhibitors, reported that oral supplementation with 600 mg/day of racemic LA appeared to stabilize cognitive function over a 1-year period.[86] This study was subsequently extended to include 43 patients with probable Alzheimer disease, who were followed up to 4 years. Patients with mild dementia or moderate-early dementia who took 600 mg/day of racemic LA, in addition to acetylcholinesterase inhibitors, experienced slower cognitive decline compared with the typical cognitive decline of patients with Alzheimer disease as reported in the literature.[87] However, the significance of these findings is difficult to assess without a control group for comparison. A randomized controlled trial found that oral supplementation with 1200 mg/day of racemic LA for 10 weeks was of no benefit in treating HIV-associated cognitive impairment.[88] Although studies in animals suggest that LA may be helpful in slowing age-related cognitive decline, randomized controlled trials are needed to determine whether LA supplementation is effective in preventing or slowing cognitive decline associated with age or neurodegenerative diseases.

Sources

Endogenous Biosynthesis

R-LA is synthesized endogenously by humans and bound to proteins (see the Bioavailability and Metabolism section above).

Food Sources

R-LA occurs naturally in foods covalently bound to lysine in proteins (lipoyllysine). Although LA is found in a wide variety of foods from plant and animal sources, quantitative information on the LA or lipoyllysine content of food is limited and published databases are lacking. Animal tissues that are rich in lipoyllysine (approx. 1–3 μg/g dry weight) include kidney, heart, and liver, while vegetables that are rich in lipoyllysine include spinach and broccoli.[89] Somewhat lower amounts of lipoyllysine (approx. 0.5 μg/g dry weight) have been measured in tomatoes, peas, and Brussels sprouts.

Supplements

Unlike LA in foods, LA in supplements is free, meaning it is not bound to protein. Moreover, the amounts of LA available in dietary supplements (200–600 mg) are likely as much as 1000 times greater than the amounts that could be obtained in the diet. In Germany, LA is approved for the treatment of diabetic neuropathies and is available by prescription.[44] LA is available as a dietary supplement without a prescription in the United States.[90] Most LA supplements contain a racemic (50/50) mixture of *R*-LA and *S*-LA (*d,l*-LA). Supplements that claim to contain only *R*-LA are usually more expensive, and information regarding their purity is not currently available.[91] Since taking LA with a meal decreases its bioavailability, it is generally recommended that LA be taken on an empty stomach (1 hour before or 2 hours after eating).

Racemic versus R-LA Supplements

R-LA is the isomer that is synthesized by plants and animals and functions as a cofactor for mitochondrial enzymes in its protein-bound form (see the Biological Activities section above). Direct comparisons of the bioavailability of oral racemic LA and *R*-LA supplements have not been published. After oral dosing with racemic LA, peak plasma concentrations of *R*-LA were found to be 40%–50% higher than *S*-LA, suggesting *R*-LA is better absorbed than *S*-LA, but both isomers are rapidly metabolized and eliminated.[11,13,16] In rats, *R*-LA was more effective than *S*-LA in enhancing insulin-stimulated glucose transport and metabolism in skeletal muscle,[49] and *R*-LA was more effective than racemic LA and *S*-LA in preventing cataracts.[92] However, virtually all of the published studies of LA supplementation in humans have used racemic LA. At present, it is not clear whether *R*-LA supplements are more effective than racemic LA supplements in humans.

Safety

Adverse Effects

In general, LA supplementation at moderate doses has been found to have few serious side effects. When used to treat diabetic peripheral neuropathy, intravenous administration of racemic LA at doses of 600 mg/day for 3 weeks[62] and oral racemic LA at doses as high as 1800 mg/day for 6 months[66] and 1200 mg/day for 2 years[65] did not result in serious adverse effects. Two mild anaphylactoid reactions and one severe anaphylactic reaction, including laryngospasm, were reported after intravenous LA administration.[45] The most frequently reported side effects of oral LA supplementation are allergic reactions affecting the skin, including rashes, hives, and itching. Abdominal pain, nausea, vomiting, diarrhea, and vertigo have also been reported, and one trial found that the incidence of nausea, vomiting, and vertigo was dose dependent.[64] Further, malodorous urine has been noted by people taking 1200 mg/day of LA orally.[76]

Pregnancy and Lactation

The safety of LA supplements in pregnant and lactating women has not been established.[93]

Drug Interactions

Because there is some evidence that LA supplementation improves insulin-mediated glucose utilization,[48] it is possible that LA supplementation could increase the risk of hypoglycemia in patients with diabetes who are using insulin or oral antidiabetic agents. Consequently, blood glucose levels should be monitored closely when LA supplementation is added to diabetes treatment regimens. Co-administration of a single oral dose of racemic LA (600 mg) and the oral antidiabetic agents, glyburide or acarbose, did not result in any significant drug interactions in one study in 24 healthy volunteers.[94]

Nutrient Interactions

Biotin

The chemical structure of biotin is similar to that of LA, and there is some evidence that high concentrations of LA can compete with biotin for transport across cell membranes.[95,96] The administration of high doses of LA by injection to rats decreased the activity of two biotin-dependent enzymes by approximately 30%–35%,[97] but it is not known whether oral or intravenous LA supplementation substantially increases the requirement for biotin in humans.[98]

Summary

- α-Lipoic acid (LA), also known as *thioctic acid*, is a naturally occurring compound that is synthesized in small amounts by humans.
- Endogenously synthesized LA is bound to protein and functions as a cofactor for several important mitochondrial enzymes.
- Supplementation with high doses of LA transiently increases plasma and cellular levels of free LA.
- Although LA is a potent antioxidant in the test tube, LA supplementation may affect health by stimulating glutathione synthesis, enhancing insulin signaling, and modulating the activity of other cell-signaling molecules and transcription factors.
- Overall, the available research indicates that treatment with 600 mg/day of intravenous racemic LA for 3 weeks significantly reduces the symptoms of diabetic peripheral neuropathy.
- Compared with intravenous administration, the effect of long-term, oral LA supplementation for diabetic peripheral neuropathy is less clear, yet some studies show that oral supplementation with at least 600 mg/day of racemic LA may be beneficial.
- It is not yet known whether LA supplementation is beneficial in the treatment of multiple sclerosis or neurodegenerative diseases like Alzheimer disease.
- For those who choose to take LA supplements, the Linus Pauling Institute recommends a daily dose of 200–400 mg/day of racemic LA for generally healthy people.

References

1. Reed LJ. A trail of research from lipoic acid to alpha-keto acid dehydrogenase complexes. J Biol Chem 2001;276(42):38329–38336
2. Carreau JP. Biosynthesis of lipoic acid via unsaturated fatty acids. Methods Enzymol 1979;62:152–158
3. Smith AR, Shenvi SV, Widlansky M, Suh JH, Hagen TM. Lipoic acid as a potential therapy for chronic diseases associated with oxidative stress. Curr Med Chem 2004;11(9):1135–1146
4. Kramer K, Packer L. R-alpha-lipoic acid. In: Kramer K, Hoppe P, Packer L, eds. Nutraceuticals in Health and Disease Prevention. New York: Marcel Dekker, Inc; 2001:129–164
5. Cicchillo RM, Iwig DF, Jones AD, et al. Lipoyl synthase requires two equivalents of S-adenosyl-L-methionine to synthesize one equivalent of lipoic acid. Biochemistry 2004;43(21):6378–6386
6. Zhao X, Miller JR, Jiang Y, Marletta MA, Cronan JE. Assembly of the covalent linkage between lipoic acid and its cognate enzymes. Chem Biol 2003; 10(12): 1293–1302
7. Cicchillo RM, Booker SJ. Mechanistic investigations of lipoic acid biosynthesis in Escherichia coli: both sulfur atoms in lipoic acid are contributed by the same lipoyl synthase polypeptide. J Am Chem Soc 2005; 127(9):2860–2861
8. Miller JR, Busby RW, Jordan SW, et al. *Escherichia coli* LipA is a lipoyl synthase: in vitro biosynthesis of lipoylated pyruvate dehydrogenase complex from octanoyl-acyl carrier protein. Biochemistry 2000; 39(49):15166–15178
9. Fujiwara K, Suzuki M, Okumachi Y, et al. Molecular cloning, structural characterization and chromosomal localization of human lipoyltransferase gene. Eur J Biochem 1999;260(3):761–767
10. Fujiwara K, Takeuchi S, Okamura-Ikeda K, Motokawa Y. Purification, characterization, and cDNA cloning of lipoate-activating enzyme from bovine liver. J Biol Chem 2001;276(31):28819–28823
11. Hermann R, Niebch G, Borbe H, et al. Enantioselective pharmacokinetics and bioavailability of different racemic alpha-lipoic acid formulations in healthy volunteers. Eur J Pharm Sci 1996;4(3):167–174
12. Teichert J, Hermann R, Ruus P, Preiss R. Plasma kinetics, metabolism, and urinary excretion of alpha-lipoic acid following oral administration in healthy volunteers. J Clin Pharmacol 2003;43(11):1257–1267
13. Gleiter CH, Schug BS, Hermann R, Elze M, Blume HH, Gundert-Remy U. Influence of food intake on the bioavailability of thioctic acid enantiomers. Eur J Clin Pharmacol 1996;50(6):513–514
14. Carlson DA, Smith AR, Fischer SJ, Young KL, Packer L. The plasma pharmacokinetics of R-(+)-lipoic acid administered as sodium R-(+)-lipoate to healthy human subjects. Altern Med Rev 2007;12(4):343–351
15. Evans JL, Heymann CJ, Goldfine ID, Gavin LA. Pharmacokinetics, tolerability, and fructosamine-lowering effect of a novel, controlled-release formulation of alpha-lipoic acid. Endocr Pract 2002;8(1):29–35
16. Breithaupt-Grögler K, Niebch G, Schneider E, et al. Dose-proportionality of oral thioctic acid—coincidence of assessments via pooled plasma and individual data. Eur J Pharm Sci 1999;8(1):57–65
17. Bustamante J, Lodge JK, Marcocci L, Tritschler HJ, Packer L, Rihn BH. Alpha-lipoic acid in liver metabo-

lism and disease. Free Radic Biol Med 1998; 24(6): 1023–1039

18. Harris RA, Joshi M, Jeoung NH, Obayashi M. Overview of the molecular and biochemical basis of branched-chain amino acid catabolism. J Nutr 2005; 135(6, Suppl):1527S–1530S

19. Packer L. alpha-Lipoic acid: a metabolic antioxidant which regulates NF-kappa B signal transduction and protects against oxidative injury. Drug Metab Rev 1998;30(2):245–275

20. Jones W, Li X, Qu ZC, Perriott L, Whitesell RR, May JM. Uptake, recycling, and antioxidant actions of alpha-lipoic acid in endothelial cells. Free Radic Biol Med 2002;33(1):83–93

21. May JM, Qu ZC, Mendiratta S. Protection and recycling of alpha-tocopherol in human erythrocytes by intracellular ascorbic acid. Arch Biochem Biophys 1998;349(2):281–289

22. Kozlov AV, Gille L, Staniek K, Nohl H. Dihydrolipoic acid maintains ubiquinone in the antioxidant active form by two-electron reduction of ubiquinone and one-electron reduction of ubisemiquinone. Arch Biochem Biophys 1999;363(1):148–154

23. Upston JM, Terentis AC, Stocker R. Tocopherol-mediated peroxidation of lipoproteins: implications for vitamin E as a potential antiatherogenic supplement. FASEB J 1999;13(9):977–994

24. Valko M, Morris H, Cronin MT. Metals, toxicity and oxidative stress. Curr Med Chem 2005;12(10):1161–1208

25. Doraiswamy PM, Finefrock AE. Metals in our minds: therapeutic implications for neurodegenerative disorders. Lancet Neurol 2004;3(7):431–434

26. Ou P, Tritschler HJ, Wolff SP. Thioctic (lipoic) acid: a therapeutic metal-chelating antioxidant? Biochem Pharmacol 1995;50(1):123–126

27. Suh JH, Zhu BZ, deSzoeke E, Frei B, Hagen TM. Dihydrolipoic acid lowers the redox activity of transition metal ions but does not remove them from the active site of enzymes. Redox Rep 2004;9(1):57–61

28. Yamamoto H, Watanabe T, Mizuno H, et al. The antioxidant effect of DL-alpha-lipoic acid on copper-induced acute hepatitis in Long-Evans Cinnamon (LEC) rats. Free Radic Res 2001;34(1):69–80

29. Suh JH, Moreau R, Heath SH, Hagen TM. Dietary supplementation with (R)-alpha-lipoic acid reverses the age-related accumulation of iron and depletion of antioxidants in the rat cerebral cortex. Redox Rep 2005;10(1):52–60

30. Hagen TM, Vinarsky V, Wehr CM, Ames BN. (R)-alpha-lipoic acid reverses the age-associated increase in susceptibility of hepatocytes to tert-butylhydroperoxide both in vitro and in vivo. Antioxid Redox Signal 2000;2(3):473–483

31. Busse E, Zimmer G, Schopohl B, Kornhuber B. Influence of alpha-lipoic acid on intracellular glutathione in vitro and in vivo. Arzneimittelforschung 1992; 42(6):829–831

32. Monette JS, Gómez LA, Moreau RF, et al. (R)-α-Lipoic acid treatment restores ceramide balance in aging rat cardiac mitochondria. Pharmacol Res 2011;63(1):23–29

33. Suh JH, Shenvi SV, Dixon BM, et al. Decline in transcriptional activity of Nrf2 causes age-related loss of glutathione synthesis, which is reversible with lipoic acid. Proc Natl Acad Sci U S A 2004;101(10):3381–3386

34. Suh JH, Wang H, Liu RM, Liu J, Hagen TM. (R)-alpha-lipoic acid reverses the age-related loss in GSH redox status in post-mitotic tissues: evidence for increased cysteine requirement for GSH synthesis. Arch Biochem Biophys 2004;423(1):126–135

35. Konrad D. Utilization of the insulin-signaling network in the metabolic actions of alpha-lipoic acid-reduction or oxidation? Antioxid Redox Signal 2005;7(7–8):1032–1039

36. Diesel B, Kulhanek-Heinze S, Höltje M, et al. Alpha-lipoic acid as a directly binding activator of the insulin receptor: protection from hepatocyte apoptosis. Biochemistry 2007;46(8):2146–2155

37. Yaworsky K, Somwar R, Ramlal T, Tritschler HJ, Klip A. Engagement of the insulin-sensitive pathway in the stimulation of glucose transport by alpha-lipoic acid in 3T3-L1 adipocytes. Diabetologia 2000;43(3):294–303

38. Estrada DE, Ewart HS, Tsakiridis T, et al. Stimulation of glucose uptake by the natural coenzyme alpha-lipoic acid/thioctic acid: participation of elements of the insulin signaling pathway. Diabetes 1996;45(12): 1798–1804

39. Zhang L, Xing GQ, Barker JL, et al. Alpha-lipoic acid protects rat cortical neurons against cell death induced by amyloid and hydrogen peroxide through the Akt signalling pathway. Neurosci Lett 2001;312(3): 125–128

40. Shay KP, Hagen TM. Age-associated impairment of Akt phosphorylation in primary rat hepatocytes is remediated by alpha-lipoic acid through PI3 kinase, PTEN, and PP2A. Biogerontology 2009;10(4):443–456

41. Zhang WJ, Wei H, Hagen T, Frei B. Alpha-lipoic acid attenuates LPS-induced inflammatory responses by activating the phosphoinositide 3-kinase/Akt signaling pathway. Proc Natl Acad Sci U S A 2007;104(10): 4077–4082

42. Smith AR, Hagen TM. Vascular endothelial dysfunction in aging: loss of Akt-dependent endothelial nitric oxide synthase phosphorylation and partial restoration by (R)-alpha-lipoic acid. Biochem Soc Trans 2003;31(Pt 6):1447–1449

43. Zhang WJ, Frei B. Alpha-lipoic acid inhibits TNF-alpha-induced NF-kappaB activation and adhesion molecule expression in human aortic endothelial cells. FASEB J 2001;15(13):2423–2432

44. Biewenga GP, Haenen GR, Bast A. The pharmacology of the antioxidant lipoic acid. Gen Pharmacol 1997; 29(3):315–331

45. Ziegler D. Thioctic acid for patients with symptomatic diabetic polyneuropathy: a critical review. Treat Endocrinol 2004;3(3):173–189

46. Jacob S, Henriksen EJ, Schiemann AL, et al. Enhancement of glucose disposal in patients with type 2 diabetes by alpha-lipoic acid. Arzneimittelforschung 1995;45(8):872–874

47. Jacob S, Henriksen EJ, Tritschler HJ, Augustin HJ, Dietze GJ. Improvement of insulin-stimulated glucose-disposal in type 2 diabetes after repeated parenteral administration of thioctic acid. Exp Clin Endocrinol Diabetes 1996;104(3):284–288

48. Jacob S, Rett K, Henriksen EJ, Häring HU. Thioctic acid—effects on insulin sensitivity and glucose-metabolism. Biofactors 1999;10(2–3):169–174

49. Streeper RS, Henriksen EJ, Jacob S, Hokama JY, Fogt DL, Tritschler HJ. Differential effects of lipoic acid stereoisomers on glucose metabolism in insulin-resistant skeletal muscle. Am J Physiol 1997;273(1 Pt 1): E185–E191

50. Schalkwijk CG, Stehouwer CD. Vascular complications in diabetes mellitus: the role of endothelial dysfunction. Clin Sci (Lond) 2005;109(2):143–159

51. Heitzer T, Finckh B, Albers S, Krohn K, Kohlschütter A, Meinertz T. Beneficial effects of alpha-lipoic acid and ascorbic acid on endothelium-dependent, nitric oxide-mediated vasodilation in diabetic patients: relation to parameters of oxidative stress. Free Radic Biol Med 2001;31(1):53–61

52. Heinisch BB, Francesconi M, Mittermayer F, et al. Alpha-lipoic acid improves vascular endothelial function in patients with type 2 diabetes: a placebo-controlled randomized trial. Eur J Clin Invest 2010; 40(2):148–154

53. Gokce N, Keaney JF Jr, Hunter LM, Watkins MT, Menzoian JO, Vita JA. Risk stratification for postoperative cardiovascular events via noninvasive assessment of endothelial function: a prospective study. Circulation 2002;105(13):1567–1572

54. Xiang G, Pu J, Yue L, Hou J, Sun H. α-lipoic acid can improve endothelial dysfunction in subjects with impaired fasting glucose. Metabolism 2011;60(4):480–485

55. Xiang GD, Sun HL, Zhao LS, Hou J, Yue L, Xu L. The antioxidant alpha-lipoic acid improves endothelial dysfunction induced by acute hyperglycaemia during OGTT in impaired glucose tolerance. Clin Endocrinol (Oxf) 2008;68(5):716–723

56. Sola S, Mir MQ, Cheema FA, et al. Irbesartan and lipoic acid improve endothelial function and reduce markers of inflammation in the metabolic syndrome: results of the Irbesartan and Lipoic Acid in Endothelial Dysfunction (ISLAND) study. Circulation 2005; 111(3):343–348

57. Haak E, Usadel KH, Kusterer K, et al. Effects of alpha-lipoic acid on microcirculation in patients with peripheral diabetic neuropathy. Exp Clin Endocrinol Diabetes 2000;108(3):168–174

58. Greene DA, Stevens MJ, Obrosova I, Feldman EL. Glucose-induced oxidative stress and programmed cell death in diabetic neuropathy. Eur J Pharmacol 1999;375(1–3):217–223

59. Obrosova IG. Diabetes and the peripheral nerve. Biochim Biophys Acta 2009;1792(10):931–940

60. The Diabetes Control and Complications Trial Research Group. The effect of intensive treatment of diabetes on the development and progression of long-term complications in insulin-dependent diabetes mellitus. N Engl J Med 1993;329(14):977–986

61. UK Prospective Diabetes Study (UKPDS) Group. Intensive blood-glucose control with sulphonylureas or insulin compared with conventional treatment and risk of complications in patients with type 2 diabetes (UKPDS 33). Lancet 1998;352(9131):837–853

62. Ziegler D, Nowak H, Kempler P, Vargha P, Low PA. Treatment of symptomatic diabetic polyneuropathy with the antioxidant alpha-lipoic acid: a meta-analysis. Diabet Med 2004;21(2):114–121

63. Ruhnau KJ, Meissner HP, Finn JR, et al. Effects of 3-week oral treatment with the antioxidant thioctic acid (alpha-lipoic acid) in symptomatic diabetic polyneuropathy. Diabet Med 1999;16(12):1040–1043

64. Ziegler D, Ametov A, Barinov A, et al. Oral treatment with alpha-lipoic acid improves symptomatic diabetic polyneuropathy: the SYDNEY 2 trial. Diabetes Care 2006;29(11):2365–2370

65. Ziegler D, Hanefeld M, Ruhnau KJ, et al. Treatment of symptomatic diabetic polyneuropathy with the antioxidant alpha-lipoic acid: a 7-month multicenter randomized controlled trial (ALADIN III Study). ALADIN III Study Group. Alpha-Lipoic Acid in Diabetic Neuropathy. Diabetes Care 1999;22(8):1296–1301

66. Reljanovic M, Reichel G, Rett K, et al. Treatment of diabetic polyneuropathy with the antioxidant thioctic acid (alpha-lipoic acid): a two year multicenter randomized double-blind placebo-controlled trial (ALADIN II). Alpha Lipoic Acid in Diabetic Neuropathy. Free Radic Res 1999;31(3):171–179

67. Ziegler D, Low PA, Litchy WJ, et al. Efficacy and safety of antioxidant treatment with α-lipoic acid over 4 years in diabetic polyneuropathy: the NATHAN 1 trial. Diabetes Care 2011;34(9):2054–2060

68. Ziegler D, Schatz H, Conrad F, Gries FA, Ulrich H, Reichel G. Effects of treatment with the antioxidant alpha-lipoic acid on cardiac autonomic neuropathy in NIDDM patients. A 4-month randomized controlled multicenter trial (DEKAN Study). Deutsche Kardiale Autonome Neuropathie. Diabetes Care 1997;20(3): 369–373

69. Marracci GH, Jones RE, McKeon GP, Bourdette DN. Alpha lipoic acid inhibits T cell migration into the spinal cord and suppresses and treats experimental autoimmune encephalomyelitis. J Neuroimmunol 2002; 131(1–2):104–114

70. Morini M, Roccatagliata L, Dell'Eva R, et al. Alpha-lipoic acid is effective in prevention and treatment of experimental autoimmune encephalomyelitis. J Neuroimmunol 2004;148(1–2):146–153

71. Schreibelt G, Musters RJ, Reijerkerk A, et al. Lipoic acid affects cellular migration into the central nervous system and stabilizes blood-brain barrier integrity. J Immunol 2006;177(4):2630–2637

72. Chaudhary P, Marracci GH, Bourdette DN. Lipoic acid inhibits expression of ICAM-1 and VCAM-1 by CNS endothelial cells and T cell migration into the spinal cord in experimental autoimmune encephalomyelitis. J Neuroimmunol 2006;175(1–2):87–96

73. Marracci GH, McKeon GP, Marquardt WE, Winter RW, Riscoe MK, Bourdette DN. Alpha lipoic acid inhibits human T-cell migration: implications for multiple sclerosis. J Neurosci Res 2004;78(3):362–370

74. Salinthone S, Schillace RV, Tsang C, Regan JW, Bourdette DN, Carr DW. Lipoic acid stimulates cAMP production via G protein-coupled receptor-dependent and -independent mechanisms. J Nutr Biochem 2011;22(7):681–690

75. Schillace RV, Pisenti N, Pattamanuch N, et al. Lipoic acid stimulates cAMP production in T lymphocytes and NK cells. Biochem Biophys Res Commun 2007; 354(1):259–264

76. Yadav V, Marracci G, Lovera J, et al. Lipoic acid in multiple sclerosis: a pilot study. Mult Scler 2005; 11(2):159–165

77. Yadav V, Marracci GH, Munar MY, et al. Pharmacokinetic study of lipoic acid in multiple sclerosis: comparing mice and human pharmacokinetic parameters. Mult Scler 2010;16(4):387–397

78. National Multiple Sclerosis Society. Progress in Research: Research Highlights Winter/Spring 2005. Available at: http://nationalmssociety.org/Highlights-Antioxidants.asp. Accessed Jan 9, 2006

79. Liu J, Head E, Gharib AM, et al. Memory loss in old rats is associated with brain mitochondrial decay and RNA/DNA oxidation: partial reversal by feeding acetyl-L-carnitine and/or R-alpha -lipoic acid. Proc Natl Acad Sci U S A 2002;99(4):2356–2361

80. Hagen TM, Liu J, Lykkesfeldt J, et al. Feeding acetyl-L-carnitine and lipoic acid to old rats significantly im-

proves metabolic function while decreasing oxidative stress. Proc Natl Acad Sci U S A 2002;99(4):1870–1875

81. Farr SA, Poon HF, Dogrukol-Ak D, et al. The antioxidants alpha-lipoic acid and N-acetylcysteine reverse memory impairment and brain oxidative stress in aged SAMP8 mice. J Neurochem 2003;84(5):1173–1183

82. Quinn JF, Bussiere JR, Hammond RS, et al. Chronic dietary alpha-lipoic acid reduces deficits in hippocampal memory of aged Tg2576 mice. Neurobiol Aging 2007;28(2):213–225

83. Shenk JC, Liu J, Fischbach K, et al. The effect of acetyl-L-carnitine and R-alpha-lipoic acid treatment in ApoE4 mouse as a model of human Alzheimer's disease. J Neurol Sci 2009;283(1–2):199–206

84. Stoll S, Hartmann H, Cohen SA, Müller WE. The potent free radical scavenger alpha-lipoic acid improves memory in aged mice: putative relationship to NMDA receptor deficits. Pharmacol Biochem Behav 1993;46(4):799–805

85. Milgram NW, Head E, Zicker SC, et al. Learning ability in aged beagle dogs is preserved by behavioral enrichment and dietary fortification: a two-year longitudinal study. Neurobiol Aging 2005;26(1):77–90

86. Hager K, Marahrens A, Kenklies M, Riederer P, Münch G. Alpha-lipoic acid as a new treatment option for Alzheimer [corrected] type dementia. Arch Gerontol Geriatr 2001;32(3):275–282

87. Hager K, Kenklies M, McAfoose J, Engel J, Münch G. Alpha-lipoic acid as a new treatment option for Alzheimer's disease—a 48 months follow-up analysis. J Neural Transm Suppl 2007; (72):189–193

88. Dana Consortium on the Therapy of HIV Dementia and Related Cognitive Disorders. A randomized, double-blind, placebo-controlled trial of deprenyl and thioctic acid in human immunodeficiency virus-associated cognitive impairment. Neurology 1998; 50(3):645–651

89. Lodge JK, Youn HD, Handelman GJ, et al. Natural sources of lipoic acid: determination of lipoyllysine released from protease-digested tissues by high performance liquid chromatography incorporating electrochemical detection. J Appl Nutr 1997;49(1 & 2):3–11

90. Hendler SS, Rorvik DR, eds. PDR for Nutritional Supplements. Montbale, NJ: Medical Economics Company, Inc; 2001

91. Alpha-Lipoic Acid Supplements. ConsumerLab.com. October 2, 2009. Available at: https://www.consumerlab.com/reviews/Alpha-Lipoic_Acid_Supplements/alphalipoic/. Accessed May 10, 2012

92. Maitra I, Serbinova E, Tritschler HJ, Packer L. Stereospecific effects of R-lipoic acid on buthionine sulfoximine-induced cataract formation in newborn rats. Biochem Biophys Res Commun 1996;221(2):422–429

93. Hendler SS, Rorvik DR. Alpha-Lipoic Acid. In: Hendler SS, Rorvik DR, eds. PDR for Nutritional Supplements. 2nd ed. Montvale, NJ: Physicians' Desk Reference Inc; 2008:25–29

94. Gleiter CH, Schreeb KH, Freudenthaler S, et al. Lack of interaction between thioctic acid, glibenclamide and acarbose. Br J Clin Pharmacol 1999;48(6):819–825

95. Prasad PD, Wang H, Huang W, et al. Molecular and functional characterization of the intestinal Na+-dependent multivitamin transporter. Arch Biochem Biophys 1999;366(1):95–106

96. Balamurugan K, Vaziri ND, Said HM. Biotin uptake by human proximal tubular epithelial cells: cellular and molecular aspects. Am J Physiol Renal Physiol 2005;288(4):F823–F831

97. Zempleni J, Trusty TA, Mock DM. Lipoic acid reduces the activities of biotin-dependent carboxylases in rat liver. J Nutr 1997;127(9):1776–1781

98. Zempleni J, Mock DM. Biotin biochemistry and human requirements. J Nutr Biochem 1999;10(3):128–138

Appendix 1   Glycemic Index and Glycemic Load

Glycemic Index

In the past, carbohydrates were classified as simple or complex, based on the number of simple sugars in the molecule. Carbohydrates composed of one or two simple sugars like fructose or sucrose (table sugar; a disaccharide composed of one molecule of glucose and one molecule of fructose) were labeled simple, while starchy foods were labeled complex because starch is composed of long chains of the simple sugar, glucose. Advice to eat fewer simple and more complex carbohydrates (i.e., polysaccharides) was based on the assumption that consuming starchy foods would lead to smaller increases in blood glucose than results from consuming sugary foods.[1] This assumption turned out to be too simplistic, since the blood glucose (glycemic) response to "complex" carbohydrates has been found to vary considerably. A more accurate indicator of the relative glycemic response to dietary carbohydrates should be glycemic load, which incorporates the relative quality and quantity of carbohydrates in the diet.

Measuring the Glycemic Index of Foods

To determine the glycemic index of a food, volunteers are typically given a test food that provides 50 g of carbohydrate and a control food (white bread or pure glucose) that provides the same amount of carbohydrate on different days.[2] Blood samples for the determination of glucose are taken prior to eating and at regular intervals after eating over the next several hours. The changes in blood glucose over time are plotted as a curve. The glycemic index is calculated as the area under the glucose curve after the test food is eaten, divided by the corresponding area after the control food is eaten. The value is multiplied by 100 to represent a percentage of the control food. For example, a baked potato has a glycemic index of 76 relative to glucose (Table A1.1) and 108 relative to white bread, which means that the blood glucose response to the carbohydrate in a baked potato is 76% of the blood glucose response to the same amount of carbohydrate in pure glucose and 108% of the blood glucose response to the same amount of carbohydrate in white bread.[3] In contrast, cooked brown rice has a glycemic index of 55 relative to glucose and 79 relative to white bread.[4] In the traditional system of classifying carbohydrates, both brown rice and potato would be classified as complex carbohydrates, despite the difference in their effects on blood glucose levels.

Physiological Responses to High-Glycemic-Index Values

By definition, the consumption of high-glycemic-index foods results in higher and more rapid increases in blood glucose levels than the consumption of low-glycemic-index foods. Rapid increases in blood glucose are potent signals to the β-cells of the pancreas to increase insulin secretion.[2] Over the next few hours, the high insulin levels induced by consumption of high-glycemic-index foods may cause a sharp decrease in blood glucose levels (hypoglycemia). In contrast, the consumption of low-glycemic-index foods results in lower but more sustained increases in blood glucose and lower insulin demands on pancreatic β-cells.[5]

Glycemic Load

The glycemic index compares the potential of foods containing the same amount of carbohydrate to raise blood glucose. However, the amount of carbohydrate consumed also affects blood glucose levels and insulin responses. The glycemic load of a food is calculated by multiplying the glycemic index by the amount of carbohydrate in grams provided by a food and dividing the total by 100 (**Table A1.1**).[1] Dietary glycemic

Table A1.1   Glycemic-index (relative to glucose) and glycemic-load values for selected foods[3,4]

Food	Glycemic Index (Glucose = 100)	Serving Size	Carbohydrate per Serving (g)	Glycemic Load per Serving
Dates, dried	103	~2 oz	40	42
Cornflakes	81	~1 cup	26	21
Jelly beans	78	1 oz	28	22
Puffed rice cakes	78	~3 cakes	21	17
Russet potato, baked	76	1 medium	30	23
Doughnut	76	1 medium	23	17
White bread	73	1 large slice	14	10
White rice, boiled	64	1 cup	36	23
Brown rice, boiled	55	1 cup	33	18
Spaghetti, white, boiled 10–15 minutes	44	~1 cup	48	21
Spaghetti, white, boiled 5 minutes	38	~1 cup	48	18
Spaghetti, whole-wheat, boiled	37	~1 cup	42	16
Rye bread	41	1 large slice	12	5
Orange, raw	42	1 medium	11	5
Pear, raw	38	1 small	11	4
Apple, raw	38	1 small	15	6
100% bran cereal	38	1 cup	23	9
Lentils, boiled	29	~1 cup	18	5
Kidney beans, dried, boiled	28	~1 cup	25	7
Pearled barley, boiled	25	1 cup	42	11
Cashews	22	~2 oz	13	3
Peanuts	14	~2 oz	6	1

load is the sum of the glycemic loads for all foods consumed in the diet. The concept of glycemic load was developed by scientists to simultaneously describe the quality (glycemic index) and quantity of carbohydrate in a meal or diet.

Disease Prevention

Type 2 Diabetes Mellitus

After a meal with a high glycemic load, blood glucose levels rise more rapidly and insulin demand is greater than after a meal with a low glycemic load. High blood glucose levels and excessive insulin secretion are thought to contribute to the loss of the insulin-secreting function of the pancreatic β-cells that leads to irreversible diabetes.[6] In several large prospective studies, high dietary glycemic loads have been associated with an in-creased risk of developing type 2 diabetes mellitus (DM). In the Nurses' Health Study (NHS), women with the highest dietary glycemic loads were 37% more likely to develop type 2 DM over a 6-year period than women with the lowest dietary glycemic loads.[7] Additionally, women with high-glycemic-load diets that were low in cereal fiber were more than twice as likely to develop type 2 DM than women with low-glycemic-load diets that were high in cereal fiber. The results of the Health Professionals' Follow-up Study (HPFS), which followed male health professionals over 6 years, were similar.[8] In the NHS II study, a prospective study of younger and middle-aged women, those who consumed foods with the highest glycemic-index values and the least cereal fiber were also at significantly higher risk of developing type 2 DM over the next 8 years.[9] The foods that were most consistently associated with increased risk of type 2 DM in the NHS and HPFS cohorts were potatoes (cooked or French-fried), white rice, white bread, and carbonated beverages.[6] The Black Women's Health study, a prospective study in a cohort of 59 000 black women in the United States, found that women who consumed foods with the highest glycemic-index values had a 23% greater risk of developing type 2 DM over 8 years of follow-up compared with those who consumed foods with the lowest glycemic-index values.[10] In the American Cancer Society Cancer Prevention Study II, which followed 124 907 men and women for 9 years, high glycemic load was associated with a 15% increased risk of type 2 DM.[11] Further, in a cohort of over 64 000 Chinese women participating in the Shanghai Women's Health Study, high glycemic load was associated with a 34% increase in risk of type 2 DM; this positive association was much stronger among overweight women.[12]

A US ecological study of national data from 1909 to 1997 found that increased consumption of refined carbohydrates in the form of corn syrup, coupled with declining intake of dietary fiber, has paralleled the increase in prevalence of type 2 DM.[13] Today, high-fructose corn syrup (HFCS) is used as a sweetener and preservative in many commercial products sold in the United States, including soft drinks and other processed foods. To make HFCS, the fructose content of corn syrup (100% glucose) has been artificially increased; common formulations of HFCS now include 42%, 55%, or 90% fructose.[13] When consumed in large quantities on a long-term basis, HFCS is unhealthful and may contribute to other chronic diseases besides type 2 DM, including obesity and cardiovascular disease.

Cardiovascular Disease

Impaired glucose tolerance and insulin resistance are known to be risk factors for cardiovascular disease and type 2 DM. In addition to increased blood glucose and insulin concentrations, high dietary glycemic loads are associated with increased serum triglyceride concentrations and decreased high-density lipoprotein (HDL) cholesterol concentrations; both are risk factors for cardiovascular disease.[14,15] High dietary glycemic loads have also been associated with increased serum levels of C-reactive protein, a marker of systemic inflammation that is also a sensitive

predictor of cardiovascular disease risk.[16] In the NHS cohort, women with the highest dietary glycemic loads had a risk of developing coronary heart disease (CHD) over the next 10 years that was almost twice as high as that of those with the lowest dietary glycemic loads.[17] The relationship between dietary glycemic load and CHD risk was more pronounced in overweight women, suggesting that people who are insulin resistant may be most susceptible to the adverse cardiovascular effects of high dietary glycemic loads.[1] A similar finding was reported in a cohort of middle-aged Dutch women followed for 9 years.[18] More recently, a prospective study in an Italian cohort of 47 749 men and women, who were followed for almost 8 years, found that a high glycemic load was associated with an increased risk of CHD in women but not in men.[19] Yet, studies to date have reported mixed results, and more research is needed to determine if diets with a low glycemic index decrease the risk for CHD.[20]

Obesity

In the first 2 hours after a meal, blood glucose and insulin levels rise higher after a meal with a high glycemic load than they do after a meal with a low glycemic load containing an equal number of calories. However, in response to the excess insulin secretion, blood glucose levels drop lower over the next few hours after a high-glycemic-load meal than they do after a low-glycemic-load meal. This may explain why 15 out of 16 published studies found that the consumption of low-glycemic-index foods delayed the return of hunger, decreased subsequent food intake, and increased satiety (feeling full) when compared with high-glycemic-index foods.[21] The results of several small, short-term trials (1–4 months) suggest that low-glycemic-load diets result in significantly more weight or fat loss than high-glycemic-load diets.[22-24] Although long-term randomized controlled trials of low-glycemic-load diets in the treatment of obesity are lacking, the results of short-term studies on appetite regulation and weight loss suggest that low-glycemic-load diets may be useful in promoting long-term weight loss and decreasing the prevalence of obesity. A recent review of six randomized controlled trials concluded that overweight or obese individuals who followed a low-glycemic-index/load diet experienced greater weight loss than individuals on a comparison diet that either had a high glycemic index or was energy restricted and low fat.[25] The length of the dietary interventions in these trials ranged from 5 weeks to 6 months.

Cancer

Evidence that high overall dietary glycemic index or high dietary glycemic loads are related to cancer risk is inconsistent. Prospective cohort studies in the United States, Denmark, France, and Australia have found no association between overall dietary glycemic index or dietary glycemic load and risk of breast cancer.[26–29] In contrast, a prospective cohort study in Italy reported a positive association between breast cancer risk and high-glycemic-index diets as well as high dietary glycemic loads.[30] A prospective study in Canada found that postmenopausal but not premenopausal women with high overall dietary glycemic-index values were at increased risk of breast cancer, particularly those who reported no vigorous physical activity,[31] while a prospective study in the United States found that premenopausal but not postmenopausal women with high overall dietary glycemic-index values and low levels of physical activity were at increased risk of breast cancer.[32] In a French study of postmenopausal women, both glycemic index and glycemic load were positively associated with risk of breast cancer but only in a subgroup of women who had the highest waist circumference (median of 84 cm [33 in]).[29] Higher dietary glycemic loads were associated with moderately increased risk of colorectal cancer in a prospective study of US men, but no clear associations between dietary glycemic load and colorectal cancer risk were observed in prospective studies of US men,[33] US women,[33–36] Swedish women,[37] and Dutch men and women.[38] However, one prospective cohort study of US women found that higher dietary glycemic loads were associated with increased risk of colorectal cancer.[39] A meta-analysis of case–control and cohort studies suggested that glycemic index and glycemic load were positively associated with colorectal cancer,[40] but a more recently published meta-analysis did not find glycemic index or load to be significantly associated with colorectal cancer.[41] Two separate meta-analyses reported that high dietary glycemic loads were associated with increased risk of

endometrial cancer.[40,42] Although there is some evidence that hyperinsulinemia (elevated serum insulin levels) may promote the growth of some types of cancer,[43] more research is needed to determine the effects of dietary glycemic load and/ or glycemic index on cancer risk.

Gallbladder Disease

Results of two studies indicate that dietary glycemic index and glycemic load may be positively related to risk of gallbladder disease. Higher dietary glycemic loads were associated with significantly increased risks of developing gallstones in a cohort of men participating in the HPFS[44] and in a cohort of women participating in the NHS.[45] Likewise, higher glycemic index diets were associated with increased risks of gallstone disease in both studies.[44,45] However, more epidemiological and clinical research is needed to determine an association between dietary glycemic index/load and gallbladder disease.

Disease Treatment

Diabetes Mellitus

Low-glycemic-index diets appear to improve the overall blood glucose control in people with type 1 and type 2 DM. A meta-analysis of 14 randomized controlled trials that included 356 patients with diabetes found that low-glycemic-index diets improved short-term and long-term control of blood glucose levels, reflected by clinically significant decreases in fructosamine and hemoglobin A_{1C} levels.[46] Episodes of serious hypoglycemia are a significant problem in people with type 1 DM. In a study of 63 men and women with type 1 DM, those randomized to a high-fiber, low-glycemic-index diet had significantly fewer episodes of hypoglycemia than those on a low-fiber, high-glycemic-index diet.[47]

Lowering Dietary Glycemic Load

Some strategies for lowering dietary glycemic load include:
- Increasing the consumption of whole grains, nuts, legumes, fruits, and nonstarchy vegetables

- Decreasing the consumption of starchy high-glycemic-index foods like potatoes, white rice, and white bread
- Decreasing the consumption of sugary foods like cookies, cakes, candy, and soft drinks

References

1. Liu S, Willett WC. Dietary glycemic load and athero-thrombotic risk. Curr Atheroscler Rep 2002;4(6):454–461
2. Ludwig DS. The glycemic index: physiological mechanisms relating to obesity, diabetes, and cardiovascular disease. JAMA 2002;287(18):2414–2423
3. Fernandes G, Velangi A, Wolever TM. Glycemic index of potatoes commonly consumed in North America. J Am Diet Assoc 2005;105(4):557–562
4. Foster-Powell K, Holt SH, Brand-Miller JC. International table of glycemic index and glycemic load values: 2002. Am J Clin Nutr 2002;76(1):5–56
5. Willett WC. Eat, Drink, and be Healthy: The Harvard Medical School Guide to Healthy Eating. New York: Simon & Schuster; 2001
6. Willett W, Manson J, Liu S. Glycemic index, glycemic load, and risk of type 2 diabetes. Am J Clin Nutr 2002;76(1):274S–280S
7. Salmerón J, Manson JE, Stampfer MJ, Colditz GA, Wing AL, Willett WC. Dietary fiber, glycemic load, and risk of non-insulin-dependent diabetes mellitus in women. JAMA 1997;277(6):472–477
8. Salmerón J, Ascherio A, Rimm EB, et al. Dietary fiber, glycemic load, and risk of NIDDM in men. Diabetes Care 1997;20(4):545–550
9. Schulze MB, Liu S, Rimm EB, Manson JE, Willett WC, Hu FB. Glycemic index, glycemic load, and dietary fiber intake and incidence of type 2 diabetes in younger and middle-aged women. Am J Clin Nutr 2004; 80(2):348–356
10. Krishnan S, Rosenberg L, Singer M, et al. Glycemic index, glycemic load, and cereal fiber intake and risk of type 2 diabetes in US black women. Arch Intern Med 2007;167(21):2304–2309
11. Patel AV, McCullough ML, Pavluck AL, Jacobs EJ, Thun MJ, Calle EE. Glycemic load, glycemic index, and carbohydrate intake in relation to pancreatic cancer risk in a large US cohort. Cancer Causes Control 2007; 18(3):287–294
12. Villegas R, Liu S, Gao YT, et al. Prospective study of dietary carbohydrates, glycemic index, glycemic load, and incidence of type 2 diabetes mellitus in middle-aged Chinese women. Arch Intern Med 2007; 167(21):2310–2316
13. Gross LS, Li L, Ford ES, Liu S. Increased consumption of refined carbohydrates and the epidemic of type 2 diabetes in the United States: an ecologic assessment. Am J Clin Nutr 2004;79(5):774–779
14. Ford ES, Liu S. Glycemic index and serum high-density lipoprotein cholesterol concentration among US adults. Arch Intern Med 2001;161(4):572–576
15. Liu S, Manson JE, Stampfer MJ, et al. Dietary glycemic load assessed by food-frequency questionnaire in relation to plasma high-density-lipoprotein cholesterol and fasting plasma triacylglycerols in postmenopausal women. Am J Clin Nutr 2001;73(3):560–566
16. Liu S, Manson JE, Buring JE, Stampfer MJ, Willett WC, Ridker PM. Relation between a diet with a high glycemic load and plasma concentrations of high-sensitivity C-reactive protein in middle-aged women. Am J Clin Nutr 2002;75(3):492–498
17. Liu S, Willett WC, Stampfer MJ, et al. A prospective study of dietary glycemic load, carbohydrate intake, and risk of coronary heart disease in US women. Am J Clin Nutr 2000;71(6):1455–1461
18. Beulens JW, de Bruijne LM, Stolk RP, et al. High dietary glycemic load and glycemic index increase risk of cardiovascular disease among middle-aged women: a population-based follow-up study. J Am Coll Cardiol 2007;50(1):14–21
19. Sieri S, Krogh V, Berrino F, et al. Dietary glycemic load and index and risk of coronary heart disease in a large italian cohort: the EPICOR study. Arch Intern Med 2010;170(7):640–647
20. Franz MJ. Is there a role for the glycemic index in coronary heart disease prevention or treatment? Curr Atheroscler Rep 2008;10(6):497–502
21. Ludwig DS. Dietary glycemic index and the regulation of body weight. Lipids 2003;38(2):117–121
22. Slabber M, Barnard HC, Kuyl JM, Dannhauser A, Schall R. Effects of a low-insulin-response, energy-restricted diet on weight loss and plasma insulin concentrations in hyperinsulinemic obese females. Am J Clin Nutr 1994;60(1):48–53
23. Bouché C, Rizkalla SW, Luo J, et al. Five-week, low-glycemic index diet decreases total fat mass and improves plasma lipid profile in moderately overweight nondiabetic men. Diabetes Care 2002;25(5):822–828
24. Spieth LE, Harnish JD, Lenders CM, et al. A low-glycemic index diet in the treatment of pediatric obesity. Arch Pediatr Adolesc Med 2000;154(9):947–951
25. Thomas DE, Elliott EJ, Baur L. Low glycaemic index or low glycaemic load diets for overweight and obesity. Cochrane Database Syst Rev 2007; (3):CD005105
26. Jonas CR, McCullough ML, Teras LR, Walker-Thurmond KA, Thun MJ, Calle EE. Dietary glycemic index, glycemic load, and risk of incident breast cancer in postmenopausal women. Cancer Epidemiol Biomarkers Prev 2003;12(6):573–577
27. Nielsen TG, Olsen A, Christensen J, Overvad K, Tjønneland A. Dietary carbohydrate intake is not associated with the breast cancer incidence rate ratio in postmenopausal Danish women. J Nutr 2005; 135(1):124–128
28. Giles GG, Simpson JA, English DR, et al. Dietary carbohydrate, fibre, glycaemic index, glycaemic load and the risk of postmenopausal breast cancer. Int J Cancer 2006;118(7):1843–1847
29. Lajous M, Boutron-Ruault MC, Fabre A, Clavel-Chapelon F, Romieu I. Carbohydrate intake, glycemic index, glycemic load, and risk of postmenopausal breast cancer in a prospective study of French women. Am J Clin Nutr 2008;87(5):1384–1391
30. Sieri S, Pala V, Brighenti F, et al. Dietary glycemic index, glycemic load, and the risk of breast cancer in an Italian prospective cohort study. Am J Clin Nutr 2007;86(4):1160–1166
31. Silvera SA, Jain M, Howe GR, Miller AB, Rohan TE. Dietary carbohydrates and breast cancer risk: a prospective study of the roles of overall glycemic index and glycemic load. Int J Cancer 2005;114(4):653–658
32. Higginbotham S, Zhang ZF, Lee IM, Cook NR, Buring JE, Liu S. Dietary glycemic load and breast cancer risk in the Women's Health Study. Cancer Epidemiol Biomarkers Prev 2004;13(1):65–70

33. Michaud DS, Fuchs CS, Liu S, Willett WC, Colditz GA, Giovannucci E. Dietary glycemic load, carbohydrate, sugar, and colorectal cancer risk in men and women. Cancer Epidemiol Biomarkers Prev 2005;14(1):138–147

34. Michaud DS, Liu S, Giovannucci E, Willett WC, Colditz GA, Fuchs CS. Dietary sugar, glycemic load, and pancreatic cancer risk in a prospective study. J Natl Cancer Inst 2002;94(17):1293–1300

35. McCarl M, Harnack L, Limburg PJ, Anderson KE, Folsom AR. Incidence of colorectal cancer in relation to glycemic index and load in a cohort of women. Cancer Epidemiol Biomarkers Prev 2006;15(5):892–896

36. Strayer L, Jacobs DR Jr, Schairer C, Schatzkin A, Flood A. Dietary carbohydrate, glycemic index, and glycemic load and the risk of colorectal cancer in the BCDDP cohort. Cancer Causes Control 2007;18(8):853–863

37. Larsson SC, Giovannucci E, Wolk A. Dietary carbohydrate, glycemic index, and glycemic load in relation to risk of colorectal cancer in women. Am J Epidemiol 2007;165(3):256–261

38. Weijenberg MP, Mullie PF, Brants HA, Heinen MM, Goldbohm RA, van den Brandt PA. Dietary glycemic load, glycemic index and colorectal cancer risk: results from the Netherlands Cohort Study. Int J Cancer 2008;122(3):620–629

39. Higginbotham S, Zhang ZF, Lee IM, et al; Women's Health Study. Dietary glycemic load and risk of colorectal cancer in the Women's Health Study. J Natl Cancer Inst 2004;96(3):229–233

40. Gnagnarella P, Gandini S, La Vecchia C, Maisonneuve P. Glycemic index, glycemic load, and cancer risk: a meta-analysis. Am J Clin Nutr 2008;87(6):1793–1801

41. Mulholland HG, Murray LJ, Cardwell CR, Cantwell MM. Glycemic index, glycemic load, and risk of digestive tract neoplasms: a systematic review and meta-analysis. Am J Clin Nutr 2009;89(2):568–576

42. Mulholland HG, Murray LJ, Cardwell CR, Cantwell MM. Dietary glycaemic index, glycaemic load and endometrial and ovarian cancer risk: a systematic review and meta-analysis. Br J Cancer 2008;99(3):434–441

43. Boyd DB. Insulin and cancer. Integr Cancer Ther 2003;2(4):315–329

44. Tsai CJ, Leitzmann MF, Willett WC, Giovannucci EL. Dietary carbohydrates and glycaemic load and the incidence of symptomatic gall stone disease in men. Gut 2005;54(6):823–828

45. Tsai CJ, Leitzmann MF, Willett WC, Giovannucci EL. Glycemic load, glycemic index, and carbohydrate intake in relation to risk of cholecystectomy in women. Gastroenterology 2005;129(1):105–112

46. Brand-Miller J, Hayne S, Petocz P, Colagiuri S. Low-glycemic index diets in the management of diabetes: a meta-analysis of randomized controlled trials. Diabetes Care 2003;26(8):2261–2267

47. Giacco R, Parillo M, Rivellese AA, et al. Long-term dietary treatment with increased amounts of fiber-rich low-glycemic index natural foods improves blood glucose control and reduces the number of hypoglycemic events in type 1 diabetic patients. Diabetes Care 2000;23(10):1461–1466

Appendix 2 Quick Reference to Diseases

Disease or Condition	Chapter Section	Food or Dietary Factor	Page(s)
Aging	Prevention	Coenzyme Q_{10}	217
		L-Carnitine	232
Alzheimer disease	Prevention	Fruits and vegetables	4
		Flavonoids	87
		Essential fatty acids	191
	Treatment	Curcumin	78
		Essential fatty acids	196
		Choline	212
		L-Carnitine	235
Angina pectoris	Treatment	Coenzyme Q_{10}	219
		L-Carnitine	234
Asthma	Treatment	Essential fatty acids	194
Athletic performance	Performance	Coenzyme Q_{10}	222
		L-Carnitine	237
Benign prostatic hyperplasia	Treatment	Phytosterols	166
Cancer (general)	Prevention	Fruits and vegetables	2
		Cruciferous vegetables	8
		Whole grains	25
		Tea	45
		Curcumin	76
		Flavonoids	86
		Isothiocyanates	111
		Indole-3-carbinol	119
		Phytosterols	165
		Resveratrol	177
		Choline	211
	Treatment	Curcumin	77
Breast cancer	Prevention	Cruciferous vegetables	9
		Legumes	16
		Soy Isoflavones	98
		Lignans	128
		Fiber	137
Colorectal cancer	Prevention	Cruciferous vegetables	9
		Coffee	33
		Fiber	137
		Organosulfur compounds (garlic)	154
Endometrial cancer	Prevention	Soy isoflavones	98
		Lignans	128

Disease or Condition	Chapter Section	Food or Dietary Factor	Page(s)
Gastric cancer	Prevention	Organosulfur compounds (garlic)	154
Liver cancer	Prevention	Coffee	33
		Chlorophyll and chlorophyllin	68
Lung cancer	Prevention	Cruciferous vegetables	8
		Carotenoids	54
Prostate cancer	Prevention	Cruciferous vegetables	9
		Legumes	15, 16
		Carotenoids	55
		Soy isoflavones	99
		Lignans	129
Cardiovascular disease (general)	Prevention	Fruits and vegetables	1
		Legumes	14
		Nuts	19
		Whole grains	25
		Tea	44
		Carotenoids	56
		Flavonoids	85
		Soy isoflavones	97
		Lignans	128
		Fiber	136
		Organosulfur compounds (garlic)	152
		Phytosterols	164
		Resveratrol	176
		Essential fatty acids	188
		Choline	211
		Coenzyme Q_{10}	217
	Treatment	Coenzyme Q_{10}	218
Angina pectoris	Treatment	Coenzyme Q_{10}	219
		Carnitine	234
Atherosclerosis	Prevention	Flavonoids	85
		Soy isoflavones	97
		Organosulfur compounds (garlic)	153
		Resveratrol	176, 177
		Essential fatty acids	190
		Coenzyme Q_{10}	217
	Treatment	Essential fatty acids	192
		Coenzyme Q_{10}	218
		Carnitine	233
Cardiac arrhythmias	Prevention	Nuts	20
		Essential fatty acids	189
	Safety	Coffee	35
Congestive heart failure	Treatment	Coenzyme Q_{10}	218

Disease or Condition	Chapter Section	Food or Dietary Factor	Page(s)
Coronary heart disease	Prevention	Fruits and vegetables	1
		Legumes	14
		Nuts	19
		Whole grains	25
		Flavonoids	85
		Fiber	136
		Phytosterols	165
		Resveratrol	176, 177
		Essential fatty acids	190
	Safety	Coffee	34
High homocysteine	Prevention	Legumes	15
		Choline	211
	Safety	Coffee	35
High total and LDL-cholesterol	Biological activities	Fiber	135
		Phytosterols	163
	Prevention	Soy isoflavones	97
		Organosulfur compounds (garlic)	153
		Essential fatty acids	189
High triglycerides	Prevention	Essential fatty acids	191
Hypertension	Treatment	Coenzyme Q_{10}	219
Intermittent claudication in peripheral arterial disease	Treatment	L-Carnitine	234
Myocardial infarction	Prevention	Fruits and vegetables	1
		Nuts	19
		Tea	45
		Fiber	136
		Essential fatty acids	190
	Treatment	Coenzyme Q_{10}	219
		L-Carnitine	233
Stroke	Prevention	Whole grains	25
		Essential fatty acids	190
Cataracts	Prevention	Fruits and vegetables	3
		Carotenoids	57
Chronic obstructive pulmonary disease	Prevention	Fruits and vegetables	4
Cognitive decline	Prevention	Soy isoflavones	100
	Treatment	Lipoic acid	247
Cystic fibrosis	Treatment	Curcumin	77
Decreased sperm motility	Treatment	L-Carnitine	236
Dental caries	Prevention	Tea	46
Depression	Treatment	Essential fatty acids	194

Disease or Condition	Chapter Section	Food or Dietary Factor	Page(s)
Diabetes mellitus, type 2	Prevention	Fruits and vegetables	2
		Legumes	14
		Nuts	20
		Whole grains	24
		Coffee	32
		Fiber	137
	Treatment	Essential fatty acids	193
		Lipoic acid	244
Diverticular disease	Prevention	Whole grains	26
		Fiber	138
Friedreich ataxia	Treatment	Coenzyme Q_{10}	222
HIV/AIDS	Treatment	L-Carnitine	235
Human papilloma virus infection	Treatment	Indole-3-carbinol	119
Huntington disease	Treatment	Coenzyme Q_{10}	221
Inflammatory bowel disease	Treatment	Essential fatty acids	193
Irritable bowel syndrome	Treatment	Fiber	139
Macular degeneration, age-related	Prevention	Fruits and vegetables	3
		Carotenoids	56
Menopausal symptoms	Treatment	Soy isoflavones	100
Mitochondrial encephalomyopathies	Treatment	Coenzyme Q_{10}	218
Multiple sclerosis	Treatment	Lipoic acid	247
Neurodegenerative diseases (general)	Prevention	Flavonoids	87
	Treatment	L-Carnitine	235
Alzheimer disease	Prevention	Fruits and vegetables	4
		Flavonoids	87
		Essential fatty acids	191
	Treatment	Curcumin	78
		Essential fatty acids	196
		Choline	212
		L-Carnitine	235
Friedreich ataxia	Treatment	Coenzyme Q_{10}	222
Huntington disease	Treatment	Coenzyme Q_{10}	221
Parkinson disease	Prevention	Coffee	32
	Treatment	Coenzyme Q_{10}	220
Osteoporosis	Prevention	Fruits and vegetables	3
		Tea	46
		Soy isoflavones	99
		Lignans	129
Parkinson disease	Prevention	Coffee	32
	Treatment	Coenzyme Q_{10}	220
Pregnancy complications	Prevention	Essential fatty acids	187
		Choline	211

Disease or Condition	Chapter Section	Food or Dietary Factor	Page(s)
Renal disease			
IgA nephropathy	Treatment	Essential fatty acids	194
Kidney failure/dialysis	Treatment	L-Carnitine	235
Kidney stones	Prevention	Tea	47
Rheumatoid arthritis	Treatment	Essential fatty acids	193
Schizophrenia	Treatment	Essential fatty acids	195
Systemic lupus erythematosus	Treatment	Indole-3-carbinol	120

Appendix 3 **Drug Interactions**

Drug classes are listed first, alphabetically, followed by specific drugs known to interact with dietary factors. Specific drugs are listed alphabetically by their generic name. A common US brand name is usually listed in parentheses after the generic name. Because there may be interactions with dietary factors that are not listed in the table below, it is important to review the prescribing or patient information of any medication prior to its use for the possibility of clinically significant interactions. This table does not address the potential for multiple interactions in individuals taking more than one medication or dietary supplement.

Drug Class	Dietary Factor	Interaction	Page(s)
Adrenergic agonists	Caffeine (coffee and tea)	Caffeine may enhance adrenergic effects and side effects	37, 48
Antibiotics	Soy isoflavones	Because soy isoflavones are metabolized by colonic bacteria, antibiotic therapy could decrease their biological activity	103
Antibiotics (pivalate-conjugated)	L-Carnitine	Pivalic acid containing antibiotics (pivampicillin, pivmecillinam, and pivcephalexin) may produce a secondary L-carnitine deficiency	238
Antibiotics (quinolones)	Caffeine (coffee and tea)	Quinolone class antibiotics impair hepatic caffeine metabolism, increasing the risk of caffeine-related side effects	36, 48
Anticoagulants and platelet inhibitors	Curcumin	Curcumin inhibits platelet aggregation in vitro, potentially increasing the risk of bleeding in people on anticoagulant therapy	79
	Flavonoids	High intakes of flavonoids from grape juice and dark chocolate may inhibit platelet aggregation, potentially increasing the risk of bleeding in people on anticoagulant therapy	90
	Soy protein (soy isoflavones)	High intakes of soy protein may interfere with the efficacy of the anticoagulant medication, warfarin (Coumadin)	103
	Garlic	Garlic supplements may inhibit platelet aggregation, potentially increasing the risk of bleeding in people on anticoagulant therapy	157
	Borage oil or evening primrose oil (omega-6 fatty acids)	High intakes of γ-linolenic acid may inhibit platelet aggregation, potentially increasing the risk of bleeding in people on anticoagulant therapy	199
	Flaxseed oil, fish oil, or EPA/DHA supplements (omega-3 fatty acids)	High intakes of omega-3 fatty acids, particularly fish oil (EPA/DHA), may inhibit platelet aggregation and increase the risk of bleeding in people on anticoagulant therapy	199
	Coenzyme Q_{10}	Concomitant use of warfarin (Coumadin) and coenzyme Q_{10} supplements has been shown to decrease the anticoagulant effect of warfarin	224

Drug Class	Dietary Factor	Interaction	Page(s)
Antidiabetic agents	Lipoic acid	Lipoic acid supplementation may improve insulin-mediated glucose utilization and thus increase the risk of hypoglycemia in people using insulin or antidiabetic agents	248
Benzodiazepines	Grapefruit juice (flavonoids)	Flavonoids and other compounds in grapefruit juice inhibit CYP3A4, increasing the bioavailability and risk of toxicity from benzodiazepines	90
Calcium channel antagonists	Grapefruit juice (flavonoids)	Flavonoids and other compounds in grapefruit juice inhibit CYP3A4, increasing the bioavailability and risk of toxicity from calcium channel antagonists	90
Estrogens	Caffeine (coffee and tea)	Estrogens impair hepatic caffeine metabolism, increasing the risk of caffeine-related side effects	36, 48
HMG-CoA reductase inhibitors (statins)	Grapefruit juice (flavonoids)	Flavonoids and other compounds in grapefruit juice inhibit CYP3A4, increasing the bioavailability and risk of toxicity from HMG-CoA reductase inhibitors (statins)	90
	Phytosterols	The LDL-cholesterol-lowering effect of plant sterols or stanols may be additive to that of HMG-CoA reductase inhibitors (statins)	168
	Coenzyme Q_{10}	Use of HMG-CoA reductase inhibitors (statins) may decrease the endogenous synthesis of coenzyme Q_{10}	224
Nucleoside analogues	L-Carnitine	Nuceoside analogues used in the treatment of HIV infection may produce a secondary L-carnitine deficiency	238
Phenothiazines	Borage oil or evening primrose oil (omega-6 fatty acids)	High doses of γ-linolenic acid may increase the risk of seizure in people on phenothiazines	199

[a] Not available in the United States.
CYP, cytochrome P450; DHA, docosahexaenoic acid; EPA, eicosapentaenoic acid; LDL, low-density lipoprotein.

Specific Drug	Dietary Factor	Interaction	Page(s)
Acetaminophen (paracetamol; Tylenol)	Caffeine (coffee and tea)	Caffeine may decrease the elimination of acetaminophen and enhance its analgesic effect	37
	Guar gum (fiber)	Guar gum may slow the absorption of acetaminophen when taken at the same time	142
Amiodarone (Cordarone, Pacerone)	Grapefruit juice (flavonoids)	Flavonoids and other compounds in grapefruit juice inhibit CYP3A4, increasing the bioavailability and risk of toxicity from amiodarone	90
Aspirin	Caffeine (coffee and tea)	Caffeine may decrease the elimination of aspirin and enhance its analgesic effect	37
Bumetanide (Bumex)	Guar gum (fiber)	Guar gum may slow the absorption of bumetanide when taken at the same time	142
Buspirone (BuSpar)	Grapefruit juice (flavonoids)	Flavonoids and other compounds in grapefruit juice inhibit cytochrome P450 CYP 3A4, increasing the bioavailability and risk of toxicity from buspirone	90
Carbamazepine (Tegretol)	Grapefruit juice (flavonoids)	Flavonoids and other compounds in grapefruit juice inhibit CYP3A4, increasing the bioavailability and risk of toxicity from carbamazepine	90
	Psyllium (fiber)	Psyllium may decrease the absorption of carbamazepine when taken at the same time	142
Ciclosporin (Neoral)	Grapefruit juice (flavonoids)	Flavonoids and other compounds in grapefruit juice inhibit CYP3A4, increasing the bioavailability and risk of toxicity from ciclosporin	90
Cimetidine (Tagamet)	Caffeine (coffee and tea)	Cimetidine impairs hepatic caffeine metabolism, increasing the risk of caffeine-related side effects	36, 48
Cisapride (Propulsid)	Grapefruit juice (flavonoids)	Flavonoids and other compounds in grapefruit juice inhibit CYP3A4, increasing the bioavailability and risk of toxicity from cisapride	90
Cisplatin	L-Carnitine	Use of cisplatin may increase the risk of secondary L-carnitine deficiency	238
Clozapine (Clozaril)	Caffeine (coffee and tea)	Caffeine may inhibit the hepatic metabolism of clozapine and increase the risk of toxicity	37, 48
Colestipol (Colestid)	Carotenoids	Colestipol may inhibit carotenoid absorption	61
Colestyramine (Questran)	Carotenoids	Colestyramine may inhibit carotenoid absorption	61
Cyclophosphamide (Cytoxan)	Curcumin	Oral curcumin administration inhibited cyclophosphamide-induced tumor regression in an animal model of breast cancer	79
Digoxin (Lanoxin)	Psyllium (fiber)	Psyllium may decrease the absorption of digoxin when taken at the same time	142
	Guar gum (fiber)	Guar gum may slow the absorption of digoxin when taken at the same time	142
Disulfiram (Antabuse)	Caffeine (coffee and tea)	Disulfiram impairs hepatic caffeine metabolism, increasing the risk of caffeine-related side effects	36, 48

Specific Drug	Dietary Factor	Interaction	Page(s)
Fluconazole (Diflucan)	Caffeine (coffee and tea)	Fluconazole impairs hepatic caffeine metabolism, increasing the risk of caffeine-related side effects	36, 48
Fluvoxamine (Luvox)	Caffeine (coffee and tea)	Fluvoxamine impairs hepatic caffeine metabolism, increasing the risk of caffeine-related side effects	36, 48
Glibenclamide (glyburide; Glynase)	Guar gum (fiber)	Guar gum may decrease the absorption of glibenclamide when taken at the same time	142
Ifosfamide	L-Carnitine	Use of ifosfamide may increase the risk of secondary L-carnitine deficiency	238
Levothyroxine	Soy protein (soy isoflavones)	Soy protein may decrease the bioavailability of levothyroxine when consumed at the same time	103
Lithium	Caffeine (coffee and tea)	Caffeine may enhance the elimination of lithium and decrease plasma lithium concentrations	37, 48
	Psyllium (fiber)	Psyllium may decrease the absorption of lithium when taken at the same time	142
Losartan (Cozaar)	Grapefruit juice (flavonoids)	Flavonoids and other compounds in grapefruit juice inhibit CYP3A4, potentially decreasing the therapeutic effect of losartan	90
Lovastatin (Mevacor)	Pectin (fiber)	Pectin may decrease the absorption of lovastatin when taken at the same time	142
Metformin (Glucophage)	Guar gum (fiber)	Guar gum may decrease the absorption of metformin when taken at the same time	142
Methotrexate	Choline	Methotrexate treatment of rats diminishes choline status, thus methotrexate may increase the choline requirement	213
Mexiletine (Mexitil)	Caffeine (coffee and tea)	Mexiletine impairs hepatic caffeine metabolism, increasing the risk of caffeine-related side effects.	36, 48
Orlistat (Xenical)	Carotenoids	Orlistat may inhibit carotenoid absorption	61
Penicillin	Guar gum (fiber)	Guar gum may decrease the absorption of penicillin when taken at the same time	142
Phenytoin (Dilantin)	Caffeine (coffee and tea)	Phenytoin increases hepatic caffeine metabolism	37
	Piperine (in some curcumin supplements)	Piperine may slow the elimination of phenytoin	79
Propranolol (Inderal)	Piperine (in some curcumin supplements)	Piperine may slow the elimination of propranolol	79
Saquinavir (Fortovase, Invirase)	Grapefruit juice (flavonoids)	Flavonoids and other compounds in grapefruit juice inhibit CYP3A4, increasing the bioavailability and risk of toxicity from saquinavir	90
	Garlic	Garlic supplements may decrease the bioavailability of saquinavir	157

Specific Drug	Dietary Factor	Interaction	Page(s)
Sertraline (Zoloft)	Grapefruit juice (flavonoids)	Flavonoids and other compounds in grapefruit juice inhibit CYP3A4, increasing the bioavailability and risk of toxicity from sertraline	90
Sildenafil (Viagra)	Grapefruit juice (flavonoids)	Flavonoids and other compounds in grapefruit juice inhibit CYP3A4, increasing the bioavailability and risk of toxicity from sildenafil	90
Tamoxifen (Nolvadex)	Soy isoflavones	Some evidence from animal studies suggests that high intakes of soy isoflavones, particularly genistein, can interfere with the antitumor effects of tamoxifen	103
Terbinafine (Lamisil)	Caffeine (coffee and tea)	Terbinafine impairs hepatic caffeine metabolism, increasing the risk of caffeine-related side effects	36, 48
Terfenadine (Seldane)[a]	Grapefruit juice (flavonoids)	Flavonoids and other compounds in grapefruit juice inhibit CYP3A4, increasing the bioavailability and risk of toxicity from terfenadine	90
Theophylline	Caffeine (coffee and tea)	Caffeine may decrease the elimination of theophylline and increase plasma theophylline levels	37, 48
	Piperine (in some curcumin supplements)	Piperine may slow the elimination of theophylline	79
Valproic acid (Depakene, Depakote, Epilim, Stavzor)	L-Carnitine	Use of the anticonvulsant, valproic acid, may produce a secondary L-carnitine deficiency	238
Warfarin (Coumadin)	Green tea	Excessive green tea intake may decrease the efficacy of warfarin	48
	Soy protein	High intakes of soy protein may decrease the efficacy of warfarin	103
	Psyllium (fiber)	Psyllium may decrease the absorption of warfarin when taken at the same time	142
	Garlic	Garlic supplements may increase the anticoagulant effects of warfarin	157
	Flaxseed oil, fish oil, or EPA/DHA supplements (omega-3 fatty acids)	High intakes of omega-3 fatty acids, particularly fish oil (EPA/DHA), may inhibit platelet aggregation and increase the risk of bleeding in people taking warfarin	199
	Coenzyme Q_{10}	Concomitant use of warfarin and coenzyme Q_{10} supplements may decrease the anticoagulant effect of warfarin	224

[a] Not available in the United States.

CYP, cytochrome P450; DHA, docosahexaenoic acid; EPA, eicosapentaenoic acid; LDL, low-density lipoprotein.

Appendix 4   Nutrient Interactions

Nutrient	Phytochemical or Dietary Factor	Interaction	Page(s)
Iodine	Cruciferous vegetables	Extremely high intakes of cruciferous vegetables may cause hypothyroidism	10
Calcium	Caffeine (coffee and tea)	Caffeine may decrease the absorption of calcium slightly	37
	Inulin and oligofructose (fiber)	Limited evidence suggests inulin and oligofructose may enhance calcium absorption	142
Iron	Flavonoids and phenolic compounds in coffee, tea, and cocoa	Flavonoids and other phenolic compounds in coffee, tea, and cocoa inhibit the absorption of nonheme iron when consumed at the same time	37, 48, 90
β-Carotene and other carotenoids	Pectin and guar gum (fiber)	Pectin and guar gum may decrease the absorption of β-carotene, lutein, and lycopene consumed at the same time	142
	Phytosterols	At doses used to lower low-density lipoprotein LDL cholesterol, plant sterols or stanols may decrease plasma α-carotene, β-carotene, and lycopene concentrations	168
Vitamin E	Omega-3 fatty acids	People on high doses of omega-3 fatty acids (EPA/DHA) may require additional vitamin E	199
	Coenzyme Q_{10}	Coenzyme Q_{10} and α-tocopherol are the principal fat-soluble antioxidants in membranes and lipoproteins	215, 216
Lysine, methionine, niacin, vitamin B_6, and iron	L-Carnitine	Endogenous biosynthesis of L-carnitine requires several nutrients, including lysine and methionine, niacin, vitamin B_6, and iron	232

DHA, docosahexaenoic acid; EPA, eicosapentaenoic acid; LDL, low-density lipoprotein.

Appendix 5 Quick Reference to Foods Rich in Phytochemicals or Other Dietary Factors

Some foods that are rich in the phytochemicals or other dietary factors discussed in this book are listed in the table below. Information about the food sources of a specific dietary factor may be found in the chapter on that phytochemical or dietary factor under "Sources."

Food	Class or Color	Examples	Phytochemicals or Dietary Factors
Vegetables	Dark green vegetables	Chard, spinach	Carotenoids (lutein and zeaxanthin), chlorophyll, fiber, lipoic acid
	Yellow and orange vegetables	Carrots, pumpkin, squash, sweet potato	Carotenoids (α-carotene, β-carotene, β-cryptoxanthin), fiber
	Cruciferous vegetables	Brussels sprouts, broccoli, garden cress, kale, mustard greens	Carotenoids (lutein and zeaxanthin), chlorophyll, isothiocyanates, indoles, lignans, fiber, phytosterols, choline, lipoic acid
	Legumes	Soy and dried beans, peas, lentils	Flavonoids (isoflavones), fiber, phytosterols, choline, lipoic acid
	Allium vegetables	Onions, leeks, chives, garlic	Flavonoids (flavonols), fiber, organosulfur compounds
Fruits	Berries	Strawberries, raspberries, blueberries	Flavonoids (anthocyanins, flavanols, flavonols), lignans, fiber, resveratrol
	Grapes	Red and purple grapes	Flavonoids (anthocyanins, flavanols, flavonols), fiber, resveratrol
	Citrus fruits	Grapefruits, oranges, lemons	Flavonoids (flavanones), fiber
	Red fruits	Apples	Flavonoids (flavanols, flavonols), fiber
		Tomatoes, watermelon	Carotenoids (lycopene), fiber lipoic acid (in tomatoes)
Nuts and seeds	Nuts	Almonds, pine nuts, walnuts	Fiber, phytosterols, essential fatty acids, coenzyme Q_{10}
	Legumes	Peanuts	Fiber, phytosterols, resveratrol, essential fatty acids, choline, coenzyme Q_{10}
	Seeds	Flaxseeds, sesame seeds	Lignans, fiber, phytosterols, essential fatty acids, coenzyme Q_{10}
Whole grains		Brown rice, barley, oats, rye, whole wheat	Lignans, fiber, phytosterols
Spices		Turmeric	Curcumin
		Parsley	Chlorophyll, flavonoids (flavones)
		Garlic	Organosulfur compounds

Food	Class or Color	Examples	Phytochemicals or Dietary Factors
Animal products	Dairy		Choline, coenzyme Q_{10}, L-carnitine
	Eggs		Choline, coenzyme Q_{10}
	Fish		Choline, coenzyme Q_{10}, L-carnitine, DHA and EPA[a]
	Poultry		Choline, coenzyme Q_{10}, L-carnitine
	Meat	Beef, pork	Choline, coenzyme Q_{10}, L-carnitine
	Organ meats	Liver	Choline, lipoic acid
		Kidney, heart	Lipoic acid

DHA, docosahaenoic acid; EPA, eicosapentaenoic acid.
[a] Not considered nutritionally essential

Appendix 6   **Glossary**

Acetylation. The addition of an acetyl group ($-COCH_3$) to a molecule.

Acidic. Having a pH less than 7.

Acute. Having a short and relatively severe course.

Adipose tissue. Specialized connective tissue that functions to store body fat as triglycerides.

Adjunct therapy. A treatment or therapy used in addition to another, not alone.

Aglycone. The nonsugar component of a glycoside. Cleavage of the glycosidic bond of a glycoside results in the formation of a sugar and an aglycone.

AI. Adequate intake. Established by the Food and Nutrition Board of the US Institute of Medicine, the AI is a recommended intake value based on observed or experimentally determined estimates of nutrient intake by a group of healthy people that are assumed to be adequate. An AI is established when an RDA (recommended dietary allowance) cannot be determined.

AIDS. Acquired immune deficiency syndrome. AIDS is caused by HIV (human immunodeficiency virus), which attacks the immune system, leaving the infected individual vulnerable to opportunistic infections.

Alkaline. Basic; having a pH greater than 7.

Alkaloid. A plant-derived compound that is biologically active, contains a nitrogen in a heterocyclic ring, is alkaline, has a complex structure, and is of limited distribution in the plant kingdom.

Alzheimer disease. The most common cause of dementia in older adults. Alzheimer disease is characterized by the formation of amyloid plaque in the brain and nerve cell degeneration. Symptoms include memory loss and confusion, which worsen over time.

Amino acids. Organic (carbon-containing) molecules that serve as the building blocks of proteins.

Amyloid plaque. Aggregates of a peptide called amyloid-β, which accumulate and form deposits in the brain in Alzheimer disease.

Anaerobic. Refers to the absence of oxygen or the absence of a need for oxygen.

Anaphylaxis. A rapidly developing and severe systemic allergic reaction. Symptoms may include swelling of the tongue, throat, and trachea, which can result in difficulty breathing, shock, and loss of consciousness. If not treated rapidly, anaphylaxis can be fatal.

Anemia. The condition of having less than the normal number of red blood cells or hemoglobin in the blood, resulting in diminished oxygen transport. Anemia has many causes, including iron, vitamin B_{12}, or folate deficiency; bleeding; abnormal hemoglobin formation (e.g., sickle cell anemia); rupture of red blood cells (hemolytic anemia); and bone marrow diseases.

Anencephaly. A birth defect, known as a neural tube defect, resulting from failure of the upper end of the neural tube to close during embryonic development. Anencephaly is a devastating and sometimes fatal birth defect resulting in the absence of most or all of the cerebral hemispheres of the brain.

Angina pectoris. Pain generally experienced in the chest, but sometimes radiating to the arms or jaw, due to a lack of oxygen supply to the heart muscle.

Angiogenesis. The development of new blood vessels.

Angiography (coronary). Imaging of the coronary arteries used to identify the location and severity of any obstructions. Coronary angiography typically involves the administration of a contrast medium and imaging of the coronary arteries using an X-ray-based technique.

Anion. A negatively charged ion.

Antagonist. A substance that counteracts or nullifies the biological effects of another, such as a compound that binds to a receptor but does not elicit a biological response.

Anticoagulant. A class of compounds that inhibit blood clotting.

Anticonvulsant. A class of medication used to prevent seizures.

Antigen. A substance that is capable of eliciting an immune response.

Antihistamine. A chemical that blocks the effect of histamine in susceptible tissues. Histamine is released by immune cells during an allergic reaction and also during infection with viruses that cause the common cold. The interaction of histamine with the mucus membranes of the eyes and nose results in "watery eyes" and the "runny nose" often accompanying allergies and colds. Antihistamines can help alleviate such symptoms.

Antimicrobial. Capable of killing or inhibiting the growth of microorganisms, such as bacteria.

Antioxidant. Any substance that prevents or reduces damage caused by reactive oxygen species (ROS) or reactive nitrogen species (RNS).

Apoptosis. Gene-directed cell death or programmed cell death that occurs when age, condition, or state of cell health dictates. Cells that die by apoptosis do not usually elicit the inflammatory responses that are associated with necrosis. Cancer cells are resistant to apoptosis.

Arrhythmia. An abnormal heart rhythm. The heart rhythm may be too fast (tachycardia), too slow (bradycardia), or irregular. Some arrhythmias, such as ventricular fibrillation, may lead to cardiac arrest if not treated promptly.

Asthma. A chronic inflammatory disease of the airways, characterized by recurrent episodes of reversible airflow obstruction.

Ataxia. A lack of coordination or unsteadiness, usually related to a disturbance in the cerebellum, a part of the brain that regulates coordination and equilibrium.

Atherogenic. Capable of producing atherosclerosis.

Atherosclerosis. An inflammatory disease resulting in the accumulation of cholesterol-laden plaque in artery walls. Rupture of atherosclerotic plaque results in clot formation, which may result in myocardial infarction or ischemic stroke.

ATP. Adenosine triphosphate. An important compound for the storage of energy in cells, as well as the synthesis of nucleic acids.

Atria. The two upper chambers of the heart that receive blood from the veins and contract to force that blood into the ventricles.

Atrial fibrillation. A cardiac arrhythmia, characterized by rapid, uncoordinated beating of the atria, which results in ineffective atrial contractions. Atrial fibrillation is known as a supraventricular arrhythmia because it originates above the ventricles.

Atrophy. Decrease in size or wasting away of a body part or tissue.

Autoimmune disease. A condition in which the body's immune system reacts against its own tissues.

Autophosphorylation. The phosphorylation by a protein of one or more of its own amino acid residues. Autophosphorylation does not necessarily occur on the same polypeptide chain as the catalytic site. In a dimer, one subunit may phosphorylate the other.

Autosomal. Refers to a trait or gene that is not located on the X or Y chromosome (not sex-linked).

Bacteria. Single-celled organisms that can exist independently, symbiotically (in cooperation with another organism), or parasitically (dependent upon another organism, sometimes to the detriment of the other organism). Examples of bacteria include acidophilus (found in yogurt); streptococcus, the cause of strep throat; and *Escherichia coli* (a normal intestinal bacteria, as well as a disease-causing agent).

Benign prostatic hyperplasia. The term used to describe a noncancerous enlargement of the prostate.

Bias. Any systematic error in an epidemiological study that results in an incorrect estimate of the association between an exposure and disease risk.

Bile. A yellow–green fluid made in the liver and stored in the gallbladder. Bile may then pass through the common bile duct into the small intestine where some of its components aid in the digestion of fat.

Bile acids. Components of bile, which are formed by the metabolism of cholesterol, and aid in the digestion of fats.

Bioavailability. The fraction of an administered compound that reaches the systemic circulation and is transported to the site of action (target tissue).

Biomarker. A physical, functional, or biochemical indicator of a physiological or disease process.

Biotransformation enzymes (phase I and phase II). Enzymes involved in the metabolism and elimination of a variety of exogenous (drugs, toxins, and carcinogens) and endogenous compounds (steroid hormones). In general, phase I biotransformation enzymes, including those of the cytochrome P450 family, catalyze reactions that increase the reactivity of fat-soluble compounds and prepare them for reactions catalyzed by phase II biotransformation enzymes. Reactions catalyzed by phase II enzymes generally increase water solubility and promote the elimination of these compounds.

Bipolar disorder. A mood disorder previously called "manic-depressive illness." Bipolar disorder is characterized by severe alterations in mood. During "manic" episodes, a person may experience extreme elevation in energy level and mood (euphoria) or extreme agitation and irritability. Episodes of depressed mood are also common in bipolar disorder.

Body mass index (BMI). Body weight in kilograms divided by height in meters squared. In adults, BMI is a measure of body fat: underweight, <18.5 kg/m^2; normal weight, 18.5–24.9 kg/m^2; overweight, 25–29.9 kg/m^2; obese, ≥ 30 kg/m^2.

Bone mineral density (BMD). The amount of mineral in a given area of bone. BMD is positively associated with bone strength and resistance to fracture, and measurements of BMD are used to diagnose osteoporosis.

Bronchitis, chronic. Long-standing inflammation of the airways, characterized by excess production of sputum, leading to a chronic cough and obstruction of air flow. Cigarette smoking is the most common cause of chronic bronchitis.

Buffer. A chemical used to maintain the pH of a system by absorbing hydrogen ions (which would make it more acidic) or absorbing hydroxyl ions (which would make it more alkaline).

C-reactive protein. A protein that is produced in the liver in response to inflammation. CRP is a biomarker of inflammation that is strongly associated with the risk of cardiovascular events, such as myocardial infarction and stroke.

Cancer. Refers to abnormal cells, which have a tendency to grow uncontrollably and metastasize or spread to other areas of the body. Cancer can involve any tissue of the body and can have different forms in one tissue. Cancer is a group of more than 100 different diseases.

Carbohydrate. Considered a macronutrient because carbohydrates provide a significant source of calories (energy) in the diet. Chemically, carbohydrates are neutral compounds composed of carbon, hydrogen, and oxygen. Carbohydrates come in simple forms known as sugars, and complex forms, such as starches and fiber.

Carcinogen. A cancer-causing agent; adjective: carcinogenic.

Carcinogenesis. The formation of cancer cells from normal cells.

Cardiomyopathy. Literally, disease of the heart muscle that often leads to abnormal function.

Cardiovascular. Referring to the heart and blood vessels.

Cardiovascular diseases. Literally, diseases affecting the heart and blood vessels. The term has come to encompass several conditions that result from atherosclerosis, including myocardial infarction (heart attack), congestive heart failure, and stroke.

Carotid arteries. The left and right common carotid arteries are the principal blood vessels that supply oxygenated blood to the head and neck. Each has two main branches, the external and internal carotid artery.

Case–control study. A study, in which exposures of people who have been diagnosed with a disease (cases) are compared with those of people without the disease (controls). The results of case–control studies are more likely to be distorted by bias in the selection of cases and controls (selection bias) and recall (recall bias) than prospective cohort studies.

Case reports. Individual observations based on small numbers of subjects. This type of research cannot indicate causality but may indicate areas for further research.

Catabolism. The breakdown of complex molecules into smaller ones, accompanied by the release of energy.

Catalyze. Increase the speed of a chemical reaction without being changed in the overall reaction process. See enzyme.

Cataract. Clouding of the lens of the eye. As cataracts progress, they can impair vision.

Cell adhesion molecules. Molecules on the outside surfaces of cells that bind to other cells or to the extracellular matrix (material surrounding cells). Cell adhesion molecules influence many important functions, including the entry of immune cells into the arterial wall.

Cell cycle. The orderly sequence of stages that a cell passes through between one cell division (mitosis) and the next. The cell cycle can be divided into four stages: the M (mitosis) phase, in which nuclear and cytoplasmic division occurs; the G1 phase or interphase; the S (synthesis) phase, in which DNA replication occurs; and the G2 phase, a quiescent period prior to the next M phase.

Cell membrane. Also called a plasma membrane, the barrier that separates the contents of a cell from its outside environment and controls what moves in and out of the cell. A mammalian cell membrane consists of a phospholipid bilayer with embedded proteins and cholesterol.

Cell signaling. Communication among individual cells to coordinate their behavior to benefit the organism as a whole. Cell-signaling systems elucidated in animal cells include cell-surface and intracellular receptor proteins and GTP-binding proteins, as well as protein kinases and protein phosphatases (enzymes that phosphorylate and dephosphorylate proteins).

Central nervous system. The brain, spinal cord, and spinal nerves.

Ceramide. A specialized type of lipid comprised of a sphingosine backbone with fatty acid side chains. Ceramides function as signaling molecules and are critical structural components in cell membranes.

Cervical intraepithelial neoplasia (CIN). A term used to describe abnormal growth of cells on the surface of the uterine cervix. CIN1 is also known as low-grade squamous intraepithelial lesion (LSIL). CIN2 and CIN3 are also known as high-grade squamous intraepithelial lesions (HSIL). Although these abnormal cells are not cancerous, they may progress to cervical cancer.

Chelate. The combination of a metal with an organic molecule to form a ring-like structure known as a chelate. Chelation of a metal may inhibit or enhance its bioavailability.

Chemotherapy. Literally, treatment with drugs. Commonly used to describe the systemic use of drugs to kill cancer cells as a form of cancer treatment.

Cholesterol. A compound that is an integral structural component of cell membranes and a precursor in the synthesis of steroid hormones. Dietary cholesterol is obtained from animal sources, but cholesterol is also synthesized by the liver. Cholesterol is carried in the blood by lipoproteins. In atherosclerosis, cholesterol accumulates in plaques on the walls of some arteries.

Chromosome. A structure in the nucleus of a cell that contains genes. Chromosomes are composed of DNA and associated proteins. Normal human cells contain 46 chromosomes (22 pairs of autosomes and two sex chromosomes).

Chronic disease. An illness lasting a long time. As defined by the US Center for Health Statistics, a chronic disease is a disease lasting 3 months or more.

Chronic obstructive pulmonary disease (COPD). A term that includes emphysema and chronic bronchitis, two chronic lung diseases that are characterized by airway obstruction.

Chylomicrons. Triglyceride-rich lipoproteins that deliver dietary triglycerides from the intestine to the tissues immediately after a meal. Chylomicrons release their triglycerides to tissue through the activity of lipoprotein lipase enzymes in tissue capillary beds. When they are depleted of most of their triglycerides, chylomicron remnants are taken up by the liver, where the lipids and cholesterol that remain are excreted in bile or incorporated into other lipoproteins.

Cirrhosis. A condition characterized by irreversible scarring of the liver, leading to abnormal liver function. Cirrhosis has several different causes, including chronic alcohol use and viral hepatitis B and C.

Clinical trial. An intervention trial generally used to evaluate the efficacy and/or safety of a treatment or intervention in human participants.

Coagulation. The process involved in blood clot formation.

Coenzyme. A molecule that binds to an enzyme and is essential for its activity but is not permanently altered by the reaction. Many coenzymes are derived from vitamins.

Cofactor. A compound that is essential for the activity of an enzyme.

Cognition. Mental process of thought, including brain functions like attention, memory, planning, developing strategies, and problem solving.

Cognitive. Referring to the processes of cognition.

Cohort. A group of people who are followed over time as part of an epidemiological study.

Cohort study. A study that follows a large group of people over a long period of time, often 10 years or more. In cohort studies, dietary information is gathered before disease occurs, rather than relying on recall after disease develops.

Collagen. A fibrous protein that is the basis for the structure of skin, tendon, bone, cartilage, and all other connective tissue.

Colon. The portion of the large intestine that extends from the end of the small intestine to the rectum. The colon removes water from digested food after it has passed through the small intestine, and stores the remaining stool until it can be evacuated.

Colorectal adenoma. A polyp or growth in the lining of the colon or rectum. Although they are not cancerous, colorectal adenomas may develop into colorectal cancer over time.

Colorectal cancer. Cancer of the colon (large intestine) or rectum.

Colostomy. The surgical construction of an artificial anus by connecting the colon to an opening in the abdominal wall.

Concomitant. Accompanying. "Concomitant intake" refers to the intake of two compounds at the same time.

Congenital malformation. Birth defect.

Congestive heart failure. A condition in which the heart loses the ability to pump blood efficiently enough to meet the demands of the body. Symptoms may include edema (swelling), shortness of breath, weakness and exercise intolerance.

Conjugation. The formation of a water-soluble derivative of a chemical by its combination with another compound, such as glutathione, glucuronate, or sulfate.

Coronary artery. One of the vessels that supply oxygenated blood to the heart muscle itself. They are called coronary arteries because they encircle the heart in the form of a crown.

Coronary artery bypass graft (CABG). A surgical procedure used to create new routes around obstructions in coronary arteries and restore adequate blood flow to the heart muscle.

Coronary heart disease (CHD). Also known as coronary artery disease and coronary disease, coronary heart disease is the result of atherosclerosis of the coronary arteries. Atherosclerosis may result in narrowing or blockage of the coronary arteries and is the underlying cause of myocardial infarction (heart attack).

Corticosteroid. Any of the steroid hormones made by the cortex (outer layer) of the adrenal gland. Cortisol is a corticosteroid. Several medications are analogs of natural corticosteroid hormones.

Crohn disease. An inflammatory bowel disease that usually affects the lower part of the small intestine or upper part of the colon but may affect any part of the gastrointestinal tract.

Crossover trial. A clinical trial where at least two interventions or treatments are applied to the same individuals after an appropriate washout period. One of the treatments is often a placebo. In a randomized crossover design, interventions are applied in a randomized order to ensure that the order of treatments does not contribute to the outcome.

Cross-sectional study. A study of a group of people at one point in time to determine whether an exposure is associated with the occurrence of a disease. Because the disease outcome and the exposure (e.g., nutrient intake) are measured at the same time, a cross-sectional study provides a "snapshot" view of their relationship. Cross-sectional studies cannot provide information about causality.

Cystic fibrosis. A hereditary disease caused by mutations in the cystic fibrosis transmembrane conductance regulator (*CFTR*) gene. Cystic fibrosis is characterized by the production of abnormal secretions, leading to the accumulation of mucus in the lungs, pancreas, and intestine. This build-up of mucus causes difficulty breathing and recurrent lung infections, as well as problems with nutrient absorption, due to problems in the pancreas and intestines.

Cytochrome P450 (CYP). A family of phase I biotransformation enzymes that play an important role in the metabolism and elimination of drugs, toxins, carcinogens, and endogenous compounds, such as steroid hormones.

Cytokine. A protein made by cells that affects the behavior of other cells. Cytokines act on specific cytokine receptors in the cells they affect.

Cytoplasm. The contents of a cell, excluding the nucleus.

Cytosol. The water-soluble contents of a cell's cytoplasm, excluding the organelles.

De novo synthesis. The formation of an essential molecule from simple precursor molecules.

Debridement. The removal of necrotic or infected tissue or foreign material from a wound.

Dementia. Significant impairment of intellectual abilities, such as attention, orientation, memory, judgment, or language. By definition, dementia is not due to major depression or psychosis. Alzheimer disease is the most common cause of dementia in older adults.

Dental caries. Cavities or holes in the outer two layers of a tooth—the enamel and the dentin. Dental caries are caused by bacteria that metabolize carbohydrates (sugars) to form organic acids, which dissolve tooth enamel.

Dermatitis. Inflammation of the skin. This term is often used to describe a skin rash.

Diabetes mellitus. A chronic metabolic disease, characterized by abnormally high blood glucose (sugar) levels, resulting from the inability of the body to produce or respond to insulin. Type 1 diabetes mellitus, formerly known as insulin-dependent or juvenile-onset diabetes, is usually the result of autoimmune destruction of the insulin-secreting β-cells of the pancreas. The most common form of diabetes is type 2 diabetes mellitus, formerly known as noninsulin-dependent or adult-onset diabetes, which develops when the tissues of the body become less sensitive to insulin secreted by the pancreas.

Dialysis. A medical procedure to filter waste products from the blood. Dialysis is needed to perform the work of the kidneys if they can no longer function effectively. Two types of dialysis are hemodialysis and peritoneal dialysis.

Diastolic blood pressure. The lowest arterial blood pressure during the heart beat cycle and the second number in a blood pressure reading (e.g., 120/80 mmHg).

Differentiation. Changes in a cell resulting in its specialization for specific functions, such as those of a nerve cell. In general, differentiation of cells leads to a decrease in proliferation.

Dimer. A complex of two molecules, usually proteins. Heterodimers are complexes of two different molecules, while homodimers are complexes of two of the same molecule.

Diverticulitis. Inflammation or infection of diverticula in the colon (see diverticulosis below), characterized by abdominal pain, fever, and constipation.

Diverticulosis. A condition characterized by the formation of small pouches (diverticula) in the colon. Although most people with diverticulosis experience no symptoms, approximately 15%–20% may develop pain or inflammation, known as diverticulitis.

DNA. Deoxyribonucleic acid; a double-stranded nucleic acid composed of many nucleotides. The nucleotides in DNA are each composed of a nitrogen-containing base (adenine, guanine, cytosine, or thymine), a 5-carbon sugar (deoxyribose), and a phosphate group. The sequence of bases in DNA encodes the genetic information required to synthesize proteins.

Double-blind. Refers to a study in which neither the investigators administering the treatment nor the participants know which participants are receiving the experimental treatment and which are receiving the placebo.

DRI. Dietary reference intake. Refers to a set of at least four nutrient-based reference values (RDA [recommended dietary allowance], AI [adequate intake], UL [upper intake limit], EAR [estimated average requirements]), each with a specific use in defining recommended dietary intake levels for individual nutrients. The DRIs are determined by expert panels appointed by the Food and Nutrition Board of the US Institute of Medicine.

Dyskinesia. Impaired control of voluntary movement. Dyskinesia is sometimes a side effect of long-term use of antipsychotic medications.

Echocardiography. A diagnostic test that uses ultrasound to make images of the heart. It can be used to assess the health of the valves and chambers of the heart, as well as to measure cardiac output.

Ecological study. An epidemiological study that examines the relationships between exposures and disease rates in a series of populations (e.g., different countries). Ecological studies often rely on published statistics, such as food-disappearance data or disease-specific death rates.

Edema. Swelling; accumulation of excessive fluid in subcutaneous tissues (beneath the skin).

Eicosanoids. Chemical messengers derived from 20-carbon polyunsaturated fatty acids, such as arachidonic acid and eicosapentaenoic acid. Eicosanoids play critical roles in immune and inflammatory responses.

Electron. A stable atomic particle with a negative charge.

Electron transport chain. A group of electron carriers in mitochondria that transport electrons to and from each other in a sequence, to generate ATP.

Emphysema. A chronic obstructive pulmonary (lung) disease, characterized by damage to the small air sacs (alveoli) and difficulty breathing. Damage to the alveoli decreases their elasticity and results in hyperinflation of the lungs, which impairs gas exchange. Smoking is the most common cause of emphysema.

Endogenous. Arising from within the body. Endogenous synthesis refers to the synthesis of a compound by the body.

Endometrium. The inner lining of the uterus.

Endothelium-dependent vasodilation. Arterial vasodilation resulting from the production of nitric oxide in the vascular endothelium.

Enterocytes. Cells that line the luminal (inner) surface of the intestine.

Enzyme. A biological catalyst; that is, a substance that increases the speed of a chemical reaction without being changed in the overall process. Enzymes are vitally important to the regulation of the chemistry of cells and organisms.

Epidemiological study. A study examining disease occurrence in a human population.

Epididymis. A system of tubules emerging from the testes, which serves as a storage site for spermatozoa during their maturation.

Epilepsy. Also known as seizure disorder. Individuals with epilepsy experience seizures, which are the result of uncontrolled electrical activity in the brain. A seizure may cause a physical convulsion, minor physical signs, thought disturbances, or a combination of symptoms.

Erythropoietin. A hormone produced by specialized cells in the kidneys that stimulates the bone marrow to increase the production of red blood cells. Recombinant erythropoietin is used to treat anemia in patients with end-stage renal failure.

Esophagus. The portion of the gastrointestinal tract that connects the throat (pharynx) to the stomach.

Ester. The product of a reaction between a carboxylic acid and an alcohol that involves the elimination of water. For example, a cholesterol ester is the product of a reaction between a fatty acid and cholesterol.

Estrogen. Hormone that binds to estrogen receptors in the nuclei of cells and promotes the transcription of estrogen-responsive genes. Endogenous estrogens are steroid hormones produced by the body. Exogenous estrogens are synthetic or natural compounds that have estrogenic activity (i.e., bind the estrogen receptor and promote estrogen-responsive gene transcription).

Etiology. The causes or origin of a disease.

Excretion. The elimination of wastes from blood or tissues.

Familial adenomatous polyposis. A hereditary syndrome characterized by the formation of many polyps in the colon and rectum, some of which may develop into colorectal cancer.

Fatty acid. An organic acid molecule consisting of a chain of carbon molecules and a carboxylic acid (COOH) group. Fatty acids are found in fats and oils and as components of several essential lipids, such as phospholipids and triglycerides. Fatty acids can be burned by the body for energy.

Fermentation. An anaerobic process that involves the breakdown of dietary components to yield energy.

Food frequency questionnaire. A type of dietary assessment in which participants are asked to report how frequently various foods are consumed over a specified period of time.

Forced expiratory volume (FEV$_1$). The volume of air that can be expelled during the first second of a forced expiration. FEV$_1$ is used to assess pulmonary (lung) function.

Fracture. A break in a bone or cartilage, often but not always the result of trauma.

Free radical. A very reactive atom or molecule, typically possessing a single unpaired electron.

Fructosamine. Describes a group of circulating proteins that have become irreversibly bound to glucose. Fructosamine assays provide information about blood glucose control 2–3 weeks prior to sample collection.

Fructose. A very sweet 6-carbon sugar abundant in plants. Fructose is increasingly common in sweeteners such as high-fructose corn syrup.

Gallbladder. A small sac adjacent to the liver. The gallbladder stores bile, which is secreted by the liver, and releases it into the small intestine through the common bile duct.

Gallstones. Crystals formed by the precipitation of cholesterol or bilirubin in the gallbladder. Gallstones may be asymptomatic (without symptoms) or they may result in inflammation and infection of the gallbladder.

Gastrointestinal. Referring to or affecting the digestive tract, which includes the mouth, pharynx (throat), esophagus, stomach, and intestines.

Gene. A region of DNA that controls a specific hereditary characteristic, usually corresponding to a single protein.

Gene expression. The process by which the information coded in genes (DNA) is converted to proteins and other cellular structures. Expressed genes include those that are transcribed to mRNA and translated to protein, as well as those that are only transcribed to RNA (e.g., ribosomal and transfer RNAs).

Genome. All of the genetic information (encoded in DNA) possessed by an organism.

Gestation. The period of time between fertilization and birth. In humans, normal gestation is around 40 weeks.

Glomerulus (plural glomeruli). A tuft of capillaries that makes up part of the filtering unit of the kidney (nephron).

Glucose. A 6-carbon sugar that plays a major role in the generation of energy for living organisms.

Glucose tolerance. The ability of the body to maintain normal glucose levels when challenged with a carbohydrate load (see impaired glucose tolerance).

Glucoside. A glycoside that contains glucose as its carbohydrate (sugar) moiety (see glycoside below).

Glutamate. An excitatory neurotransmitter. Under certain circumstances, glutamate may become toxic to neurons. Glutamate excitotoxicity appears to play a role in nerve cell death in some neurodegenerative disorders.

Glutathione. A tripeptide consisting of glutamate, cysteine, and glycine. Glutathione is an endogenous intracellular antioxidant and is also required for some phase II biotransformation reactions.

Glycemic index. An index of the blood-glucose-raising potential of the carbohydrate in different foods. The glycemic index is calculated as the area under the blood glucose curve after a test food is eaten, divided by the corresponding area after a control food (glucose or white bread) is eaten. The value is multiplied by 100 to represent a percentage of the control food.

Glycemic load. An index that simultaneously describes the blood-glucose-raising potential of the carbohydrate in a food and the quantity of carbohydrate in a food. The glycemic load of a food is calculated by multiplying the glycemic index by the amount of carbohydrate in grams provided by a food and dividing the total by 100.

Glycoside. A compound containing a sugar molecule that can be cleaved by hydrolysis to a sugar and a nonsugar component (aglycone).

Glycosylated hemoglobin. Glucose-bound hemoglobin. A test for glycosylated hemoglobin measures the percentage of hemoglobin that is glucose bound. Since glucose remains bound to hemoglobin for the life of a red blood cell (approx. 120 days), glycosylated hemoglobin values reflect blood glucose control over the past 4 months.

Gout. A condition characterized by abnormally high blood levels of uric acid (urate). Urate crystals may form in joints, resulting in inflammation and pain. Urate crystals may also form in the kidney and urinary tract, resulting in kidney stones. The tendency to develop elevated blood uric acid levels and gout is often inherited.

Gray matter. The darker-colored tissue in the central nervous system that contains mostly cell bodies and dendrites.

GTP. Guanosine triphosphate. A high-energy molecule, required for several biochemical reactions, including nucleic acid and protein synthesis (formation).

HDL. High-density lipoprotein. HDLs transport cholesterol from the tissues to the liver, where it can be eliminated in bile. HDL cholesterol is considered good cholesterol, because higher blood levels of HDL cholesterol are associated with lower risk of cardiovascular disease.

Heme. Compounds of iron complexed in a characteristic ring structure known as a porphyrin ring.

Hemodialysis. The process of removing blood from an artery, removing waste products from the blood through dialysis, and returning it to the body through a vein. Hemodialysis is used to treat end-stage renal failure.

Hemoglobin. The oxygen-carrying pigment in red blood cells.

Hemoglobin A$_{1C}$. The main fraction of glycosylated (glucose-bound) hemoglobin. Since glucose remains bound to hemoglobin for the life of a red blood cell (approx. 120 days), hemoglobin A$_{1C}$ values reflect blood glucose control over the past 4 months.

Hemorrhage. Excessive or uncontrolled bleeding.

Hemorrhagic stroke. A stroke that occurs when a blood vessel ruptures and bleeds into the brain.

Hepatitis. Literally, inflammation of the liver. Hepatitis caused by a virus is known as viral hepatitis. Other causes of hepatitis include toxic chemicals and alcohol abuse.

Hepatocellular carcinoma. The most common type of primary liver cancer.

Heterozygous. Possessing two different forms (alleles) of a specific gene.

Histone. Protein that binds to DNA and packages it into compact structures to form nucleosomes.

HIV. Human immunodeficiency virus; the virus that causes AIDS.

Homocysteine. A sulfur-containing amino acid, which is an intermediate in the metabolism of another sulfur-containing amino acid, methionine. Elevated homocysteine levels in the blood have been associated with increased risk of cardiovascular disease.

Homologous. Having the same appearance, structure, or evolutionary origin.

Homozygous. Possessing two identical forms (alleles) of a specific gene.

Hormone. A chemical released by a gland or a tissue, which affects or regulates the activity of specific cells or organs. Complex bodily functions, such as growth and sexual development, are regulated by hormones.

Hot flushes. Sensations of heat in the skin, particularly the face, neck and chest, also known as hot flashes. Hot flushes are most often related to declining estrogen levels during the perimenopause (time period surrounding menopause).

Human papilloma virus (HPV). A group of viruses that may cause papillomas (growths or warts) on the skin or other parts of the body, including the genitals and the larynx (voice box). Infection with particular strains of HPV is associated with increased risk of cervical cancer.

Huntington disease. An inherited degenerative disorder of the brain. Its symptoms include movement disorders and impaired cognitive function. Symptoms of Huntington disease, previously known as Huntington chorea, typically develop in the fourth decade of life and progressively deteriorate over time.

Hydrolysis. Cleavage of a chemical bond by the addition of water. In hydrolysis reactions, a large compound may be broken down into smaller compounds when a molecule of water is added.

Hydrophobic. A molecule that repels water and thus will not dissolve in water.

Hydroxylation. A chemical reaction involving the addition of a hydroxyl (-OH) group to a compound.

Hypertension. High blood pressure. Hypertension is defined by the US Joint National Committee on Prevention, Detection, Evaluation and Treatment of High Blood Pressure as a systolic blood pressure of 140 mmHg or higher and/or a diastolic blood pressure of 90 mmHg or higher.

Hypoglycemia. An abnormally low blood glucose concentration. Symptoms may include nausea, sweating, weakness, faintness, confusion hallucinations, headache, loss of consciousness, convulsions, or coma.

Hypothesis. An educated guess or proposition that is advanced as a basis for further investigation. A hypothesis must be subjected to an experimental test to determine its validity.

Hypothyroidism. A deficiency of thyroid hormone that is normally made by the thyroid gland, located in the front of the neck.

Idiopathic. Of unknown cause.

Ileostomy. A surgically created connection between the ileum (small intestine) and an opening in the abdominal wall (stoma) that allows for the evacuation of feces when a portion of the bowel has been removed.

Impaired glucose tolerance. A metabolic state between normal glucose regulation and overt diabetes. Impaired glucose tolerance is defined medically as a plasma glucose concentration between 140 mg/dL and 199 mg/dL (7.8–11.0 mmol) 2 hours after the ingestion of 75 g of glucose during an oral glucose tolerance test.

Incontinence. Inability to control the evacuation of urine or feces.

Induction. Initiation of or increase in the expression of a gene in response to a physical or chemical stimulus (inducer).

Inflammation. A response to injury or infection, characterized by redness, heat, swelling, and pain. Physiologically, the inflammatory response involves a complex series of events, leading to the migration of white blood cells to the inflamed area.

Inflammatory bowel disease. A group of autoimmune diseases that affect the small and large intestines.

Insoluble. Not dissolvable. With respect to bioavailability, certain substances form insoluble complexes that cannot be dissolved in digestive secretions and therefore cannot be absorbed by the digestive tract.

Insulin. A peptide hormone secreted by the β-cells of the pancreas, required for normal glucose metabolism.

Insulin resistance. Diminished responsiveness to insulin.

Insulin sensitivity. The ability of tissues to respond to insulin.

Intermittent claudication. A condition characterized by leg pain or weakness on walking that diminishes or resolves with rest. It is usually associated with peripheral arterial disease.

International normalized ratio (INR). The preferred method for reporting prothrombin time, a measure of coagulation status that may be used to evaluate the therapeutic efficacy of anticoagulants, such as warfarin. The INR is a method for standardizing prothrombin time results, in order to minimize variability between laboratories.

Intervention trial. An experimental study (usually a clinical trial) used to test the effect of a treatment or intervention on a health- or disease-related outcome.

In vitro. Literally "in glass," referring to a test or research done in the test tube, or research done in cell cultures, outside a living organism.

In vivo. "Inside a living organism." An in vivo assay evaluates a biological process occurring inside the body.

Ion. An atom or group of atoms that carries a positive or negative electric charge as a result of having lost or gained one or more electrons.

Ion channel. A protein, embedded in a cell membrane, that serves as a crossing point for the regulated transfer of an ion or a group of ions across the membrane.

Ischemia. A state of insufficient blood flow to a tissue.

Ischemic stroke. A stroke resulting from insufficient blood flow to an area of the brain, which may occur when a blood vessel supplying the brain becomes obstructed by a clot.

Isomers. Compounds that have the same numbers and kinds of atoms but that differ in the way the atoms are arranged.

Kidney stones. Solid masses resulting from the crystallization of minerals and other compounds found in urine. Common types of kidney stones include those composed of calcium oxalate, calcium phosphate, and urate. Kidney stones may form in the kidneys, ureters, or urinary bladder.

Larynx. The area of the throat (pharynx) that contains the vocal cords.

LDL. Low-density lipoprotein. LDLs transport cholesterol from the liver to the tissues of the body. Elevated serum LDL cholesterol is associated with increased cardiovascular disease risk.

Lens. The transparent structure inside the eye that focuses light rays onto the retina (the nerve cells at the back of the eye).

Leukocyte. A white blood cell. Leukocytes are part of the immune system. Monocytes, lymphocytes, neutrophils, basophils, and eosinophils are different types of leukocytes.

Leukotrienes. Cell-signaling molecules involved in inflammation. Lipoxygenases catalyze the formation of leukotrienes from eicosanoids, such as arachidonic acid and eicosapentaenoic acid (EPA).

Lipid peroxidation. The process by which lipids are oxidatively modified, so named because lipid hydroperoxides are formed in the process.

Lipids. A chemical term for fats. Lipids found in the human body include fatty acids, phospholipids, and triglycerides.

Lipoproteins. Particles composed of lipids and protein that allow the transport of lipids through the bloodstream. A lipoprotein particle is composed of an outer layer of phospholipids, which renders it soluble in water, and a hydrophobic core that contains triglycerides and cholesterol esters. Different types of lipoproteins are distinguished by their surface proteins (apoproteins), their size, and the types and amounts of lipids they contain.

Lumbar spine. The portion of the spine between the chest (thorax) and the pelvis. It is commonly referred to as the small of the back.

Lumen. The channel within a tube, such as a blood vessel or the intestine.

Lupus. See Systemic lupus erythematosus (SLE).

Lymphocytes. Leukocytes (white blood cells) that play important roles in the immune system. T lymphocytes (T cells) differentiate into cells that can kill infected cells or activate other cells in the immune system. B lymphocytes (B cells) differentiate into cells that produce antibodies.

Lysosome. A cellular organelle containing hydrolytic enzymes specialized for breaking down cellular debris. Lysosomal enzymes are separated from the rest of the cell by a lysosomal membrane and function optimally at an acid pH.

Macrophage. A white blood cell that engulfs and degrades pathogens (bacteria) and cellular debris. Macrophages are activated or transformed monocytes.

Macula. A small area of the retina where vision is the sharpest. The macula is located in the center of the retina and provides central vision.

Malignant. Cancerous.

Meta-analysis. A statistical technique used to combine the results from different studies to obtain a quantitative estimate of the overall effect of a particular intervention or exposure on a defined outcome.

Metabolic syndrome. A combination of medical conditions that places one at risk for cardiovascular diseases and type 2 diabetes. (Metabolic syndrome is also called metabolic syndrome X, syndrome X, and insulin resistance syndrome.) Diagnostic criteria include the presence of three or more of the following conditions:

- Abdominal obesity (waist circumference: ≥40 in [102 cm] for men, ≥35 in [88 cm] for women)

- Elevated triglycerides (≥150 mg/dL)

- High blood pressure (≥130/85 mmHg)

- Glucose intolerance/insulin resistance (fasting blood glucose ≥110 mg/dL)

- Decreased HDL cholesterol (<40 mg/dL for men, <50 mg/dL for women).

Metabolism. The sum of the processes (reactions) by which a substance is assimilated and incorporated into the body or detoxified and excreted from the body.

Metabolite. A compound derived from the metabolism of another compound is said to be a metabolite of that compound.

Methionine. A sulfur-containing amino acid, required for protein synthesis and other vital metabolic processes. It can be obtained through the diet in protein or synthesized from homocysteine.

Methylation. A biochemical reaction resulting in the addition of a methyl group ($-CH_3$) to another molecule.

Micelle. An aggregate or cluster of amphipathic molecules in water. Amphipathic molecules have a polar or hydrophilic end and a nonpolar or hydrophobic end. In micelles, amphipathic molecules orient with their hydrophobic ends in the interior and their hydrophilic ends on the exterior surface, exposed to water.

Mineral. Nutritionally significant element. Elements are composed of only one kind of atom. Minerals are inorganic, that is, they do not contain carbon, unlike vitamins and other organic compounds.

Mitochondria. Energy-producing structures within cells. Mitochondria possess two sets of membranes, a smooth continuous outer membrane and an inner membrane arranged in folds. Among other critical functions, mitochondria convert nutrients into energy via the electron transport chain.

mmHg. Millimeters of mercury. The unit of measure for blood pressure.

Moiety. A portion of something, such as a functional group of a molecule.

Mole. The fundamental unit for measuring chemical compounds (abbreviated mol). One mole equals the molecular weight of a compound in grams. The number of molecules in a mole is equal to 6.02×10^{23} (Avogadro's number).

Monocyte. A white blood cell that is the precursor to a macrophage.

Monomer. A molecule that can be chemically bound as a unit of a polymer.

Monounsaturated fatty acid. A fatty acid with only one double bond between carbon atoms.

Multifactorial. Refers to diseases or conditions that are the result of interactions between multiple genetic and environmental factors.

Multiple sclerosis (MS). An autoimmune disorder in which the myelin sheaths of nerves in the brain and spinal cord are damaged, resulting in progressive neurological symptoms.

Mutation. A change in a gene; in other words, a change in the sequence of base pairs in the DNA that makes up a gene. Mutations in a gene may or may not result in an altered gene product.

Myocardial infarction (MI). Death (necrosis) of heart muscle tissue due to an interruption in its blood supply. Commonly known as a heart attack, an MI usually results from the obstruction of a coronary artery by a clot in people who have coronary atherosclerosis (heart disease).

Myocytes. Muscle cells.

Myopathy. Any disease of muscle.

Necrosis. Unprogrammed cell death, in which cells break open and release their contents, promoting inflammation. Necrotic cell death may be the result of injury, infection, or infarction.

Nephropathy. Kidney damage or disease.

Nerve impulse. The electrochemical signal transmitted in the cell membrane of a neuron or muscle cell. Also called an action potential.

Neural tube defect (NTD). A birth defect caused by abnormal development of the neural tube, the structure that gives rise to the central nervous system. Neural tube defects include anencephaly and spina bifida.

Neurodegenerative disease. Disease resulting from the degeneration or deterioration of nerve cells (neurons). Alzheimer disease and Parkinson disease are neurodegenerative diseases.

Neurological. Or neurological; involving nerves or the nervous system (brain, spinal cord, and all sensory and motor nerves).

Neuron. Cell of the nervous system that conducts nerve impulses. Also called a nerve cell.

Neuropathy. Nerve damage or disease.

Neurotransmitter. A chemical that is released from a nerve cell and results in the transmission of an impulse to another nerve cell or organ (e.g., a muscle). Acetylcholine, dopamine, norepinephrine (noradrenaline), and serotonin are neurotransmitters.

Neutrophil. A white blood cell that internalizes and destroys pathogens, such as bacteria. Neutrophils are also called polymorphonuclear leukocytes because they are white blood cells with multilobed nuclei.

NIH. National Institutes of Health. Administered under the US Department of Health and Human Services, the NIH includes more than 20 separate institutes and centers devoted to medical research.

Nitric oxide. A gaseous signaling molecule synthesized from the amino acid arginine by enzymes called nitric oxide synthases. In the vascular endothelium, nitric oxide promotes arterial vasodilation.

Nucleic acids. DNA (deoxyribonucleic acid) and RNA (ribonucleic acid); long polymers of nucleotides.

Nucleotides. Subunits of nucleic acids. Nucleotides are composed of a nitrogen-containing base (adenine, guanine, cytosine, uracil, or thymine), a 5-carbon sugar (ribose or deoxyribose), and one or more phosphate groups.

Nucleus. A membrane-bound cellular organelle, which contains DNA organized into chromosomes.

Obesity. A condition of increased body fat; defined as a body mass index (BMI) ≥ 30 kg/m^2 for adults.

Observational study. A study in which no experimental intervention or treatment is applied. Participants are simply observed over time.

Organelles. Specialized components of cells, such as mitochondria or lysosomes, so named because they are analogous to organs.

Organic. Refers to carbon-containing compounds, generally synthesized by living organisms.

Oropharynx. A term used to describe the mouth and throat.

Osteoblasts. Bone cells that are responsible for the formation of new bone mineral in the bone-remodeling process.

Osteoclasts. Bone cells that are responsible for the breakdown or resorption of bone in the bone-remodeling process.

Osteoporosis. A condition of increased bone fragility and susceptibility to bone fracture due to a loss of bone mineral density (BMD).

Oxidant. Reactive oxygen species (ROS).

Oxidation. A chemical reaction that removes electrons from an atom or molecule.

Oxidative damage. Damage to cells caused by reactive oxygen species (ROS).

Oxidative stress. A condition in which the effects of pro-oxidants (e.g., free radicals and reactive oxygen and reactive nitrogen species) exceed the ability of antioxidant systems to neutralize them.

Pancreas. A small organ located behind the stomach and connected to the duodenum (small intestine). The pancreas synthesizes enzymes that help digest food in the small intestine and hormones, including insulin, that regulate blood glucose levels.

Parkinson disease. A disease of the nervous system caused by degeneration of a part of the brain called the basal ganglia, as well as by low production of the neurotransmitter dopamine. Symptoms include muscle rigidity, tremors, and slow voluntary movement.

Pathogen. Disease-causing agent, such as a virus or a bacterium.

Peptide. A chain of amino acids. A protein is made up of one or more peptides.

Peptide hormone. A hormone that is a protein, as opposed to a steroid hormone, which is made from cholesterol. Insulin is an example of a peptide hormone.

Percutaneous transluminal coronary angioplasty. A nonsurgical technique, in which a balloon catheter is inserted into a peripheral artery and passed into an occluded coronary artery, where the balloon is inflated to dilate the artery.

Perinatal. The period of time just before and after birth (varyingly defined as the time period starting between 20–28 weeks' gestation and ending 1–4 weeks after birth).

Peripheral arterial disease (PAD). Atherosclerosis of the arteries of the extremities.

Peripheral neuropathy. A disease or degenerative state affecting the nerves of the extremities (arms and legs). Symptoms may include numbness, pain, and muscle weakness.

Peripheral vascular disease. Atherosclerosis of the vessels of the extremities, which may result in insufficient blood flow or pain in the affected limb, particularly during exercise.

pH. A measure of acidity or alkalinity.

Pharmacokinetics. The study of the absorption, distribution, metabolism, and elimination of drugs and other compounds.

Pharmacological dose. The dose or intake level of a nutrient many times the level associated with the prevention of deficiency or the maintenance of health. A pharmacological dose is generally associated with the treatment of a disease state and considered to be a dose at least 10 times greater than that needed to prevent deficiency.

Phase I clinical trial. A clinical trial in a small group of people aimed at determining bioavailability, optimal dose, safety, and early evidence of the efficacy of a new therapy.

Phase II clinical trial. A clinical trial designed to investigate the effectiveness of a new therapy in larger numbers of people and to further evaluate short-term side effects and safety of the new therapy.

Phenolic compounds. A class of chemical compounds consisting of a hydroxyl functional group (-OH) attached to an aromatic hydrocarbon group. An aromatic hydrocarbon has a ring structure like that of benzene. Polyphenolic compounds contain more than one phenolic group.

Phospholipids. Lipids in which phosphoric acid as well as fatty acids are attached to a glycerol backbone. Phospholipids are important structural components of cell membranes.

Phosphorylation. The creation of a phosphate derivative of an organic molecule. This is usually achieved by transferring a phosphate group ($-PO_4$) from ATP to another molecule.

Physiological dose. The dose or intake level of a nutrient associated with the prevention of deficiency or the maintenance of health. A physiological dose of a nutrient is not generally greater than that which could be achieved through a conscientious diet, as opposed to the use of supplements.

Phytochemicals. Biologically active, non-nutrient compounds synthesized by plants.

Phytoestrogens. Compounds with estrogenic activity derived from plants.

Pigment. A compound that gives a plant or animal cell color by the selective absorption of different wavelengths of light.

Placebo. An inert treatment that is given to a control group, while the experimental group is given the active treatment. Placebo-controlled studies are conducted to make sure that the results are due to the experimental treatment, rather than another factor associated with participating in the study.

Placenta. The organ that connects the fetus to the pregnant woman's uterus, allowing the exchange of oxygen, carbon dioxide, nutrients, and waste between the woman and fetus.

Plasma. The liquid portion of blood, in which the cells are suspended. Plasma is separated from blood cells using a centrifuge. Unlike serum, plasma retains clotting factors because it is obtained from blood that is not allowed to clot.

Platelets. Irregularly shaped cell fragments that assist in blood clotting.

Polymer. A large molecule formed by combining many similar smaller molecules (monomers) in a regular pattern.

Polymorphism. A variant form of a gene. Most polymorphisms are harmless and are part of normal human genetic variation, but some polymorphisms affect the function of the gene product (protein).

Polyp. A benign (non-cancerous) mass of tissue that forms on the inside of a hollow organ, such as the colon.

Polyunsaturated fatty acid. A fatty acid with more than one double bond between carbons.

Postprandial. After eating or after a meal.

Precursor. A molecule that is an ingredient, reactant, or intermediate in a synthetic pathway for a particular product.

Preeclampsia. A condition characterized by a sharp rise in blood pressure during the third trimester of pregnancy. High blood pressure may be accompanied by edema (swelling) and proteinuria (protein in the urine). In some cases, untreated preeclampsia can progress to eclampsia, a life-threatening situation for the woman and child.

Prevalence. The proportion of a population with a specific disease or condition at a given point in time.

Procarcinogen. A carcinogen precursor that must be modified or metabolized to become an active carcinogen.

Prognosis. Predicted outcome based on the course of a disease.

Proliferation. Rapid cell division.

Promoter. DNA sequence to which RNA polymerase binds to initiate transcription.

Pro-oxidant. An atom or molecule that promotes oxidation of another atom or molecule by accepting electrons. Examples of pro-oxidants include free radicals, reactive oxygen species (ROS), and reactive nitrogen species (RNS).

Prophylaxis. Prevention, often refers to a treatment used to prevent a disease.

Prospective cohort study. An observational study in which a group of people—known as a cohort—are interviewed or tested for risk factors (e.g., nutrient intake), and then followed up at subsequent times to determine their status with respect to a disease or health outcome.

Prostaglandins. Cell-signaling molecules involved in inflammation. Cyclooxygenases catalyze the formation of prostaglandins.

Prostate. A gland in men, located at the base of the bladder and surrounding the urethra. The prostate produces fluid that forms part of semen. If the prostate becomes enlarged, it may exert pressure on the urethra and cause urinary symptoms. Prostate cancer is one of the most common types of cancer in men.

Prostate-specific antigen (PSA). A compound normally secreted by the prostate that can be measured in the blood. If prostate cancer is developing, the prostate secretes larger amounts of PSA. Blood tests for PSA are used to screen for prostate cancer and to follow up on prostate cancer treatment.

Protein. A complex organic molecule composed of amino acids in a specific order. The order is determined by the sequence of nucleic acids in a gene coding for the protein. Proteins are required for the structure, function, and regulation of the body's cells, tissues, and organs, and each protein has unique functions.

Proton. An elementary particle identical to the nucleus of a hydrogen atom, which, along with neutrons, is a constituent of all other atomic nuclei. A proton carries a positive charge equal and opposite to that of an electron.

Psoriasis. A chronic skin condition often resulting in a red, scaly rash located over the surfaces of the elbows, knees, and scalp and around or in the ears, navel, genitals, or buttocks. Approximately 10%–15% of patients with psoriasis develop joint inflammation (psoriatic arthritis). Psoriasis is thought to be an autoimmune condition.

Quartile. One-fourth of a sample or population.

Quintile. One-fifth of a sample or population.

Racemic mixture. A mixture of equal amounts of isomers that are mirror images of each other (enantiomers).

Randomized controlled trial. A clinical trial with at least one active treatment group and a control (placebo) group. In randomized controlled trials, participants are chosen for the experimental and control groups at random and are not told whether they are receiving the active or placebo treatment until the end of the study. This type of study design can provide evidence of causality.

Randomized design. An experiment in which participants are chosen for the experimental and control groups at random, to reduce bias caused by self-selection into experimental and control groups. This type of study design can provide evidence of causality.

RDA. Recommended dietary allowance. Established by the Food and Nutrition Board of the US Institute of Medicine, the RDA is the average daily dietary intake level of a nutrient sufficient to meet the requirements of nearly all healthy individuals in a specific life stage and gender group.

Reactive nitrogen species (RNS). Highly reactive chemicals, containing nitrogen, that react easily with other molecules, resulting in potentially damaging modifications.

Reactive oxygen species (ROS). Highly reactive chemicals, containing oxygen, that react easily with other molecules, resulting in potentially damaging modifications.

Receptor. A specialized molecule inside or on the surface of a cell that binds a specific chemical (ligand). Ligand binding usually results in a change in activity within the cell.

Recessive trait. A trait that is expressed only when two copies of the gene responsible for the trait are present.

Rectum. The last portion of the large intestine, connecting the sigmoid colon (above) to the anus (below). The rectum stores stool until it is evacuated from the body.

Redox reaction. Another term for an oxidation–reduction reaction. A redox reaction is any reaction in which electrons are removed from one molecule or atom and transferred to another molecule or atom. In such a reaction, one substance is oxidized (loses electrons) while the other is reduced (gains electrons).

Reduction. A chemical reaction in which a molecule or atom gains electrons.

Renal. Refers to the kidneys.

Residue. A single unit within a polymer, such as an amino acid within a protein.

Resorption. The process of breaking down or assimilating something. With respect to bone, resorption refers to the breakdown of bone by osteoclasts, resulting in the release of calcium and phosphate (bone mineral) into the blood.

Response element. A sequence of nucleotides in a gene that can be bound by a protein. Proteins that bind to response elements in genes are sometimes called transcription factors or binding proteins. Binding of a transcription factor to a response element regulates the production of specific proteins by inhibiting or enhancing the transcription of genes that encode those proteins.

Restenosis. With respect to the coronary arteries, restenosis refers to the reocclusion of a coronary artery after it has been dilated using coronary angioplasty.

Retina. The nerve layer that lines the back of the eye. In the retina, images created by light are converted to nerve impulses, which are transmitted to the brain via the optic nerve.

Retrospective study. An epidemiological study that looks back in time. A retrospective study begins after the exposure and the disease have occurred. Most case–control studies are retrospective.

Rheumatoid arthritis. A chronic autoimmune disease characterized by inflammation of the synovial lining of the joints. Rheumatoid arthritis may also affect other organs of the body, including the skin, eyes, lungs, and heart.

Ribonucleotide. A molecule consisting of a 5-carbon sugar (ribose), a nitrogen-containing base, and one or more phosphate groups.

RNA. Ribonucleic acid; a single-stranded nucleic acid composed of many nucleotides. The nucleotides in RNA are composed of a nitrogen-containing base (adenine, guanine, cytosine, or uracil), a 5-carbon sugar (ribose) and a phosphate group. RNA functions in the translation of the genetic information encoded in DNA to proteins.

Saturated fatty acid. A fatty acid with no double bonds between carbon atoms.

Scavenge (free radicals). To combine readily with free radicals, preventing them from reacting with other molecules.

Schizophrenia. A debilitating brain disorder that affects approximately 1% of the world's population. Symptoms may include hallucinations, delusions, thought disorders, disorders of movement, cognitive deficits, flat affect, lack of pleasure, or impaired ability to speak, plan, or interact with others. Although its cause is not known, schizophrenia is thought to result from a combination of genetic and environmental factors.

Seizure. Uncontrolled electrical activity in the brain, which may produce a physical convulsion, minor physical signs, thought disturbances, or a combination of symptoms.

Serotonin. 5-Hydroxytryptamine. Serotonin is a neurotransmitter that may also function as a vasoconstrictor (substance that causes blood vessels to narrow).

Serum. The liquid portion of blood, in which the cells are suspended. Serum is separated from blood cells using a centrifuge. Unlike plasma, serum lacks clotting factors because it is obtained from blood that has been allowed to clot.

Signal transduction pathway. A cascade of events that allows a signal outside a cell to result in a functional change inside the cell. Signal transduction pathways play important roles in regulating numerous cellular functions in response to changes in a cell's environment.

Small intestine. The part of the digestive tract that extends from the stomach to the large intestine. The small intestine includes the duodenum (closest to the stomach), the jejunum, and the ileum (closest to the large intestine).

Spina bifida. A birth defect, also known as a neural tube defect, resulting from failure of the lower end of the neural tube to close during embryonic development. Spina bifida, the most common cause of infantile paralysis, is characterized by a lack of protection of the spinal cord by its membranes and vertebral bones.

Status. The state of nutrition of an individual with respect to a specific nutrient. Diminished or low status indicates inadequate supply or stores of a specific nutrient for optimal physiological functioning.

Stenosis. Obstruction or narrowing of a passage. Coronary stenosis refers specifically to obstruction or narrowing of a coronary artery, which supplies blood to the heart muscle (myocardium).

Steroid. A molecule related to cholesterol. Many important hormones, such as estrogen and testosterone, are steroids.

Steroid hormone receptor. A protein within a cell that binds to a specific steroid hormone. Binding of the steroid hormone changes the shape of the receptor protein and activates it, allowing it to activate gene transcription. In this way, a steroid hormone can activate the synthesis of specific proteins.

Stroke. Damage that occurs to a part of the brain when its blood supply is suddenly interrupted (ischemic stroke) or when a blood vessel ruptures and bleeds into the brain (hemorrhagic stroke). A stroke is also called a cerebrovascular accident.

Subcutaneous. Under the skin.

Substrate. A reactant in an enzyme-catalyzed reaction.

Supplement. A nutrient or phytochemical supplied in addition to that which is obtained in the diet.

Synergistic. When the effect of two treatments together is greater than the sum of the effects of the two individual treatments, the effect is said to be synergistic.

Synthesis. The formation of a chemical compound from its elements or precursor compounds.

Systematic review. A structured review of the literature designed to answer a clearly formulated question. Systematic reviews use systematic and explicitly predetermined methods to identify, select, and critically evaluate research relevant to the question, and to collect and analyze data from the studies that are included in the review. Statistical methods, such as meta-analysis, may be used to summarize the results of the included studies.

Systemic lupus erythematosus (SLE). A chronic autoimmune disease, characterized by inflammation of the connective tissue. SLE is more common in women than men and may result in inflammation and damage to the skin, joints, blood vessels, lungs, heart, and kidneys.

Systolic blood pressure. The highest arterial pressure measured during the heart-beat cycle, and the first number in a blood pressure reading (e.g., 120/80 mmHg).

Thyroid. A butterfly-shaped gland in the neck that secretes thyroid hormones. Thyroid hormones regulate several physiologic processes, including growth, development, metabolism, and reproductive function.

Topical. Applied to the skin or other body surface.

Total parenteral nutrition. Intravenous feeding that provides patients with essential nutrients when they are too ill to eat normally.

Transcription. The process by which one strand of DNA is copied into a complementary sequence of RNA.

Transcription factor. A protein that functions to initiate, enhance, or inhibit the transcription of a gene. Transcription factors can regulate the formation of a specific protein encoded by a gene.

Translation. The process by which the sequence of nucleotides in a messenger RNA molecule directs the incorporation of amino acids into a protein.

Tremor. Trembling or shaking of a part or all of the body.

Tricarboxylic acid (TCA) cycle. The metabolic pathway in the mitochondria that oxidizes acetyl compounds from food to carbon dioxide and water. Also referred to as the Krebs cycle and the citric acid cycle.

Triglycerides. Lipids consisting of three fatty-acid molecules bound to a glycerol backbone. Triglycerides are the principal form of fat in the diet, although they are also synthesized endogenously. Triglycerides are stored in adipose tissue and represent the principal storage form of fat. Elevated serum triglycerides are a risk factor for cardiovascular disease.

Trimethylaminuria. A hereditary disorder characterized by increased urinary excretion of trimethylamine, a compound with a "fishy" or foul odor.

UL. Tolerable upper intake level. Established by the Food and Nutrition Board of the US Institute of Medicine, the UL is the highest level of daily intake of a specific nutrient likely to pose no risk of adverse health effects in almost all individuals of a specified age.

Ulcerative colitis. A chronic inflammatory disease of the colon and rectum. Symptoms of ulcerative colitis include abdominal pain, cramping, and bloody diarrhea.

Unsaturated fatty acid. A fatty acid with at least one double bond between carbons.

Uric acid. An antioxidant produced by the body.

Vascular endothelium. The single cell layer that lines the inner surface of blood vessels. Healthy endothelial function promotes vasodilation and inhibits platelet aggregation (clot formation).

Vasodilation. Relaxation or opening of a blood vessel.

Ventricles. The two lower chambers of the heart that pump blood to the body (left) and the lungs (right).

Virus. A microorganism that cannot grow or reproduce apart from a living cell. Viruses invade living cells and use the synthetic processes of infected cells to survive and replicate.

Vitamin. An organic (carbon-containing) compound necessary for normal physiological function that cannot be synthesized in adequate amounts and must therefore be obtained from the diet.

Xenograft. A transplant of tissue from a donor of one species to a recipient of another species.

Index

Page references in *italics* refer to illustrations